Atlas of
Small Animal Wound Management and Reconstructive Surgery

Third Edition

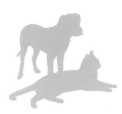

Atlas of
Small Animal Wound Management and Reconstructive Surgery

Third Edition

Michael M. Pavletic DVM

Diplomate American College of Veterinary Surgeons
Director of Surgical Services
Angell Animal Medical Center
Boston, Massachusetts

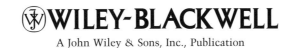

A John Wiley & Sons, Inc., Publication

First edition first published 1993, W.B. Saunders Company.
Second edition first published 1999, W.B Saunders Company.
Third edition first published 2010.
© 2010 Michael M. Pavletic

Blackwell Publishing was acquired by John Wiley & Sons in February 2007. Blackwell's publishing program has been merged with Wiley's global Scientific, Technical, and Medical business to form Wiley-Blackwell.

Editorial Office
2121 State Avenue, Ames, Iowa 50014-8300, USA

For details of our global editorial offices, for customer services, and for information about how to apply for permission to reuse the copyright material in this book, please see our Website at www.wiley.com/wiley-blackwell.

Library of Congress Cataloging-in-Publication Data
Pavletic, Michael M.
    Atlas of small animal wound management and reconstructive surgery / Michael M. Pavletic. – 3rd ed.
        p. ; cm.
    Rev. ed. of: Atlas of small animal reconstructive surgery / Michael M. Pavletic. 2nd ed. c1999.
    Includes bibliographical references and index.
    ISBN-13: 978-0-8138-1124-6 (alk. paper)
    ISBN-10: 0-8138-1124-4 (alk. paper)
  1. Dogs–Surgery–Atlases. 2. Cats–Surgery–Atlases. 3. Veterinary plastic surgery–Atlases. I. Pavletic, Michael M. Atlas of small animal reconstructive surgery. II. Title.
    [DNLM: 1. Dogs–surgery–Atlases. 2. Animals, Domestic–surgery–Atlases. 3. Cats–surgery–Atlases. 4. Reconstructive Surgical Procedures–veterinary–Atlases. 5. Surgical Flaps–veterinary–Atlases. 6. Wounds and Injuries–veterinary–Atlases. SF 991 P338ab 2010]
    SF991.P38 2010
    636.089'71–dc22

                                                                                    2009021678

A catalog record for this book is available from the U.S. Library of Congress.

Set in 9.5/12 pt Palatino by Toppan Best-set Premedia Limited.
Printed in Singapore by Markono Print Media Pte Ltd

Disclaimer
The contents of this work are intended to further general scientific research, understanding, and discussion only and are not intended and should not be relied upon as recommending or promoting a specific method, diagnosis, or treatment by practitioners for any particular patient. The publisher and the author make no representations or warranties with respect to the accuracy or completeness of the contents of this work and specifically disclaim all warranties, including without limitation any implied warranties of fitness for a particular purpose. In view of ongoing research, equipment modifications, changes in governmental regulations, and the constant flow of information relating to the use of medicines, equipment, and devices, the reader is urged to review and evaluate the information provided in the package insert or instructions for each medicine, equipment, or device for, among other things, any changes in the instructions or indication of usage and for added warnings and precautions. Readers should consult with a specialist where appropriate. The fact that an organization or Website is referred to in this work as a citation and/or a potential source of further information does not mean that the author or the publisher endorses the information the organization or Website may provide or recommendations it may make. Further, readers should be aware that Internet Websites listed in this work may have changed or disappeared between when this work was written and when it is read. No warranty may be created or extended by any promotional statements for this work. Neither the publisher nor the author shall be liable for any damages arising herefrom.

5   2016

Dedication

This book is dedicated to my wife Adria; my daughters Afton and Maylin; my parents Merle and Gerry; my mother-in-law Mary; my brothers Frank, Jeff, Mark, and Briant; and my sister Eileen for their love, help, encouragement and support. Gone, but not forgotten, I also dedicate this book to my late father-in-law Frank.

Contents

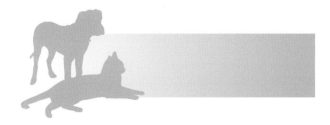

Preface

Once considered a small niche of veterinary medicine, plastic and reconstructive surgery has expanded dramatically over the past three decades.

This third edition of my Atlas includes additional wound management and reconstructive surgical techniques that have evolved since the 1999 edition. I have expanded the text to include the most current information on the management of problematic wounds and wound care products available to the small animal surgeon. Information boxes are included throughout the text to emphasize important points and to add personal observations based on my 35 years of experience and insight in wound management and reconstructive surgery.

The reader will also note the expanded number of case-based photographs that are now in color to complement both the text and the plate illustrations. Forty additional plates have been added, including new sections on bandage/splint techniques, reconstructive surgery of the prepuce, and the management of problematic skin fold conditions. I trust that the reader will find this book a practical, informative, and single-source reference for the surgical restoration of our small animal patients.

I would again like to thank my artist, Sandra Durant, for her invaluable assistance in creating this third edition.

Atlas of Small Animal Wound Management and Reconstructive Surgery

Third Edition

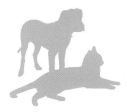

The Skin

SKIN FUNCTION

The integument is the largest organ of the body and serves as the body's first line of defense against microorganisms. It comprises 24% of body weight of the puppy but only 12% of that of an adult dog. The outer horny layer, the stratum corneum, provides protection against desiccation and hydration.

The skin is a sensory receptor for touch, pressure, vibration, pain, heat, and cold. Its multiple functions include vitamin D production; storage of water, fat, electrolytes, carbohydrates, and proteins; a barrier against chemicals and radiation; and along with the subcutaneous fat, insulation.

SKIN STRUCTURE

The skin is composed of an outer stratified epithelium (epidermis) and an underlying fibrous dermis (corium). The epidermis is derived from ectoderm, whereas the dermis is of mesenchymal origin. Each of these two layers will be discussed separately.

Epidermis

The epidermis originates as a single layer of cuboidal ectodermal cells that becomes stratified as the fetus matures. In hair-bearing areas, the epidermis of hairy skin, consists of three major layers: the stratum cylindricum (stratum basale), the stratum spinosum (stratum malpighii or prickle cell layer), and the stratum corneum. The combined stratum cylindricum and stratum spinosum layers form the *stratum germinativum*. Mitotic activity in both layers is responsible for proliferation of epidermal cells.

Surgical Relevance

In full-thickness skin wounds, the stratum germinativum along the viable skin margin is the source of epithelial cells to cover the exposed vascularized wound bed.

Melanocytes, which originate from the neural crest of the embryo, are located in the stratum cylindricum and the lower layer of the stratum spinosum. In a few hairy areas, the stratum granulosum and stratum lucidum are found where keratinization is retarded, such as around the hair follicle orifices. These two layers are well developed in the footpads, but are absent in the planum nasale. Epidermal pegging, evident in the footpads, planum nasale, and lip of the dog, is not present in the hairy skin. In contrast, the dermal-epidermal junction of hairy skin is thrown into folds that parallel the skin surface. Small tactile elevations termed *epidermal papillae* are found over hairy skin surfaces of the dog and cat. The epidermis is generally thicker in areas that lack a thick hair coat and thinner in regions with a dense hair growth (Fig. 1-1 and 1-2). The nose and digital pads have the thickest epidermis.

The Dermis

The dermis (corium) is composed of collagenous, reticular (precollagen), and elastic fibers within a mucopolysaccharide ground substance. This ground substance is composed of hyaluronic acid and chondroitin sulfuric acid; it is the major component of the dermis. Ninety percent of the dermal fibers are composed of collagen. Fibroblasts, macrophages, plasma cells, and mast cells present throughout the dermis are more numerous in the superficial dermal layer. Occasionally chromatophores and fat cells are noted. The dermis contains the cutaneous capillary network, lymphatics, nerve components, arrector pili muscles, hair follicles, and glandular structures.

The dermis of the dog and cat is divided into the superficial stratum papillare and the deep stratum reticulare. The stratum papillare has fine elastic and reticular fibers in densely interwoven collagenous bundles. The basement membrane is formed from reticular fibers and a viscous ground substance, and the stratum cylindricum is attached to the basement membrane via cytoplasmic processes. The stratum reticulare is composed of coarse, densely interwoven collagen bundles.

The most pliable skin (axilla, flank, dorsum of the neck) has small and more loosely woven dermal collagen bundles and greater numbers of elastic fibers in the papillary layer (Fig. 1-3). Less pliable skin (tail, ear, digital pads) have wider, more closely packed collagen bundles with fewer elastic fibers. Collagen fibers in areas of thick skin (head, dorsal body surfaces) are roughly parallel to the cutaneous surface.

Skin of animals essentially is a nonhomogenous viscoelastic tissue with the combined characteristics of a viscous fluid and elastic solid. The inherent elasticity of the skin describes the natural ability of skin to stretch or deform during normal activities.

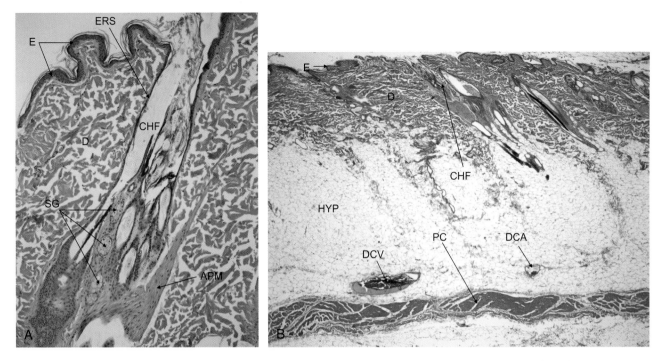

FIG. 1-1 (A, B) Histologic slide of canine skin identifying the following structures: E, epidermis; D, dermis; HYP, hypodermis; CHF, compound hair follicle; ERS, external root sheath; SG, sebaceous glands; DCA, direct cutaneous artery; DCV, direct cutaneous vein; PC, panniculus carnosus muscle; APM, arrector pili muscle. (Slides courtesy of Melanie A. Buote, DVM, DACVP.)

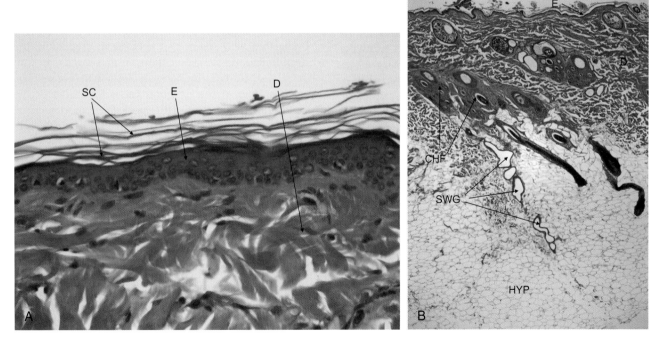

FIG. 1-2 (A, B) Histologic slide of feline skin identifying the following structures: SC, stratum corneum; E, epidermis; D, dermis; HYP, hypodermis; CHF, compound hair follicles; SWG, sweat glands. (Slides courtesy of Melanie A. Buote, DVM, DACVP.)

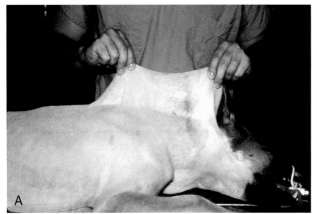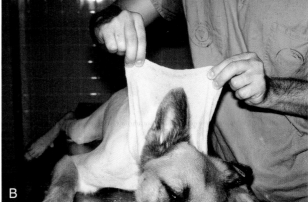

FIG. 1-3 (A) Lateral and (B) anterior view of a German shepherd demonstrating the inherent elasticity of the skin in the cervical region.

> **Surgical Relevance**
>
> Surgeons normally assess the *inherent elasticity* of skin by grasping and lifting the skin or by pushing the skin with the index finger toward the direction of the proposed surgical site. Potential lines of tension are assessed, better allowing the surgeon to decide on how to close the surgical defect. (See Plates 11, 12, and 28.)

The skin's extensibility or ability to stretch is dependent upon three factors occurring consecutively as a load (stretching force), applied to the skin, is progressively increased: (1) convolutions in dermal collagen progressively straighten; (2) dermal collagen fibers align parallel to each other in the direction of the applied load; and (3) fully aligned collagen fibers extend only upon application of great increases in tension. As a result, it is possible to mechanically stretch skin sufficiently to facilitate wound closure by the processes of *mechanical creep* and *stress relaxation*. (See Chapter 10.)

> **Surgical Relevance**
>
> Skin can be manipulated to stretch beyond the limits of its inherent elasticity by the application of a force that stretches skin progressively over time. This newly recruited skin can be used to close problematic wounds. Examples include presuturing (Plate 30), skin stretchers (Plates 24, 31, 32), and tissue expanders (Plate 33). Details are discussed in Chapters 9 and 10.

Cat skin contains collagen bundles, which are generally coarser and denser than canine skin. The arrec-

tor pili muscles also are larger than those in the dog. The stratum papillare of feline skin contains fine, more uniform collagenous fibers, which usually parallel the epidermis. In the stratum reticulare, these fibers are dense, irregularly arranged, and three times larger than those of the papillary layer. In the most flexible cutaneous areas of the cat—the dorsal neck, scapular region, and lateral upper forelimb—the collagen bundles are smaller and more loosely arranged.

The thickness of the skin is directly related to the thickness of the dermal layer and varies according to body area, sex, breed, and species. In thick skin, the dermis usually is thicker than 1 mm, whereas in thin skin, the dermal thickness is less than 1 mm. The thickest skin of the dog and cat is located over the head and the dorsum of the neck, back, and sacrum. The thinnest skin is located along the ventral body surface, the medial surface of the limbs, and the inner pinna.

> **Surgical Relevance**
>
> The durability of fur-bearing skin is primarily the result of the dermal thickness. Skin thickness is taken into consideration when closing wounds in body areas more subject to direct trauma, including skin overlying bony prominences. Dense hair growth also affords some degree of protection.

The Extracellular Matrix

The tissue component outside the cellular walls of organs is referred to as the *extracellular matrix* (ECM): the noncellular components of the dermis are the ECM of the skin. Tissues cells and the ECM are in a state of "dynamic reciprocity." In embryonic development, their interaction plays an essential role in cellular differentiation and function. Cells in turn secrete macromolecules into their immediate environment, forming a matrix between the developing cells. The regional embryonic mesenchymal tissue induces epithelial cell differentiation: epithelial cells, in turn, influence the development and structure of the mesodermal tissues. The ECM includes the fibrillar proteins and glycosaminoglycans (GAGS) that attach to core proteins, forming proteoglycans. The dermal ECM can be described as a network of fibrillar proteins organized within a hydrated gel of proteoglycans. The two principal types of the skin's ECM are the *basement membrane* (or *basal lamina*) in contact with the basal epithelial cells and the underlying *stromal* or *connective tissue*. The stromal tissue provides structural integrity and support to the cellular components of the skin. Collagens are the major proteins of the ECM. However, the ECM comprises a variety of extracellular proteins that may be classified on a functional basis: structural (basal lamina and connective tissue) or adhesive (fibrin and fibronectin); remodeling or counteradhesive (thrombospondin, tenascin, SPARC—*secreted protein acidic and rich in cysteine*); proteolytic (serine proteases, matrix metalloproteases [MMPS]) and antiproteolytic (serpins, plasminogen activator inhibitor-1, tissue inhibitors of metalloproteases [TIMPs]). These proteins have a complex interrelationship during wound healing that will be discussed in Chapter 2.

CUTANEOUS ADNEXA

The cutaneous appendages (adnexa) of hairy skin include the hair follicles, sweat glands, and sebaceous glands. Other cutaneous glandular structures include the mammary glands, supracaudal (tail) glands, anal sacs, superficial circumanal glands, and perianal (deep circumanal) glands. All these structures are ectodermal in origin.

Hair

The hair follicles are the units of hair production. They are located in the lower portions of the dermis but also extend into the subcutaneous tissue (subcutis, hypodermis). The wall of the hair follicle is continuous with the epidermis and is divided into inner and outer root sheaths. During fetal development hair follicles originate from clusters of germinative cells in the epidermis. These ectodermal cells sink into the dermis and form a cylindrical epidermal peg, the base of which

develops into the hair bulb. The hair bulb molds around a mesenchymal papilla. These germinative cells give rise to the inner epithelial root sheath and the hair shaft. The outer epithelial root sheath, which encircles the hair shaft, is a continuation of the stratum cylindricum.

Surgical Relevance

In partial thickness skin losses, both the epidermis and variable portions of the dermis have been destroyed. The epithelial cells comprising the external root sheath of the compound hair follicles are the primary source of epithelial cells required for reepithelialization of partial thickness skin defects. (See Fig. 1-4.)

Sebaceous glands develop as extensions of the outer root sheath at the upper part of the follicle. In dogs and cats, an apocrine sweat gland develops with each hair follicle and extends into the hypodermis. The duct empties into the common portion of the follicle complex between the skin surface and sebaceous gland orifice.

The arrector pili muscles originate in the dermal papillary layer and insert in the connective tissue of the hair follicle. They are anchored by elastic fibers at their attachments and are innervated by the autonomic nervous system. The arrector muscles are especially well developed along the back of the dog and cat, causing the hair to bristle upon their contraction.

In the newborn animal, hair follicles develop from a simple follicle containing a single hair to a compound follicle containing 7–10 hairs emerging from a common follicle orifice. This occurs at 28 weeks of age as a result of accessory buds arising from the original follicle. Sebaceous glands also become compound, emptying where the hairs are contained as a single tubular follicle. The compound follicle contains a main or guard hair surrounded by a number of finer, woolly lanugo, or underhairs. Although the hair shafts share the same external follicular orifice, they branch into their own respective hair follicles below the level of the sebaceous glands. The guard hair follicle is larger and penetrates into the subcutaneous tissue.

Feline hairs are arranged in clusters of two, three, four, and five, grouped around a central guard hair. Clusters of two and three are more common on the dorsal aspect of the feline body; clusters of four and five usually occur on the ventral body and lower extremities. Each lateral group contains 3 primary hairs surrounded by 6 to 12 lanugo hairs. In adult dogs, 3 to 15 hairs are noted in each compound follicle, whereas in cats, the compound follicles contain 12 to 20 hairs.

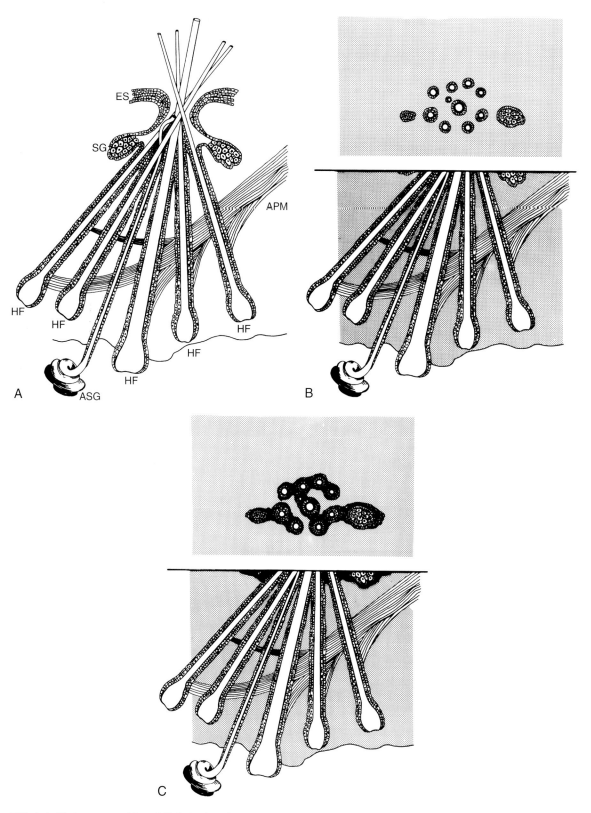

FIG. 1-4 (A) A compound hair follicle (HF) with its associated sebaceous gland (SG), apocrine sweat gland (ASG), and arrector pili muscle (APM). Note the epidermal cellular components of these cutaneous adnexa, which are continuous with the epidermal surface (ES). (Pavletic MM. 1993. The integument. In: Slatter DH, ed. *Textbook of Small Animal Surgery*, 2nd ed. Philadelphia: WB Saunders). (B) Loss of the epidermis and superficial dermal surface. (C) Note epithelial cell migration primarily originating from the external root sheath of each hair follicle.

Vibrissae are larger, more prominent tactile or sinus hairs involving the muzzle and facial area. They allow dogs and cats to locate and assess the proximity of adjacent objects.

Hair growth rates vary seasonally among breeds. Hair growth in male beagles has been noted to be 0.4 mm/day in the winter and 0.34 mm/day in the summer, whereas greyhounds have a growth rate of 0.18 mm/day in the fall and 0.04 mm/day in the summer. Hair growth is more rapid in the winter. As a rule, short canine hair coats take approximately 130 days to regrow. However, as long as 18 months is required for regrowth of the hair coat in long-haired breeds such as the Afghan. These facts must be taken into account prior to clipping a patient, particularly when dealing with show dogs and cats.

The characteristics of the hair coat in dogs and cats vary with the location on the body. The hair coat is usually thicker over the back and sides of the body, whereas the hair inside the ears and on the flanks, ventral abdomen, and underside of the tail is thinner. Cosmetic wound closure should account for variations in growth patterns and direction of growth of the coat.

Cutaneous Glands

The glandular structures of the skin include the sebaceous glands, sweat glands, supracaudal (tail) glands, anal sacs, circumanal glands, and mammary glands. These ectodermally derived structures form by the downgrowth of epidermal cells into the dermis during embryonic development.

Sebaceous Glands

Sebaceous glands commonly originate from the external root sheath. They produce an oily secretion that exits through the pilosebaceous canal to keep the skin and hair soft and pliable and to protect them from excessive moisture and drying. Sebaceous glands are well developed over the neck, back, and tail of the dog, particularly in the tail gland area.

The sebaceous gland complex in the cat is smaller and simpler in structure than that of the dog. Larger sebaceous glands are found in association with the hair follicles of the upper jaw, prepuce, and dorsal tail surface. Sebaceous glands not associated with hair follicles include the meibomian, or tarsal, glands of the eyelids and glands of the labia, vulva, anus, prepuce, glans penis, and external ear canal. These holocrine glands empty directly onto the epithelial surface.

Circumanal glands (superficial sebaceous glands) and perianal glands (deep sebaceous glands) are modified sebaceous glands located at the mucocutaneous junction of the anus. Perianal glandular tissue also can be found in the skin of the prepuce and groin. Circumanal glands have well-defined ducts and contain fat. Perianal glands have solid ducts and show no secretory activity. Circumanal glands contain fat, unlike the deeper perianal glands. Perianal gland cells are filled with proteinaceous cytoplasmic granules.

Sweat Glands

Sweat (sudoriferous) glands are apocrine and merocrine (eccrine) in nature. Cutaneous apocrine sweat glands are large, simple, saccular or tubular structures with a coiled secretory portion and a straight duct. The glands may be tortuous or serpentine. The apocrine sweat gland duct opens at the external root sheath between the skin surface and pilosebaceous canal. Merocrine glands are coiled, simple, tubular glands found mainly in the footpads of the dog and empty directly onto the epidermal surface. Sweat glands are better developed in the long, fine-haired dog breeds.

Sweat glands in the hairy skin of dogs and cats do not participate actively in the central thermoregulatory mechanism but protect the skin from an excessive rise in temperature. This is in contrast to human beings, in whom the cutaneous sweat glands are vital for vaporizational heat loss to cool the body at high temperatures.

A number of apocrine glands have specialized structures and functions. These include Moll's glands of the eyelids, the ceruminous glands of the external ear canal, the anal sac, and the glands of the prepuce, vulva, and circumanal region.

The mammary glands of the skin are compound tubuloalveolar apocrine glands resembling sweat glands in their mode of development. They undergo conspicuous changes during pregnancy and during and after lactation in the female. They remain rudimentary in the male dog and cat.

Anal sacs have a thin, stratified squamous epithelial lining that includes sebaceous and apocrine sweat glands. Sebaceous glands tend to line the neck of the sac, whereas the apocrine glands are concentrated in the fundus.

> ### Surgical Relevance
> Increased secretory function of the sebaceous and aprocrine sweat glands is noted with inflammatory processes involving the skin, especially where a large number of these glandular structures are assembled. During these inflammatory processes, more frequent bandage changes may be expected. Wound care is important to the prevention of tissue maceration and infection secondary to moisture accumulation.

THE HYPODERMIS

The hypodermis (subcutis) is associated with the overlying dermis. This subcutaneous tissue is composed primarily of fat with loose collagenous trabeculae and elastic fibers. It varies in thickness regionally but is poorly developed beneath the eyelids, ears, and scrotum, and other areas where the skin is closely attached to underlying structures.

The inherent elasticity of the skin; its lack of firm attachments to bone, muscle, and fascia; and the length and extensibility of the direct cutaneous vessels account for the high degree of mobility of skin over the head, neck, and trunk of the dog and cat. In one histological study, two distinct layers of the hypodermis were reported: the stratum adiposum subcutis (containing fat) and a deeper stratum fibrosum subcutis, which includes the panniculus muscle layer.

The hypodermis is closely associated with normal skin function. Direct cutaneous vessels must traverse this layer to supply the overlying skin. In this respect, the panniculus muscles play an important role during the surgical elevation of the skin (Fig. 1-1 and 1-2).

Panniculus Muscles

The *panniculus muscle* (panniculus carnosus) is a collection of thin muscles beneath some cutaneous areas in the dog and cat (Fig. 1-1 and 1-2). The panniculus muscles in the head and neck regions are the platysma, sphincter colli superficialis, and sphincter colli profundus. The cutaneous trunci is the major cutaneous muscle of the body, extending from the gluteal region cranial and ventral to the pectoral region. It is not present beneath the skin over the middle and lower portions of the limbs. Fibers from this muscle make up the preputialis muscle in the male dog and the supramammarius muscle in the female dog.

The cat has a similar cutaneous muscle distribution. The cutaneous trunci (cutaneous maximus) of the cat extends over the thoracic and abdominal regions of the body. The platysma in the cat covers the head and neck. In the cervical region, the platysma can be subdivided into the supercervicocutaneous muscle and cervicofacial muscle along a line of attachment to the skin. The associated sphincter colli superficialis muscle is smaller and of irregular occurrence. The feline panniculus muscle is a component of the stratum fibrosum subcutis, the deep connective tissue layer of the hypodermis.

Panniculus muscle fibers are very irregular and tend to run transversely. Fibers penetrate the dermis and allow voluntary movement of the skin. The cutaneous trunci is used to shake the skin in response to irritating or noxious stimuli. Repeated contraction (shivering) of this muscle can increase heat production in cold animals. The platysma muscle moves the vibrissae and gives expression to the face. The preputial muscle in dogs helps to draw the prepuce over the glans penis after erection. The supramammary muscle aids in the support of the mammary glands and perhaps in milk ejection in the bitch.

> ### Surgical Relevance
> The direct cutaneous vascular supply and associated subdermal plexus of the skin are closely associated with the panniculus muscle layer, where present. Preservation of this thin muscle layer with the overlying skin helps preserve cutaneous circulation during the surgical manipulation of the skin (e.g., skin flaps, tissue undermining). See Figures 1-5 and 1-6.

CUTANEOUS CIRCULATION

The cardiovascular system is the first major system to function during embryonic development. The hemangioblast is believed to be the precursor to blood vessels and blood cells during embryonic development. Blood vessels are constructed by two processes: *vasculogene-*

sis and *angiogenesis*. In vasculogenesis, blood vessels are created *de novo* from the lateral plate mesoderm. Hemangioblasts formed from these splanchnic mesodermal cells condense into "blood islands." The inner cells of these blood islands become hematopoetic stem cells, the precursors of blood cells. The outer cells become angioblasts, the precursors of blood vessels. Angioblasts differentiate into endothelial cells. Endothelial tubes form and interconnect to form the *primary capillary plexus.* Angiogenesis is the process in which this primary capillary network is remodeled and pruned into distinct arteries, veins, and capillary beds. The developing vascular network is essential to supplying the tissues with the necessary oxygen and nutrients essential to fetal development. *Cytokines* or growth factors play a central role in the initiation of vasculogenesis.

The cutaneous vascular system is divided into three interconnected levels:

1. The deep, subdermal, or subcutaneous plexus
2. The middle, or cutaneous plexus
3. The superficial, or subpapillary plexus

This general vascular arrangement is present in the hairy skin. Variations in the arrangement are noted in the canine external ear, footpad, nipple, and the mucocutaneous junctions of the nostril, lip, eyelid, prepuce, vulva, and anus.

The Subdermal Plexus

The subdermal plexus is the major vascular network to the overlying skin. The vessels of this plexus generally run in the subcutaneous fatty and areolar tissue on the deep face of the dermis of the middle to distal portions of the limbs where no panniculus muscle is present. Where there is a layer of cutaneous muscle, the subdermal plexus lies both superficial and deep to it (Fig. 1-5). An experimental study (Pavletic) on the misapplication of subcutaneous pedicle flaps in the dog demonstrated the vital relationship between the panniculus muscle and the overlying skin. Complete severance of the panniculus muscle results in necrosis of the island flap, whereas preservation of the muscular layer assures its survival by preserving the subdermal plexus. The skin should always be undermined in the fascial plane beneath the cutaneous musculature to preserve the integrity of the subdermal plexus. In areas devoid of this muscle layer, one should undermine in the fascial plane well below the dermal surface to preserve it (Fig. 1-6).

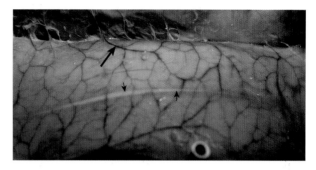

FIG. 1-5 Skin reflected from the back of a cat cadaver. Blue latex has been injected into the arterial system to highlight the direct cutaneous arteries. The thin cutaneous trunci (panniculus) muscles on each side of the cat join over the dorsal midline (small arrows). A direct cutaneous artery can be seen approaching the panniculus muscle and overlying skin in parallel fashion (large arrow). As it arborizes, terminal branches "form" and supply the subdermal plexus. Note the "mirror" image formed by the direct cutaneous vasculature on each side of the midline. (Pavletic MM. 2003. The integument. In: Slatter DH, ed. *Textbook of Small Animal Surgery*, 3rd ed., 250–9. Philadelphia: WB Saunders.)

Cutaneous (Middle) and Superficial Plexuses

The subdermal plexus supplies the hair bulb and follicle, tubular glands, and deeper portions of the ducts as well as the arrector pili muscle. Branches of the subdermal plexus ascend into the dermis to form the middle, or cutaneous plexus located at the sebaceous glands. Branches from the cutaneous plexus ascend and descend into the dermis to supply the sebaceous glands and reinforce the capillary networks around the hair follicles, tubular gland ducts, and arrector pili muscle. The middle plexus shows developmental and positional variations according to the distribution of the hair follicles in the skin. Radicals from the middle plexus ascend to supply the superficial plexus. The superficial plexus lies in the outer layer of the dermis. Capillary loops from this plexus project into the dermal papillary bodies to supply the epidermal papillae and adjacent epidermis. However, the capillary loop system and papillary bodies are poorly developed in the dog and cat, unlike the human, anthropoid ape, and pig, all of which have well-developed capillary loops. This anatomical difference explains why canine skin generally does not normally blister with superficial burns.

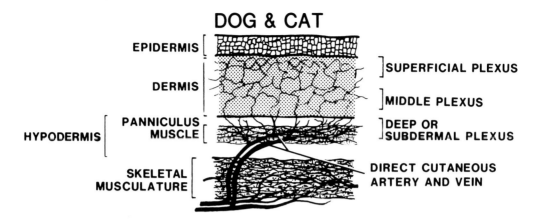

FIG. 1-6 Cutaneous circulation in the dog and cat. The subdermal plexus is supplied by terminal branches of direct cutaneous vessels at the level of the panniculus muscle in the dog and cat. Note the parallel relationship between the direct cutaneous vessels and the overlying skin. This is unlike the perpendicular orientation of musculocutaneous vessels in the human. (Pavletic MM. 2003. The integument. In Slatter DH, ed. *Textbook of Small Animal Surgery,* 3rd ed., 250–9. Philadelphia: WB Saunders.)

Surgical Relevance

Split-thickness skin grafts are normally harvested with the use of a dermatome. The depth of the dermal incision will expose different levels of the dermal vascular network. For example, thinner grafts expose the finer, numerous vascular channels of the superficial plexus. Exposure of the graft's vascular channels increases the probability of successful revascularization. For this reason, thin split-thickness skin grafts reportedly have a higher probability of revascularization when compared to thicker skin grafts. The bleeding pattern on the cut dermal surface will reflect the depth of the graft harvested.

Cutaneous Arteries

Segmental vessels arising from the aorta, well beneath the body muscle mass, give off perforator branches that traverse the skeletal muscle to supply the subdermal plexus. Two types of arteries supply the cutaneous circulation in the human: musculocutaneous arteries and direct cutaneous arteries. Musculocutaneous arteries are the primary vascular supply to the skin of humans, apes, and swine. Perforator arteries send several branches to the overlying muscle mass before terminating as musculocutaneous arteries perpendicular to the skin. Direct cutaneous arteries arise from perforator arteries that send few branches to the over-

lying muscle mass before ascending to the subdermal plexus. Direct cutaneous arteries run parallel to the skin and supply a greater area of the skin compared with a single musculocutaneous artery but play a secondary role in the total cutaneous circulatory pattern in the human (Fig. 1-5 and 1-6).

Hughes and Dransfield divided arteries supplying the canine skin into two groups: mixed cutaneous arteries and simple cutaneous arteries. Mixed cutaneous arteries run through a muscle mass and supply a significant number of branches to it before emerging and supplying the skin. Simple cutaneous arteries give few branches to muscles, between which they run, before supplying the skin. Despite the descriptive similarities to the perforator-musculocutaneous and perforator-direct cutaneous systems of humans, all vessels in the skin of dogs and cats approach and travel parallel to the skin and are direct cutaneous arteries (Figs. 1-7 and 1-8). Standard anatomy texts illustrate the superficial arteries of the canine trunk (Fig. 1-9).

Clinical Relevance

By far, the single most important consideration in reconstructive surgery is preservation of the circulation. Because of differences in skin circulation, care must be taken when attempting to adapt human reconstructive surgical techniques to the dog and cat.

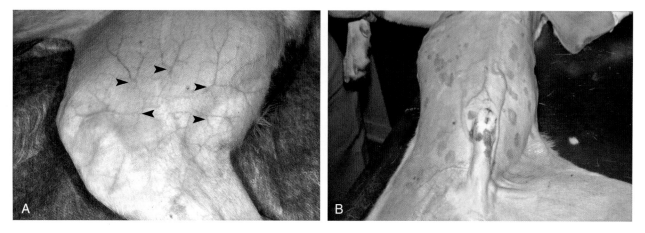

FIG. 1-7 (A) Inner thigh of a greyhound illustrating several direct cutaneous vessels traveling parallel to the overlying skin surface. (B) Ventral abdomen in a thin-skinned retriever, demonstrating prominent caudal and cranial superficial epigastric vessels.

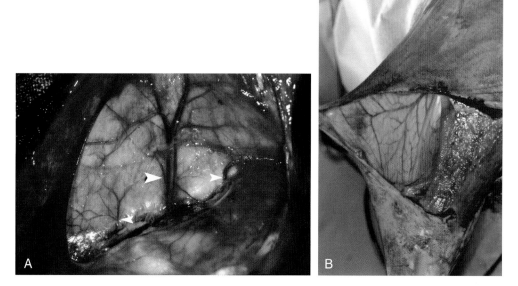

FIG. 1-8 (A) Elevation of a skin flap illustrating a large direct cutaneous artery and vein (large arrow). Small direct cutaneous vessels (small arrows) also are noted. (B) Intraoperative view of the ventral branch of the deep circumflex iliac artery and vein in a cat. The skin is being elevated to close a skin defect involving the left mid-thigh region.

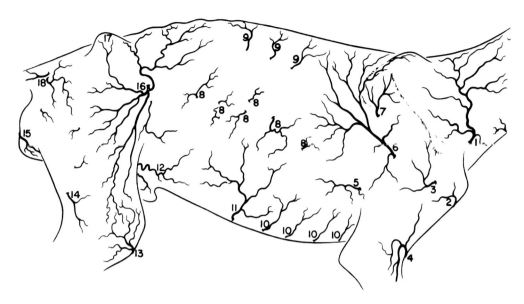

FIG. 1-9 Superficial arteries of the canine trunk. 1, Superficial cervical branch of omocervical; 2, cranial circumflex humeral; 3, caudal circumflex humeral; 4, proximal collateral radial; 5, lateral thoracic; 6, cutaneous branch of thoracodorsal; 7, cutaneous branch of subscapular; 8, distal lateral cutaneous branches of intercostals; 9, proximal lateral cutaneous branches of intercostals; 10, ventral cutaneous branches of internal thoracic; 11, cranial superficial epigastric; 12, caudal superficial epigastric; 13, medial genicular; 14, cutaneous branch of caudal femoral; 15, perineal; 16, deep circumflex iliac; 17, tubera coxae; 18, cutaneous branches of superficial lateral coccygeal (Evans HE. 1993. *Miller's Anatomy of the Dog*, 3rd ed. Philadelphia: WB Saunders).

CONGENITAL SKIN DISORDERS

Cutaneous Asthenia

Cutaneous asthenia is a congenital hereditary collagen defect in humans and animals that is highlighted by fragile, hyperextensible skin. The condition is analogous to *Ehlers-Danlos Syndrome* (EDS), an eponym for eight variations (EDS I–VIII) of this disorder in humans. Other names include *dermatosparaxis* and *dermatosparaxis* and *collageneous tissue dysplasia* in sheep, cats, sheep, and cattle, a condition similar to EDS I in humans. The disease is generally considered autosomal dominant with incomplete penetrance in dogs, cats, and mink. Dematosparaxis in some cats, cattle, and sheep may be a recessive trait. (In humans, EDS I, II, III, and VIII are considered autosomal dominant; EDS V X-linked recessive; EDS VI and VII autosomal recessive.)

Canine breeds affected with cutaneous asthenia include springer spaniels, beagles, Manchester terriers, Welsh corgis, German shepherds, dachshunds, boxers, St. Bernards, and mixed breeds. It has been reported in Persian, Himalayan, and domestic short-haired cats.

Documented biochemical disorders in humans have included type III collagen synthesis (EDS IV), lysyl oxidase deficiency (EDS V), lysyl hydroxylase deficiency (EDS VI), a type I collagen defect (EDS I, II, III), and a procollagen peptidase deficiency (EDSVII).

In humans, EDS can result in joint hypermobility, congenital vascular fragility, bowel ruptures, ocular lesions, and hernias. Hernia repairs in human patients normally require the use of reinforcement mesh. However, increased skin fragility with hyperelasticity and laxity is the primary clinical feature of EDS in humans. Extracutaneous collagen fragility has been noted in the mesentery, intestinal wall, aorta, and muscle attachments in dogs.

Hyperlaxity may increase with age in dogs: the skin may appear excessive, hanging in folds, especially around the limbs. Affected animals usually have a history of lacerations and abscesses. The skin tears easily with comparatively minor trauma. Scars appear tissue paper–thin (onion-skin scars). "Pseudotumor" formation secondary to vascular fragility may be noted.

Histologically, the dermis and epidermis may have variable thickness. The most notable alteration is the size, shape, and orientation of the collagen bundles. Many collagen fibers appear smaller in diameter than normal, and larger collagen fibers may be fragmented. Collagen bundles may be dissociated and haphazardly arranged and lack the normal characteristic interwoven appearance seen in normal skin. Abnormalities in dermal collagen packing into fibrils and fibers have been noted in mixed-breed dogs. A decrease in acid glycosaminoglyan also has been reported without histological evidence of collagen fiber disorders. The collagen may also lack normal staining uniformity. A skin extensibility index greater than 17% correlates consistently with collagen packing defects.

The prevention and management of skin injuries is of primary concern in dogs and cats. Care is required to prevent trauma to the skin from clippers. Use of atraumatic or reverse-cutting needles are used to help prevent suture pull-out. Combining an intradermal pattern with a vertical mattress suture pattern may be advisable to reduce the risk of dehiscence. In cats, declawing the patient can reduce self-inflicted trauma from scratching. An Elizabethan collar also should be considered to prevent licking and chewing at any surgical area. Interestingly, wounds can heal readily by second intention, and the stages of healing appear similar to unaffected skin. Tensile strength of healed wounds appears comparable to the surrounding skin. The hereditary nature of this disorder would preclude breeding affected animals.

Epitheliogenesis Imperfecta

Epitheliogenesis imperfecta is a heritable condition highlighted by areas of skin and mucosa lacking an epidermis. It has been reported in cats, lambs, and horses. Skin ulcerations are susceptible to infection. If the condition is limited to a few areas, wound closure techniques may be considered. Breeding of affected animals is inadvisable.

Suggested Readings

Al-Bagdadi F. 1993. The integument. In: Evans HE, ed. *Miller's Anatomy of the Dog*, 3rd ed. Philadelphia: WB Saunders.

Gilbert ST. 2006. *Developmental Embryology*, 8th ed. Sunderland, Massachusetts: Sinauer Associates.

Hughes HV, Dransfield JW. 1959. The blood supply of the skin of the dog. *Brit Vet J* 115:1–12.

Lanza PP, Langer R, Chick WL. 1997. *Principles of Tissue Engineering*. Austin, Texas: RB Landes Company.

Moore KL, Persaud TVN. 1998. *The Developing Human*, 6th ed. Philadelphia: WB Saunders.

Pavletic MM. 1980. The vascular supply to the skin of the dog: a review. *Vet Surg* 9:77–82.

Pavletic MM. 1982. Misapplication of subcutaneous pedicle flaps in the dog. *Vet Surg* 11:18–22.

Pavletic MM. 1991. Anatomy and circulation of the canine skin. *Microsurg* 12:103–107.

Pavletic MM. 1994. Surgery of the skin and management of wounds. In: Sherding RG, ed. *The Cat: Diseases and Clinical Management*, 2nd ed., 1601–1629. New York: Churchill Livingstone.

Pavletic MM. 2000. Use of an external skin-stretching device for wound closure in dogs and cats. *J Am Vet Med Assoc* 217(03):350–354.

Pavletic MM. 2003. The integument. In: Slatter DH, ed. *Textbook of Small Animal Surgery*, 3rd ed., 250–259. Philadelphia: WB Saunders.

Sadler TW. 2004. *Langmann's Medical Embryology*, 9th ed. Philadelphia: Lippincott Williams, Wilkins.

Scott DW. 1980. Normal integument (feline dermatology). *J Am Anim Hosp Assoc* 16:333–339.

Taylor GI, Minabe T. 1992. The angiosomes of the mammals and other vertebrates. *Plast Reconstr Surg* 89:181–215.

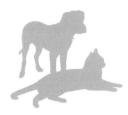

2

Basic Principles of Wound Healing

INTRODUCTION

By definition, a wound is a break or loss of cellular and anatomic continuity. Trauma, by definition, is a physical injury or wound caused by external force or violence. In common usage, *trauma* is used to indicate the general aspects of a physical injury, whereas *wound* is used to describe a more specific lesion.

Wounds to the skin, subcutis, and underlying muscle are among the most common injuries treated by veterinarians. The causes are many, including bites; automobile accidents; lacerations from sharp objects; penetration by bullets, sticks, metal objects; and thermal injuries. Surgical wounds are created in the process of resecting diseased or damaged skin regions.

All wounds are the result of the absorption of energy transferred to the body, whether it is from a projectile, electrical current, or a surgeon's scalpel blade. The severity of the insult depends upon the strength of the energy source, how it is dispersed to the body, and the specific tissue(s) absorbing it. Understanding the processes of wound repair is essential to a thoughtful approach to wound care.

WOUND HEALING

Significant advances in cellular and molecular biology over the past several years have improved our understanding of the processes of wound healing and tissue regeneration. Wound healing is a complex dynamic process that integrates the functions of formed blood elements, the extracellular matrix (ECM) (see Chapter 1), parenchymal cells, and soluble mediators. In uncomplicated wounds, the repair process follows a fairly consistent time sequence. There are a number of factors that are capable of delaying healing, and these will be discussed in detail in Chapter 6.

For the sake of simplicity, healing can be divided into three phases: the inflammatory phase, the proliferative phase, and the maturation/remodeling phase. However, these phases are not mutually exclusive, but overlap in time.

Each phase of wound healing is regulated in large part by mediators termed *cytokines*. Cytokines can act on the cells responsible for their release (autocrine), adjacent cells (paracrine), or distant cells (endocrine). *Intracrine* refers to intracellular cytokines that exert their effect within the cell. Cytokines can direct cells to produce proteins, enzymes, proteoglycans, attachment glycoproteins, and other components required in the repair of the extracellular tissues.

Prostaglandins and leukotrienes also appear to play a role in the healing processes. Prostaglandins of the E series may be involved in the inflammatory phase of healing, while the later anti-inflammatory effects may be due to prostaglandins of the F and possibly A series.

Cytokines and Wound Healing

As noted, cytokines play a major role in regulating the processes of wound repair. *Growth factors* are cytokines that bind to cell surface receptors and serve as important regulators of cell function and growth. These extracellular proteins originate from a variety of tissues and often exist as several isoforms. The most notable growth factors include the following:

- Platelet derived growth factor (PDGF)
- Epidermal growth factor (EGF)
- Fibroblast growth factor (FGF)
- Keratinocyte growth factor (KGF)
- Connective tissue growth factor (CTGF)
- Vascular endothelial growth factor (VEGF)
- Nerve growth factor (NGF)
- Insulin-like growth factor-1 (IGF-1)
- Transforming growth factor-alpha (TGF-α)
- Transforming growth factor-beta (TGF-β)

Other cytokines include tumor necrosis factor (TNF), interleukins, interferons, and colony-stimulating factor. Cytokines generally have more than one effect on the healing processes. Their cellular effects include chemotaxis, promoting mitosis (mitogenic properties), cellular stimulation and activation, and regulatory properties on different components of the wound-healing process.

Growth factors hold promise in the management of nonhealing wounds. In experimental rabbit and rat studies, PDGF significantly accelerated the healing response: there was an increased rate of granulation tissue formation and the formation of procollagen-laden fibroblasts in a dose-dependent manner. Challenges in their clinical use include the manufacturing of specific growth factors while providing a stable and effective vehicle for their application to problematic wounds. Selection and application of exogenous growth factors may be an oversimplistic approach to problematic wounds due to the complex interrelationship between the cytokines. Regranex (becaplermin; manufactured by Ortho-McNeil Pharmaceutical, Inc, Raitan, NJ) has had variable results in the management of diabetic ulcers in humans. Regranex is a human recombinant platelet-derived growth factor in a gel vehicle for application. The author has been encouraged by its use in problematic extremity wounds in a few small exotic animals, both in its stimulation of a healthy granulation tissue and subsequent epithelialization of the slow-healing cutaneous defects. Controlled studies are needed to determine its efficacy compared to other modalities of wound management. Instead of exogenous sources of growth factors, a great deal of research has focused on topical agents that are capable of stimulating cytokine production by the patient.

PDGF, for example, is strongly chemotactic for monocytes, neutrophils, fibroblasts, and smooth muscle cells. It has mitogenic properties, promoting the mitosis of fibroblasts, endothelial cells, and smooth muscle cells. It stimulates angiogenesis, wound contraction, granulation tissue formation, and wound remodeling. PDGF also stimulates the production of fibronectin, hyaluronic acid, and matrix metalloproteinases (MMPs). It also inhibits platelet aggregation and regulates integrin expression. Originally isolated from platelets, other cells produce PDGF, including tissue macrophages, endothelial cells, keratinocytes, and smooth muscle cells.

Transforming growth factor-beta (TGF-β), and its three isoforms, are derived from platelets, T lymphocyctes, macrophages, endothelial cells, keratinocytes, smooth muscle cells, hepatocytes, eosinophils, and fibroblasts. TGF-β has similar chemotactic properties to PDGF, including lymphocytes. It has a powerful mitogenic effect on macrophages, smooth muscle cells, and osteoblasts. Like PDGF, it stimulates angiogenesis and fibroplasia as well as keratinocyte migration. It also stimulates TIMP (tissue inhibitor of matrix metalloproteinase) synthesis and regulates integrin (see Proliferative Phase below) expression and other cytokines. TGF-β has an inhibitory effect on the production of MMP, keratinocyte proliferation, endothelial cell growth, lymphocytes, and epithelial cells.

Epidermal, keratinocyte, connective tissue, endothelial cell, and fibroblast growth factors have mitogenic properties for their named cell lines, but they also have stimulatory properties for other aspects of wound healing. EGF (derived from platelets, and macrophages), for example, stimulates keratinocyte migration and granulation tissue formation. KGF (derived from fibroblasts) stimulates keratinocyte migration, proliferation, and differentiation. KGF may stimulate progenitor cells within the hair follicles and sebaceous glands. Thus, it may play an important role in adnexal reepithelialization of partial-thickness skin wounds. FGF (derived from macrophages, mast cells, T lym-

phocytes, endothelial cells, fibroblasts, and other tissues) also stimulates keratinocyte migration as well as angiogenesis, wound contraction, and matrix deposition. FGF appears to be mitogenic for cells of mesenchymal and neuroectodermal origin. CTGF (derived from endothelial cells and fibroblasts) has chemotactic and mitogenic properties for various connective tissue cells. Insulin-like growth factors IGF-1 and IGF-2 (derived from macrophages, fibroblasts, liver, pancreas, and other tissues) stimulate the synthesis of collagen, sulfated proteoglycans, fibroblast proliferation, and keratinocyte migration. Tumor necrosis factors TNF-α and TNF-β (derived from macrophages, monocytes, mast cells, T lymphocytes) activate macrophages and stimulate angiogenesis and fibroblast mitosis, but also have a regulatory effect on other cytokines. TNF appears to play a role in collagen remodeling by stimulating collagenase production. Colony-stimulating factor (CSF) (derived from a variety of cells) modulates monocyte and macrophage function and promotes differentiation and proliferation of granulocytes. Nerve growth factor (derived from neural and glial cells) is a neurotrophic factor that modulates neuronal cell survival.

Interleukins (IL-1) (derived from macrophages, mast cells, keratinocytes, lymphocytes, etc.) are chemotactic for fibroblasts and polymorphonuclear cells. They also stimulate angiogenesis, MMP-1, and TIMP synthesis. They play a regulatory role with other cytokines. Interferons (IFN) (derived from lymphocytes and fibroblasts) activate macrophages; they play an inhibitory role in fibroblast proliferation and the synthesis of MMPs. Like interleukins, they also regulate other cytokines.

The exact mechanisms that lead to cessation of healing in problematic wounds occasionally remains elusive. There are a number of recognizable factors (poor nutritional support, improper wound care, etc.) that negatively impact wound healing. When all identifiable causes are eliminated, concern is directed at the possibility of healing deficiencies at the cellular level. A lack of, or an imbalance of cytokines may be a factor in these challenging cases.

Phases of Wound Healing

Inflammatory Phase

The inflammatory phase is occasionally referred to as the *lag phase* or *preparatory phase* of healing. Severe tissue trauma causes the disruption of blood vessels with the extravasation of blood constituents. Vasoconstriction is the immediate response to injury, lasting for 5–10 minutes, followed by vasodilatation. Blood clotting within the vessel lumen reestablishes hemostasis, whereas the extravascular clot will later provide a provisional matrix or scaffold for cellular migration. The extravascular clot is an important component of the inflammatory response. Platelets facilitate the formation of this hemostatic plug while secreting vasoactive mediators and chemotactic factors to recruit leukocytes. Fibrin in concert with fibronectin will later serve as a provisional matrix for the migration of monocytes, fibroblasts, and endothelial cells. Cell migration is dependent upon the formation of integrin receptors on the surface of each cell. Integrin receptors recognize and attach to the molecular structure of fibrin, fibronectin, and vitronectin. Proteolytic enzymes (proteases) later assist in removing these proteins in preparation for the proliferative phase of wound healing. Two major classes of proteases of the extracellular matrix include serine proteases and MMPs. MMPs require calcium or zinc for activation. Some proteases (certain collagenases) can be highly specific in their lytic activity, whereas others (including stromelysins) are more general. Protease inhibitors (anti-proteases), including serine protease inhibitors (serpins) and TIMPs bind directly to the proteolytic enzyme to block its activity. Thus, normal wound healing involves the proper balance between proteolytic enzymes and their inhibitors.

Within 30–60 minutes after injury, leukocytes adhere to the endothelium (termed *margination*) of the vessels at the injury site; this especially is evident along the venules. Gaps between endothelial cells allow for the escape of tissue fluid and macromolecules including plasma proteins, complement, antibodies, water, electrolytes, and circulating humoral substances. Histamines, serotonin, and kinins released primarily from mast cells act on the venous side of capillary loops of 20 to 30 microns in size, resulting in a separation of contacts between endothelial cells: this in turn allows blood components to escape from the vascular lumen. Transudation increases in magnitude for approximately 72 hours. Damaged endothelial cells release phospholipids from the cell membrane and are subsequently converted into arachidonic acid. Arachidonic acid is an important mediator in platelet aggregation, and vascular tone.

Leukocytes pass through the basement membrane of the vessel wall by diapedesis. Endothelial cell surface receptors (selectins) assist neutrophil adherence to the endothelium, whereas integrin receptors on the neutrophil cell surfaces assist in their binding to the extracellular matrix. Activated neutrophils release elastase and collagenase molecules, which facilitate their penetration through the blood vessel basement membranes. Both neutrophils and monocytes emigrate to the injured tissues, but neutrophils arrive in greater numbers due to their abundance in the circulation. Chemotactic substances (complement factors, IL-1, TNF-α, PDGF, TGF-β, platelet factor-4, fibrinopeptides, fibrin degradation products, and bacterial products) stimulate neutrophil migration. PDGF, collagen fragments, elastin, fibronectin, enzymatically active thrombin, and TGF-β serve as chemoattractants for monocytes. Monocytes entering the wound progressively become activated, transforming into tissue macrophages.

Neutrophils release proteinases to degrade necrotic tissue, which in turn serves as a chemoattractant for additional neutrophil migration. Neutrophils at the wound site destroy contaminating bacteria via phagocytosis and enzymatic and oxygen radical mechanisms. Neutrophils also remove damaged cells and denatured extracellular matrix. Interestingly, provided that infection is not present, neutrophils are not essential to the healing process.

Neutrophils within the tissue undergo programmed cell death (apoptosis) within a few days. These effete neutrophils are subsequently phagocytosed by tissue macrophages. However substantial contamination (bacteria, foreign debris, necrotic tissue) can propagate a neutrophil-rich wound environment until particle clearance has been completed. Macrophages continue to survive and begin to dominate numerically by the fifth day in uncomplicated wounds.

Pus is the liquid product of inflammation and is composed of tissue fluid, dead and degenerated neutrophils, and albuminous substances. An abscess is the localized collection of pus in any part of the body. Although most abscesses are associated with bacterial infection, they can form under sterile conditions in the presence of a foreign irritant. Prompt medical and surgical intervention in acute injuries can reduce the likelihood of infection.

The macrophage has been described as the "digestive tract" of the wound. It also has been referred to as the "grand maestro" of the wound-healing process. Macrophages are capable of surviving in an oxygen-depleted environment, removing bacteria, contaminants, and tissue debris by phagocytosis. They also release proteases (including collagenase, elastase, and plasminogen activator), facilitating wound debridement: excessive release of these enzymes is also capable of damaging healthy tissues. In uncomplicated wounds, the macrophage population will decline as the inflammatory phase subsides. In the face of extensive foreign debris, contaminants, and necrotic tissue, macrophage numbers will persist in the wound, a "cellular indicator" associated with chronic inflammatory conditions.

Wound debridement and lavage can significantly reduce the volume of necrotic tissue and contaminants, thereby facilitating the healing processes. The removal of dead tissue and debris also plays an important role in preventing and controlling infection.

Macrophages may coalesce to form multinucleated giant cells designed for the phagocytosis of foreign debris. Macrophages also have the capacity to differentiate into epitheloid cells and histiocytes. Some macrophages appear to be primarily involved with host defense and cell-mediated immunity, whereas other cells are involved in tissue growth and repair. Thus, activated macrophages serve in a "director capacity" and play a pivotal role in the transition between inflammation and repair. Macrophage-derived growth factors are essential to the initiation and propagation of new tissue formation, including fibroplasia and angiogenesis. The macrophages also release lactate into the wound environment which stimulates fibroplasia and subsequent collagen production.

The inflammatory, or lag, phase lasts for approximately 5 days in experimental wounds.

The classic signs of inflammation (redness, swelling, heat, pain) are the result of vasodilation, fluid escape, and obstruction of the local lymphatic channels. Lymphatics are fragile and easily injured; fibrin formed at the wound site can plug these channels and enhance local fluid retention. Pressure, chemical stimulation, and stretching of nerve endings results in pain. Circulatory compromise will lower wound pH due to accumulation of lactic acid. This wound environment is ideal for bacterial infection. Rough handling of these compromised tissues may be the factor that "tips the scale" in favor of tissue necrosis and subsequent infection.

Proliferative Phase

The proliferative phase is usually considered to be 5–20 days after injury.

The term *granulation tissue* is derived from the granular appearance of newly forming tissue when incised and its edge is visually examined. The surface of a well-developed granulation bed often assumes a fine pebble-grain or granular appearance

In a simple wound, the acute inflammatory reaction subsides and early repair commences in 3–5 days after the initial insult. Approximately 4 days after an uncomplicated injury, early granulation tissue begins to form.

Macrophages, fibroblasts, and capillary buds migrate into the wound as a unit or "wound module," underscoring their interdependence during tissue repair. The cytokines secreted by the macrophages play a key role in stimulating fibroplasia and angio-

genesis. The blood clot (specifically the fibrin and fibronectin network) serves as a provisional extracellular matrix. The fibrin and fibronectin form a scaffold to support and guide low-impedance cell migration (macrophages, fibroblasts) and collagen deposition. As noted, integrins are cell membrane receptors necessary for cell binding or adherence to specific glycoproteins of the ECM matrix. The fibronectin receptor complex binds the cell wall to fibronectin as well as cytoskeletal proteins on the inside of the cell. As a result, contraction of intracellular actin microfilaments can move the cell through anchorage to the fibronectin and other ECM proteins. Thus, integrins are receptor proteins that integrate the extracellular and intracellular scaffolds, allowing them to work in concert. Once fibroblasts and endothelial cells express the proper integrin receptors under stimulation of cytokines and provisional matrix proteins, they are capable of moving into the wound environment.

The four key processes associated with the proliferative phase of wound healing will be discuss as subsets, including (1) neovascularization/angiogenesis; (2) fibroplasia and collagen deposition; (3) epithelialization; and (4) wound contraction (Fig. 2-1).

(1) Neovascularization: Angiogenesis

A key event in the healing process is new blood vessel formation, termed *angiogenesis*. Without adequate circulation, fibroblasts cannot survive in the wound environment: in short, no fibroblasts, no collagen. Epithelialization also is dependent on the presence of a vascularized ECM.

Angiogenesis is a complex process and depends on four interrelated phenomena, including (1) cell phenotype alteration, (2) chemoattractant-driven migration, (3) mitogenic stimulation, and (4) the local development of a supportive extracellular matrix. Growth and chemotactic factors within the wound prompt local endothelial enzyme release. The local wound environment also potentiates angiogenesis, including the presence of low oxygen tension, biogenic amines, and lactic acid. The low oxygen tension likely stimulates macrophages to produce and secrete angiogenic factors.

Plasminogen activator and collagenase released from endothelial cells (located at the venule side closest to the angiogenic stimulus) transit through the degraded basement membrane. Endothelial cells project pseudopodia through the weakened basement membrane and migrate into the perivascular space. Endothelial cells from the parent vessels proliferate by the second or third day after injury and serve as a cell source during angiogenesis. Capillary buds extend into the matrix, where their tips eventually branch and

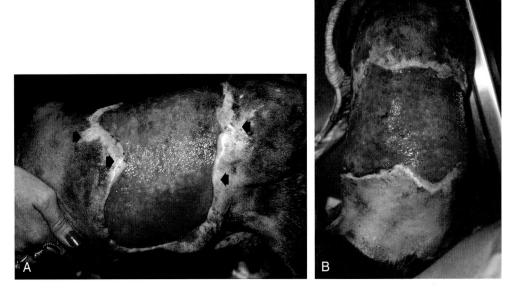

FIG. 2-1 (A, B) Granulation bed involving the canine trunk. Early wound epithelialization (arrows) is noted along the wound margins. Note the distinct "pebble-grain" or granular surface composed of outgrowths of capillaries by budding from existing capillaries. Fibroblasts surround these capillary loops forming individual granules that coalesce to form granulation tissue.

connect, forming capillary loops. New branches extend from the loops to form a capillary plexus.

The ECM has a strong influence on endothelial cell morphology and function. A rich fibronectin matrix around the endothelial buds helps support and guide endothelial cell movement. This neovasculature deposits its own matrix of proteoglycans and fibronectin, ultimately forming its own basement membrane.

(2) Fibroplasia and Collagen Deposition

Fibroplasia is the component of granulation tissue that includes the fibroblasts and the associated ECM. Fibroblasts originated from the viable "peri-wound" tissues, although other viable mesenchymal cells are capable of differentiating into fibroblasts. Cytokines and the provisional matrix stimulate proliferation of fibroblasts, express the formation of integrin receptors, and ultimately migrate into the wound space. Fibrin adheres to fibrin, and fibronectin cell receptors allow fibroblasts to move through the filamentous scaffold. Fibroblasts also have integrin receptors allowing them to attach directly to fibrin and other protein strands. Fibroblasts will advance toward the chemotactic gradient by extending lamellipodia toward the stimulus. The integrin bonds will release and reform as the fibroblast creeps forward. Fibroblasts release proteolytic enzymes—plasminogen activator, interstitial collagenase (MMP-1), gelatinase (MMP-2), and stromelysin (MMP-3)—to facilitate their migration through this filamentous fibrin-linked jungle. After migration into the wound, fibroblasts gradually shift to protein synthesis. Initially, fibroblasts secrete large quantities of fibronectin, forming a loose ECM: a collagenous matrix follows.

Collagen is a glycoprotein arranged in three alpha chains forming a spiral or helix. The collagen molecule is composed of 33% glycine, 33% proline, and the remaining 33% is a variety of other amino acids. The amino acids proline and lysine must be hydroxylated when they are incorporated into the alpha chains by the fibroblast. The enzymes propyl hydroxylase and lysyl hydroxylase are necessary for this essential step in collagen formation. Oxygen, ferrous iron, alpha ketoglutarate, and a reducing agent such as ascorbate (vitamin C) or light-activated riboflavin are necessary for the enzymatic hydroxylation process. Vitamin C is essential for optimum collagen production. If the hydroxylation process is not completed, the collagen molecule cannot be excreted from the fibroblast. Although the dog and cat generally possess adequate levels of vitamin C, it is worthy to consider its supplementation in severely stressed patients that have a poor nutritional status.

Upon hydroxylation, a galactose molecule is attached to the assembled intracellular collagen molecule, which is then excreted. This extracellular molecule is termed *procollagen*. Terminal or registration peptides are cleared from this molecule by procollagen C-proteinases and procollagen N-proteinases. When this occurs, the procollagen molecule aggregates to form tropocollagen fibers. The tropocollagen molecules in turn assemble to form fibrils. This assembly or aggregation, due to lysine-lysine amino acid cross-linkage, is responsible for a major portion of the strength in the collagen fibril. A variety of diseases and drugs can alter this orderly process, resulting in potentially serious wound healing and functional complications.

During the wound remodeling process previously discussed, a primitive collagen gel (collagen III) or matrix initially is deposited only to be resorbed by collagenase enzymes as a stronger collagen (collagen I) is laid down over a period of weeks to months following an injury (see the Maturation and Remodeling Phase discussion, below). Sources of collagenase in the wound are inflammatory cells, endothelial cells, fibroblasts, and keratinocytes. Collagenase activity is closely controlled by cytokines. As noted, the net result of the process is less collagen compared to the original closely packed collagen, but a collagen network of greater tensile strength due to its structurally superior basket-weave design. Collagen generally realigns to form sheets parallel to physiologic tension lines using increasingly firm cross-linkage of collagen strands or bundles. This is readily evident in the normal controlled healing process during tendon repair.

Day 4–5 after surgery is a critical juncture in surgical wound repair. Prior to this, sutures primarily maintain alignment of the tissues. Day 4–5 is the time at which fibroplasia and early collagen deposition are noted. Tensile strength increases rapidly after this point.

Although wound dehiscence can occur at any point of the healing process, it is the author's clinical experience that most cases of wound dehiscence occur 3–5 days postoperatively. For problematic wound closures, the first 5 days of healing (inflammatory phase) requires the surgeon's closest attention.

Collagen is directly responsible for the tensile strength of a healing wound. A lack of collagen or its improper formation can lead to wound dehiscence.

As collagen is deposited by fibroblasts, fibrin strands are removed. Net collagen synthesis is increased for at least 4–5 weeks after wounding, spanning the proliferative and maturation phases of healing. Increased collagen deposition is due to increased fibroblast numbers and increased collagen deposition from each cell. Collagenase activity in advancing epithelial cells and in adjacent fibroblasts is important in controlling collagen deposition. This

fibroplastic phase lasts for 2–4 weeks, depending on the wound size. The termination of this phase is noted by a decline in the number of capillaries and fibroblasts and by a greater deposition of collagen.

Over time, chronic granulation tissue will form in a nonhealing open wound. Older scar beds are laden with collagen, while the fibroblast and the capillary populations have declined. As a result, chronic granulation tissue does not support epithelialization or wound contraction without surgical intervention.

(3) Epithelialization

Wound healing is incomplete without restoration of the epithelial surface. One or two days after injury, epithelial cells begin to proliferate in the basal zone and overlying prickle cell layer along the viable border of the skin defect. The epithelial cells dissect clot and damaged stroma by secreting proteolytic enzymes (collagenase, plasminogen activator) as they attempt to repave the viable tissue surface.

Epithelial cells undergo a marked phenotypic alteration. They lose their tenacious binding with the dermis and lose their apical-basal polarity. They advance over the viable tissue surface by extending pseudopods along the basolateral sides of the wound. Epithelial cells will enlarge and flatten during migration over the vascular wound bed as they lose their attachments to the basement membrane and adjacent epithelial cells. Chalone (water-soluble glycoproteins) found in the epidermis normally inhibits mitosis; it is diminished in wounds, allowing epithelial cells at the perimeter of the wound to undergo mitosis and migrate onto the adjacent granulation tissue (or viable vascular tissue). As the cells slide forward, collagenase is released to facilitate their migration beneath any scab present on the wound surface. Integrin receptors facilitate their movement over the wound surface and the bed of fibrinogen, fibronectin, and type 1 collagen. Epithelial migration is guided by collagen fibers.

In sutured wounds with a minimal dermal gap, epithelial cells can bridge the minor gap by 48 hours.

In moderate to large wounds, epithelial migration may take weeks or may never completely cover the open wound. Thus, the process of epithelialization can extend from the proliferative phase well into the maturation phase of healing in problematic wounds.

The surface of epithelialized wounds (scar epithelium) is normally characterized by thinness and fragility. The initial epithelial layer is only one cell layer thick, but gradually thickens to a variable degree as additional cell layers form. On "protected" areas of the animal, the durability of scar epithelium may be satisfactory. In body areas subject to periodic trauma,

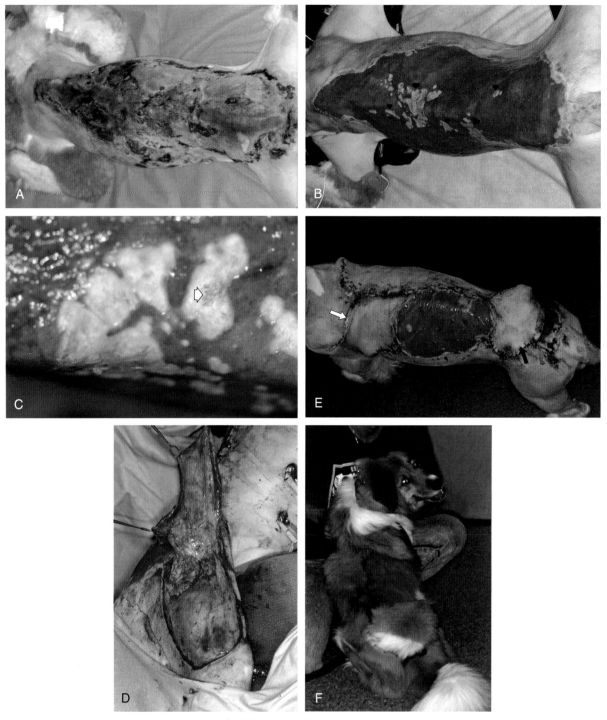

FIG. 2-2 *See legend on opposite page.*

abrasive surfaces, or solar exposure, the same scar surface may ulcerate. Hair growth is minimal within the epithelialized scar. Given these considerations, coverage with full-thickness skin (flaps, grafts, skin advancement) may be advisable, depending upon the location and magnitude of the cutaneous defect, the durability required to withstand wound breakdown, and the cosmetic results desired.

The source of epithelial cells varies according to the thickness of the skin defect (see Chapter 1.) The viable skin perimeter is the source of epithelial cells in full-thickness skin defects. Partial-thickness wounds (loss of the epidermis and portions of the dermis) can predominately reepithelialize from viable dermal adnexa, especially the external root sheaths of the compound hair follicles. (See Chapter 3) (Fig. 2-2).

Partial-thickness loss of skin is commonly seen with deep dermal abrasions and second-degree burns. Despite the loss of the epidermis, adnexal reepithelialization is considerably faster than comparable full-thickness skin defects. In the more superficial injuries, healing may occur with little scarring and surprisingly good cosmetic results.

PSEUDO-HEALING

Sutured wounds can appear healed after epithelialization has occurred at the junctional gap of apposed skin margins. However, without appropriate collagen deposition below the epidermal surface, the wound has a low tensile strength and is subject to dehiscence with premature suture removal.

This has been noted in dogs on high levels of corticosteroids over a prolonged period of time. Pseudo-healing also has been reported in cats as a result of the comparatively slower healing processes. When a delay in wound healing is suspected, sutures should be retained for a longer period of time (3 weeks suggested) to reduce this risk. Additionally, intradermal sutures can be used to support incisional healing, followed by skin sutures. The intradermal pattern can reduce incisional tension and provide additional support after skin suture removal. Another cautionary measure can be used in problematic healing cases: alternate skin sutures can be removed, followed by the remaining half 2–3 days later.

(4) Wound Contraction

By definition, wound contraction is the process in which the skin peripheral to a full-thickness defect advances in a centripedal fashion toward the center of the wound. Wound contraction spans both the proliferative and maturation phases of healing (Fig. 2-2). After migration into the ECM, fibroblasts change to a profibrotic phenotype during which collagen (type I

FIG. 2-2 (A) Extensive thermal wound in a dog, maliciously set on fire using a flammable agent.

(B) Large granulation bed formed after aggressive debridement of an extensive full-thickness burn to the trunk, 1 week later. Islands of epithelium are forming in the central area of the wound bed (arrows).

(C) Close-up view of these epithelial islands demonstrate that hair follicles (arrow) surviving in deep dermal and hypodermal tissue after debridement are the source of these epithelial cells. Combined cutaneous closure techniques were necessary to cover this massive defect.

(D) Intraoperative view of deep circumflex iliac island arterial flap (ventral branch). The flap was rotated 180 degrees to cover the dorsal pelvic portion of this sizeable skin defect.

(E) Combined closure employing a thoracodorsal axial pattern flap (open arrow), deep circumflex iliac island arterial flap (ventral branch) (solid arrow), and advancement of the lateral thoracic skin using "walking sutures." Islands of epithelium (noted in C, above) were harvested and reimplanted as punch grafts in the remaining granulation bed.

(F) The patient, 6 weeks after surgery. The remaining open wounds primarily closed by wound contraction, with epithelialization playing a secondary role in this instance. (From Pavletic MM. 1990. Massive trunk wound secondary to thermal trauma. *Vet Med Report* 2:59.)

and III) is deposited. During the second and third week of repair, fibroblasts develop smooth muscle properties as contracile proteins (F-actin microfilaments) develop along the cytoplasmic face of the basement membrane. These contractile fibroblasts are called myofibroblasts.

Myofibroblast integrins link the cells to the fibronectin network and the collagenous fibrils in the ECM. Collagen bundles in turn interlink within the granulation tissue and the dermal layer of the bordering skin margins. These cell-cell, cell-matrix, and matrix-matrix interconnections result in the ability of myofibroblasts to apply a traction force onto this pericellular matrix. This force is exerted as myofibroblasts align with the wound contraction lines. As the myofibroblasts extend and contract their pseudopods, the collagen bundles align and condense in concert. Cytokines (especially PDGF from macrophages) likely are involved in activation of these processes. Earlier reports suggest fibroblasts also are capable of contributing to the process of wound contraction in the appropriate ECM components, and cytokine signals are present.

The cross-linkage of collagen and fibronectin with myofibrolastic attachments is analogous to a fishnet used in commercial fishing. Traction on the net draws or drags anything trapped or attached to the fishnet. In wound contraction, the skin margins interlinked with the collagen network are literally dragged toward the center of the granulation bed.

The timing of wound contraction has been reported to be between the 3rd and 42nd day in experimental rabbits. By contrast, the lag phase in dogs is 5–9 days. As the skin is stretched in a centripetal fashion, both the epidermis and dermis narrow in response to the tension. The term *intussceptive* growth describes the process of epithelial proliferation and collagen deposition that occurs within the stretched skin to bolster and restore cutaneous areas that are under significant tension. As will be discussed in Chapter 10, skin also is capable of stretching beyond its inherent or natural elasticity by application of external forces, including the use of skin stretchers and tissue expanders.

WOUND CONTRACTION: CLINICAL CONSIDERATIONS

Experimentally, wound contraction proceeds at a rate of 0.6–0.75 mm per day. Wound contraction appears to decline after 42 days in experimental rabbits; it also decreases in other animals over time. Therefore, 6 weeks is a general guideline on what to expect for wounds in which wound contraction is considered the best option to close a problematic wound. After 6 weeks, any remaining skin defect will need to close by epithelial cell migration (without surgical intervention). In some cases, the surgeon may elect to manage a problematic wound by promoting the process of wound contraction. If the wound closes significantly during this time, any remaining defect will be smaller and more amenable to a simpler closure technique.

Contracture is the loss or inhibition of motion or function as a result of excessive scar tissue or muscle atrophy or fibrosis. Wound contraction also can contribute to contracture formation when skin tension secondary to this healing process limits function (especially involving the extremities). This will be discussed in greater detail in Chapter 6.

Puppies and kittens have the remarkable ability to close wounds primarily by the process of wound contraction (Fig. 2-3). Provided with a healthy diet and proper wound care, surprisingly large skin wounds can close within weeks after injury. During this process it is important to assess the patient periodically for signs of wound contracture.

Wound contraction is remarkably effective in loose-skinned, fur-bearing animals compared to the human. As a result, surgical intervention using skin grafts and flaps is more common for larger wounds in humans, whereas wound contraction may be considered a useful option in many veterinary patients. Interestingly, square and rectangular wounds contract more effectively than circular skin defects, based on animal studies. The linear edges favor the linear traction forces of the myofibroblasts. By contrast, circular wound margins are pulled simultaneously, with the skin margin binding from the offset or angular contractile forces applied to its edge. From a wound management standpoint, any remaining skin defect would need to heal by epithelial cell migration. (For this reason, a circular skin wound is used to accommodate a colostomy stoma in humans. A linear incision or square skin defect created at the stoma is more likely to contract and form a constriction.)

The independent healing processes of wound contraction and epithelialization will affect the cosmetic outcome in wound closure. Skin wounds that close primarily by contraction will have a relatively small, hairless epithelialized scar. Adjacent hair growth may cover over this hairless area. In contrast, wounds that heal to a significant degree by epithelialization will have a comparatively large, thin, hairless surface. From a cosmetic and functional standpoint, this is less favorable.

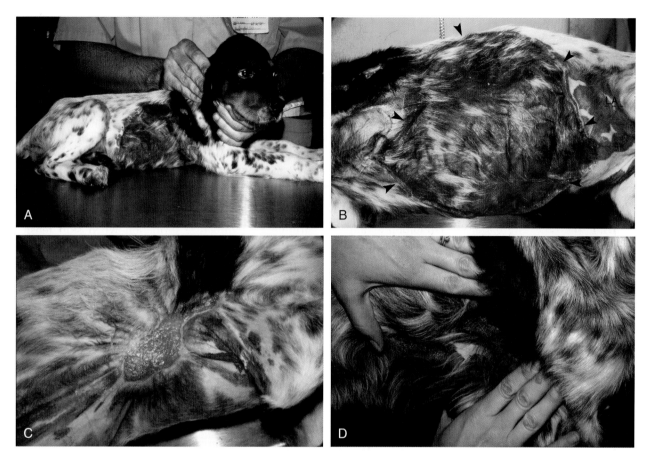

FIG. 2-3 (A) Extensive thermal burn as a result of an electrical heating pad in this retriever puppy.

(B) Close-up view of the lower thorax and abdomen. Wound contraction progressed during the next 6 weeks by centipedal advancement of peripheral loose skin. Serial debridement was performed; silver sulfadiazine was used on the burn.

(C) The thermal wound closed predominately by contraction.

(D) A small epithelialized scar eventually can be seen after parting the hair. (From Parritz DL, Pavletic MM. 1992. Physical and chemical injuries: heatstroke, hypothermia, burns and frost bite. In: Murtaugh R, Kaplan P, eds. *Veterinary Emergency and Critical Care Medicine.* St. Louis: Mosby-Yearbook.)

Maturation and Remodeling Phase

During the transition from granulation tissue to scar maturation, collagen remodeling occurs, with a balance between collagen deposition and collagen catabolism. Type III collagen gradually decreases as type I collagen increases. Specific collagenase enzymes (metalloproteinases) from macrophages, fibroblasts, and epidermal cells cleave type I, II, III, X, and XIII collagens. Balancing the degradation of collagen are tissue inhibitors of metalloproteinases (TIMPs). Cytokines and the ECM play an important role in this process. Nonfunc-

tional collagen fibers are broken down by these proteolytic enzymes within the ECM.

Collagen deposition is directly related to the tensile strength of a wound. Three weeks after injury, the scar has 20% of its final strength. Thereafter, gains of tensile strength occur at a much slower rate. Over the next several weeks, a scar will achieve only 70%–80% of the tensile strength of normal skin. Tensile strength is primarily associated with collagen remodeling, resulting in larger collagen bundles and intermolecular cross-links with adjacent collagen fibers. In the end, there is less collagen than initially noted in the early healing process but with a structurally superior configuration. As maturation progresses, the dense capillary network of healthy granulation tissue progressively declines.

The maturation and remodeling phase is generally considered to take place from day 20 to approximately 1 year after injury.

As noted, chronic, nonhealing wounds develop a fibrotic matrix highlighted by collagen deposition and a decline in the capillary population. Chronic wound beds usually lack the vascularity to support epithelialization or the application of a skin. Tangential excision of the chronic granulation bed down to the otherwise healthy underlying tissue plane can induce formation of a healthy vascular granulation bed. In less than 1 week, the reconstituted granulation bed usually is able to support free graft application.

SPECIES VARIATIONS IN WOUND HEALING

Differences in the anatomy and circulation to the skin have been well recognized both in mammals and other species. Variations in wound healing also can be expected. One study in cats indicated that formation of granulation tissue is slower in cats compared with dogs (7.5 days in dogs versus 19 days in cats). Granulation tissue appeared to originate from the entire wound bed in dogs whereas granulation tissue appeared to develop along the wound border and progressively advance over the wound in a centripetal fashion. Overall, the development of granulation tissue, wound contraction, and epithelial cell migration in cats lagged behind dogs. Wound epithelialization and total healing were greater for the dog than the cat over a 21-day period. Wound contraction was greater in dogs than cats at day 7, but not at days 14–21. As a result, the tensile strength of feline incisions was substantially less (approximately 50%) than canine subjects in this study. Furthermore, removal of the subcutaneous tissues at wound closure may slow the processes of healing, especially in cats. Due to the limitations of this study, additional research is required to explain these physiologic differences in healing.

As discussed, when there is a concern regarding the completeness in wound healing, skin sutures can be retained well beyond the time sutures are normally removed. Prolonged retention of skin sutures can result in more prominent suture scars, which is not a major concern in fur-bearing animals.

Intradermal skin sutures can provide supplemental support to skin closures and significantly reduce the risk of wound dehiscence after external skin sutures are removed.

ARTIFICIAL SKIN

Research has focused on the creation of a three-dimensional synthetic collagen weave similar to the ECM of the dermis. This matrix allows tissue cells, including fibroblasts and macrophages, to assemble and develop in this synthetic stroma to form a more normal dermal structure. As discussed, the ECM has a critical influence in cells and serves in a "director capacity," in cellular function and the deposition of collagen, elastin, fibronectin, laminin, and proteoglycans. Endothelial cells enter the matrix to revascularize the forming ECM. In turn, this revascularized "neodermis" will support epithelial coverage. Reformation of a basement membrane over the neodermis improves the likelihood that the epidermis will reform in a manner similar to normal skin. By contrast, wounds lacking this artificial lattice (such as extensive burns) will deposit collagen that lacks any similarity to normal dermal architecture. Because dermal integrity plays an important role in epidermal cell attachment and orientation, epithelialized scars are less durable and more prone to epidermal trauma.

In humans Dermagraft™ and Skin2™ have been designed to replace the loss of the dermis in persons sustaining serious thermal injuries or suffering from chronic skin ulcers. Human diploid fibroblasts are grown on a polymer scaffold to which growth factors and matrix proteins are added. Once developed, the artificial dermis is packaged and kept frozen (−70 °C) until needed. Because of the low antigenic properties of Dermagraft, there is no rejection of this neodermis. Application of epithelial cells from the patient will repopulate the surface. Although studies are not complete, dermagrafts may improve the cosmetic and functional outcomes in those patients with problematic skin wounds.

Suggested Readings

Bohling MW, Henderson RA. 2006. Differences in cutaneous wound healing between dogs and cats. *Vet Clin No Am* 36:687–692.

Bohling MW, Henderson RA, Swaim ST, et al. 2004. Cutaneous wound healing in the cat: a macroscopic description and comparison with cutaneous wound healing in the dog. *Vet Surg* 33:579–587.

Bohling MW, Henderson RA, Swaim ST, et al. 2006. Comparison of the role of the subcutaneous tissues in cutaneous wound healing in the dog and cat. *Vet Surg* 35:1–12.

Bucknall TE, Ellis H. 1984. *Wound Healing for Surgeons*. Philadelphia, PA: Bailliere Tindall.

Epstein FH. 1999. Cutaneous wound healing. *N Eng J Med* 341:738–746.

Gilbert SF. 2006. *Developmental Embryology*, 8th ed. Sunderland, Massachusetts: Sinauer Associates, Inc.

Fitch RB, Swaim SF. 1995. The role of epithelialization in wound healing. *Compend Contin Edu Pract Vet* 17(2): 167–177.

Hosgood G. 1993. The role of platelet derived growth factor and transforming growth factor beta. *Vet Surg* 22: 490–495.

Hosgood G. 2002. Wound repair and specific tissue response to injury. In: Slatter D, ed. *Textbook of Small Animal Surgery*, 3rd ed., 66–86. Philadelphia, PA: Saunders Elsevier Sciences.

Hosgood G. 2006. Stages of wound healing and their clinical relevance. *Vet Clin No Am* 36:667–685.

Hunt TK, Dunphy JE. 1979. *Fundamentals of Wound Management*. New York: Appleton & Lange.

Johnston DE. 1990. Wound healing in skin. *Vet Clin No Am* 20:1–25.

Lanza PP, Langer R, Chick, WL. 1997. *Principles of Tissue Engineering*. Austin, TX: RG Landes Company.

Pavletic MM. 1985. Introduction to wound healing and wound management. In Proceedings of the American Animal Hospital Association. Lakewood, CO: AAHA.

Pavletic MM. 1993. Surgery of the skin and management of wounds. In: Sherding RG, ed. *The Cat: Diseases and Clinical Management*, 2nd ed. New York: Churchill Livingstone.

Peacock EE. 1984. *Wound Repair*. 3rd ed. Philadelphia, PA: WB Saunders.

Probst CW. 1993. Wound healing and specific tissue regeneration. In Slatter DH, ed. *Textbook of Small Animal Surgery*, 2nd ed. Philadelphia, PA: WB Saunders.

Robson MC. 1997. The role of growth factors in the healing of chronic wounds. *Wound Repair Regen* 5(1):12–17.

Sadler TW. 2004. *Langman's Medical Embryology*, 9th ed. Philadelphia, PA: Lippincott Williams Wilkins.

Schilling JA. 1976. Wound healing. *Surg Clin No Am* 5:859–874.

Steed DL. 1997. The role of growth factors in wound healing. *Surg Clin No Am* 77:575.

Swaim SF, Henderson RA. 1997. *Small Animal Wound Management*, 2nd ed. Philadelphia, PA: Lippincott Williams and Wilkins.

Tredget EE, Nedelec B, Scott PG, et al. 1997. Hypertrophic scars, keloids, and contractures. *Surg Clin No Am* 77:701–730.

Witte MB, Barbul A. 1997. General principles of wound healing. *Surg Clin No Am* 77:509–528.

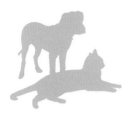

3

Basic Principles of Wound Management

INTRODUCTION

The principles of wound management have not significantly wavered from those advocated by Esmarch and Halsted decades ago (Tables 3-1 and 3-2). Although many of the wounds seen by the clinician are not life-threatening, proper assessment and management of the wounds will have a significant impact on their outcome. Many smaller wounds can heal despite the misguided efforts of disinterested clinicians. Careless wound management of more serious injuries can promote multiple wound complications, including tissue necrosis, infection, and wound dehiscence. More importantly, further trauma by the veterinarian may be the "death blow" to a body region already suffering from circulatory compromise secondary to disease or injury. The tissue death that follows may result in the need to amputate an affected limb, precipitate the need for costly treatments, or result in the death of the animal (Fig. 3-1).

Consistently, successful results in wound management require practice, attention to small details, and adherence to the basic principles of wound care.

PATIENT PRESENTATION

When a traumatized patient is first presented to the surgeon-practitioner, a complete medical history must be obtained, including specific details pertaining to the cause of the injuries. A detailed physical examination is performed on all patients. Patients with minor trauma require no emergency treatment on presentation. Patients that present with severe trauma are best managed with a simultaneous team approach employing the critical care, surgical, and radiology staff. Assessment of the critical care patient's airway, breathing, and circulatory status is performed as supportive care is instituted, including the insertion of one or more intravenous catheters. Collection of samples to determine the baseline complete blood count, serum chemistry profile, and urinalysis should be considered for each patient. Subsequent or serial reassessments are predicated on a patient's intraoperative and postoperative status.

Some injuries may require immediate emergency surgery following initial efforts to stabilize the patient. For unstable patients with nonthreatening open wounds, basic wound care and bandage application can suffice until definitive wound exploration and closure can be attempted. Analgesics and sedation should be considered, provided that medication does not impair the ability to fully assess the critical patient. In general, analgesics and/or sedation should be initiated as soon as patient assessment is complete. Specific details on wound care are discussed later in this chapter.

MECHANISMS OF INJURY AND WOUND TERMINOLOGY

In humans, three basic forces have been described that result in injury to the skin: shearing, compression, and tension. Shearing injuries are the result of sharp objects,

---

TABLE 3-1
Halsted's principles of surgery.

A. Minimal surgical trauma (gentle tissue handling)
B. Accurate hemostasis
C. Preservation of an adequate blood supply
D. Aseptic surgical technique
E. No tension on tissues
F. Careful tissue approximation
G. Obliteration of dead space

TABLE 3-2
Esmarch's principles of wound management.

A. Nonintroduction of anything harmful
B. Tissue rest
C. Wound drainage
D. Avoidance of venous stasis
E. Cleanliness

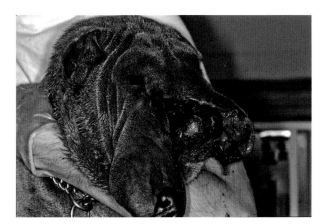

FIG. 3-1 Shar-Pei with massive facial injury secondary to vehicular trauma. Despite the shearing wound to the face, the excellent blood supply to the head maintained tissue viability. Atraumatic surgical technique is important to minimize further circulatory compromise to these traumatized tissues.

including knives, glass, and other cutting surfaces. Because energy is dispersed along a more finite area, minimal tissue destruction may be noted. Tension injuries arise from the tangential or angular impact from a blunt or semiblunt object or surface. The skin is under tension at the point of impact, and the skin splits. Partial avulsion of skin or traumatic flap formation may be noted. Large avulsion wounds often result in the tearing of regional circulation: a variable degree of tissue necrosis should be anticipated. Compression injuries occur when an object or surface strikes the skin at a right angle, resulting in a ragged edge to the skin. The effects of tissue compression or crushing may result in significant circulatory compromise to the area, with an increased risk of necrosis and infection. Bite wounds, for example may have compression and tension forces applied to regional tissues. Circulatory compromise and tissue necrosis, combined with the introduction of oral bacterial flora, is an invitation to infection.

There are several terms generally used to describe specific wounds (Table 3-3). They are useful for accurately describing this subset of injuries commonly seen in small animal practice.

WOUND CLASSIFICATION

Four Basic Wound Classifications

The surgeon is faced with a variety of issues when managing an open wound. Clearly, the severity of tissue trauma, degree of contamination, and the presence of or potential for infection are factors in determining the most appropriate wound care. The intraoperative assessment of the wound after exploration, debridement, and lavage is the best time to determine if wound closure should be attempted now or at a later time.

Thorough debridement of necrotic tissue and cleansing—lavage to remove contaminants—may convert a contaminated wound to a surgically clean wound that is suitable for primary closure.

From the information gathered from the history and physical examination, a wound can be classified into one of four basic categories according to its condition. These four categories, in their increasing order of severity, are the following:

- Clean
- Clean-contaminated
- Contaminated
- Dirty and Infected

TABLE 3-3
Descriptive terminology in wound management.

Abrasion
- Skin wounds caused by tangential trauma to the epidermis and dermis.
- Skin is rubbed against a resistant surface in a rubbing or scraping fashion.

Note: Minor abrasions to the skin also may be noted with removal of an adhesive agent (adherent bandage, surgical adhesive, etc.)

Avulsion
- *Complete avulsion:* Complete displacement or tearing of a tissue segment or portion of the body
- *Partial avulsion:* Partial detachment of a tissue segment or portion of the body (for example, traumatic skin flap)
- *Degloving injury:* Traumatic partial avulsion of skin from an extremity in a circumferential fashion, resembling the peeling off or removal of a glove

Incision
- A cut of orderly depth with a sharp instrument

Laceration
- An irregular cut of nonorderly depth; a jagged wound or cut

Puncture Wound
- A hole or wound created by a sharp pointed object.
- Penetrating wound: A puncture wound in which the object enters a given tissue plane or structure but does not emerge beyond it
- Perforating wound: A puncture wound in which the object enters and exits a given tissue plane or structure (a "through-and-through" wound to the involved tissue plane or structure)

Contusion (Bruise)
- An injury in which the skin is not broken, usually exemplified by swelling, pain, and discoloration (capillary rupture with escape of blood)

It is occasionally difficult to accurately select the exact category based on gross assessment of the degree of contamination and the time that transpired after injury. When in doubt, it is best to downgrade the wound's classification and treat it accordingly. Clean, clean-contaminated and contaminated wounds would generally be considered to have fewer than 100,000 bacteria per gram of tissue. Because bacterial counts increase for every hour of neglect, early intervention can reduce the likelihood of infection. See the section, Age of the Wound: Clinical Significance below.

The basic question on the mind of the doctor is: Can I close the wound primarily or should the wound be managed as an open wound for a variable period of time? Wound classifications are a useful guideline for determining how a given wound is best managed. Selection of the most appropriate method of closure is best determined after definitive wound exploration and initial management of the wound.

Clean Wounds

A clean wound is a nontraumatic, uninfected operative wound in which neither the oro-pharyngeal cavities nor the respiratory, alimentary, or genitourinary tracts are entered. Clean wounds are made under aseptic conditions. They are usually primarily closed (Fig. 3-2).

Clean-Contaminated Wounds

Clean-contaminated wounds are operative wounds in which the respiratory, alimentary, or genitourinary tract is entered without unusual contamination. Wounds with minor contamination or a clean wound with a "minor" break in sterile surgical technique may be classified in this category (Fig. 3-3).

Contaminated Wounds

Contaminated wounds include open traumatic wounds, wounds made in operations during which there was a major break in sterile technique, and incision wounds made in areas of acute, nonpurulent inflammation or made in or near contaminated or inflamed skin. Unless the procedure is performed without a breech in sterile surgical technique, wounds made for access to the lumen of the colon may belong in this category (Fig. 3-4).

Dirty and Infected Wounds

Dirty and infected wounds include old traumatic wounds and those involving clinical infection or perforated viscera. The definition of this classification suggests that greater than 100,000 organisms per gram of tissue are present in the wound before the operation, or that pus has contaminated the wound (Fig. 3-5).

Age of the Wound: Clinical Significance

Many pet owners have no exact knowledge of the time a given injury occurred, especially in those unsupervised animals allowed to roam outdoors for extended periods of time. In those cases, the clinician must rely on his/her clinical assessment of the patient to determine the best method to manage the open wound.

Clean-contaminated wounds generally are considered a wound less than 6 hours old. Wounds less than 6 hours old also are referred to as class 1 wounds. Some subdivide contaminated wounds into wounds 6–12 hours old (class 2) and greater than 12 hours old (class 3). However, time in and of itself is not an accurate guideline in determining the classification of a given wound and the appropriate method of closure.

The time frame of less than 6 hours has been referred to as the "golden period" of wound healing in the literature: the bacterial inoculum is likely to be below the threshold of infection ($<10^6$ per gram of tissue). Intervention within this grace period can reduce the risk of establishing infection. Research has indicated that bacteria can proliferate from 100 organisms per gram of tissue to over 100,000 organisms per gram within 6 hours.

There are a variety of factors that influence the risk of infection. Surgeons experienced in wound management know that the severity of wound contamination, body region involved, presence of necrotic tissue, and circulatory compromise are greater considerations than time, both in classifying a wound and selecting the appropriate method of closure.

To reduce the likelihood of wound infection, early medical and surgical intervention is preferable to unnecessary delays in open wound management.

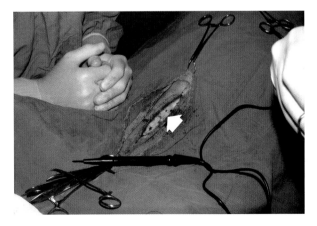

FIG. 3-2 A clean wound (arrow) is one created under sterile surgical conditions.

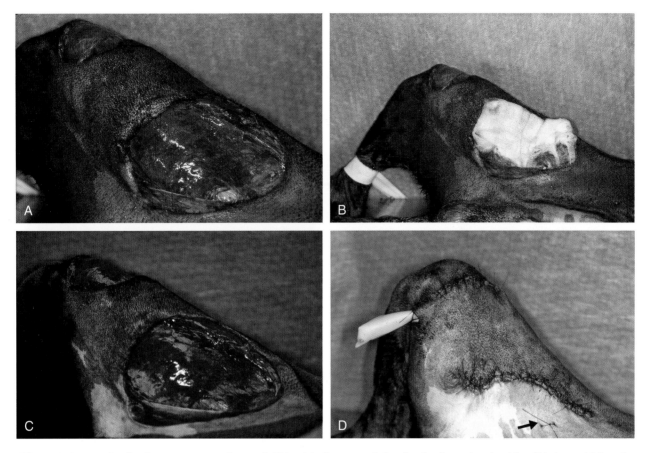

FIG. 3-3 (A) Example of a clean-contaminated wound. This pit bull presented shortly after lacerating the skin of his inner thigh and knee while leaping over a cyclone fence. Minimal contamination was evident in this fresh wound.

(B) The wound was protected with a sterile, moistened saline gauze pack prior to the liberal removal of fur and surgical preparation.

(C) Damaged and devitalized tissue was excised upon removal of the gauze sponges. The wounds were lavaged under pressure with sterile saline.

(D) The wound was closed primarily; a Penrose drain was used to control dead space and prevent serum accumulation. Note only the distal portion of the drain is exposed. The proximal end is secured with a single suture placed through the skin (arrow).

The body region involved in the injury also impacts whether primary closure or delayed closure options should be considered. For example, the head has a superior blood supply compared with the distal extremities. Primary closure may be a suitable option for many older head wounds whereas a similar wound involving the lower extremities may be better suited to open wound management for a variable period of time before wound closure is contemplated.

Any wound (regardless of the time of injury) after aggressive cleansing, irrigation, and debridement can be considered for primary closure if:

- all devitalized tissue is removed;
- all contaminants and debris are removed;
- the tissues appear healthy with a viable circulation; and
- there is no evidence of infection.

OPTIONS FOR WOUND CLOSURE

Classification of a wound will enable the clinician to logically decide on the proper method of management.

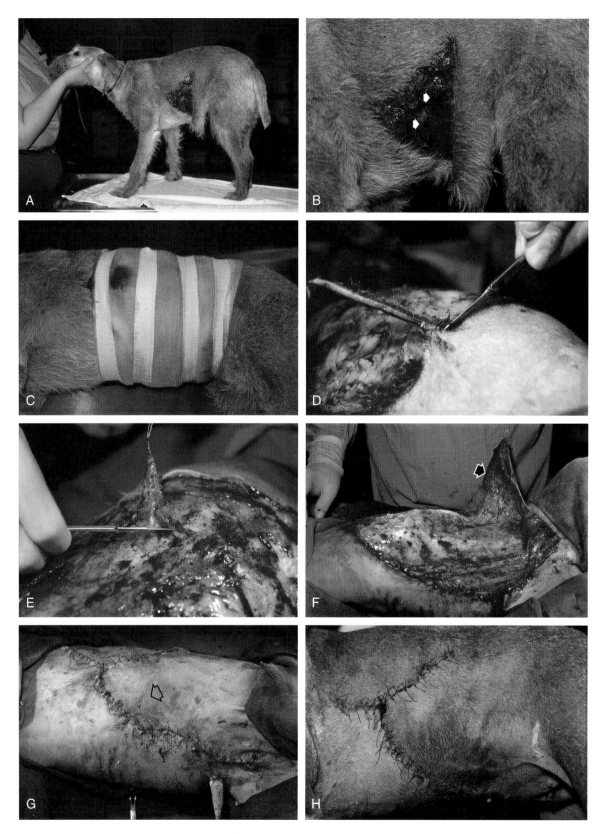

FIG. 3-4 *See legend on opposite page.*

For a given wound, there may be more than one option to achieve closure. The four basic options for closure of an open wound include:

1. primary closure,
2. delayed primary closure,
3. secondary closure, and
4. healing by second intention.

A variation of second intention healing is adnexal re-epithelialization of partial-thickness skin losses. The choice among these four basic methods of closure depends upon the wound size, location, and condition.

Over the years, one factor stands out as a major reason to avoid primary closure in favor of open wound management: the presence of dying or devitalized tissue. Wound healing is impaired with its presence, and bacteria thrive on the retention of this substrate.

Primary Closure

Primary closure or healing by first intention is the direct closure of a recently created wound. Wounds considered for primary closure include the following:

- Wounds with little or no contamination and minimal tissue trauma
- Contaminated wounds converted to "clean" wounds with judicious debridement and copious lavage with sterile isotonic solutions (Fig. 3-4)
- Skin defects after complete excision of smaller, localized areas of contamination and infection
- Adjacent skin available to close the wound without undue tension (see Chapter 9, Tension-Relieving Techniques; Chapter 11, Local Flaps)

FIG. 3-4 (A) Example of a contaminated wound involving the lateral thorax and abdomen. The skin was avulsed when it was hooked on a metallic object as the dog was running.

(B) The avulsion wound involving this dog's lateral thorax and abdomen was contaminated with bark and dried leaves adhered to the exposed subcutaneous tissues (arrows).

(C) A sterile wet (saline-chlorhexidine) dressing was temporarily applied to the wound prior to anesthetic induction.

(D) Irregular skin edges were excised to facilitate closure. Although it is desirable to note vigorous bleeding to the cut skin edge, the presence or lack of bleeding is not consistently accurate in determining skin viability at the time of surgery. More aggressive skin excision can be performed when ample loose skin is present to facilitate closure.

(E) Contaminated subcutaneous fat overlying the skeletal muscle was excised tangentially.

(F) Debridement was followed by copious pressure lavage. Contaminants that adhered to the partially avulsed skin segment (arrow) were carefully removed with forceps in order to avoid further circulatory compromise. The avulsed skin flap was partially debrided back to a bleeding skin margin, providing sufficient skin for surgical closure.

(G) Primary closure of this contaminated wound was successfully accomplished after prompt surgical intervention and attention to thorough removal of contaminants and necrotic tissue. A Penrose drain was used in this case; a closed suction unit would have been more appropriate to control this wide area of dead space.

(H) Healed wound. The thin skin of the lower abdomen readily shows subcutaneous hemorrhage.

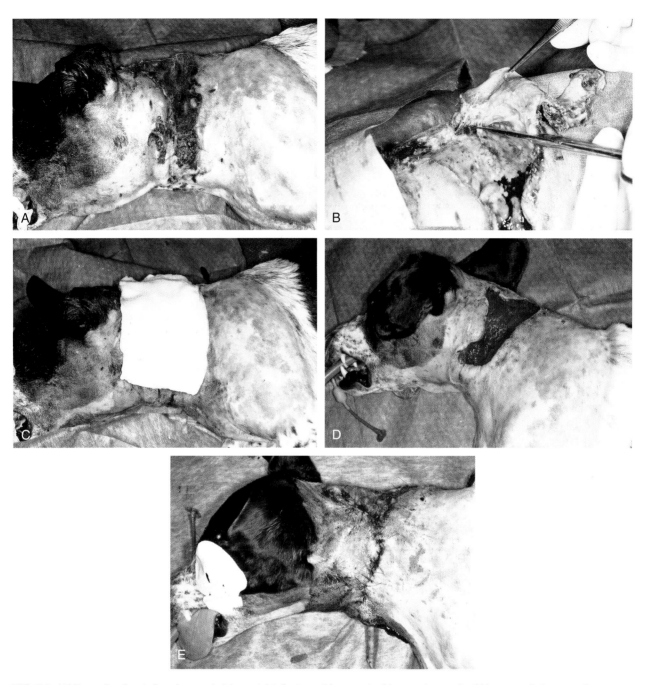

FIG. 3-5 (A) Example of an infected wound. A bacterial infection with necrotic skin was the result of bite wounds improperly managed 4 days prior to presentation.

(B) Wound debridement of the necrotic skin and subcutis.

(C) Wet–to-dry dressings, changed twice daily, were used to mechanically debride residual necrotic tissue for 3 days. This was followed by the topical application of an enzymatic debriding agent (trypsin).

(D) Six days following surgical debridement, a healthy granulation bed has formed.

(E) Because the owner had no desire to manage the wound at home, secondary closure was performed. Portions of the granulation bed and fibrotic skin borders were excised to facilitate accurate skin apposition with sutures. A Penrose drain exits ventral to the wound. Healing proceeded without incident.

Delayed Primary Closure

As the term implies, wound closure is delayed for a 3- to 5-day period in order to manage and reassess the wound during daily bandage changes. Sterile dressings/topical agents are inserted into the wound cavity and changed one to three times per day, depending on the condition of the wound. Delayed closure provides optimal drainage to the area, time for inflammation to subside, and circulation to improve before closure. Consequently, tissue resistance to infection improves dramatically, thereby reducing the likelihood of infection after closure. Common wounds considered for delayed primary closure include the following:

- Wounds with borderline contamination despite initial wound exploration, debridement, and lavage

- Wounds with moderate tissue trauma or considered at risk of infection after wound exploration, debridement, and lavage

- Wounds in which there is a question as to the tissue viability at the wound site

- Wounds that require additional (serial) debridement beyond initial wound cleansing and debridement

- Wounds in which significant tissue swelling precludes primary closure

By day 4–5 after injury, capillary buds, fibroplasia, tissue macrophages, and associated cytokines are present within the wound. As a result, tissues are more resistant to infection at this time. If the tissues are viable and swelling has declined without evidence of infection, successful closure is likely (Fig. 3-6).

Secondary Closure

Secondary closure is attempted between the fifth and tenth day after injury. By this point, a healthy granulation bed normally is developing over the open wound surface.

Secondary closure is reserved for problematic wounds in which

- delayed primary closure is not possible, usually as a result of persistent infection;

- persistence of necrotic tissue requires additional serial debridement and wound care beyond 5 days; and

- there is persistence of a moderate to severe inflammatory response.

Secondary closure can be attempted by one of two methods: (1) direct suture apposition of the two granulation surfaces (healing by third intention) or (2) granulation tissue excision and primary closure. The latter technique is preferred by many surgeons for humans because of the relative ease in mobilization of the wound edges for closure, the better cosmetic results, and the lower incidence of infection after excision of the granulation tissue (Fig. 3-5). The author uses a combination of both variations by removing sufficient scar tissue to facilitate closure of the defect. Complete excision of a healthy granulation bed generally is unnecessary.

Second-Intention Healing: Contraction and Epithelialization

Healing by second intention or contraction and epithelialization is a commonly employed method to close problematic wounds in veterinary medicine. With appropriate management, the processes of myofibroblastic wound contraction and epithelial cell migration over the external surface of granulation tissue is promoted (see Chapter 1). Second intention healing is generally reserved for the following wounds:

- Dirty and infected wounds in which closure by the previous three techniques is unadvisable.

- Cutaneous defects that cannot be closed adequately using conventional surgical techniques. This is particularly true for skin defects located in areas lacking a source of loose elastic skin to facilitate primary closure (mid- to lower extremities, tail wounds, large trunk wounds, etc.).

- Wounds that would benefit from surgical closure, but could heal by second intention. In many cases, financial constraints preclude surgery in favor of open wound management until contraction and epithelialization is complete.

- Many moderate to large trunk wounds in puppies and kittens have a remarkable ability to heal by second intention.

Skin tension around a wound (inherent elasticity of the skin) can be assessed by manually pushing the wound border to determine the degree of laxity required for wound contraction to occur unimpeded. Skin tension is best assessed only after tissue swelling

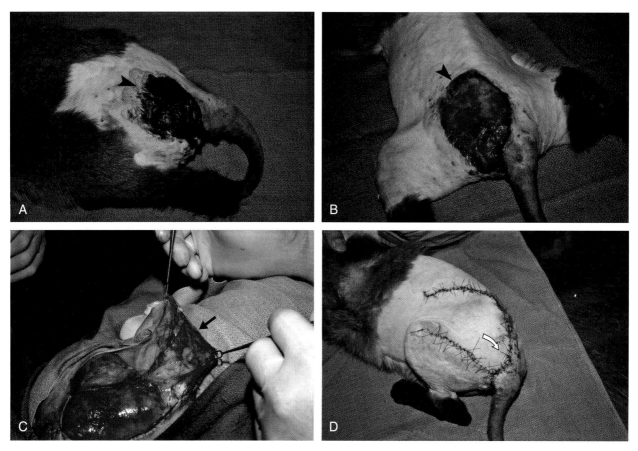

FIG. 3-6 (A) Delayed primary closure of a burn. This thermal wound was sustained when the cat contacted an automobile muffler. (B) The burn eschar was excised and the wound treated with topical medicated wet dressings to facilitate debridement. (C) A transposition flap was elevated on day 4 from the lateral abdominal wall prior to its placement (arrow) on the recipient bed. (D) The flap was rotated (arrow) and sutured into the wound bed. (From Pavletic MM. 1993. Surgery of skin and management of wounds. In Sherding RG, ed. *The Cat: Disease and Clinical Management*, 2nd ed. New York: Churchill Livingstone.)

subsides. If sufficient peripheral skin laxity is present, unimpeded wound contraction can be expected in many cases. Otherwise, epithelialization must cover the remaining deficit once contraction ceases (Fig. 3-7). This may be an impossible task in large defects.

The clinical question, "Can this wound heal by second intention?" can be partially answered by assessing the skin tension (inherent skin elasticity) bordering the defect. As will be discussed in Chapter 6, Common Complications in Wound Healing, a lack of mobile skin can effectively neutralize the centripetal force exerted on the skin by myofibroblastic contraction. This is particularly evident when assessing moderate-sized defects involving the lower extremities.

Skin tension is best assessed only after tissue swelling subsides. (Edema separates the dermal collagen and elastin fibers. The collagen and elastin fibers also retract away from the wound, exaggerating the magnitude of the skin defect in the early days of injury.)

Skin tension around the wound can be determined by lifting or pushing the local skin toward the center of the defect. If the opposing skin edges can be compressed into the defect, a variable degree of wound contraction is likely to occur. In irregularly shaped wounds, narrower areas are more likely to heal by second intention before the widest part of the wound defect.

Experimentally, wound contraction normally slows 42 days (6 weeks) after injury. Epithelial cell

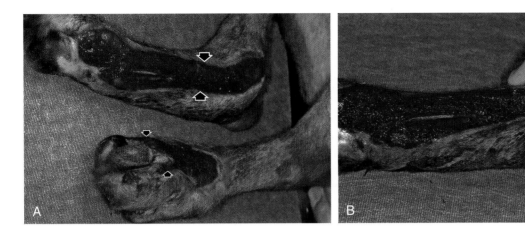

FIG. 3-7 (A) Full-thickness skin loss sustained in an automobile accident. A healthy granulation bed has formed. Edema has subsided, allowing for assessment of peripheral skin tension. Narrow areas of the wound bed (arrows) are expected to epithelialize and contract rapidly; the widest area of the wound will be the last to heal. (B) Gently grasping the wound borders and displacing skin toward the central defect indicates sufficient skin laxity is present to promote wound contraction. Epithelialization will cover the remaining portions of the wound.

migration must cover the remaining open wound at this point, unless surgical intervention is considered (see Chapter 2).

In many cases, second intention healing is a practical and economical method of effecting closure, provided that adequate wound care is administered. There are cases, however where healing is prolonged, and the attendant costs of hospital visits, bandage materials, and topical medications meet or exceed the cost of surgical closure.

Not all wounds expected to heal by second intention will close in optimal fashion. Wounds that heal primarily by epithelialization will have a larger hairless scar compared to those defects that close primarily by myofibroblastic contraction. Fragile epithelialized scars exposed to mild external trauma may abrade or split. As noted in Chapter 2, excessive scarring or contraction resulting in restricted motion to a limb or other body region is called wound contracture (see also Chapter 6). Cosmetic and functional results may be unsatisfactory.

Preliminary studies by Bohling et al. suggest that cutaneous wound healing proceeds more slowly in cats than in dogs. Slower gains in tensile strength and healing by second intention is also noted in cats when compared to dogs. The authors speculate that loss of subcutaneous tissues appears to retard healing in cats more so than in dogs (see Chapter 2.)

Second intention healing can be used as a means of reducing the size of some problematic wounds that may not necessarily heal to completion. Wound contraction can direct regional elastic skin centripetally to reduce the size of a wound substantially. When contraction slows or stops, and epithelialization is not likely to close the remaining defect, surgical closure may be attempted. By delaying surgery, a smaller skin flap or skin graft may now used, thereby reducing the cost associated with final closure. This technique is not used for closing large regional wounds that have little or no likelihood of partial closure by second intention healing. In these more problematic cases, definitive surgical closure becomes the first choice of managing the wound.

Healing by Adnexal Re-Epithelialization

Not all wounds involve the entire thickness of the skin. Tangential loss of a portion of the skin layers may result in the partial loss of the epidermis or complete loss of the epidermis and a variable degree of dermal destruction. Examples of partial thickness skin losses include the following:

- Superficial burns (first-degree burns)
- Partial-thickness burns (second-degree burns)
- Abrasions or scrapes of varying depth

- Chemical burns (including turpentine and other chemical irritants)
- Split-thickness skin graft donor site

Cutaneous burns and abrasions of the skin may be categorized as superficial, partial-thickness, or full-thickness according to the depth of injury (see Chapter 7). Superficial cutaneous loss includes loss of the epithelium but sparing of the germinal layer. Re-epithelialization originates from this surviving epithelial layer. A partial-thickness loss results in the loss of the entire epithelial surface and a variable portion of the dermis. In this case, surviving adnexal structures (hair follicles, sebaceous glands, sweat glands) located in the remaining dermis and subcutaneous tissue are the source of epithelial cells for healing (see Chapter 2.) The donor site from which a split-thickness graft is harvested will heal as a partial-thickness wound. Similarly, the donor site, however, has the advantage of minimal tissue injury because the wound is made under aseptic conditions with minimal trauma. One must remember that any partial-thickness injury may be converted to a full-thickness loss by infection or improper wound management (Fig. 3-8).

"POINTERS" IN SELECTING THE PROPER CLOSURE TECHNIQUE

Clean wounds and wounds with minimal surface contamination are natural candidates for primary closure,

provided that sufficient skin is available. Most lightly contaminated wounds with minor tissue necrosis can be closed primarily after single-stage debridement and wound lavage.

Local skin flaps or tension-relieving techniques may be used to close wounds where incisional tension may be problematic. If edema and contusions are evident, delayed primary closure may be advisable, allowing time for the circulation and lymphatic drainage to improve in this 4- to 5-day period.

Small contaminated or infected wounds can be completely excised and the area closed primarily. This is a useful technique for wounds located in body regions with sufficient skin laxity to facilitate "en bloc" resection of the area.

The most important factor in determining the best method of closure is the final assessment of the wound after proper exploration, debridement, and copious pressure lavage of the wound.

Many of the larger grossly contaminated and infected wounds are not difficult to assess: the poor state of the regional tissues clearly precludes primary closure. Whether the wound can be handled by delayed primary closure, secondary closure, or healing by second intention is determined as wound management progresses.

Those wounds that require closer assessment are grossly contaminated wounds. Infection may not be evident, but contamination with grit, dirt, and organic matter has been present in the wound for a variable period of time. Close postoperative assessment for infection is necessary. If there are any doubts, the wound should be managed as an open wound (delayed

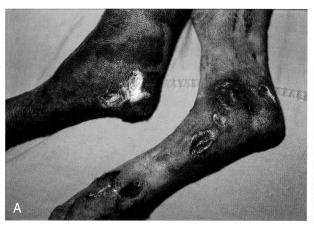
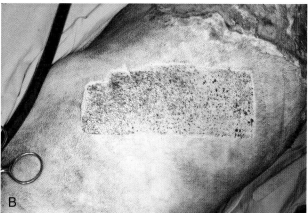

FIG. 3-8 (A) Partial-thickness abrasions to the lower extremities of a Doberman secondary to being struck by an automobile. Partial- and full-thickness skin wounds are evident. (B) Donor site after harvesting a split-thickness skin graft. This partial-thickness wound will heal readily by adnexal reepithelialization.

primary closure, secondary closure, second intention healing).

The surgeon must determine the probable viability of the tissues in the wound. If tissue survivability cannot be accurately assessed at this time, open wound management is advisable. Otherwise, aggressive debridement can be considered for those traumatized tissues considered expendable.

If small areas of necrotic tissue cannot be excised without causing unnecessary tissue injury, open wound management is again advisable. Serial (scalpel, scissors) or mechanical debridement (wet-to-dry dressings) techniques are used to remove necrotic tissue remnants, provided that significant collateral tissue trauma can be avoided. More selective forms of debridement (autolytic, enzymatic) are very useful once the bulk of necrotic tissue is removed. Selective debridement should be considered in wounds where delicate tissue structures may be otherwise damaged by surgical/mechanical debridement techniques. The presence of necrotic tissue is particularly problematic since the risk of infection increases. Timely removal of dead tissue can dramatically reduce the bacterial population in a wound.

It is important to note that secondary closure is the next step if delayed primary closure is not advisable. In turn, second intention healing is the next option if secondary closure is not feasible. Surgical closure is considered for those cases in which contraction and epithelialization cannot close a wound effectively. Surgical intervention can be performed at the point at which there is an absence of infection and tissue viability is assured.

Granulation tissue is a key indicator of tissue viability. Granulation tissue forms only from the viable vascularized tissues comprising the base and the margins of the wound. Its presence over the surface of the wound is the "surgeon's indicator" that necrotic tissue has been eliminated.

Granulation tissue is a natural barrier to invasive infection. Once granulation tissue covers the wound, systemic antibiotics can be eliminated in favor of topical antimicrobial agents. Exceptions to this general rule would include those patients with other underlying infections or health issues that require continued systemic antibiotic therapy.

With partial-thickness skin wounds, gentle cleansing of the wounds with sterile saline/lactated Ringer's or a commercial wound cleansing agent (Chapter 4), followed by an appropriate topical dressing and topical agent, can support the epithelial remnants necessary for reepithelialization of the area. Depending on the depth of injury, this process usually occurs within 2 to 3 weeks after injury. However, the veterinarian may elect excision and primary closure of small partial thickness wounds when sufficient skin is present.

Most wound contaminants can be eliminated with debridement and pressure lavage. Complete tissue viability and the elimination of necrotic tissue are the two key points in determining whether early wound closure can be attempted. Wounds closed with the presence of necrotic tissue are candidates for infection, dehiscence, and drainage. Removal of dead tissue dramatically reduces the primary source of nutrition and shelter of bacteria. However, with the presence of infection at the time of intervention, open wound management for a variable period of time is the safest method to reduce or eliminate the risk of perpetuating an infection once final closure is attempted. Open wound management provides optimal drainage and allows the surgeon to inspect the wound daily.

BASIC WOUND MANAGEMENT IN SIX SIMPLE STEPS

Establishment of a healthy vascular wound bed, free of necrotic tissue and infection, allows the surgeon to consider all options for final wound closure. Initial management of open wounds can be summarized in six simple steps (see Fig. 3-4):

1. Prevent further wound contamination
2. Debride dead and dying tissue
3. Remove foreign debris and contaminants
4. Provide adequate wound drainage
5. Establish a viable vascular bed
6. Select the appropriate method of closure

Preventing Further Wound Contamination

On admission, the patient's wounds should be temporarily protected from further trauma and hospital-borne bacteria with a topical antimicrobial, sterile dressing, and protective wrap (Figs. 3-3 and 3-4; see also Chapters 4 and 5). Sterile gauze moistened with saline that contains an antibiotic or a nonirritating antimicrobial agent are useful, especially to maintain tissue hydration and control infection until definitive wound repair can be performed later in the day.

Stock povidone iodine solution can be diluted to 1 part solution to 9 parts saline. This 0.1% solution has antimicrobial properties and will not cause tissue injury. Stock chlorhexidine diacetate solution can be diluted to a 0.05% solution by adding 1 part solution to 40 parts sterile saline. This solution also has antimicrobial properties and will not cause tissue injury.

In preparation for definitive wound cleansing and surgical management, the exposed wound is covered with sterile gauze pads impregnated with sterile K-Y Jelly (Johnson & Johnson, Langhorne, PA), sterile saline, or an antimicrobial solution prior to liberally clipping the skin and preparing the defect for surgery. Sterile K-Y Jelly can be applied to the fur along the wound borders before clipping (No. 40 clipper blades). The gel facilitates clumping of the fur and reduces airborne hair fragments from being deposited onto the adjacent wound surface. The temporary wound cover minimizes further open wound contamination from clipped hair fragments and topical debris when preparing the area for surgery.

Fur should be liberally removed around the wound area. A circumferential clip is recommended when managing extremity wounds. Fur adjacent to wounds has a tendency to retain discharge from the wound surface, potentiating tissue maceration and bacterial proliferation: its removal also facilitates periodic wound cleansing and bandage reapplications. Water-impermeable drapes are ideally used to drape off the surgery site; the temporary protective dressing is then removed.

Debridement: Selective versus Nonselective

There are two broad categories of wound debridement: selective and nonselective. Selective forms of wound debridement more specifically target the presence of necrotic tissue. Nonselective debridement is considered less precise, since it inadvertently damages viable tissue to a variable degree within the wound. Forms of selective debridement include the use of gels and dressings that create an ideal medium for autolytic debridement. Enzymatic debridement is a second form of selective debridement, using exogenous proteolytic enzymes to separate nonviable tissues. Biotherapy, using maggots, is a third form of selective debridement. (See Chapters 4 and 5 for details pertaining to selective debridement techniques and products.)

Nonselective debridement is a more aggressive and faster method of removing necrotic tissue. The downside is that nonselective debridement may traumatize viable tissues in the wound to a variable degree. The two forms of nonselective debridement include

1. surgical (scalpel, tissue excision) and
2. mechanical (wet-to-dry dressings) debridement.

Selective debridement is a less aggressive and slower method for removing necrotic tissue. The upside is that necrotic tissue is targeted and viable tissue trauma is minimized. The three basic forms of selective debridement are

1. autolytic (use of topical gels, dressings),
2. enzymatic (use of topical enzymes), and
3. biotherapeutic (maggot debridement therapy).

Surgical and mechanical debridement are two forms of nonselective debridement. Surgical debridement normally employs the use of scalpel blades, surgical scissors, and forceps to lift and excise the tissue. The most common form of mechanical debridement is the use of wet-to-dry dressings: serial dressing changes pull or lift attached necrotic tissue that is adhered to the gauze. If overused, this technique also irritates and damages local tissue (see Chapter 5). However, both methods are able to quickly and effectively remove necrotic tissue. The judicious use of nonselective debridement in the first few days of wound management causes minimal collateral damage. The rapid removal of necrotic tissue facilitates granulation tissue formation and opens the possibility of early wound closure. Small areas of necrotic tissue may be effectively managed with many of the topical agents promoting autolytic debridement. Indeed, surgeons may disagree on which method to use on a given wound containing necrotic tissue. It is the author's contention that large areas of necrotic tissue are best excised; wet-to-dry dressings can be used to remove residual areas of necrotic tissue for an additional 3- to 5-day period. Alternatively, topical autolytic debridement agents and dressings can be substituted for wet-to-dry dressings when minimal amounts of necrotic tissue are present, according to the preference of the clinician. In general, selective debridement techniques alone are not ideally suited for the removal of large areas of dead tissue.

Surgical Debridement

The surgeon's ability to remove necrotic and severely compromised tissues is a major determinant for whether primary closure should be considered. Areas of questionable viability may be excised if the tissue is not essential to healing or function (see Fig. 3-4). Areas of the body with loose, elastic skin permit a more aggressive approach to debridement, whereas extremity wounds warrant a more cautious approach when tissue viability cannot be determined on presentation.

It is not always possible, however, to accurately assess tissue viability at the time of initial wound exploration, and it may take 24 hours or longer to clearly delineate devitalized tissues. It would be appropriate to consider delayed primary closure until tissue survival is assured, especially when important structures are involved. Daily wound assessment and serial surgical debridement can be used to remove devitalized tissue as it becomes identifiable.

Is this skin viable? Assessment of skin viability, in the early stages of trauma can be difficult. Black to an ashen gray are the characteristic colors of necrotic skin, although pale (pearl) white is noted in skin devoid of circulation. Skin pigmentation can obscure color assessment. Deeply contused (bruised) skin may precede skin necrosis, although circulation may recover in some cases. Keep in mind that hemorrhage beneath thin skin (especially the lower abdominal skin) is easily visualized and may not reflect skin viability.

When large amounts of devitalized tissue are present, removal of the tissue is facilitated by locating a definable underlying fascial plane. Debridement of full-thickness skin necrosis is facilitated by undermining at the level of the hypodermis. In turn, necrotic hypodermal tissues are resected; the underlying muscle fascia (epimysium) and muscle tissues are assessed for viability and managed accordingly. This stepwise, downward excisional technique is occasionally referred to as "layered debridement."

Exposed contaminated and compromised subcutaneous fat overlying skeletal muscle can be safely excised, thus removing the devitalized tissue and the embedded debris. However, excision of subcutaneous fat and portions of panniculus muscle attached to the dermal surface of traumatized skin is best avoided if possible: debridement under these circumstances may further compromise the traumatized skin's blood supply (subdermal plexus and associated direct cutaneous vessels). Wound lavage and careful removal of topical debris (with forceps) from partially avulsed skin is preferable. The area can be reassessed with subsequent bandage changes.

Although bleeding along the skin margins is considered a desirable intraoperative clinical sign of adequate cutaneous arterial circulation, it provides no information as to venous return when dealing with traumatized skin (Fig. 3-4). It is also no guarantee that blood is not being shunted away from the nutrient circulation of the skin. Vasospasm and pronounced hypotension may cause a temporary drop in local cutaneous circulation with a misleading decline in bleeding from the wound edge. Furthermore, the presence of circulation within a skin area at the time of initial examination also is no assurance that trauma, edema, infection, venous compromise, or progressive thrombosis will not subsequently obstruct the circulation. Feline skin generally bleeds less than canine skin when incised.

Early visual indicators play a role in assessing skin viability after initial injury. For example, large avulsion wounds in which significant loss of segmental direct cutaneous vessels is noted would suggest a variable portion of the terminal "traumatic flap" will undergo necrosis. Additionally, stripping of the underlying subcutaneous tissues is an indicator of vascular compromise via loss of the subdermal plexus and supporting direct cutaneous vasculature. The options are to wait and reassess the skin over the next 4 to 5 days or to consider partial resection of the compromised tissue.

Restrained debridement is initiated by excising the terminal edge of the traumatized skin, looking for indications of edge bleeding. The excision is performed in a stepwise fashion. Excision is stopped at the point at which primary closure can still be accomplished with minimal tension. Excision obviously can be stopped before this point, if bleeding is noted at the incised edge of the traumatic flap. At this point, the wound may be closed or left open and reassessed over the next 4–5 days for final debridement and wound closure. During the next few days, the remaining skin is assessed for viability before final closure (see Chapter 1 regarding circulation to the skin.)

Removing Foreign Debris and Contaminants

Dirt, clay particles, and organic debris promote infection and delay wound healing. Radiographs can be used to locate radiopaque materials including glass fragments, grit and gravel, and metallic objects. Ultrasonography is useful in detecting radiolucent objects and abscesses.

Gross contaminants adhered to adipose tissue overlying muscle surfaces may be removed more easily by excising this tissue tangentially (Fig. 3-4). As previously noted, debris adhered to the subcutis of skin should be manually removed to better preserve cutaneous circulation. Manual removal of gross debris followed by pressure lavage with isotonic solutions will remove additional microscopic contaminants remaining after the initial debridement. Small- to moderate-sized wounds are generally lavaged with 500 to 1000 ml normal saline or lactated Ringer's solutions. Additional lavage solution is employed for large wounds. The author has had excellent clinical results with the use of isotonic solutions in contaminated wounds under pressure, using an 18-gauge needle attached to a 35-ml syringe. Full force of the plunger will effectively deliver 8 pounds per square inch (psi) to the wound surface when the needle is placed immediately perpendicular to the wound surface. This is considered the appropriate pressure for wound lavage. The addition of a three-way stopcock attached to a sterilized intravenous fluid line will enable the surgeon to refill the syringe more quickly during lavage. Funnel tip syringes also can be adapted to pressure lavage with a catheter adaptor (Fig 3-9). The surgeon should cup a hand around the area to minimize overspray. Commercial lavage units also are available for clinical use for those practices that have a caseload capable of supporting their cost. Stryker Corporation sells a disposable pressure lavage unit (Surgilav) that connects to intravenous fluid bags (Fig 3-10).

It is important for the surgeon to separate and elevate the wound edges gently to examine adjacent fascial planes that are likely to be harboring debris. However, indiscriminant dissection is to be avoided in the interest of preventing additional tissue trauma and contamination to uninvolved areas.

It is best to avoid or minimize the use of deep dermal or subcutaneous sutures in those wounds in

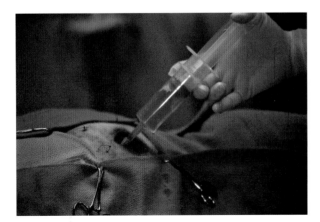

FIG. 3-9 Funnel-tip syringe, with catheter tip adaptor, for pressure lavage. A gunshot wound over the left scapula is being lavaged with a chlorhexidine-saline solution after debridement.

which residual contamination may precipitate infection with their use.

Provision of Adequate Wound Drainage

As a general rule, leaving a wound open provides optimal drainage for problematic wounds with the presence of contaminants/infection. At the time of closure, drains may be used to control dead space and provide an outlet for the removal of tissue fluids that may accumulate in the area. In the face of infection without devitalized tissue and foreign debris, drains can provide an outlet for purulent discharges that otherwise may accumulate or spread into adjacent tissues.

Drains can be divided into two basic types: passive drain systems and active drain systems. Each system has specific advantages and disadvantages. (See the discussion in Chapter 4 regarding wound drainage systems.)

Promotion of a Viable Vascular Bed

Removal of necrotic tissue, debris, and contaminants minimizes the risk of infection and delayed healing. Similarly, adequate postoperative wound drainage provides a route for the escape of debris and tissue fluid, and this can further reduce the likelihood of abscessation. Dressings and bandages help protect the wound from additional contaminants and trauma. Under these circumstances, circulation to the remaining viable tissues can improve and support the development of a granulation bed. Thus, the veterinarian's major effort in the management of most dirty and infected wounds is to promote a healthy vascular (granulation) bed. At this point, the appropriate method for closing the wound can be chosen.

Exposed Bone

Although exposed bone stripped of the periosteum cannot easily support a granulation bed, the adjacent viable soft tissue will often form healthy granulation tissue that creeps over the bone surface (Fig. 3-11). Small holes may be drilled into the cancellous layer of the bone to promote granulation tissue coverage of the exposed cortical surface. This technique is usually reserved for large exposed bone surfaces or smaller areas in which healing is delayed. Care must be taken

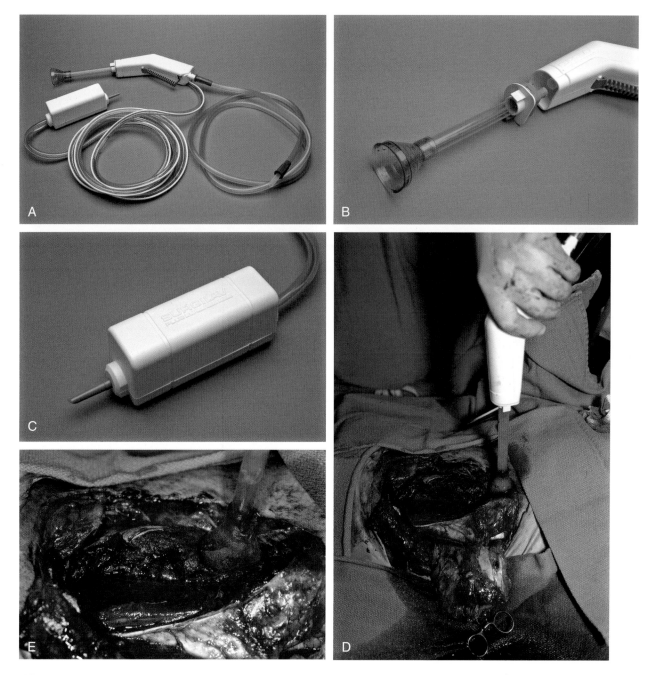

FIG. 3-10 (A) Surgilav debridement unit (Stryker Instruments, Kalamazoo, MI). Note the hand piece connected to the battery-powered motor unit. The blue-tipped tubing is connected to a vacuum canister.

(B) Detachable funnel tip with spray jets.

(C) The motor unit is inserted into an intravenous fluid bag.

(D) Surgilav unit being used to clean a contaminated avulsion wound involving the left lateral lumbar region.

(E) Close-up view of the funnel tip in contact with the tissue surface. The cone prevents overspray from the fluid nozzle; a vacuum port in the attachment simultaneously sucks fluid away from the wound and into the vacuum canister.

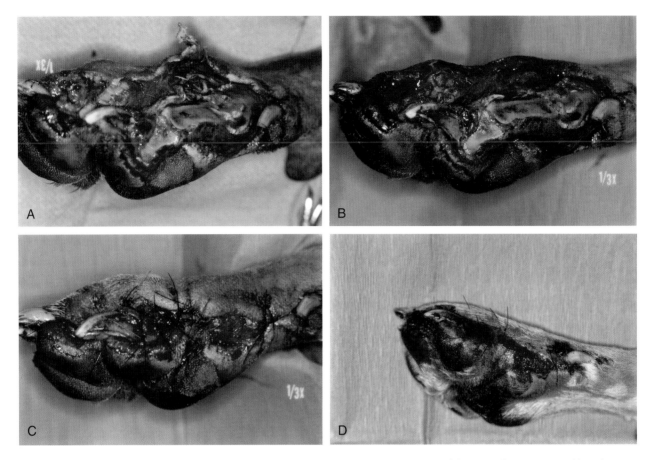

FIG. 3-11 (A) Shearing wound to the left rear paw secondary to vehicular trauma. The size of the wound is exaggerated by edema and elastic retraction of the cutaneous borders. (B) Debridement and copious lavage were used to remove necrotic tissue and contaminants. (C) Skin borders were tacked to adjacent fascia. (D) After 2 weeks, the edema has subsided, and the small remaining wound will heal by second intention.

to avoid fracturing narrow, compromised bone segments such as the metacarpal or metatarsal bones. In some areas, muscle flaps can be rotated over an exposed bone to improve circulation to the wound area and provide a vascular surface, if needed. (See Chapter 6 for additional details in managing exposed bone.)

Selection of Appropriate Method of Closure

The true magnitude of the defect is best determined once tissue swelling subsides and the wound is devoid of necrotic tissue. This is particularly evident when managing open wounds of the lower extremities. At this stage (generally 7 to 10 days after the initial injury),

the surgeon may note that the wound is considerably smaller than originally ascertained and that it may heal by contraction and epithelialization without further surgical intervention (Fig. 3-11). Secondary closure may be attempted if there is adequate skin adjacent to the wound. Skin flaps or free grafts should be considered for larger defects, for which healing by second intention may be prolonged or expensive. These reconstructive techniques also are advisable when wound contracture or a fragile epithelialized scar may occur. As discussed, surgeons will occasionally manage some open wounds for a few weeks to determine whether healing by second intention will reduce the magnitude of the wound before final surgical closure is attempted. This option often is considered for some small- to moderate-sized skin wounds (not located in a critical area), in which sufficient peripheral skin is present to help promote contraction and epithelialization.

Suggested Readings

Bohling MW, Henderson RA. 2006. Differences in cutaneous wound healing between dogs and cats. *Vet Clin No Am* 36:688–692.

Bohling MW, Henderson RA, Swaim ST, et al. 2004. Cutaneous wound healing in the cat: a macroscopic description and comparison with cutaneous wound healing in the dog. *Vet Surg* 33:579–587.

Bohling MW, Henderson RA, Swaim SF, et al. 2006. Comparison of the role of the subcutaneous tissue in cutaneous wound healing in the dog and cat. *Vet Surg* 35:1–12.

Dernell WS. 2006. Initial wound management. *Vet Clin No Am* 36:713–738.

Hosgood G. 2006. Stages of wound healing and their clinical relevance. *Vet Clin No Am* 36:667–685.

Hunt TK, Dunphy JE. 1979. *Fundamentals of Wound Management*. New York: Appleton & Lange.

Hunt TK, Hopf HW. 1997. Wound healing and wound infection: what surgeons and anesthesiologists can do. *Surg Clin No Am* 77:587–606.

Pavletic MM. 1985. Introduction to wound healing and wound management. In Proceedings of the American Animal Hospital Association. Lakewood, CO: AAHA.

Pavletic MM. 1993. Surgery of the skin and management of wounds. In: Sherding RG, ed. *The Cat: Diseases and Clinical Management*, 2nd ed. New York: Churchill Livingstone.

Pavletic MM. 1995. *Bite Wound Management in Small Animals*. American Animal Hospital Association, Professional Library Series. Lakewood, CO: AAHA.

Peacock EE. 1984. *Wound Repair*, 3rd ed. Philadelphia, PA: WB Saunders.

Robson MC. 1997. Wound infection. *Surg Clin No Am* 77:637–650.

Swaim SF. 1980. *Surgery of Traumatized Skin: Management and Reconstruction in the Dog and Cat*. Philadelphia, PA: WB Saunders.

Swaim SF, Henderson RA. 1993. *Small Animal Wound Management*. Philadelphia, PA: Williams & Wilkins.

Trott AT. 2005. *Wounds and Lacerations*. Philadelphia, PA: Elsevier Mosby.

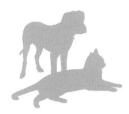

4

Wound Care Products and Their Use

WOUND DRAINAGE SYSTEMS

Passive Drains

The simplest and most economical of the passive drains employed in small animal surgery is the Penrose drain (Tyco/Kendall Healthcare, Mansfield, MA), a soft tubular strip of radiopaque latex that is sold in various widths. In small animal practice, only the 1/4-inch Penrose drain is considered useful; larger drains are rarely needed (Fig. 4-1). Penrose drains allow for the passage of fluids by capillary action over the outer surface of the drain. Fluid then gravitates downward and out of the dependently placed exit incision. Cutting holes in a Penrose drain does not improve drainage and has the added disadvantage of increasing the drain's susceptibility to tearing if traction is applied to the exposed end. The

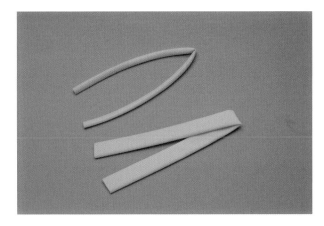

FIG. 4-1 Penrose drains are composed of radiopaque latex. They come in a variety of sizes. Examples include the 1/4-inch and 3/8-inch Penrose drain. In small animal surgery, the 1/4-inch Penrose drain is the preferred size.

FIG. 4-2 (A) Method for inserting Penrose drains into dead-space pockets and seromas using Allis tissue forceps. The Penrose drain is grasped at its end with the forceps. A portion of the drain is tucked into the space between the jaws of this instrument.

(B) The Allis forceps and drain are inserted through a stab incision created in the dependent area of the surgical site. The forceps are inserted into the cavity. The forceps are palpable beneath the skin. As a suture needle is inserted through the skin, the Allis forceps are rotated slightly, allowing the needle to pass through the instrument gap where the drain has been tucked. The end of the needle is then pushed partially through the skin. Leaving the needle in position, the Allis tissue forceps are removed. The drain is gently tugged to confirm the suture needle has captured or secured the drain.

(C) The drain is sutured into position, including a suture placed at the exit wound. This technique is both simple and effective in blind placement of Penrose drains.

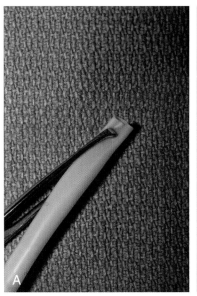

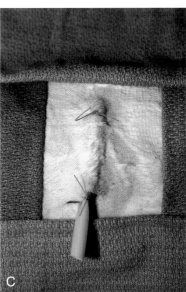

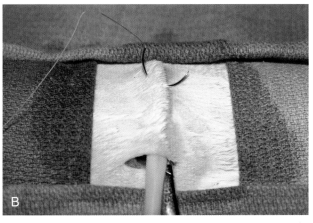

dorsal/proximal end of the buried drain is secured with a single skin suture; a second suture is used to secure the drain to the skin as it exits ventrally/distally (Fig. 4-2).

> There are surgeons who prefer to secure the dorsal/proximal drain in the deeper tissues, using a fine absorbable suture (usually 4-0 chromic catgut). When the drain is no longer required, a firm tug is used to break the retention suture and remove the drain. The author does not advise using this technique for one simple reason: there is a risk of tearing the drain, with retention of a fragment in the wound. Retrieval of retained drain fragments can be surprisingly difficult. Blind retrieval can be attempted by inserting forceps through the exit wound; fluoroscopy also has been used to locate problematic drain fragments. Partially reopening the original surgical incision or using a smaller access incision over the location of the drain fragment is a last resort.

In general, placement of a Penrose drain beneath the incision line or across the suture line is best avoided. The drain may irritate the tissues in contact with the drain and possibly interfere with healing of the closed incision. Healing of the skin incision to the underlying tissue plane also may be impaired. More commonly, careless suturing of the skin may inadvertently snag the underlying drain, making subsequent drain removal difficult. [*Note:* tugging on the drain usually will "wiggle" the offending suture(s).] In practice, the location of the incision or wound in relation to the necessary dependent exit site of a drain can make the above rule of thumb impossible to follow. Despite the potential problems noted, the author has **not** found that having a drain cross an incision line poses a significant problem to wound healing.

Penrose drains are adequate for the drainage of smaller dead-space areas but are less than ideal for larger areas, especially when prolonged drainage is anticipated. Penrose drains are normally retained for 3 to 5 days, depending upon the volume of fluid exiting the area. They can be removed by the second day if drainage is minimal. In general, the longer the drain is retained, the greater the likelihood of ascending infection from contamination at the drain exit (Fig. 4-3). When possible, the exposed end of a Penrose drain should be covered with a sterile dressing and a topical antimicrobial agent, although this is not easily accomplished in some body regions (e.g., inguinal and axillary areas). If left exposed, it is advisable to gently cleanse the exit area with sterile saline (with the addition of povidone-iodine or chlorhexidine) followed by a topical antimicrobial agent three times daily (Fig. 4-4). Using an Elizabethan collar is advisable to prevent the patient from chewing or removing the drain. If a patient should tear a portion of the drain, radiographs may be necessary to confirm retention of the radiopaque fragment.

Penrose drains function suboptimally in body areas where gravitational drainage cannot be provided. Moreover, they permit the entry of air into a wound area and cannot be used in thoracic wounds in which pneumothorax may occur. In flank wounds, the exit site of the drain occasionally can create a sucking

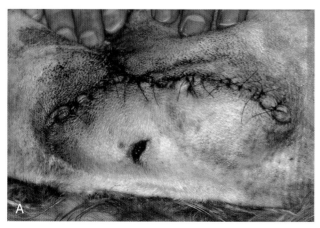 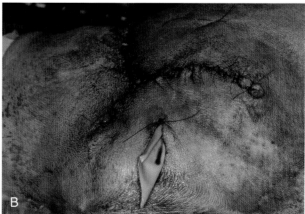

FIG. 4-3 (A) Forelimb amputation; premature removal of a surgical drain resulted in seroma formation. (B) Allis tissue forceps were used to replace a Penrose drain, followed by an external bandage to help control dead space.

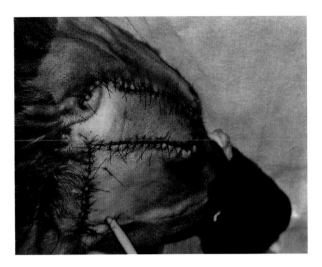

FIG. 4-4 For smaller dead space areas, Penrose drains can be used very effectively. In this example, a 1/4-inch drain is used to control the dead space below the transposed flap and the donor area.

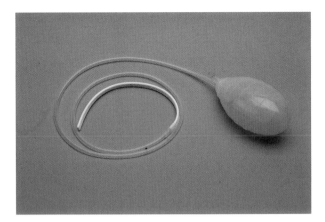

FIG. 4-5 Example of the Jackson-Pratt 100-ml vacuum reservoir and attached drain tubing. Composed of silicone, the reservoir and tubing can be cleaned and autoclaved. Several companies supply this economical vacuum drain system.

wound, with subsequent development of subcutaneous emphysema to a variable degree. Closed suction drainage systems are best employed in these situations.

> There are two common errors noted with the use of Penrose drains: (1) improper placement (a "mental disorientation" error) of the **exit** site associated with the position of the surgical patient and (2) having both the proximal/dorsal and distal/ventral ends of the Penrose drain exit the skin.
>
> In the former, a patient is in dorsal recumbency and the surgeon accidentally directs the **exit** wound in the inappropriate (dorsal/proximal) location. This placement error usually is discovered only after the patient is being placed in lateral recumbency during anesthetic recovery.

Active Drains

Closed suction drainage devices are active drain systems that operate on the principle of creating a vacuum in a chamber that draws fluid from the body area through a rigid fenestrated drain placed beneath the skin. Most chambers are collapsible plastic canisters that rely on an internal spring mechanism or the inherent tendency of the chamber wall to expand outward in order to create a vacuum. A one-way (antireflux) valve prevents reflux of fluid from the chamber back to the wound. Milliliter markings on the

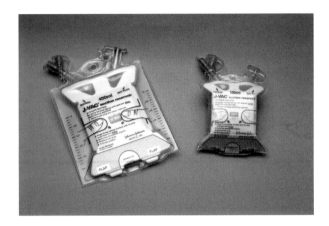

FIG. 4-6 Examples of the Johnson & Johnson J-Vac closed drainage system (450-ml and 150-ml reservoir capacity.) J-Vacs cannot be resterilized in the autoclave. The larger reservoir is too large for routine small animal usage.

canister allow the surgeon to determine the relative amount of fluid accumulated. A spout permits emptying of fluid or any air accumulated in the vacuum chamber; the reservoir is collapsed and closed to reinstitute this active drainage system (Figs. 4-5 and 4-6). The Jackson-Pratt Active Drain System (Cardinal Health, McGaw Park, IL) is one of the more common systems currently used in veterinary surgery (Fig. 4-5).

The best wound drains are silastic (silicone) materials with multiple holes and recessed grooves to minimize obstruction. The fenestrated portion of the drain is placed in the wound; the nonfenestrated portion exits the area through a small stab wound in the skin. The fenestrated tubing can be shortened to accommodate to the wound space. A purse-string skin suture provides an airtight seal, and the suture strands are then looped around the drain and tied to prevent tube displacement (sometimes called the "Roman sandal" knot or "Chinese finger-trap knot"). Redundant external tubing is cut off with scissors before attaching this nonfenestrated segment to the vacuum canister. The canister or reservoir is secured to a bandage or an adhesive band placed around the trunk or cervical area. Closed suction units can be used for several days with minimal risk of ascending infection. In general, they are used for 3 to 5 days.

Vacuum drains have several advantages over Penrose drains:

- They function independent of gravity.

- They allow the surgeon to quantify fluid volume.

- They eliminate the need for bandages and nursing care associated with the external drainage associated with Penrose drains.

- With basic instructions, they are easy for most owners to manage at home.

- The risk of ascending infection is minimal.

- They are very useful for draining deep wound pockets and abscess cavities devoid of necrotic tissue and contaminants.

- The vacuum draws tissue planes together, thereby eliminating the need for internal "tacking" sutures to eliminate subcutaneous dead space.

- If so desired, silicone drains and reservoirs can be cleaned and autoclaved for additional usage.

Vacuum drainage systems are remarkably effective in removing fluid from wide surface areas (Fig. 4-7). Most owners are capable of managing vacuum drains at home (see Table 4-1 for instructions). The author also has used vacuum drain systems for managing mild cases of peritonitis and various abdominal abscesses over the past 20 years and has found them quite effective.

In the presence of active bleeding, clotted blood can obstruct the drain holes. Tissue debris occasionally obstructs the drain. In many cases this problem can be remedied by removing the drain from the reservoir and flushing it with several milliliters of sterile saline to clear tube fenestrations. The vacuum is reactivated and watched closely for any future obstructions.

TABLE 4-1
Vacuum drain instructions for pet owners.

1. The oval reservoir holds 100 ml (about 3 oz) of fluid. A milliliter scale is marked on the side of the reservoir.

2. To open the reservoir, remove the attached stopper from the spout. Next, look at the scale and note the volume of fluid in the chamber.

3. Record in a notebook the fluid volume and the date and time of removal.

4. To empty the reservoir canister, pour the liquid into a disposable container (e.g., a Dixie cup). This fluid can then be flushed down the toilet and the paper cup can be discarded.

5. To reactivate the vacuum inside the reservoir chamber, squeeze the air out of the chamber and insert the stopper back into the spout. The reservoir will appear to be collapsed.

6. The entire drain system (reservoir and tube) can be removed when the amount of drainage decreases significantly. Contact your doctor to determine when to removed the drain.

7. The surgeon can remove the drain on an outpatient basis: in most cases drain removal will take less than 5 minutes.

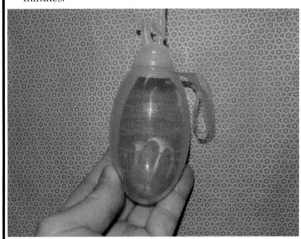

The milliliters of fluid removed, as well as its color and clarity, are recorded along with the time the reservoir is emptied by the owner. The drain can be removed when the volume declines to several milliliters over a 24-hour period.

On occasion, obstruction of the fenestrated drain can be misread as a decline in fluid volume. One indication of tube obstruction is any visible/palpable accumulation of fluid at the surgical area. As noted, "retro-flushing" of the drain can be used to clear obstructed channels and reinvigorate the vacuum system. If this maneuver fails, drain replacement may be necessary.

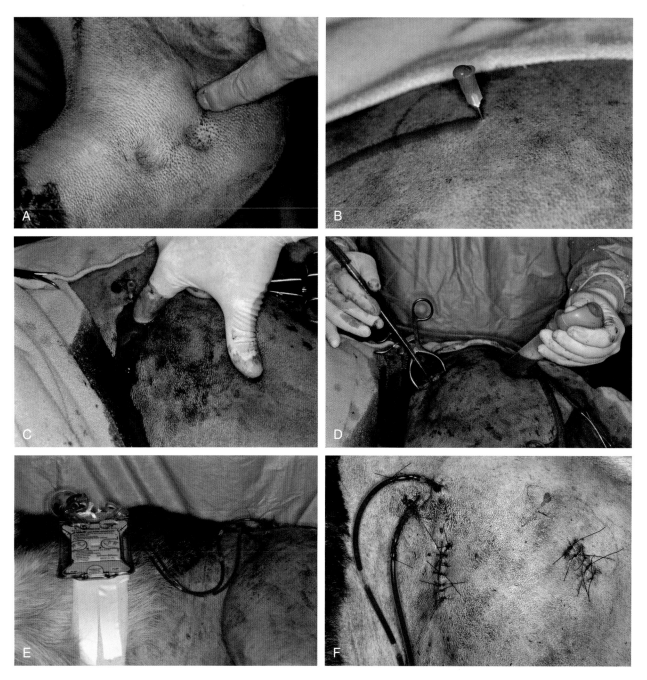

FIG. 4-7 (A) Massive abscess of the left femoral area. The exact cause of this infection was unknown, although a penetrating wound was suspected in this farm dog. Note the pitting edema of the lower extremity. Ultrasonography outlined a deep U-shaped abscess cavity, curving from the hip down the femoral shaft area.

(B) The depth and location of the abscess was determined with a syringe needle. When the abscess cavity was located, pus can be seen exiting the needle hub. A scalpel blade is used to incise down to the cavity, using the intact needle as a depth guide. Blunt dissection with Metzenbaum scissors was performed to approach this long abscess cavity from two sites.

(C) A finger was inserted into the depth of the abscess: aerobic and anaerobic cultures were obtained from the deep abscess cavity.

(D) All pus was aspirated and flushed from the abscess pocket. The interconnecting access incisions facilitated drainage and visual inspection of the cavity.

(E) The drain tubes exited through two small, separate stab incisions and were secured to the skin with a purse-string suture and Roman sandal suture.

(F) Close-up view of the surgical area. Access incisions were closed, and the reservoirs were attached to the drain tubes. The drains were left in the area for 6 days after insertion.

A common complication noted in the immediate postoperative period is air entering the wound through the closed skin incision, inactivating the reservoir vacuum required to remove fluid. The chamber expands with air when there is an incisional leak, loose connection, or hole in the external drain tubing/reservoir. The skin incision, exit site of the drain, the exter-nal tubing, and the reservoir must be examined to locate the source of the air leak. On occasion, a few drops of surgical soap can be applied to confirm the potential site of an the air leak in the external tube segment. When the vacuum chamber is activated, the area is assessed for bubbles, signifying a source of air entry.

Long incisions are more prone to cumulative air entry between individual skin sutures or staples, until a fibrin seal forms along the incision line hours after surgery. Air entry negates the vacuum within the reservoir, necessitating its evacuation and vacuum reactivation. To prevent this, the author has used a few techniques that can be effective in sealing air entry along an incision line (Fig. 4-8).

- Apply a "caulking bead" of ointment over the incision line and repeat as necessary. (Usually a fibrin seal will be noted by the following day.)

- Depending on the length of the incision, a surgical cyanoacrylate glue may be applied over the suture/staple line.

- If an exact area of air leakage is seen between sutures, additional reinforcing sutures or skin staples may be applied.

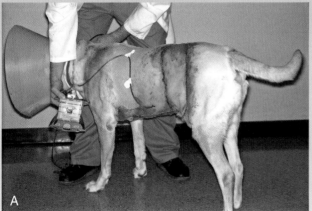
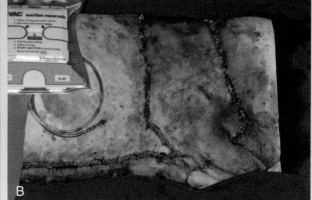
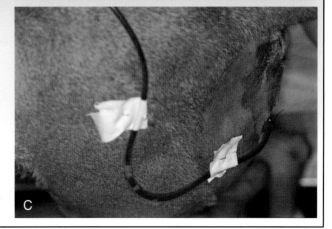

FIG. 4-8 (A) J-Vac used to control dead space beneath a caudal superficial epigastric axial pattern flap used to reconstruct the flank area after wide tumor resection.

(B) The combined closure of the long donor and recipient areas increases the probability of air seepage between skin sutures/staples. Until a fibrin seal forms, application of an incisional sealant may be needed to prevent inactivation of the reservoir vacuum. Topical ointment or the application of a surgical glue over the closed incisions can be effective for this purpose. Adhesive plastic drapes can be used, although the cost of maintaining them may be greater.

(C) Close-up view of a drain tube leading to a reservoir. To maintain the position of the tubing, tape strips can be applied to the tube and sutured or stapled to the skin.

Although closed suction devices are somewhat more expensive than Penrose drains, they are considered indispensable for the proper treatment of many of the larger, more serious wounds encountered in veterinary practice today. There are many models available for use with variable prices: silicone models are capable of being cleaned and resterilized.

Noncommercial Active Drain Systems

A small vacuum collection system can be made from a 35- to 60-cc syringe to manage small wounds. A vacuum chamber is created from the syringe by drawing and securing the inner syringe plunger to the outer cylinder, thereby creating a static vacuum chamber. Commercial tubing can be partially fenestrated with scissors and inserted into the wound (Fig. 4-9). This device can be used effectively for small wounds, especially when a comparatively small volume of fluid is anticipated.

Originally reported for use in human pediatric surgery, Vacutainer tubes can be adapted for draining small dead space pockets. A partially fenestrated drain is created with a butterfly catheter, removing the syringe hub and partially fenestrating a portion of the tube. The tubing is secured to the surgical area and the needle is inserted into the Vacutainer. As fluid accumulates, the Vacutainer suctions the fluid into its chamber. The author has found this to be unreliable, largely due to the narrow-diameter tubing frequently plugging. The reservoir capacity also is quite small. As a result, its routine use is inadvisable.

Vacuum-Assisted Closure (VAC) Systems

Vacuum-assisted wound drainage systems (KCI USA, Inc., San Antonio, TX; Venturi, Talley Medical, Lansing, MI) have been developed to manage problematic wounds in humans. The KCI system includes (1) a polyurethane open cell foam sheet (three sizes) that can be trimmed with sterile scissors to conform to the wound surface; (2) a firm plastic tube that attaches to the foam pad; (3) a vacuum pump with a fluid reservoir; and (4) a plastic sheet with a topical adhesive that overlaps the foam and tubing, forming an air-tight seal over the entire wound area. Lastly, the external tube is connected to the vacuum pump that applies subatmospheric pressure to the foam chamber created (Fig. 4-10). The Talley Medical Venturi system utilizes a gauze matrix placed under negative pressure. Gauze

coated with PHMB (polyhexamethylene biguanide) is considered an ideal material.

Foam or gauze serve as a platform for distributing the vacuum force uniformly to the surface of the wound, both drawing and retaining fluid (wound discharge, tissue fluid–edema) into its matrix. Pressures can be adjusted (−50 to −200 mm Hg) and applied continuously or intermittently. Intermittent application of the vacuum (3 minutes on, 5 minutes off) was demonstrated to have beneficial effects on blood flow, granulation tissue formation, and skin flap survival in experimental animals. Removal of the extracellular fluid, in particular, can significantly improve microcirculation to edematous tissues.

During the "off period" of the pump, the foam reexpands, and this motion does cause pain in human patients. In most cases, continuous suction is used without adverse results. A negative pressure of −125 mm Hg is most commonly used in human and veterinary patients. A lower negative pressure of −50 mm Hg is selected for wounds with excessive serous drainage and the postoperative prevention of fluid accumulation (seroma, edema). The polyurethane foam or gauze variation usually is replaced every 2–3 days with the patient under heavy sedation.

Increased bacterial clearance from the wound bed is an advantage to vacuum-assisted closure. However, these systems are not a replacement for surgical debridement of devitalized tissues. Removal of necrotic tissue is necessary before using these negative pressure systems. Highly contaminated and infected wounds may require daily changes. Malodorous changes would indicate more frequent bandage changes are needed. In many cases the bandage is changed a total of 2–3 times before the wound is ready for surgical closure.

The vacuum systems (−125 mm Hg) also can be used as a dressing to secure free grafts. However, care is required when changing the foam or gauze in order to avoid displacement of the graft. Application of a nonadherent petroleum dressing (Adaptic, Johnson & Johnson, Langhorne, PA) over the graft may prevent polyurethane foam or cotton gauze adherence to exposed granulation tissue.

Complications associated with vacuum systems include the ingrowth of granulation tissue and superficial tissue trauma associated with the embedment of the foam or gauze into the wound surface. Forceful removal usually results in minor bleeding. This is more commonly noted if the bandage is left in place for more than 3 days. Large air leaks can negate the vacuum; small air leaks may cause the adjacent skin to dry from the continuous passage of air over the area. Negative pressure systems are expensive: the vacuum

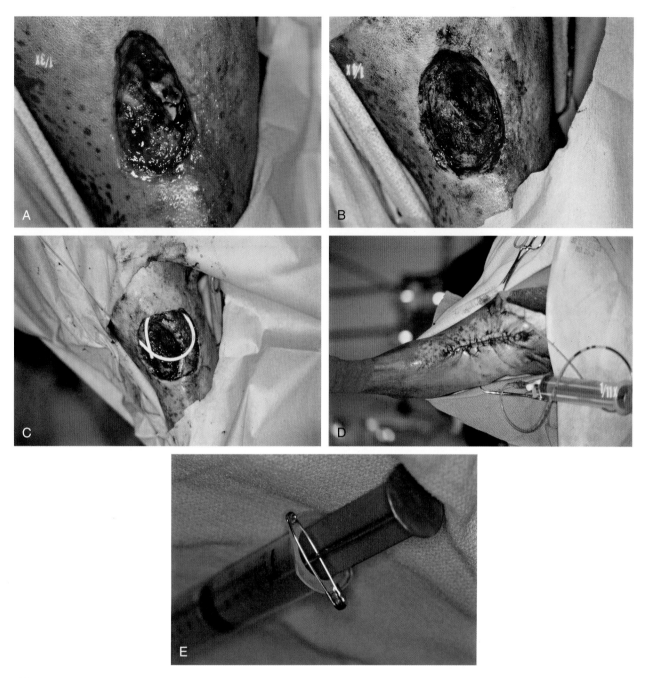

FIG. 4-9 (A) Chronic radiation ulcer in the popliteal area of a dog, secondary to ortho-voltage therapy for mast cell tumor.

(B) Surgical debridement and lavage. The skin borders were partially undermined to facilitate wound closure.

(C) Insertion of 5-mm round fenestrated tube; the tube was shortened to fit into the small dead space pocket prior to skin closure.

(D) A purse-string suture and Roman sandal knot were used to secure the drain tube exiting the small stab incision. Skin closure with intradermal sutures followed by a vertical mattress tension suture pattern. A syringe vacuum was used to collapse the wound pocket and prevent seroma formation in this clean-contaminated wound. Use of a three-way stopcock facilitates use of this simple drainage system.

(E) Safety pins are useful to maintain the vacuum chamber. This "lock" pin can be shifted eccentrically to empty the syringe without its removal.

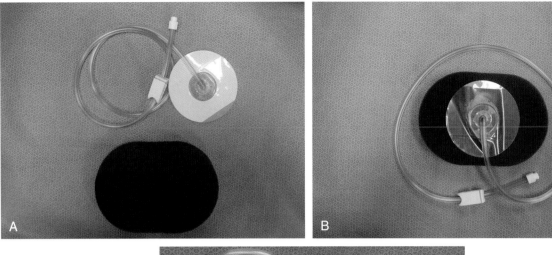

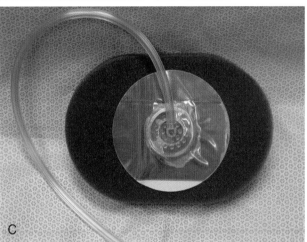

FIG. 4-10 (A, B) The VAC or vacuum-assisted closure system. The system comprises sterile polyurethane (open cell) foam, an attachable vacuum tube, and an adherent plastic drape designed to envelope the foam and adjacent wound margins. Foam pads come in different sizes and can be trimmed to fit a specific wound bed.

(C) Close-up view of perforated adhesive disc that attaches to the foam surface. The opposite end of the tube is attached to the VAC pump, which provides continuous or intermittent subatmospheric pressure to the foam. A plastic adhesive drape overlaps the peripheral skin and forms an airtight canopy over the foam, tubing, and wound. Activation of the vacuum pump removes air beneath the plastic cover, collapsing the foam. Fluid accumulating on the wound surface (wound discharge, serum, edema-tissue fluid accumulation) is drawn into the foam. Excess fluid is collected in the pump reservoir. As discussed, gauze-based systems appear to have comparable clinical results.

pumps can be leased or purchased. Patients normally require continuous supervision during their hospitalization to assure proper function. (There are veterinarians who have used rigid tubing, commercial polyurethane foam or gauze, plastic adhesive drapes, and commercial vacuum pumps to create an economical alternative to the VAC. It must be kept in mind that this alternative may involve patent infringement.) However, changes staged every 2–3 days will reduce the costs otherwise associated with wound care techniques that require daily bandage replacements. It is possible to change the foam or gauze through a small central access incision in the overlying plastic seal, thereby eliminating the need to redo the entire replacement process: after its replacement, a second adhesive sheet can be used to seal the area. In general, two or three changes may be needed before wound closure can be performed.

As noted, negative pressure wound therapy systems are not a substitute for the proper surgical debridement and lavage of contaminated and infected open wounds. They may be most useful for large, deep-pocketed contaminated and infected wounds. These systems must be used with caution if thoracic or abdominal viscera risk contact with the foam. Thin and compromised skin can be traumatized with negative pressure therapy. Lastly, they should not be used on wound surfaces containing cancerous tissue (see Plate 1).

TOPICAL WOUND CARE PRODUCTS

Overview

Historically, a variety of topical agents have been used in managing open wounds, and the list of these products is rather long. Some of the more unusual remedies noted by Rudolph and Noe in their book, *Chronic Problem Wounds* (see Suggested Readings) have included carrots, turnips, bread, egg white, gold leaf, aluminum foil, linseed oil, pectin paste, silicone spray, chlorophyll, tannic acid, yeast extract, wine and vinegar, frankincense and myrrh, mud, oil and grease, beer, dung, fresh meat, heavy metals, saliva, sesame oil, willow leaves, rust, soot, onion, garlic, cinnamon and other aromatic spices, licorice root, and rose water. Although not advocated for use, there is some scientific basis underlying the variable benefits of these products.

There is a renewed interest in the use of honey and sugar for topical wound care. In more recent years, Preparation-H (Wyeth Pharmaceuticals, Richmond, VA; live yeast cell derivative, phenylephrine HCl, shark liver oil) anecdotally has been used for open wound care, reportedly with beneficial results. Sterilized (boiled) potato peelings have been used as a poultice in burn management. Unfortunately, the true efficacy of all topical products cannot be accurately assessed without well-designed comparative studies.

Wound care products are a multi-billion dollar industry in human health care: the veterinary market is a mere fraction of this burgeoning market. In veterinary medicine, most information pertaining to wound care products is largely based on professional experience. The lack of well-designed comparative studies of wound-healing products in dogs and cats is in large part due to a lack of research funding. Most pharmaceutical research uses rats, rabbits, and pigs. Variations in research protocols make accurate comparisons of products difficult. Although clinical applicability of studies between species is open to debate, research results can serve as general guidelines regarding the use of wound care products in veterinary patients. *In vitro* study results may not correlate with *in vivo* efficacy of a given product.

Problems with Veterinary Medicine and Current Research on Wound Healing
- Species differences
- Variations in wound depth, size, and body location
- *In vivo* vs. *in vitro*
- Experimental vs. clinical wounds
- Clinical case variables
- Research design flaws
- Limited number of subjects

There is a true need for evidence-based medicine, allowing us to incorporate new information and technology and allowing veterinarians to integrate the best research evidence with our clinical expertise.

Wound-healing models for assessment of epithelialization normally are based on the creation of partial-thickness skin wounds in research animals using a dermatome. (Most wound closure in humans relies more heavily on epithelialization than wound contraction.) Partial-thickness skin defects epithelialize in a fashion different from full-thickness wounds (see Chapter 2).

In fur-bearing animals, second intention healing is often dominated by myofibroblastic contraction. Because epithelialization occurs independent of wound contraction (and vice versa), research pertaining to rates of epithelialization often fails to address rates of wound contraction.

Providing an optimal environment for epithelialization may not necessarily be ideal to wound contraction. For example, rigid adherent dressings may impair the centripetal movement of skin (splinting the skin margins) but provide a moist environment for epithelialization.

> To date, there is insufficient evidence to suggest whether a given wound care product is superior to others in open wound care.

As discussed in Chapter 3, initial wound management is directed at removing devitalized tissue and contaminants, thereby improving the likelihood that earliest possible wound closure can be achieved. In turn, veterinary clinicians seek out the simplest effective means of closing the wound and restoring function to the injured area. Most open wounds in small animals in fact heal using basic wound care principles outlined in Chapter 3. Confusion often arises when attempting to select the best wound care product for more problematic wounds from an array of topical agents currently available in the health-care market. The variety of topical products available adds to the confusion regarding which products to select. Brochures demonstrating the superior "before and after" benefits on clinical cases do not always hold up to closer clinical scrutiny. With a lack of accurate comparative research, veterinarians are naturally inclined to use products they have had success with in the past, but look for other options only when results are suboptimal for a given patient.

In determining the most appropriate topical wound product, there are a few basic questions to ask.

1. Is there devitalized tissue or tissue of questionable viability?
2. Is the skin wound partial or full-thickness?
3. Is infection present, or is it a significant concern?
4. What stage of wound healing is present?
5. Is wound healing progressing normally?

These questions will help direct you to selecting the most appropriate topical agents to consider for managing an open wound. Devitalized tissue will require removal surgically or by the use of topical debridement agents (discussed later in this section.) Infection must be managed or prevented, often with topical/ systemic antibacterial medications. Otherwise healthy wounds normally require a protective moist environment to support the normal healing processes leading to wound contraction and epithelialization of the defect. Delayed healing dictates elimination of potential causes, and the possible use of topical agents to "jump start," enhance, or supplement the processes of wound healing. In a number of cases, surgical closure of the wound can preclude the cumulative expense of topical agents, dressings, bandage materials, appointments, and transportation costs in more problematic wounds.

General Definitions to Remember

Aerosols: Medicinal agents incorporated in a suitable solvent and packaged under pressure with a propellant. Wide, uniform dispersion and ease of application are advantages to the use of aerosol compounds.

Cleansing agents: A broad class of agents used to facilitate the removal of debris and contaminants from the surface of the skin or open wounds. Agents may contain surfactants, antibacterials, or particulate materials to facilitate wound cleansing prior to open wound management or surgical closure.

Cream: A water-oil emulsion containing a drug or chemical. Evaporation of the water leaves an oily film. Creams often are easier to apply than ointments.

Collodion: A drug in an ethereal solution of cellulose acetate. After application, the ether evaporates, leaving a flexible coating on the skin surface.

Gel: A clear, jellylike topical agent, usually with a greaseless water-soluble base. Medicinal agents may be dispersed in the base.

Liniments (braces): Liquid or semisolid preparations to be applied to the skin with rubbing (inunction). Most contain counterirritants to relieve muscle or tendon pain. Liniments are more commonly employed in horses.

Lotion: A solution or suspension of soothing substances applied to the skin without friction.

Ointment (salve, unguent): A semisolid greasy preparation in which the drug is dispersed in a suitable base; the base may be an oleaginous substance (petroleum, lard, or lanolin) to which the medication is added. Ointments also may have a water-soluble base, such as polyethylene glycol. Ointments normally are denser and less easily spread over the skin or wound surface than are creams and gels.

Topical Enzymatic Debridement Agents

Enzymatic debridement usually refers to the topical application of proteolytic enzymes to degrade nonviable proteins within the wound, facilitating its separation from the underlying viable tissues (see Table 4-2). Collagen fibers form attachments between the viable wound bed and overlying necrotic tissue; degradation of these collagen bonds facilitates separation of the necrotic tissue. Maggot (biologic) debridement therapy is another option to consider in problematic cases (see below).

TABLE 4-2
Enzymatic debridement agents.

Papain-urea	Accuzyme Ointment, Accuzyme SE, Healthpoint Ltd., Fort Worth, TX; Ethezyme, Ethex Corp., St. Louis, MO; Kovia Ointment, Stratus Pharmaceuticals, Sonar Products Inc., Carstadt, NJ. Cost: Accuzyme 30-g ointment tube[++++] *Application*: Papain is derived from the papaya (pawpaw) *Carica papaya*. The proteolytic enzymes papain and chymopapain are present in this fruit. Activity level is over a pH range of 3 to 12. Urea molecules disrupt cross-linking bonds in collagen, allowing the proteins to unfold. Unfolding of the collagen fibrils allows the enzyme papain to digest the exposed proteins. Cross-hatching of a thick eschar is necessary to facilitate penetration into the deeper tissues. A layer of ointment is applied to the wound and covered with a dressing. Debris is flushed from the wound and the ointment reapplied once or twice daily. Papain may be inactivated by salts of heavy metals (lead, mercury, silver). Hydrogen peroxide also inactivates this enzyme.
Papain-urea, chlorophyllin copper complex sodium	Panafil, Panafil SE, Healthpoint Ltd; Ziox Ointment, Stratus Pharmaceuticals, Sonar Products, Inc. Cost: Panafil 30-g tube* *Application*: In addition to papain-urea, chlorophyllin copper complex (CCC) reduces fibrin formation, reportedly facilitating macrophage migration and fibroblast activation for collagen deposition. Copper reportedly enhances structural integrity of the deposited collagen matrix. CCC also is reported to promote healthy granulation tissue, control local inflammation, and reduce wound odors. CCC inhibits the hemagglutination and inflammatory properties of protein degradation products in the wound, including the products of enzyme digestion. Wound cleansing precedes application of the ointment, once or twice daily. Longer intervals between redressings (2–3 days) also may prove to be satisfactory, depending on the condition of the wound.
Trypsin, balsam of Peru, castor oil	Granulex-V, Pfizer Animal Health, Exton, PA; Xenaderm, Healthpoint Ltd (Fig. 4-11). Cost: Granulex V, 1-oz bottle[+]; 4-oz spray[++] *Application*: Balsam of Peru is a capillary bed "stimulant" and has mild antibacterial properties. Castor oil forms an oily barrier, providing a moist environment for promoting epithelialization. Providing a moist environment also reduces local wound pain. Trypsin is the mild enzymatic debriding agent.
Collagenase	Santyl, Healthpoint Ltd. Gladase, Smith & Nephew Inc., St Petersburg, FL. Cost: Santyl 15-g ointment tube[+++] *Application*: Enzyme is derived from the fermentation of *Clostridium hemolyticum*. Optimal pH range is 6–8. Avoid use with heavy metal ions, detergents. Compatible with Dakin's solution, hydrogen peroxide. Apply once per day. Thick eschars should be incised (cross-hatched) with a scalpel blade to facilitate penetration. Remove as much loosened necrotic tissue as possible to facilitate enzymatic debridement. Wounds are cleansed prior to application of ointment. Topical antibiotic powder may be applied to the wound prior to ointment application. The medicated wound is covered with a dressing. The bandage is changed on a daily basis.
Desoxyribonuclease, with fibrinolysin	Elase; Astellas, Deerfield, IL. Cost: 15-g tube[+++]; Elase-Chloromycetin 15-g tube[+++] *Application*: Fibrinolysin derived from bovine plasma; desoxyribonuclease derived from bovine pancreas. Combined actions include breakdown of fibrinous material and nucleoprotein (DNA). Fibrinolytic activity is primarily directed at denatured protein. The wound is cleansed prior to application once or twice daily. Elase would appear to be less commonly employed than other enzymatic debriding agents noted.

Cost: + <$10.00; ++ <$20.00; +++ <$30.00; ++++ <$40.00; +++++ <$50.00; *>$50.00; **>$75.00; ***>$100.00.

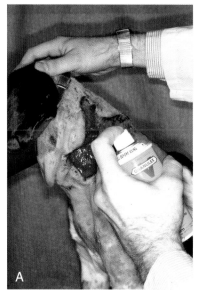
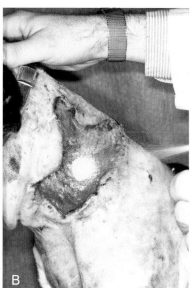

FIG. 4-11 (A) Application of Granulex enzymatic spray, containing trypsin, balsam of Peru, and castor oil.

(B) The spray is easy to apply without contaminating the nozzle for future use. Granulex was used to remove a small area of residual necrotic tissue and provide a moisture barrier to prevent wound desiccation. A nonadherent dressing and light bandage were used to help keep the medication in continuous contact with the wound surface. There are other enzymatic agents available for more aggressive removal of necrotic tissue (see text).

> Enzymatic debridement is considered a selective method of debridement since it specifically targets devitalized tissue only, sparing the adjacent viable tissues. (As a comparison, wet-to-dry dressings are considered nonselective, since this technique can remove viable tissues adjacent to the necrotic tissues.)
>
> Advantages of selective debridement include little or no hemorrhage or pain, and the avoidance of any trauma to important tissue structures during surgical debridement. However, careful surgical debridement can rapidly eliminate major amounts of devitalized tissue: this may enhance the efficacy of enzymatic agents or eliminate their need.

In the natural healing process (autolytic debridement), collagenase and other proteolytic enzymes within the wound break the peptide bonds in collagen to facilitate its detachment from the wound surface. Some topical agents are designed to facilitate autolytic debridement by providing an optimal wound environment for this to occur.

Enzymatic debridement is most commonly reserved for use in patients that are not suitable candidates for surgical debridement. Because these enzymatic agents do not damage viable tissues, they can be used in areas where bleeding, pain, and collateral damage associated with surgical debridement are best avoided. Removal of a necrotic eschar can be facilitated with the use of collagenase, papain, or trypsin. Fibrinolysin is useful for the removal of fibrin or blood. Incising or cross-hatching the surface of necrotic eschars can facilitate topical enzyme penetration.

Surgical debridement is more effective than enzymatic debridement for the rapid removal of large areas of necrotic tissue, especially in septic patients. The more potent enzymatic debriding agents can be expensive (see Table 4-1) to use and normally require a dressing or bandage wrap to assure their prolonged contact with the exposed wound surface.

Pharmaceutical websites are available for readers interested in these products.

Topical Products Promoting Autolytic Debridement

Autolytic debridement (necrotic tissue autolysis) refers to the body's natural process of debridement at the cellular level within the wound. Moisture-retaining gels and dressings can be used to promote this form of selective debridement by optimizing the softening or maceration of devitalized tissues, facilitating phagocytic cells, and proteolytic enzyme liquefaction of the nonviable tissues.

> Autolytic debridement is considered a selective or gentler method of debridement since it specifically targets nonviable tissues only, sparing adjacent viable tissues. Advantages include less hemorrhage, pain, and collateral trauma that may be associated with surgical debridement. However, there is a risk of promoting infection with autolytic debridement, particularly with the presence of significant amounts of devitalized tissue.

Many of these topical gel-like compounds also have been laminated to synthetic membranes, forming a dressing platform for easier application to flat wound surfaces. Similarly, other moisture-retaining barrier dressings (occlusive and semiocclusive) can be used to promote proteolysis within the wound (see Dressings, Chapter 5). There are a variety of topical hydrophilic wound gel products available for use in humans, most of which are applicable to animals (see Wound Gels below.)

When possible, performing surgical debridement can dramatically reduce the volume of necrotic tissue and better control bacterial proliferation. In turn, both enzymatic and autolytic debridement are more effective when the devitalized tissue burden is significantly reduced by surgical debridement.

Wet-to-dry dressings or *mechanical* debridement of residual necrotic tissue is an economical alternative to enzymatic and autolytic debridement, especially after surgical debridement has been performed to reduce the volume of necrotic tissue (see Chapter 5). Wet-to-dry dressings are considered a form of *non-selective debridement*: both necrotic tissue and local viable tissue (epithelium, granulation tissue) may be inadvertently removed during the process of removing the gauze packing. For this reason, the author uses wet-to-dry dressings for no more than 3–5 days. If minimal necrotic tissue remains, products promoting autolytic debridement can be substituted for wet-to-dry dressings.

It is the author's opinion that, in many cases of open wound management (in healthy patients), the combination of surgical debridement and the short-term use of wet-to-dry dressings (3–5 days) is one of the fastest and most economical methods of establishing a healthy wound bed. Thereafter, other topical agents may be used or surgical closure attempted after development of a healthy wound bed.

Wound Gels

There are a variety of gel-like products on the market for wound management.

Hydrogels are compounds containing water (80%–90%); hydrogel dressings are a glycerin-based gel laminated onto a synthetic membrane (see Chapter 5).

Hydrogels provide a moist substrate to hydrate wounds but normally have modest capacity to absorb and retain discharge from the wound (Fig. 4-12).

Gel application is restricted to the wound surface since prolonged exposure to the adjacent skin can cause skin softening secondary to overhydration. A topical dressing and light bandage usually are required to help maintain gel contact with the wound bed. Gels will soften and may drain from beneath the overlying wrap, depending on the location of the wound. Depending on the condition of the wound, gels normally are applied once or twice daily.

Gels can be used for autolytic debridement as described above, or as a topical agent on healthy granulation beds or partial thickness skin wounds. The following is a partial list of gels available on the market:

Curafil Wound Gel (Tyco/Kendall Healthcare): 0.5-, 1-, 3-oz tubes[++]

Curasol Gel Wound Dressing (Healthpoint Ltd., Fort Worth, TX): 90-g tube[++]

Intrasite Hydrogel (Smith & Nephew Inc., St Petersburg, FL): 15-g tube[+]

NuGel Collagen Wound Gel (Johnson & Johnson/Ethicon, Cornelia, GA): 90-g tube[++]

Other agents, such as the following, can be added to a gel base to enhance its healing properties:

Maltodextrin (Intracell Gel, Macleod Pharmaceuticals Inc., Fort Collins, CO): 3-oz tube[++]

Acemannan (CarraVet, Carrington Laboratories Inc., Irving, TX): 3-oz tube[++] (see Fig. 4-12)

Acemannan (Carra Sorb M, Carrington Laboratories Inc.): 4-inch tube[+]

Collagen (Collagen Hydrogel, Coloplast Corp., Minneapolis, MN): 3-oz tube[++]

Collagen (Medifil Collagen Gel, BioCore Medical Technologies Inc., Elkridge, MD): 9-cc syringe[++++]

Tripeptide copper complex (Iamin Hydrating Gel, ProCyte Corp., Kirkland, WA): 0.5-oz tube[++]

Chitosan (Ultrasan, BioSyntech Inc., Laval, Quebec)

Bercaplermin (Regranex, Ortho–McNeil Pharmaceuticals, Raritan, NJ): 15-g tube (0.01%)[***]

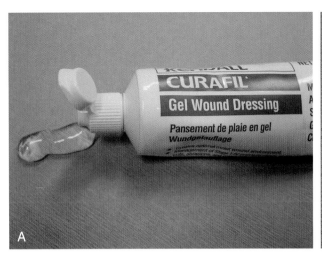

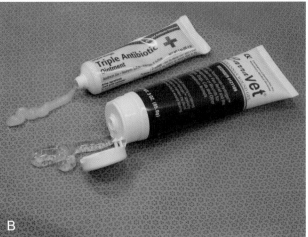

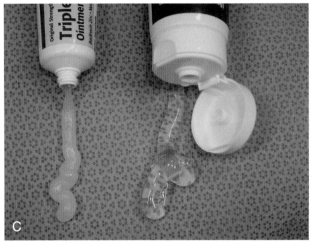

FIG. 4-12 (A) Curafil hydrogel. Hydrogels are applied liberally to the wound and usually are covered with a nonadherent dressing and bandage wrap. Hydrogels will have a greater tendency to drain into the secondary bandage layer and may require more frequent application, especially during early wound management.

(B, C) Example of a hydrogel (Carravet) with a tube of generic triple-antibiotic ointment. Hydrogels will hydrate tissues but have limited ability to absorb significant amounts of discharge. Triple-antibiotic ointment has a white petrolatum base, combined with the antibiotics bacitracin zinc, neomycin sulfate, and polymyxin B sulfate. The oily film helps provide moisture retention (semiocclusive effect). The ointment and wound discharge will be wicked into the secondary bandage layer over time.

(See the price code included in Table 4-2 to determine the cost associated with the products listed above.)

These products and their uses will be discussed below. The above list is not exclusive: there are a number of companies now incorporating collagen, maltodextrin, aloe vera (acemannan), and tripeptide copper complex in their individual product lines. An Internet search can locate these products.

Hydrophilic Pastes and Powders

Hydrophilic pastes and powders are available to fill *exudative* wound cavities or pockets. As they absorb discharge from the wound surface they form a gel. Like the hydrogels noted above, they facilitate autolytic debridement. Examples include Duoderm Hydroactive Sterile Paste (Convatec, Skillman, NJ), Coloplast Comfeel Sterile Paste, Avalon Copolymer Flakes (Summit Hill Lab, Tinton Falls, NJ),and Coloplast Comfeel Sterile Powder (Coloplast Corp.).

Topical Wound-Healing Enhancers

While the term *enhancers* may be a debatable description for some of these agents, the following have been reported to accentuate components of the wound healing process: maltodextrins, acemannan, collagen, tripeptide copper complex, chitosan, and bercaplermin.

Wound Care Products: Do They Enhance, Accelerate, or Promote Wound Healing?

By definition, the word *enhance* means to increase, make greater, or augment. *Accelerate* means to increase the speed of, to cause to occur sooner than expected, to cause to develop or progress more quickly. The term *promote* means to contribute to the progress or growth of something. These terms are often used in describing the benefits of many wound-healing products, not always accurately. Most wounds managed in practice heal uneventfully using basic wound care techniques. Delays in healing may be the result of a variety of factors that are discussed in greater detail in Chapter 6.

Maltodextrin is a D-glucose polysaccharide derived from the hydrolysis of corn or potato starch. It absorbs moisture, forming a protective cover on wound surfaces. It is reported to have chemoattractant properties, attracting neutrophils, macrophages, and lymphocytes into the wound; this in turn increases cytokine levels. Maltodextrin also has been reported to have antibacterial and bacteriostatic properties. Hydrolysis of this polysaccharide may provide a source of glucose to the cells. As a powder (Multidex, De Royal Industries, Powell, TN) or incorporated into a gel (Intracell, Techni-Vet Inc., Burnswick, ME; McLeod Pharmaceuticals Inc.), it can be used for enhancing autolytic debridement and may be used as a topical agent in the latter phases of wound healing. It can reduce odor, swelling, and infection and may enhance epithelialization. A topical dressing and supportive bandage is necessary to maintain contact of a 5- to 10-mm layer of maltodextrin compounds with the wound surface. Saline is used to flush residual gel from the wound prior to reapplication on a daily basis (See Absorptive Beads and Powers for Exudative Wounds, below).

Acemannan (acetylated mannan or mannose) is derived from the aloe vera plant. It reportedly serves as a growth factor and increases levels of the cytokines (interleukin-1, tumor necrosis factor-α). These factors in turn are known to stimulate fibroblast proliferation, epidermal growth and motility, neovascularization, and collagen deposition. It may also bind growth factors, prolonging their stimulating effect on granulation tissue. Acemannan in gel or dry wafer form (Carravet, Carra Sorb M, Carrington Laboratories Inc.) can be used for autolytic debridement and throughout the management of open wounds (Fig. 4-12). Its greatest effect may be during the first 7 days of application (See Absorptive Beads and Powders for Exudative Wounds, below.)

Bovine collagen gels, powders, sheets, wafers, and sponges have been employed in open wound management (Kollagen, Medifil, BioCore Medical Technologies Inc.; Collamend, Genitrix Ltd., Billingshurst, UK; Collasate, PRN Pharmacal, Pensacola, FL; Hycure, HyMed Group, Bethlehem, PA; FasCure, KenVet, Greeley, CO, etc.). The hydrophilic property of topical collagen products helps maintain a moist wound environment for autolytic debridement while possibly providing a protective environment for epithelialization in the latter phases of healing (Fig. 4-13 and 4-14). It may initiate an inflammatory response, stimulating fibroplasia and providing a scaffold for fibroblast migration. Hydrolyzed collagen may provide a substrate for fibroblasts and subsequent collagen deposition. Like other topical agents, a dressing and outer bandage are required to help maintain product contact with the wound: bandages are changed daily. (See Absorptive Beads and Powders for Exudative Wounds, below.)

Tripeptide copper complex (glycyl-L-histidyl-L-lysine-copper) has been reported to stimulate several mechanisms essential to wound healing, including

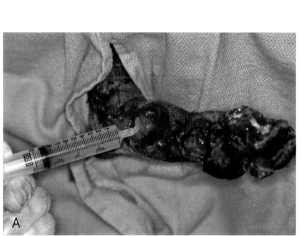
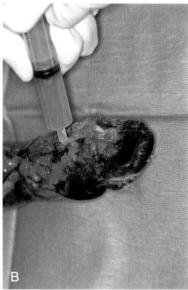

FIG. 4-13 (A, B) Application of collagen gel to shearing wounds using a dispensing syringe. Following application, a nonadherent dressing and light bandage were used to keep the gel in continuous contact with the wound surface.

stimulating neovascularization, collagen deposition, wound contraction, and epithelialization. It is a chemoattractant for mast cells, monocytes, and macrophages. Copper is needed by enzymes involved in collagen cross-linking. It can be applied in a hydrogel base (Iamin, ProCyte Corp.). Only one study in dogs demonstrated greater granulation tissue formation with its use at day 7 compared to the vehicle/base and control. However, by day 14 and 21, there was no notable difference in the contraction and epithelialization of the four groups. (Despite early granulation tissue formation, another interpretation of the results would suggest that tripeptide copper complex did not improve the final outcome of wound healing.)

Chitosan (glucosamine, polysaccharide) is primarily derived from the chitin exoskeleton of shellfish. It is a linear copolymer of linked beta glucosamine and *n*-acetyl-d glucosamine that is usually derived from the chitin-rich crab shell. Topically, it is reported to enhance the function of inflammatory cells (neutrophils, macrophages), fibroblasts, and cytokines (transforming growth factor, platelet-derived growth factor). There is one small study using three research dogs that claims beneficial healing results. There is one chitosan dressing currently available for wound care (HemCon, HemCon Medical Technologies Inc., Portland, OR)

Bercaplermin (Regranex, Ortho-McNeil Pharmaceuticals) is a recombinant human platelet–derived growth factor for topical management of lower extrem-

ity diabetic neuropathic ulcers in humans that extends into the subcutaneous tissues or the viable tissues beyond. It is an adjunct to ulcer management. Clinical studies have demonstrated increased neovascularization, epithelialization, and wound contraction in humans when applied on a daily basis, although its overall efficacy in humans is variable. The cost of a 15-g tube is over $100 to the doctor. The over-the-counter price at pharmacies is substantially greater. The author and exotic medicine clinicians at Angell Animal Medical Center have used it in a long-standing, nonhealing lower-extremity ulcer in a chinchilla and a wing wound in a cockatoo (secondary to feather picking). Healing was complete within six weeks of initiation of therapy in both patients. There is one small study in two dogs that indicated beneficial results in promoting epithelialization. Bercaplermin may be worth considering for use in small problematic wounds in which surgical alternatives are not feasible or ideal.

Natural Products

Honey and Sugar

Unpasteurized honey and sugar are ancient remedies in the management of open wounds. Both honey and sugar are hygroscopic agents that have been used to reduce local tissue edema. Both have the capacity to

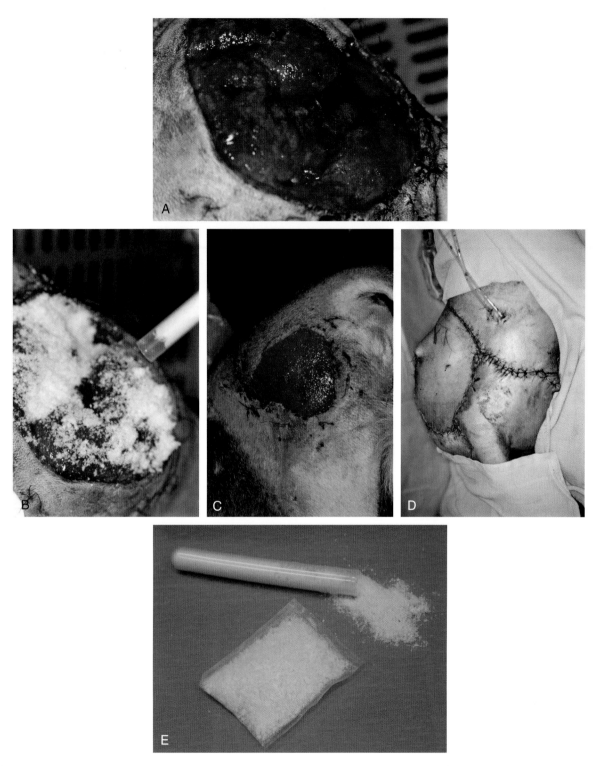

FIG. 4-14 (A) Skin loss secondary to vehicular trauma. The large skin wound was overlying the left trochanteric area in this dog.
(B) Following surgical debridement of the necrotic skin, collagen powder was applied to this moist wound surface, followed by a nonadherent dressing secured with a padded tie-over dressing.
(C) Development of a healthy granulation bed.
(D) Closure with a left deep circumflex iliac axial pattern flap (dorsal branch).
(E) Collagen powder also can be applied to cavitated wounds in a packet form: a clear, perforated Telfa membrane contains the collagen medication.

draw and retain tissue fluid, facilitating autolytic debridement. The gram-positive and gram-negative antibacterial properties of honey may be related to its natural hydrogen peroxide (inhibine) content (glucose oxidase in honey resulting in hydrogen peroxide production) as well as its high osmolarity and acidity (pH 3.6–3.7). There are a variety of unpasteurized honeys available in the world, and their antibacterial properties can vary considerably. Manuka honey, derived from the flowers of the Manuka or tea tree (*Leptospermum scoparium*) is considered the most useful of the topical honey products.

Glucose content in honey (40% glucose, 40% fructose, 20% water) provides an alternate source of energy both to the viable tissues and bacteria. Bacteria may utilize glucose over the amino acids present in the wound and may in turn produce lactic acid rather than malodorous discharge from putrefaction of the nonviable tissue. In contrast, sugar primarily reduces bacterial proliferation due to its high osmolarity, thereby reducing moisture content in the wound. Other wound-healing attributes of honey include its reported stimulation of macrophage migration, angiogenesis, and fibroplasias as a result of hydrogen peroxide production. Sugar also is reported to enhance macrophage migration, granulation tissue formation, and epithelialization. Like honey, sugar may serve as a nutrient substrate for bacteria, reducing the malodorous bacterial putrefaction of devitalized tissues.

Comvita Medical (USA distributor, Derma Sciences Inc., Princeton, NJ) offers a natural honey–based barrier dressing that does not stick to the wound. Apinate dressings contain manuka honey in an alginate base. Besides the presence of hydrogen peroxide, Comvita's Woundcare 18+ manuka honey contains a very high level of an antibacterial agent UMF (unique manuka factor) with an antiseptic potency equivalent to an 18% solution of phenol. Manuka honey is commercially available for oral consumption and topical use and has a variety of UMF ratings, some of which have a 25+ rating.

APPLICATION

Large areas of necrotic tissue are best surgically debrided prior to application of honey and sugar. Both should be applied liberally to the wound, followed by the application of a dressing and a thick outer absorptive layer to help retain discharge from the wound surface. Bandage changes two to three times daily may be necessary to assure the wounds are continuously covered with these hygroscopic agents. Wounds are lavaged and inspected prior to reapplication. Gauze soaked in honey can be used to simplify application to the wound, keeping in mind the gauze may adhere to viable tissues and cause pain and irritation during its removal. Sugar can be poured into the wound with a 1-cm plus layer over the wound surface, followed by a topical dressing and bandage wrap. Bandage changes are typically performed two to three times per day.

Because some human patients complain of discomfort during application of sugar, a less painful sugar paste has been used to facilitate its application to open wounds. The product comprises 400 g castor sugar, 600 g icing sugar, 480 ml glycerin BP, and 7.5 ml of 3% hydrogen peroxide. Reports on its use in animals are lacking.

When a healthy granulation bed forms, surgical closure can be considered or open wound management continued with other topical products. Caution is required when using honey and sugar on large surface areas. Loss of fluid, protein, and electrolytes can be considerable, necessitating close assessment of the patients.

Live Yeast Cell Derivative

Live yeast cell extract (brewer's yeast, *Saccharomyces cerevisiae*) contained in Preparation H (Whitehall Laboratories, New York, NY), may stimulate oxygen consumption, epithelialization, and collagen production in wounds. (Note: Not all formulations of Preparation H contain live yeast extract.) No research study has demonstrated its clinical efficacy, although anecdotally it has been purported to enhance epithelialization.

Aloe Vera

Aloe vera extract has antithromboxane and antiprostaglandin properties. It is useful to reduce inflammation (superficial burns), but may negatively alter the inflammatory phase when managing an open wound. Aloe vera is commonly added to a variety of commercial products.

Absorptive Beads and Powders for Exudative Wounds

These products are generally used with exudative wounds; they are contraindicated in wounds with minimal discharge, since they would have a drying effect on the wound. The wounds normally have been debrided of most devitalized tissues and cleansed prior to their application.

Debrisan (Pharmacia & Upjohn Ltd., Milton Keynes, UK) comprises small polysaccharide beads that are 0.1–0.3 mm in diameter. The dextranomer beads will absorb four times their weight in tissue fluid and exudates. A minimum 3-mm-thick layer is applied to the wound and covered with a retention dressing. At the time of dressing change, the beads are flushed from the wound surface prior to application of an additional layer of beads. As a result, Debrisan is used on moist, exudative wounds to draw tissue fluid and debris from the wound surface: a form of "internal flushing." Dressings are changed once or twice per day. As the wound improves, changes can be extended to alternate day treatments.

There are several manufacturers of particulate or powdered bovine collagen (Kollagen, Medifil, Biocore Medical Technologies Inc.; Collamend particles, Bio-Vet Inc, Blue Mounds, WI; Genitrix Ltd., etc.). These dry collagen materials may be applied in a fashion similar to Debrisan. The collagen material is highly absorptive: Collamend is reported to absorb up to 60 times its weight in fluid. The wound surface is cleansed and slightly dabbed of excess moisture before applying the collagen powder. A layer up to 1/4-inch thick may be used, depending on the amount of exudates. Highly exudative wounds may be covered with gauze to help retain the fluid. A retention dressing is used to maintain contact with the wound bed. The collagen powder may be flushed and the wound dabbed of excess moisture before reapplication on a daily basis. Less frequent changes are required as the condition of the wound improves.

Maltodextrin powder with 1% ascorbic acid (Multidex [DeRoyal Industries]) also can be used as a hydrophilic powder in exudative wounds. The gel form of this product is used for dry wounds. A 1/4-inch layer of powder is secured with a nonadherent, nonocclusive dressing. Dressing changes are similar to those using Debrisan and collagen powders.

Freeze-dried acemannan powder (Carra Sorb M, Carrington Laboratories) can be applied to wounds. This hydrophilic powder is used in exudative wounds in a manner similar to that of the other products in this section.

Biologic Debridement: Maggot Debridement Therapy

Small animal veterinarians normally encounter maggots (fly larvae) infesting open wounds, primarily in warm weather. Facultative or opportunistic myiasis is in contrast to obligatory myiasis, in which a portion of a fly's life cycle is dependent on the animal host for its development. *Cuterebra* sp. is one example of obligatory myiasis (Fig. 4-15).

Maggots ingest only dead cells, exudates, secretions, and debris. The release of proteolytic enzymes facilitates the liquefaction and subsequent consumption of necrotic tissue. Second- and third-stage larvae of myiasis-producing flies have mouthparts capable of rasping the skin and inflicting considerable damage. Tissue trauma and secondary infection can result in extensive tissue destruction (Fig. 4-15).

Not all larvae have an adverse effect on the processes of wound healing. As early as the 16th century, maggots were used as a form of *biotherapy* to remove gangrenous tissue, thereby facilitating the process of wound healing. Each maggot may consume up to 75 mg of necrotic tissue per day. Monarch Labs (Irvine, CA, www.MonarchLabs.com) is the exclusive supplier of disinfected, medical-grade maggots (*Phaenicia sericata*, or green blow fly) in the United States. Maggot debridement therapy (MDT) has been used in veterinary medicine to a limited degree. This technique may be particularly useful for chronic, problematic wounds in which effective debridement is difficult.

APPLICATION

Medical maggots arrive in a sterile container. If they have not hatched, they can be placed in a warming incubator (37°C). Normally, maggots should be used within 24 hours of receipt. A specialized dressing is needed to confine the maggots to the wound. The shape of the wound or ulcer is cut out of the center of a hydroactive dressing (Duoderm, Convatec). This is applied over the wound, leaving the ulcer exposed. Maggots are applied by removing (with a moistened sponge) five to ten larva per square centimeter of wound surface area and applying them to the wound surface. A patch of Dacron chiffon mesh (or nylon stocking) is applied over the hole, followed by a semipermeable transparent adhesive dressing (Tegaderm, Tegapore, 3M, St. Paul, MN). A central hole is provided in this last dressing layer to provide aeration for the maggots. A light layer of gauze sponges is applied over this containment dressing with tape. The outer gauze pads absorb discharge from the wound via the central opening in this specialized dressing; they are changed as needed. Maggots are removed every 48 hours (maximum 72 hours) as a general rule. The maggots are removed with moistened sponges and cotton swabs; the maggots and bandage material are secured in a plastic bag prior to disposal. The wound is gently cleansed and inspected before reapplication

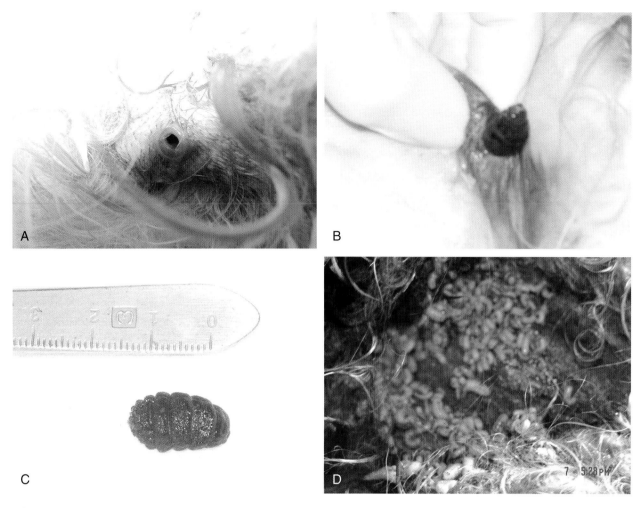

FIG. 4-15 (A) *Cuterebra* sp. in a young dog, located beneath the cervical skin. Note the small sinus opening.

(B, C) The stout larva can be gently expressed from its cavity facilitated by the use of surgical forceps. The small subcutaneous pocket created by this larva is flushed with an antiseptic solution: the wound normally heals uneventfully.

(D) Infected skin wounds containing maggots. Tissue necrosis, infection, and invasive fly larva can result in life-threatening sepsis in small animal patients. Maggots can wander or migrate into other body regions; on rare occasions they also may invade adjacent body orifices, including the anus and vulva.

of additional maggots. Normally three to five replacement cycles are used to manage the average problematic wound. Medical maggots (250–500) cost approximately $80.00; Monarch Labs sells the "Creature Comforts" sterile Dacron chiffon dressings ($4.00 to $8.00 each) and sterile nylon stocking dressings ($10.00). Shipping costs are $40.00–$80.00, depending on the method used. Current costs can be determined at the company's website.

Common Topical Antiseptic Solutions

Chlorhexidine Diacetate

Chlorhexidine diacetate is an effective gram-positive and gram-negative antibacterial agent used both as a surgical scrub and topical solution (Fig 4-16). It maintains bactericidal activity in the presence of blood or pus. A 0.05% solution was compared to a 0.1% povidone-iodine solution in one study. The *in vivo* study indicated that chlorhexidine diacetate had greater bacterial activity over a longer time frame (6 hours) compared with povidone-iodine. The addition of Tris EDTA (see below) reportedly enhances bacterial susceptibility to destruction by 1000-fold, compared to 0.05% chlorhexidine alone. It reportedly lyses *Pseudomonas aeruginosa*, *Escherichia coli* and *Proteus vulgaris* on contact. Like chlorhexidine alone, it will pre-

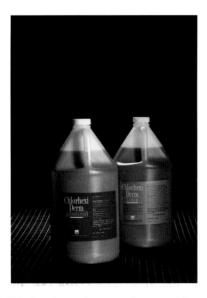

FIG. 4-16 Chlorhexidine solution, with a 1:40 dilution with sterile saline, is an effective and economical cleansing agent for open wounds. It also can be used in wet-to-wet and wet-to-dry dressings.

cipitate in electrolyte solutions and will not affect its potency.

APPLICATION

Stock chlorhexidine solution can be diluted (1 part chlorhexidine to 40 parts sterile water or saline) for use as a wound lavage solution, wet-to-wet dressings, and wet-to-dry dressings. The resultant 0.05% concentration is effective against bacteria without causing damage to viable tissue.

Povidone-Iodine Solution

Povidone-iodine is a commonly used surgical scrub and prep solution that has the bactericidal activity of iodine. Iodine is slowly released from this polymer: a 7.5% povidone-iodine solution releases 0.75% iodine. It is effective against gram-positive and gram-negative bacteria, fungi, viruses, yeasts, and protozoa. The presence of organic material does not affect the efficacy of povidone-iodine. Povidone-iodine has less bacterial activity and a shorter duration of efficacy compared to chlorhexidine diacetate in a previous study.

Application

A dilution of 1 part povidone-iodine solution to 9 parts sterile saline can be used as a lavage solution without causing significant harm to viable tissues. This solution can be used in wet-to-wet and wet-to-dry dressings.

Tris [Hydroxymethyl] Aminomethane-EDTA

Tris buffer (tris [hydroxymethyl] aminomethane buffer) enhances the antimicrobial properties of EDTA (disodium-calcium salt of ethylenediaminetetraacetic acid). Tris-EDTA in sterile water readily lyses *P. aeruginosa*, *E. coli*, and *Proteus vulgaris*. Tris-EDTA synergism against *E. coli* is noted with penicillin, oxytetracycline, and chloramphenicol. Similarly, it has synergistic properties against *P. vulgaris* when combined with gentamycin, oxytetracycline, polymyxin B, nalidixic acid, and trip sulfonamide.

Application

This broad spectrum lavage solution is inexpensive and easily prepared (1.2 g of EDTA with 6.05 g of tris added to one liter of sterile water for injection). The pH is adjusted to 8.0 with a dilute solution of sodium hydroxide. The solution is autoclaved for 15 minutes after mixing.

Wound-Cleansing Solutions

A variety of solutions have been advocated for cleansing wounds. Tap water, although hypotonic and potentially harmful to exposed tissues, has been advocated by some for the removal of gross contaminants adhering to open wounds. A comparison of tap water versus sterile saline in irrigating experimental wounds in rats indicated both were similar in their ability to reduce bacterial counts. However, an *in vivo* study demonstrated that tap water (hypotonic, alkaline pH) is notably cytotoxic to fibroblasts. Sterile saline (0.9% NaCl, unbuffered, acidic pH) also displayed cytotoxic effects to fibroblasts; no negative effects were associated with phosphate-buffered saline and Ringer's lactate.

Sterile saline is most commonly used to swab or flush wounds in veterinary medicine; under pressure (8 psi is ideal), it can be effective in displacing microscopic contaminants. Antiseptic solutions (listed above) are frequently used to cleanse wounds. Although uncommonly used in veterinary medicine, hydrotherapy is used to facilitate the removal of devitalized tissue, primarily in human burn patients with large surface thermal injuries.

There are a number of commercially available wound-cleansing agents used to facilitate the removal of surface contaminants and wound exudate. They are most commonly used to clean a wound prior to the reapplication of a topical agent and dressing.

Wound cleansers basically contain water, surfactants (sodium lauryl sulfate, etc.), salt, and a preservative. Some cleansers include antimicrobial agents (triclosan, chlorhexidine gluconate, chloxylenol, etc.). Humectants may be added for their moisturizing property (glycerin, methyl glucose esters, lactates, lanolin derivatives, mineral oil, etc.). Various alcohols may be added for their antibacterial properties and to serve as an emollient or thickening agent. Common wound-cleansing products include CuraKlense and Constant Clens (Kendall Co., Mansfield, MA), Allclenz (HealthPoint Co.), Sur-Clens (Convatect), UltraKlenz and CarraKlenz (Carrington Laboratories Inc.), and Dermagran (Derma Sciences Inc.). In one study, Constant Clens was considered the most biocompatible. Most wound-cleansing products come in a convenient pump spray or squeeze bottle for application to the wound surface (Fig. 4-17).

Topical Antimicrobial Agents

Topical antimicrobial agents are used both to prevent and to manage infections in open wounds. The oint-

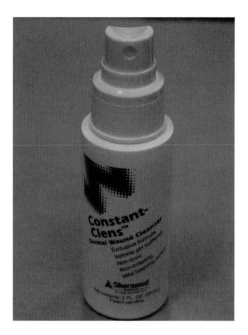

FIG. 4-17 One example of a wound-cleansing agent. Many come in a convenient pump-spray bottle. Wound cleansers commonly contain water, a surfactant, humectants, and an antimicrobial agent.

ment or cream base can provide a moisture-retaining barrier to prevent tissue desiccation, promoting epithelialization. They are capable of delivering concentrated amounts of the antibacterial agent directly to the wound surface.

Removal of debris and necrotic tissue will enhance their efficacy both in preventing and treating wound infections.

There are a variety of economical topical antimicrobial agents on the market

Chlorhexidine ointment (Nolvasan 1%, Fort Dodge Labs, Fort Dodge, IA)

Gentamycin ointment

Nitrofurazone cream/ointment

Povidone-iodine ointment

Silver sulfadiazine (see Fig. 4-18)

Triple antibiotic ointment

Note that there are a variety of manufacturers for most of these products.

Chlorhexidine ointment is currently manufactured by Fort Dodge Labs (Nolvasan 1%). Chlorhexidine, silver sulfadiazine, and povidone-iodine ointment are hydrophilic (water-miscible) ointments that are easily flushed from the wound surface to facilitate inspection. Oil-based (hydrophobic) topical antimicrobials, including gentamycin ointment and triple-antibiotic ointment, form a greasy film that may repel lavage solutions. The author finds water-miscible agents useful in cases of delayed primary closure: they are easily flushed from the wound surface, allowing for easier assessment of the tissues during subsequent bandage changes. In turn, oil-based products are preferred on healthy granulation beds for their better ability to maintain a protective film on the wound surface. In most routine cases, triple-antibiotic ointment is both effective and economical to use.

In practice, the use of "community jars" of ointment is best discouraged due to the potential of introducing contaminants. The author has witnessed a number of occasions when busy veterinarians use an index finger to dispense a dollop of the medication directly onto a wound or dressing. Jars are best used exclusively for a single patient. Autoclaved tongue depressors can be used for removing the ointment, especially when dealing with large open wounds (burns). Individual tubes of topical antimicrobials reduce the risk of contamination and can be devoted to individual patients with smaller wounds.

Chlorhexidine has a broad spectrum of activity against microorganisms. Gentamycin has efficacy against gram-negative microorganisms, including

Pseudomonas spp. and *Staphylococcus* spp. Nitrofurazone has both gram-positive and gram-negative activity. It has broad-spectrum antibacterial properties, but has little effect against *Pseudomonas* spp. Its hydrophilic polyethylene base enables it to draw and retain body fluid and discharge from the wound surface. Topical povidone-iodine ointment also has a broad-spectrum of activity against a variety of microorganisms.

Triple antibiotic ointment (neomycin sulfate, bacitracin zinc, polymyxin-B sulfate) is both economical and readily available in pharmacies and veterinary supply houses. The combination of these three antibiotics has a synergistic effect against a variety of bacteria, although less so against *Pseudomonas* spp. Triple-antibiotic ointment can enhance reepithelialization but may have a slight retardant effect on contraction.

Silver sulfadiazine is effective against a variety of microorganisms including *Pseudomonas* spp. The author normally reserves its use for burns (Chapter 7). *In vitro* studies indicate it has toxicity to human keratinocytes and fibroblasts and an inhibitory effect on neutrophils and lymphocytes that can be reversed with aloe vera. Clinically, it remains one of the most effective topical agents in the management of thermal injuries.

Triple antibiotic ointment is economical, easily accessible, and economical. The author commonly uses it for smaller wounds and for the protection of free grafts. The sticky petroleum base provides protection against tissue desiccation. Combined with a nonadherent dressing and protective bandage, it has a semiocclusive effect on the grafted area.

Prior to the closure of a granulation bed, the liberal application of a topical broad-spectrum antibiotic 24–48 hours before surgery can substantially reduce the residential bacterial population prior to the final surgical preparation of the area.

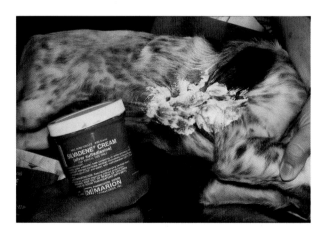

FIG. 4-18 Application of water-miscible silver sulfadiazine ointment to a burn. Silver sulfadiazine is most commonly used in the management of burn wounds.

Topical antimicrobial agents can have variable effects on the processes of wound contraction and epithelialization. In general, comparative studies are lacking to determine which ointment or cream has the greatest wound-healing benefits: it is unlikely there is a dramatic difference between these products.

ALTERNATIVE FORMS OF WOUND THERAPY

Hyperbaric Oxygen

Chronic wounds may lack the circulation required to deliver oxygen to the ischemic tissues. Hypoxic tissues cannot heal optimally and are more susceptible to infection. Oxygen tension above 40 mm Hg promotes healing; chronic wounds may have oxygen tensions below 20 mm Hg. Traumatic and infected wounds typically have oxygen tension values less than 30 mm Hg. Considering that active cell division requires a minimum of 30 mm Hg, the normal processes of healing are jeopardized in chronic nonhealing wounds. Hyperbaric oxygen increases dissolved oxygen in plasma, stimulating the growth of new capillaries, and may have special use in the management of ischemic wounds. Hyperbaric oxygen has been used to salvage skin compromised by external trauma, disease, or surgery (e.g., skin flaps, skin grafts, muscle flaps). In two animal studies, however, hyperbaric oxygen therapy failed to improve flap and graft survival.

Hyperbaric oxygen therapy has been used with some success for problematic wounds in humans. Smaller units are available for small animal patients. Although detailed information pertaining to their clinical efficacy in veterinary medicine is lacking, the main deterrent to their use is their high cost in relation to the comparatively low numbers of animals that would possibly benefit from hyperbaric oxygen therapy.

Mechanical Stimulants

Low-intensity laser light (phototherapy) and pulse electromagnetic fields (0.5–18 Hz) have been used experimentally to stimulate the normal healing processes. Low-level laser therapy reportedly induces the proliferation of fibroblasts. It reportedly can shorten the inflammatory phase of healing and enhance the release of factors that stimulate the proliferative phase of healing. There was a synergistic effect reported when laser therapy was combined with photosensitizer drugs in experimental rats.

Electrical stimulation, including the use of pulsed electromagnetic fields, has been demonstrated to improve microvascular flow while activating fibroblasts. One study indicated that pico-tesla electromagnetic field treatment improved wound strength and speeded contraction of open wounds in rats. Another study reported enhancement of wound epithelialization in dogs. Similarly, microwave irradiation has been used to induce hyperthermia, thereby improving epithelialization in wounds involving rabbits and humans.

Evidence of the true clinical efficacy of using laser, photodynamic, electromagnetic, and microwave irradiation is lacking. The reader is reminded that the vast majority of wounds seen in veterinary practice can be managed successfully without the use of these devices. Additional research is needed to prove their clinical worth.

CONCLUDING REMARKS

Wound drainage is an important component of managing wounds. Penrose drains, vacuum drains, and more recently vacuum-assisted closure are options to consider, depending on the size, location, and condition of the wound.

There are a variety of topical agents that may be employed in the management of open wounds. They often have multiple effects on wound healing. Removal of necrotic tissue is a vital step in reducing the presence or risk of infection; its removal also promotes the formation of a healthy granulation bed in most cases. Both selective and nonselective debridement techniques may be used in veterinary patients. Surgical debridement remains the quickest means of removing major areas of devitalized tissue. Topical agents may be used to facilitate the removal of smaller areas of necrotic tissues (topical enzymatic debridement, autolytic debridement). Infection can be managed with a variety of topical antibacterial agents, depending on the condition of the wound. Topical agents that reportedly enhance or accelerate healing are worth closer scrutiny by the veterinary clinician. The bottom line is the final point of wound closure; early benefits seen in a comparative study mean little if the final outcome is the same. Without well-designed research models and clinical data, the selection of topical wound products is largely based on the information provided by the company and the experience of the clinicians who use a given product. Fortunately, most wounds heal with basic surgical and medical care.

Suggested Readings

Adkesson MJ, Travis EK, Weber MA, et al. Vacuum-assisted closure for treatment of a deep shell abscess and osteomyelitis in a tortoise. *J Am Vet Med Assoc* 231:1249–1254.

American Pediatric Surgical Nurses Association. All about Dressings. Available at: http://www.apsna.org/mc/page.do?sitePageId=24204.

Armstrong DG, Mossel J, Nixon BP, et al. 2002. Maggot debridement therapy—a primer. *J Am Podiatr Med Assoc* 92:398–401.

Ashworth CD, Nelson DR. 1990. Antimicrobial potentiation of irrigation solutions containing tris [hydroxymethyl] aminomethane-EDTA. *JAVMA* 197:1513–1514.

Ben-Amotz R, Lanz OI, Miller JM, et al. 2007. The use of vacuum-assisted closure therapy for the treatment of distal extremity wounds in 15 dogs. *Vet Surg* 36:684–690.

Braakenburg A, Obdeijn MC, Feltz R, et al. 2006. The clinical efficacy and cost effectiveness of the vacuum-assisted closure technique in the management of acute and chronic wounds: a randomized controlled trial. *J Plast Reconstr Surg* 118(2):390–397.

Buffa EA, Lubbe AM, Verstraete FJM, et al. 1997. The effects of wound lavage solutions on canine fibroblasts: an in vitro study. *Vet Surg* 26:460–466.

Canapp SO, Farese JP, Schultz GS, et al. 2003. The effect of topical tripeptide-copper complex on healing of ischemic open wounds. *Vet Surg* 32:515–523.

Elkins AD. 1997. Hyperbaric oxygen therapy: potential veterinary applications. *Compend Contin Edu Pract Vet* 19:607–612.

Fahie MA, Shettko D. 2007. Evidence-based wound management: a systematic review of therapeutic agents to enhance granulation and epithelialization. *Vet Clin No Amer* 37:559–577.

Guille AE, Tseng LW, Orsher RJ. 2007. Use of vacuum-assisted closure for management of a large skin wound in a cat. *J Am Vet Med Assoc* 230(11):1669–1673.

Hendrix CM. 1991. Facultative myiasis in dogs and cats. *Compend Contin Edu Pract Vet* 13:86–93.

Hosgood, G. 1993. The role of platelet-derived growth factor and transforming growth factor beta. *Vet Surg* 22:490–495.

Hosgood G. 2003. Wound repair and specific tissue response to injury. In: Slatter D (ed). *Textbook of Small Animal Surgery*, 3rd ed. Philadelphia, PA: WB Saunders.

Jonsson K, Jenson JA, Goodson WH III, et al. 1991. Tissue oxygenation, anemia, and perfusion in relation to wound healing in surgical patients. *Ann Surg* 214(5):605–613.

Kerwin SC, Hosgood G, Strain GM, Vice CC, et al. 1993. The effect of hyperbaric oxygen treatment on a compromised axial pattern flap in the cat. *Vet Surg* 22:31–36.

Krahwinkel DJ, Boothe HW. 2006. Topical and systemic medications for wounds. *Vet Clin No Am* 36:739–758.

Lee AH, Swaim SF, Yang ST, et al. 1984. Effects of gentamicin solution and cream on the healing of open wounds. *Am J Vet Res* 45:1487–1492.

Lee AH, Swaim SF, Yang ST, et al. 1986. The effects of petrolatum, polyethylene glycol, nitrofurazone, and a hydroactive dressing on open wound healing. *J Am Anim Hosp Assoc* 22:443–451.

Lemarie RJ, Hosgood G, VanSteenhouse J, et al. 1998. Effect of hyperbaric oxygen on lipid peroxidation in free skin grafts in rats. *Am J Vet Res* 59(7):913–917.

Lucroy MD, Edwards BJ, Madewell BR. 1999. Low-intensity laser light-induced closure of a chronic wound in a dog. *Vet Surg* 28:292–295.

Mathews K, Binnington A. 2002. Wound management using sugar. *Compend Contin Edu Pract Vet* 24:41–50.

Mathews K, Binnington A. 2002. Wound management using honey. *Compend Contin Edu Pract Vet* 24:53–59.

Morykwas M, Argenta L, Shelton-Brown E, et al. 1997. Vacuum-assisted closure: a new method for wound control and treatment: animal studies and basic foundation. *Ann Plast Surg* 38:553–652.

Moscati R, Mayrose J, Fincher L. 1998. Comparison of normal saline with tap water for wound irrigation. *Am J Emerg Med* 16:379–381.

Rodeheaver GT. 2001. Wound cleansing, wound irrigation, wound disinfection. In: Krasner DL, Rodeheaver GT, Sibbald GR, eds. *Chronic Wound Care: a Clinical Source Book for Healthcare Professionals*. Wayne, PA: HMP Communications.

Rudolph R, Noe JM. 1983. *Chronic Problem Wounds*. Boston: Little, Brown and Co.

Sartipy U, Lockowandt U, Gabel J, et al. 2006. Cardiac rupture during vacuum-assisted closure therapy. *Ann Thorac Surg* 82:1110–1111.

Scardino MS, Swaim SF, Sartin EA, et al. 1998. Evaluation of treatment with a pulsed electromagnetic field on wound healing, clinicopathologic variables, and central nervous system activity in dogs. *Am J Vet Res* 59(9):1177–1181.

Sherman RA. 1997. A new dressing design for treating pressure ulcers with maggot therapy. *Plast Reconstr Surg* 100:451–456.

Sherman RA. 2002. Maggot versus conservative debridement therapy for the treatment of pressure ulcers. *Wound Repair Regen* 10:208–214.

Subrahmanyam M. 1996. Honey dressing versus boiled potato peel in the treatment of burns: a prospective randomized study. *Burns* 22:491–493.

Swaim SF, Bradley DM, Spano JS, et al. 1993. Evaluation of multipeptide-copper complex medications on open wound healing in dogs. *J Am Anim Hosp Assoc* 29:519–525.

Swaim SF, Gillette RL. 1998. An update on wound medications and dressings. *Compend Contin Edu Pract Vet* 20:1133–1145.

Swaim SF, Gillette RL, Sartin EA, et al. 2000. Effects of a hydrolyzed collagen dressing on the healing of open wounds in dogs. *AJVR* 61:1574-1578.

Swaim SF, Riddell KP, McGuire JA. 1992. Effects of topical medications on the healing of open pad wounds in dogs. *J Am Anim Hosp Assoc* 28:499–502.

Tibbles PM, Edelsberg JS. 1996. Hyperbaric-oxygen therapy. *N Eng J Med* 334(25):1642–1648.

Trostel CT, McLaughlin RM, Lamberth JG, Cooper RC, et al. 2003. Effects of pico-tesla electromagnetic field treatments on wound healing in rats. *Am J Vet Res* 64:845–854.

Ueno H, Mori T, Fujinaga T. 2001. Topical formulations and wound healing applications of chitosan. *Adv Drug Deliv Rev* 52(2):1005–1015.

Ueno H, Yamada H, Tanaka I, et al. 1999. Accelerating effects of chitosan for healing at early phase of experimental open wound in dogs. *Biomaterials* 20:1407–1414.

Webb LX. 2002. New techniques in wound management: vacuum-assisted wound closure. *J Am Acad Orthop Surg* 10:303–311.

Wheeler JL. 2007. Vacuum-assisted wound closure and initial experience in small animal surgery. North American Veterinary Conference Post Graduate Institute, pp 170–174.

Plate 1   **Vacuum-Assisted Closure**

DESCRIPTION

Vacuum-assisted closure (VAC, KCI, USA) refers to a simple drainage system comprising open cell polyurethane foam that is connected to a vacuum pump with rigid plastic tubing. Discharge from the wound surface is partially retained in the foam, whereas excess tissue fluids are retained in the vacuum pump reservoir. The VAC is best considered for large, deep, or cavitated wounds; it may also be used to secure skin grafts to a recipient bed. VAC is capable of reducing edema during open wound management. A similar alternative is a gauze-based system (Venturi, Talley Medical) more recently introduced into the veterinary market.

TECHNIQUE

(A₁) Example of a large cavitated wound involving the left flank and lateral abdominal area. The skin has been widely clipped of fur and cleaned with a surgical scrub and isopropyl alcohol swabs: the skin must be completely dry.

(A₂) After initial surgical management of the wound (removal of necrotic tissue and debris), the VAC foam pad is trimmed to the size of the wound. An adhesive medallion secures the flexible plastic tubing to the surface of the polyurethane foam. Alternatively, gauze can be used in place of the plastic foam sheet. Gauze sponges impregnated with PHMB may be most useful.

(B) Prior to application of the adherent plastic drape over the entire wound site, a thick bead of adhesive sealant paste used for colostomy bags (Stoma Paste, Salts Healthcare, Birmingham, UK; Stomadhesive, Convatec; Adapt Paste, Hollister Inc., Libertyville, IL) can be applied to better secure the perimeter against an air leak.

(C) The adherent plastic drape is applied to seal the entire area. A spray adhesive may be used on the skin to improve adherence of the plastic drape to the skin (Vi-Drape, Medical Concepts Development, St Paul, MN; Vi-Drape, The Clinipad Corp, Norwich, CT). The exit tube is inserted into the vacuum pump/reservoir. A continuous vacuum pressure of −125 mm Hg is most commonly used. (See text for additional details on the use of negative pressure systems.) The foam or gauze is changed and the wound inspected every 2–3 days. Normally two to three changes are required to manage problematic wounds. (See details in the chapter text). Some clinicians will incise the center of the plastic drape to remove the foam or gauze and inspect the wound. Following reapplication of a new foam or gauze dressing, a second plastic drape is applied over the hole created in the first plastic cover: the vacuum is then reactivated. Patients are normally kept in an intensive care ward for continuous monitoring of the negative pressure wound therapy.

COMMENTS

KCI USA Inc. (San Antonio, TX) sells the components of this wound drainage system and leases the pump apparatus. Talley Medical (Lansing, MI) sells their pump and its components. Although the basic components of the system are commercially available, including polyurethane open cell foam, gauze rigid tubing, plastic surgical drapes, and standard vacuum pumps, using them in this manner may be in violation of a company's patent rights. Veterinarians are encouraged to contact company representatives for the purchase and use of their devices.

The primary question regarding negative pressure wound therapy is its real niche in veterinary surgery. Most of the wounds noted in lectures and journal articles have been (and can be) handled by other means that are often more economical. Necrotic tissue and debris still must be removed from the wound prior to the use of these systems. It is the author's impression that the systems would be most effective in deep, cavitated wounds (e.g., large flank wounds extending into the medial thigh region) where drainage and wound care are especially problematic. Both systems have been reported to be effective means of

Plate 1

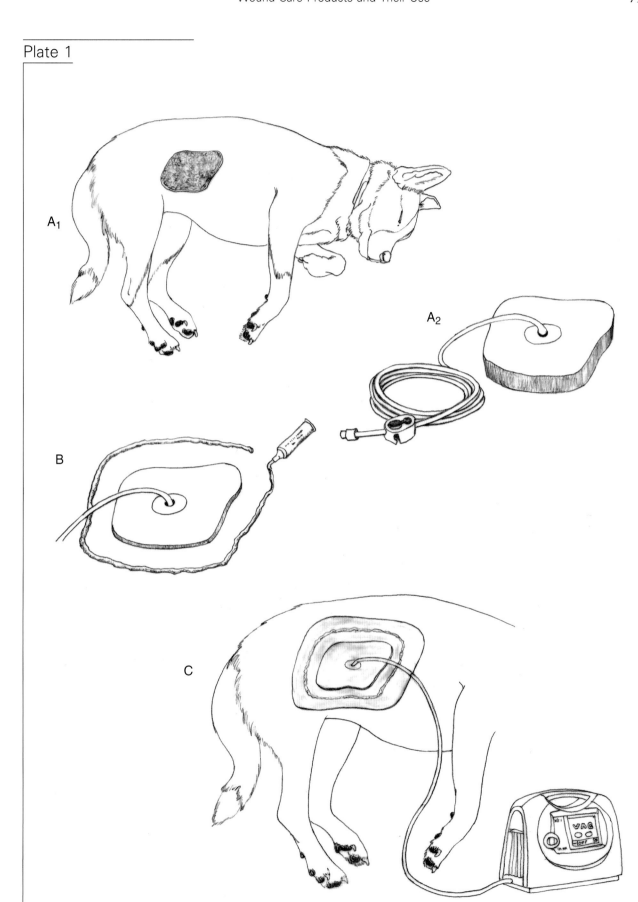

Plate 1

(Continued)

immobilizing free grafts in a problematic body region: when used for this purpose, a nonadherent dressing is applied over the graft to prevent the foam or gauze from adhering to the surgical area. They also would be useful for reducing edema in open wounds with extensive soft tissue swelling. The surgeon must assess the advantages of negative pressure wound therapy versus other methods of wound care based on (1) wound size, location, and classification and (2) all costs (including time and labor) associated with the use of these systems versus alternative methods. Clinicians are often enamored of new products and technology: only by their clinical use will veterinarians determine the long-term merits of vacuum-assisted closure.

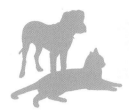

5

Dressings, Bandages, External Support, and Protective Devices

INTRODUCTION

Bandages are an integral part of wound management. A bandage is a wrap primarily used to hold plain and medicated dressings in place, support or immobilize a body part, apply pressure to control hemorrhage, obliterate dead-space or cavities, and protect a wound from external trauma and contamination (Fig. 5-1).

A dressing refers to a material that is applied directly to the surface of the wound. Some dressings are designed for direct application to a wound without the need for an outer supportive wrap. Most dressings require the added support of a bandage to prevent their displacement, optimize their contact with the wound bed, and potentially serve as an outer absorptive layer for retention of any discharge. As a result, the dressing is part of the anatomy of a bandage.

Bandages have three defined layers: the primary (contact dressing) layer, the secondary (intermediate) layer, and the tertiary (outer) layer.

COMPOSITION OF A BANDAGE

The Primary Layer: Wound Dressings

The primary layer lies in direct contact with the wound. Most commonly, this involves the application of a topical wound dressing. The term *dressing* has changed somewhat in its usage over the past several years. Wound dressings are normally considered topical membranes, gauze materials, or pads designed for direct application to a wound. Some companies refer to their topical agents (pastes, gels, etc.) as *wound dressings.* No single dressing is suitable for all types of wounds. Different dressings may be needed during the various phases of wound management. In general, dressings perform one or more of the following functions: absorb and retain discharge from the wound, provide a moist environment to promote healing, provide a product that promotes the healing process, provide protection from bacteria and other contaminants, absorb wound odor, provide insulation and mechanical protection, and facilitate wound debridement.

Is there a perfect wound dressing? The answer is no: different dressings may be useful for different phases of the wound healing process.

If the ideal dressing existed, it would have all of the following properties:

Is safe (nontoxic, nonirritating)

Maintains a moist environment

Has low or nonadherence*

Provides thermal Insulation

Provides protection from external contaminants

Provides mechanical protection

Has good absorptive properties (exudative wounds)

Provides comfort to the patient

Is easy to use and change

Conforms easily to the wound surface

Requires infrequent changes

Is affordable and cost-effective to use

*Adherent dressings are used as a form of mechanical debridement.

Dressings will be discussed in the following categories:

Adherent dressings

Nonadherent dressings

Absorptive dressings

Semiocclusive dressings

Occlusive dressings

Moisture-retaining dressings

These broad categories overlap to a variable degree: a given dressing can have more than one property and function. Moreover, as discussed in Chapter 4, various topical agents can have an effect on wound healing similar to the dressings discussed in this section. For

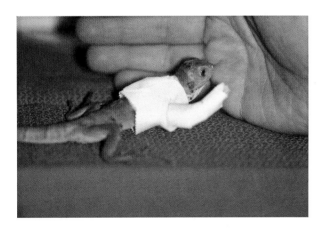

FIG. 5-1 Spica bandage for a lizard. Bandages can be a critically important component to wound management in small animals.

example, a topical gel applied to a wound may have the same basic properties as a hydrogel dressing. The primary difference is the external membrane of the dressing with its adherent gel compared to the use of a gel and the retention layer (gauze or dressing) placed over it. In deeper wounds, gel may be preferable to a hydrogel dressing whereas shallower wounds may be managed more easily by using a hydrogel dressing. Watery gels will tend to gravitate from beneath a topical dressing or bandage, thus requiring more frequent application.

> The rapid proliferation of a variety of "designer dressings" by multiple manufacturers has added an element of confusion to the process of selecting the best dressing for a given set of circumstances. Alginates, collagen, and starch copolymers alone or in combination have been added to moisture -retentive dressings. Which hydrogel or hydrocolloid dressing is best? It is impossible to say. How one dressing compares to another dressing cannot be ascertained without comparative studies.

Dressings either play a relatively passive protective function (passive products, such as plastic membranes, nonadherent dressings) vis-à-vis the wound or play an interactive role in promoting wound healing (interactive products, such as hydrogels, foam dressings, etc.). Such "interactive dressings" can provide a substrate or microenvironment supportive of the wound-healing process (e.g., bioactive products, such as hydrocolloids, alginates, collagens, chitosan, etc.).

Adherent Dressings

Adherent dressings are used for the mechanical debridement of necrotic tissue and the absorption of discharge from the wound surface. Wet-to-dry and dry-to-dry bandages fall into this category. Both bandages use coarse or wide-mesh cotton gauze as the contact layer with the wound surface.

> Mechanical debridement refers to the removal of necrotic tissue and foreign material from a wound by physical force. This includes the use of wet-to-dry dressings: removal of the adherent gauze also removes necrotic tissue and topical debris adhering to its surface. Hydrotherapy and wound irrigation also are forms of mechanical debridement. These modes of debridement are considered "nonselective" since their use can indiscriminately damage local healthy tissues at the same time they remove devitalized tissues.

Wet-to-dry dressings are gauze pads moistened with Ringer's lactate or sterile saline and applied directly to the wound surface. (A 0.05% chlorhexidine diacetate or 0.1% povidone iodine solution may be used; see Chapter 4). The moist sponges initially hydrate the wound environment and dilute the purulent discharge, facilitating its absorption into the gauze.

> Comprised of readily available surgical gauze and sterile isotonic fluids, wet-to-dry dressings are economical to use. Cost is primarily determined by the frequency and duration of dressing changes.
>
> Wet-to-dry dressings can be used effectively in wounds with low to high amounts of exudates: they hydrate, dilute tenacious exudates, and have a high capacity to wick and retain the discharge.

Over several hours, moisture partially evaporates through the outer surface of the dressing. As it (partially) dries, the gauze has a tendency to adhere to the wound surface and necrotic tissue in contact with its surface. As the gauze is lifted from the wound, adherent necrotic tissue is stripped from the viable tissues. The process is repeated, ideally two to three times per day (Fig. 5-2).

> Sponges impregnated with the antimicrobial agents polyhexamethylene biguanide (PHMB; The Kendall Co.) can be moistened with Ringer's lactate or sterile saline for immediate application to the open wound. These sponges also have been used in conjunction with negative pressure wound therapy. See Chapter 4.
>
> To reduce the risk of wicking bacteria into the wound (strike-through) an outer wrap should be applied to a wet dressing. The author commonly uses surgical paper drapes secured with tape to cover the wet-to-dry dressing.

Wet-to-dry dressings have been criticized primarily for causing a variable degree of trauma to the adjacent viable tissues. Removal can be transiently painful to the patient.

It is the author's contention that *surgical* debridement should be used to reduce the bulk of devitalized tissue in problematic wounds; wet-to-dry dressings, *used for no more than 3–5 days*, is an easy and economical method of removing the residual necrotic tissue in the wound. Short-term use, as described, does not significantly interfere with the emerging granulation tissue and has minimal effect on epithelialization. Thereafter, other topical agents or dressings are used on the wound.

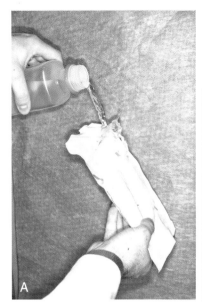

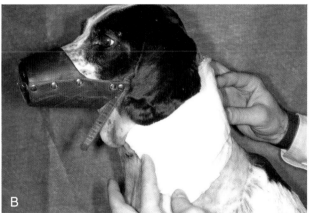

FIG. 5-2 (A) Applying saline to a package of sterile gauze pads prior to dressing an open wound. An antimicrobial agent can be added to the solution to treat a bacterial infection (see Chapter 4). (B) Application to a cervical bite wound.

Judicious surgical debridement, combined with wet-to-dry dressings, is one of the faster methods of preparing wounds for eventual closure. There is no indication for their use on healthy wound beds.

Wet-to-dry dressings are often used for unreasonably long periods of time by many veterinarians. Short-term use, for no more than 3–5 days, is strongly recommended to avoid prolonged trauma to the emerging granulation tissue and epithelialization noted during the proliferative phase of wound healing.

The negative effects of wet-to-dry dressings have been seriously overstated both in the literature and by the manufacturers of wound dressings. The key to the effective use of wet-to-dry dressings is that application should be limited to the first few days of managing the problematic wound containing necrotic tissue. Prolonged use clearly is detrimental to the overall healing process.

exudative wound. The gauze absorbs the tissue fluids, and moisture is lost from evaporation from the bandage surface. Gauze sponges are removed (partially) dry. It is the author's opinion that wet-to-dry dressings are used only when mechanical debridement is required to remove adherent residual necrotic tissue. In the absence of necrotic tissue, adherent dressings serve no practical purpose in open wound care over other dressings discussed below. Moisture-retaining dressings can be used to facilitate autolytic debridement once most of the necrotic tissue has been removed surgically or mechanically. They should not be applied in the presence of moderate amounts of devitalized tissue.

Dry-to-dry dressings are not commonly used in open wound management. Technically a dry-to-dry dressing would describe simple gauze application to a closed wound. In practice, dry-to-dry describes the application of dry sponges to a low-viscosity, highly

Warm sterile saline or lactated Ringer's solution can be used to reduce gauze adherence to the wound. Keep in mind, however, that adherence is necessary to optimize mechanical debridement. Oversoaking should be avoided.

Alternatively, 2% lidocaine can applied topically to the gauze. Lidocaine also can be diluted with sodium bicarbonate (9:1 mixture ratio) to reduce the stinging sensation occasionally noted with the subcutaneous injection of 2% lidocaine as a local block.

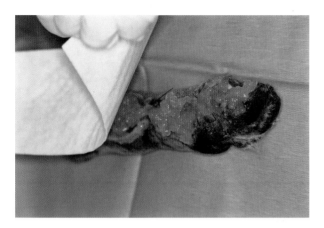

FIG. 5-3 Application of nonadherent Telfa pad over a wound. A collagen gel has been applied to the wound surface before its application. An outer bandage wrap is required to maintain the position of the dressing.

Nonadherent or Low Adherent Dressings

Nonadherent (or more properly, low adherent) dressings are most commonly applied over a healthy wound or skin graft to facilitate dressing removal with minimal disturbance to the underlying tissue. These dressings are usually comprised of a treated fabric mesh impregnated with paraffin or petrolatum. Examples include cotton leno-weave fabric impregnated with paraffin, such as tulle gras dressings, including Jelonet and Bactigras dressings (Smith & Nephew) and Sofra-Tulle (Hoechst Marion Roussell Ltd., Uxbridge, UK); knitted acetate fabric impregnated with a petrolatum emulsion (Adaptic, Johnson & Johnson); and a fine mesh gauze impregnated with petrolatum and 3% bismuth tribromophenate (Xeroform, Kendall Co.). Telfa (Kendall Co.) consists of a thin layer of absorbent cotton fibers enclosed in polyethylene terephthalate. This perforated plastic film has reduced adherence to the wound surface while allowing the passage of exudates into the cotton backing of the dressing (Fig. 5-3). The author finds Telfa nonadherent strips and Adaptic nonadherent dressings the most flexible and useful of the nonadherent dressings.

Nonadherent dressings are commonly used in conjunction with topical wound healing ointments, creams, and gels to help maintain their contact with the wound surface (see Chapter 4). This combined effect can create a partial- or semiocclusive dressing that helps provide moisture retention while protecting the area from desiccation. The porous or perforated surface of the nonadherent dressing allows for the passage of tissue fluids and exudates into the overly-ing secondary (absorptive) layer of a protective bandage. Over time, as the topical medication and discharge pass into the overlying absorptive layer, its occlusive properties diminish.

> Despite their name, nonadherent dressings do occasionally adhere to portions of the wound surface. Fibrin and dried exudate can "glue" the dressing matrix to the wound surface. Granulation tissue can imbed into the open channels, forming "keys" that make removal difficult without causing a small amount of bleeding. Warm saline can be applied to soften the fibrin and dried discharge to facilitate their removal. More frequent dressing changes can reduce this complication. Dressings such as Telfa have smaller pores than Adaptic and may reduce granulation tissue embedment. However, the large openings in Adaptic provide superior drainage. The clinician must judge which dressing is most useful for a particular wound.

Other dressings, including occlusive dressings, may have nonadherent or low adherent properties, but they are more appropriately discussed separately.

Absorptive Dressings

In the first week of wound management, wounds tend to be more transudative or exudative as a result of inflammation, infection, venous congestion, and local lymphatic compromise. The volume of fluid released can be retained and controlled by the use of an absorptive dressing and/or the overlying secondary (absorptive) layer of a bandage.

Both wet-to-dry and dry-to-dry cotton dressings are highly absorptive; as noted, wet-to-dry dressings can hydrate and dilute thick exudates and facilitate their absorption into the gauze matrix. In the presence of necrotic tissue, they provide mechanical debridement. However, there are other dressings that may be used to withdraw and retain discharge from the wound and are better suited to promote the natural process of (selective) autolytic debridement of residual devitalized tissue.

POLYURETHANE FOAM

Polyurethane foam is highly absorbent and able to retain several times its weight in fluid. It can be very useful in managing wounds releasing large volumes of tissue fluid. Foam can be used in conjunction with an overlying absorptive layer of bandage material.

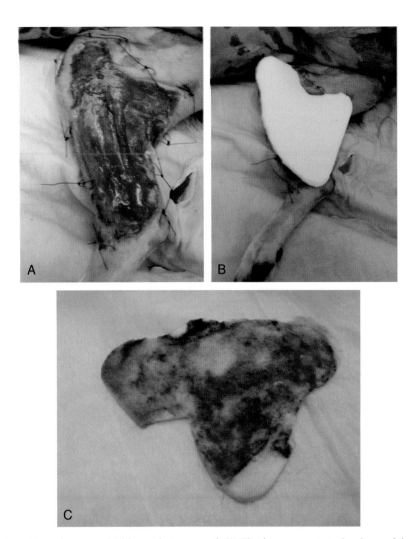

FIG. 5-4 (A) Use of polyurethane foam on a highly exudative wound. (B) The foam was cut to the shape of the wound and secured with a tie-over dressing. (C) Dressing change 24 hours later: note the high absorptive capacity of this dressing.

Because of its fine porous surface, it is basically non-adherent. Foams are less effective in debridement compared to alginate and hydrocolloid dressings (e.g., promoting autolytic debridement). Polyurethane foam can be moistened and applied to hydrate dry wounds. Because of their partial retention of moisture, they can be considered *semiocclusive* in nature. Hydrosorb (Tyco/Kendall Co.) has a smooth, soft, nonirritating surface. It can be useful in protecting the skin over flexion surfaces from the abrasive effects of bandage material during ambulation. Because of their elastic nature, they do not readily contour to irregular surface wounds without the application of an outer wrap to maintain their position. They can be used to cover a healthy granulation bed, although other products may be more useful for this purpose. Based on the physical properties of the material, polyurethane is a nonadher-

ent dressing, absorptive dressing, semiocclusive dressing, and moisture-retentive dressing, depending on the wound environment (Fig. 5-4). Examples of this product include Hydrosorb, Flexipore (Advanced Medical Solutions, Cheshire UK), Allevyn (Smith & Nephew), and Sof-Foam (Johnson & Johnson).

Polyurethane foam is most useful for highly exudative wounds. In low exudative wounds, it also may be premoistened before application.

Frequency of dressing changes will depend on the volume of discharge absorbed by the dressing. As a healthy granulation bed forms, the frequency of dressing changes normally declines.

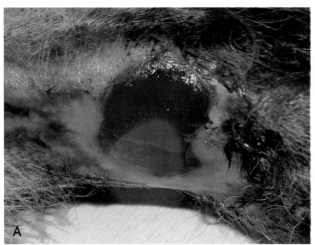 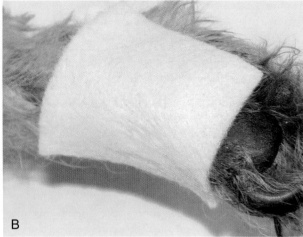

FIG. 5-5 (A) Feline paw wound managed with an alginate dressing. Note the excellent granulation bed and peripheral epithelialization. (B) A single alginate pad can be divided into smaller pads as second intention healing progresses.

ALGINATE DRESSINGS

Alginate dressings are comprised of alginic acid derived from algae (Phaeophyceae) found in various varieties of seaweed. Alginic acid consists of a polymer containing mannuronic and guluronic residues. Alginates rich in mannuronic acid form soft flexible gels, whereas those rich in guluronic acid form firmer gels. Zinc, sodium, and calcium salts are added to the alginic acid polymer. Silver ions also have been added to alginate dressings to enhance their antibacterial property (see Antimicrobial Dressings, below). Alginate-maltodextrin dressings have been introduced to the wound-healing market (Caligtrol DX, Magnus Biomedical, Pasadena, CA).

Retained alginate is broken down by the cells into sugars without eliciting a foreign body reaction. Alginate dressings (especially containing zinc) have a topical hemostatic effect by activating prothrombin. Alginate dressings are commonly used in flat sheets, although a rope form is available for packing deeper wounds. Alternatively, the flattened sheet can be rolled and inserted into narrow cavities.

> Because of their highly absorptive nature (20–30 times their weight), they are very useful for moderately exudative wounds.
> If applied to low exudative wounds, they can be premoistened before application.

It is common to cover alginate dressings with an outer absorptive bandage to maintain the position of the dressing and assist in the absorption of excessive discharge from a wound surface. Alginates and collagen commonly are added to various moisture-retentive dressings. Upon absorption of moisture, the dressings tend to soften into a gel-like compound that has the capacity to trap and store bacteria to a variable degree. With loss of moisture, alginate dressings can dry, forming a sticky plaque that requires traction with forceps during removal. Saline can be used to facilitate separation. Because of their absorptive properties, they can dehydrate the surface of low exudative wounds. The author has also used lightly moistened alginate dressings to cover healthy granulation beds. Contrary to one report, the author has seen no adverse effects to the skin peripheral to a wound if an alginate dressing overlaps the area. The flat dressings however can be trimmed to better conform to the surface of a wound. Dressings normally are changed every 3–4 days. In heavily exudating wounds, changes one or twice a day are advisable. It is the author's opinion that alginate dressings are best used in wounds after early formation of a granulation bed (Fig. 5-5.). Examples include Curasorb ZN (Tyco/Kendall Co.), Nu-Derm (Johnson & Johnson), Sorbsan (PharmaPlast Ltd., Alexandria, Eygpt), and Tegaderm alginate (3M). Alginate dressings that include an absorbent backing also are available for heavy exudative wounds (Sorbsan Plus; Pharmplast Ltd.). Alternatively, an absorbent layer of gauze or absorbent pads can be applied over the alginate dressing to help retain the anticipated wound drainage. Apinate dressings, made by Comvita

Medical (distributed by Derma Sciences) is a combination of a calcium alginate dressing and manuka honey. (See Chapter 4 regarding manuka honey).

HYPERTONIC SALINE DRESSINGS

Hypertonic saline dressings are cotton gauze sponges saturated with 20% sodium chloride. The hypertonic saline has an absorptive osmotic effect on the wound and can be useful in reducing edema secondary to trauma. In drawing water from the wound, it can facilitate the hydration of devitalized tissue and its subsequent mechanical debridement during bandage changes. The hypertonic saline also blunts the ability of bacteria to proliferate. Unfortunately, these dressings also have the potential to dehydrate viable tissue in the wound. As moisture is drawn into the dressing, the salt concentration will progressively decline, necessitating periodic bandage changes every 3 days or less, depending on the volume of fluid. Curasalt (Kendall Co.) is marketed to veterinarians. (In essence, hypertonic saline–impregnated gauze dressings are a variation of the wet-to-dry dressing previously discussed.)

Moisture-Retentive Dressings and Occlusive Dressings

Providing a protected, moist wound environment can optimize the processes of wound healing. The moisture-retentive dressings are soothing to sensitive wound surfaces and reduce patient discomfort. These properties also may be accomplished with topical medications (see Chapter 4) or by using specialized moisture-retentive dressings.

There is a broad range of dressings that fall into the category of "moist dressings." As noted, some absorptive dressings also may have variable moisture-retentive properties.

> Hydrocolloid and hydrogel dressings have a moisture-retaining matrix applied to an outer synthetic membrane. In effect, they are similar to comparable topical agents designed to provide a moist environment for optimal healing. This group of dressings may be easier to apply and change compared to the reapplication of a comparable topical gel for shallow wounds. Topical gels may be more useful for more cavitated defects with a dressing and bandage applied to help maintain their prolonged contact with the wound surface.

Many moisture-retaining dressings are occlusive or semiocclusive by nature. The outer synthetic membranes of occlusive dressings prevent or minimize penetration of contaminants. Low oxygen tension beneath an occlusive dressing stimulates macrophage activity, fibroblast proliferation, and neovascularization. The rate of epithelialization is reportedly twice as fast as for wounds left exposed to the air. Partially occlusive dressings may be gas permeable or moisture vapor permeable—allowing moisture beneath the dressing to escape from the membrane. Because they retain and hydrate tissues, these dressings facilitate natural autolytic debridement of residual necrotic tissue adhered to the underlying viable wound surface. Hair should be clipped from around the wound liberally to improve their adherence to the adjacent skin to facilitate wound care.

Dressings with a low moisture vapor transmission have a higher retention of water and are better able to maintain a moist wound environment. Moisture is typically lost through normal skin, and this can be quantified as transepidermal water loss. Intact human skin has a transepidermal water loss of $4–9 g/m^2/h$, whereas water loss increases dramatically in partial and full-thickness skin wounds ($80–90 g/m^2/h$). Dressings that have a low moisture vapor transmission value less than $35 g/m^2/h$ are considered moisture retentive. Dressings that retain the tissue fluids also help contain both the cellular and extracellular components (cytokines, etc.) of wound healing (see Chapter 3) that naturally support the healing process.

> ### Moisture Transmission Values of Common Dressings in g/m²/h
> Normal skin: 4.0–9.0
>
> Hydrocolloid dressing: <12.5
>
> Polyurethane film: 12.5–33
>
> Polyurethane foam: 33.4–208
>
> Cotton gauze: 67

WET-TO-WET DRESSINGS

Wet-to-wet dressings are particularly useful to hydrate dry or mummified necrotic tissue, thereby facilitating its removal. This normally can be accomplished in 24 hours. A wet-to-wet dressing includes the application of moistened gauze sponges secured to the wound with an outer wrap or "tie-over" dressing (see below). Sponges are periodically moistened with Ringer's lactate or saline during this time. An antimicrobial solution (chlorhexidene or povidone-iodine) may be used, or antimicrobial polyhexamethylene biguanide–impregnated gauze sponges can be substituted for standard cotton sponges (Kendall Co.; see Antimicro-

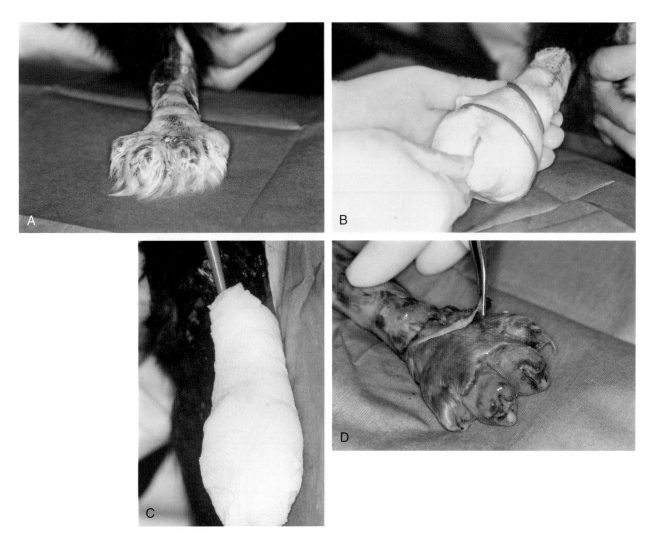

FIG. 5-6 (A) Extensive skin loss involving the hind paw of a cat. A wet-to-wet dressing was applied to hydrate the mummified necrotic skin overlying the metatarsal area.

(B) Saline-moistened cotton gauze sponges were wrapped over the entire paw, followed by the spiral application of a fenestrated rubber catheter. An additional layer of sponges was wrapped over the tubing, followed by a layer of self-adherent roll gauze and autoclaved Vetrap.

(C) Approximately 10 ml of saline was injected into the funnel-tipped catheter end exiting the bandage. This was repeated every 6 hours.

(D) After 24 hours, the patient was sedated and the bandaged removed. The hydrated necrotic tissue easily peeled off the paw with forceps. The foot was closed with a mesh graft a few days later.

bial Dressings, below). The author prefers to insert sterile fenestrated tubing between gauze layers to facilitate injecting additional fluid into the bandage every 6 hours in order to maintain a high moisture level (Fig. 5-6 and 5-7). Alternatively, fluid can be injected or trickled into the bandage with a syringe.

When the wet-to-wet dressing is removed, the necrotic skin and underlying tissues are invariably softened from the absorption of water, facilitating their surgical removal. Heavy sedation or general anesthesia facilitates the bulk removal of devitalized tissue. If residual necrotic tissue remains, wet-to-dry dressings,

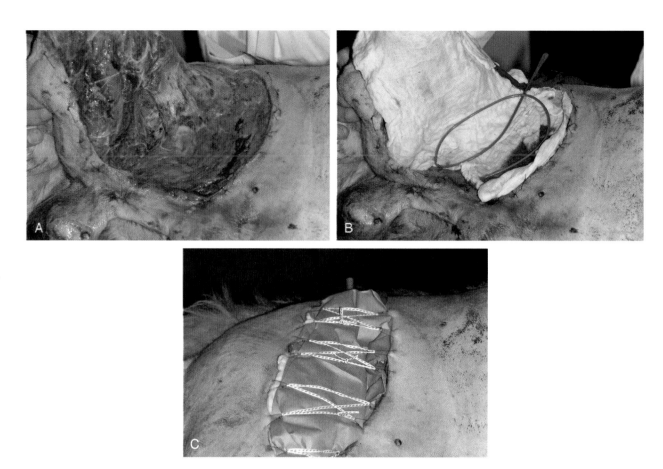

FIG. 5-7 (A) Large right flank and thigh wound extending to the knee due to secondary vehicular trauma.

(B) After initial surgical debridement, a wet-to-wet dressing was used to facilitate subsequent removal of residual necrotic tissue. Saline-moistened laparotomy pads were applied to the wound, followed by a fenestrated red rubber tube. A second moistened pad was applied over the coiled tubing.

(C) The wet-to-wet dressing was secured to the area with a tie-over. A caudal superficial epigastric flap was later used to close this large skin defect.

hydrating topical agents (see Chapter 4), or a moisture-retaining dressing (below) can be used to facilitate its removal.

HYDROGEL DRESSINGS

Hydrogel dressings are primarily comprised of water (70%–95%) that is retained in a fiber network of humectants, and various superabsorbent hydrophilic polymers (carboxy-methyl-cellulose, polyethylene oxide, starch-grafted copolymer, polyvinyl alcohol copolymers, etc.) that absorb aqueous solutions by hydrogen bonding with water. However, SentrX Animal Care (see below) makes a product line of gel dressings containing cross-linked hyaluronic acid-based films (hyaluronan hydrogel). In general, hydrogel dressings essentially are sheets of cross-linked polymer gels. (*Note:* superabsorbent polymers are also used in many personal hygiene products, including baby diapers.) Many of these dressings are semitransparent, which facilitates initial wound inspection (Fig. 5-8 and 5-9). Some hydrogel dressings contain other products: Nu-Gel (Johnson & Johnson) and Purilon (Coloplast Corp.), for example, also contain alginate in their hydrogel matrix. Nu-Gel also comes in a dressing containing collagen in order to enhance the otherwise modest absorptive capacity of the dressing. Antimicrobial agents, such as silver, metronidazole, and silver sulfadiazine, have been added to hydrogel dressings to prevent or manage low-grade infections (see Antimicrobial Dressings, below). Most hydrogel dressings require an outer bandage or wrap to secure them to the wound surface. Hydrogels are relatively easy to apply to flat wound surfaces. Overlapping the adjacent skin margins of a wound should be minimized, since the skin may contribute to maceration.

> Unstable dressings can be secured to a wound surface with surgical staples or sutures. This is particularly useful in assuring the dressing will not slip off the wound surface when infrequent dressing changes are necessary.

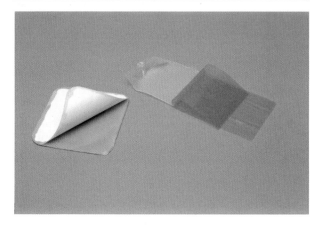

FIG. 5-8 Examples of a hydrocolloid (left) and hydrogel dressing (right). A protective cover is peeled off the dressing, exposing the sticky contact surface of the dressing for placement over an open wound.

Hydrogel dressings form a protective gel covering with a somewhat limited capacity to absorb exudates. They can be considered an "interactive dressing." Their ability to hydrate a wound facilitates autolytic debridement of residual necrotic tissue. They support healing by second intention and reduce patient discomfort. In one experimental study (Ramsey et al. 1995), they appeared to promote wound contraction on extremity wounds, but less so for trunk wounds in dogs. They are best employed for wounds free of infection and excessive necrotic tissue. Dressings are normally changed every 3 or 4 days for most noninfected wounds. Saline or a wound-cleansing agent (see Chapter 4) can be used to prepare the wound for the replacement dressing. Because of their occlusive properties, their use in infected wounds is not advisable. In one study, wounds covered with hydrogel dressings displayed greater wound contraction compared to hydrocolloid and polyethylene dressings. A few examples of hydrogel dressings include Biodress (DVM Pharmaceuticals, Miami, FL), Vigilon (Bard Medical Division, Covington, GA), Tielle (Johnson & Johnson), Aquasorb (DeRoyal Industries), Curagel (Tyco/Kendall Co.), Curity Conforma Gel (Kendall Canada), and Nu-Gel Dressings (Johnson & Johnson).

SentrX Corporation (Salt Lake City, UT) has a product line of disulfide cross-linked hyaluronan (hyaluronic acid-based films) hydrogel dressings for use in small animals (canitrX, felitrX) and horses (equitrX). Control studies between the various hydrogel products are lacking.

FIG. 5-9 (A) Mesh graft application to a problematic inner thigh defect. (B) In this case a hydrogel dressing was stapled over the grafted area to maintain hydration of the area and promote epithelialization. The hydrogel was successfully used, but was not considered any better than the customary use of a nonadherent dressing (Adaptic) combined with triple antibiotic ointment.

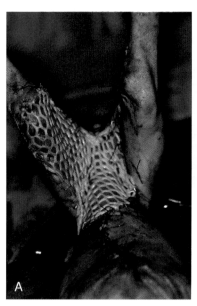
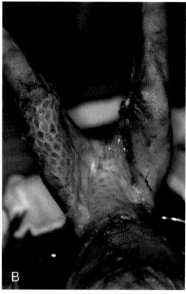

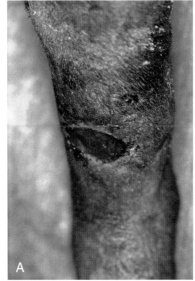 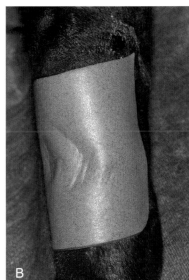

FIG. 5-10 (A) Application of a hydrocolloid dressing (Duoderm, ConvaTec) to a lower extremity wound. (B) The dressing overlaps the skin and adheres fairly well to the area. Tape strips or a light wrap can be used to assure the dressing does not shift. The rigidity of this type of dressing may impede wound contraction.

HYDROCOLLOID DRESSINGS

Hydrocolloid dressings contain a variety of constituents, including sodium carboxymethylcellulose, gelatin, pectin, and polyisobutylene. Gelatin, pectin, elastomers, alginates, silver, and other materials can be added to these substrates. The tacky matrix is affixed to a polyurethane film or foam backing for easy application to flat wound beds. The outer cover forms a protective barrier against external moisture and contaminants (Fig. 5-8 and 5-10). Hydrocolloid dressings tend to be stiffer than most hydrogel dressings: they will soften to some degree when warmed by simply compressing the dressing between the hands for a couple minutes before application. Hydrofiber pads or ribbons can be formed from sodium carboxymethylcellulose fibers.

Hydrocolloid dressings have some capacity to absorb exudates from the wound surface, forming a gel over time. For this reason, they are also considered to be an interactive dressing. Hydrocolloid dressings may vary in their performance as it pertains to their individual absorbency, fluid-handling characteristics, and physical properties. The moist environment facilitates autolytic debridement. However, they are best used for wounds with minimal necrotic tissue; they should be avoided in the presence of wound infection. Hydrocolloid dressings are normally applied to a wound by slightly overlapping the skin that makes up the perimeter of the wound. Excessive overlapping may overhydrate the adjacent skin. Most dressings are changed every 3–4 days. Saline or wound-cleansing agents (see Chapter 4) may be used to remove the somewhat tenacious gel-exudative debris that forms on the wound surface during their use. Hydrocolloid dressings may adhere to the wound without a secondary wrap. When used on the lower extremity, tape strips can be used for added security. The relative stiffness of these dressings may "splint" the wound, thereby impeding myofibroblastic contraction of the skin bordering the wound (Fig. 5-11). A few examples of hydrocolloid dressings include Duoderm or Granuflex (Convatec), Restore Hydrocolloid Dressing (Hollister Inc.), Nu-Derm (Johnson & Johnson), Tegaderm Hydrocolloid Dressing (3M Health), Replicare Hydrocolloid Dressing (Smith & Nephew), and Invacare Hydrocolloid Dressing (Invacare Corp., Cleveland, OH).

In early wound care, considerable effusion may be noted, and overwhelm the fluid retaining capacity of hydrogel and hydrocolloid dressings. More absorptive dressings would be advisable until capillary stability and fluid reduction is noted. This is usually associated with the development of a healthy granulation bed. This general rule of thumb also would be applicable to highly exudative wounds. As a result, the use of these dressings may be more suitable for granulation beds free of excess necrotic tissue and contaminants.

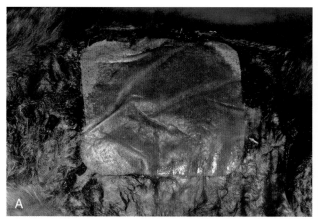 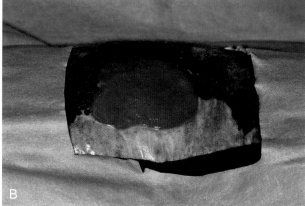

FIG. 5-11 (A) Application of a hydrocolloid dressing (Duoderm) to a problematic skin defect in a cat. Note the hydrocolloid discharge onto the lower adjacent skin surface.

(B) The wound remained unchanged after 4 weeks. A transposition flap was later used to successfully close this defect. This example underscores the fact that many wounds will remain challenging despite the development of multiple wound dressings and topical agents designed to promote healing.

VAPOR-PERMEABLE FILMS

Vapor-permeable films generally allow for the passage of water vapor and oxygen. However, vapor permeability, adhesiveness, and conformability vary with a given product. The term *film dressings* refers to thin, transparent polyurethane membranes coated with a layer of adhesive to secure it to the bordering skin surface. The film can be used as a protective membrane over minimal exuding wounds or as a protective barrier (e.g., closed incisions).

Polyurethane is the most commonly used transparent plastic film barrier to protect wounds. Polyurethane is permeable to gas, but protects the wound from external contaminants (water, bacteria). Polyurethane films are considered semiocclusive, allowing water vapor to escape from their surface. They have no absorptive capacity, and moisture can accumulate beneath polyurethane, potentially promoting the proliferation of skin organisms.

The film may be applied to superficial wounds with minimal exudates and it has an adhesive to secure the dressing to the skin surrounding the wound borders (minimum 1 inch overlap). Removal of fur, followed by cleansing and drying the skin, will facilitate its adherence. In general, film does not adhere and conform well to mobile body regions and skin folds. The use of film alone should be avoided in the presence of infection, necrotic tissue, or highly exudative wounds. Some polyurethane films contain a light gauze dressing and can be used as protective barriers over a sutured incision (Tegaderm from 3M; OpSite Post-OP from Smith & Nephew). Polyurethane dressings also are used as protective containment barriers to secure other dressings (e.g., alginates, gauze, etc.) and topical medications. Tegaderm and Opsite are two examples of polyurethane dressings (Fig. 5-12). These film dressings are frequently used to protect a skin incision from moisture and topical contaminants postoperatively, rather than as a dressing for open wounds.

Plastic drapes primarily used in orthopedic procedures can be adapted to maintaining dressings and bandages in problematic body areas. Ioban (3M), Vi-Drape (Medical Concepts Development, Woodbury, MN), and Opsite Incise Drapes (Smith & Nephew) are examples of plastic drapes used in surgery. Surgical drape adhesives can be used sparingly to enhance the adherence of these plastic films to the skin (Vi-Drape). They may be useful for securing dressings and bandages to the lateral surfaces of small animals. Subsequent dressing changes may be facilitated simply by splitting the plastic drape to gain access to the wound. The drape opening is retaped after changing the dressing.

Miscellaneous Dressings

ANTIMICROBIAL DRESSINGS

It has long been recognized that silver ions possess broad-spectrum antimicrobial properties, including efficacy against *Pseudomonas aeruginosa* methicillin-resistant *Staphylococcus aureus* and vancomycin-resistant *Enterococcus*, and *Candida sp.* Silver ions also may mitigate inflammation by inhibiting matrix metalloproteinase activity.

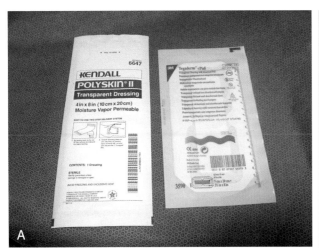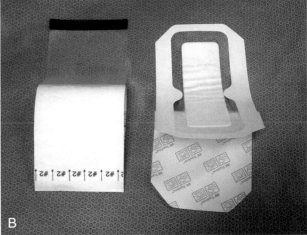

FIG. 5-12 (A, B) Tegaderm + Pad (3-M) and PolyskinII (Kendall Co.) dressings. The coated paper backing is peeled off the adhesive surface and applied over the surgical site. Note the Tegaderm (B) has a thin gauze pad embedded into the center of this plastic dressing. These dressings are useful for protecting surgical incisions from moisture and topical contaminants postoperatively.

Silver-impregnated dressings are available in a variety of forms. Examples include the following antimicrobial alginate dressings: Silvercel (Johnson & Johnson), Algicell (Derma Sciences Inc.), Calgitrol (Magnus Biomedical), Seasorb-Ag (Coloplast Corp.), Sorbsan Silver (Unomedical Ltd., Reddich, UK), Silverlon CA (Argentum Medical LLC, Geneva, IL), and Maxorb Extra Ag (Medline Industries Ltd., Mundelein, IL); 90% collagen-10% alginate wound dressing (Fibracol, Johnson & Johnson) collagen-oxidized regenerated cellulose dressing containing 1% silver (Prisma, Johnson & Johnson); Actisorb silver antimicrobial binding dressing using an activated charcoal woven fabric containing 0.15% silver by weight (Johnson & Johnson); hydrogel dressing containing silver (Silvasorb, Medline Industries Ltd.); nylon impregnated dressings (Silverlon Negative Pressure Dressing, Argentum Medical LLC); and foam products Algidex AG (DeRoyal Industries), Polymem Silver (Ferris Manufacturing Co., Burr Ridge, IL); and a highly absorbent sodium carboxymethylcellulose hydrofiber dressing, Aquacel (Convatec).

As noted previously, gauze impregnated with the antimicrobial agent polyhexamethylene biguanide (PHMB), can be used to manage or help prevent infection. PHMB is a cationic surface-active agent (related to chlorhexidine) that irreversibly destabilizes cytoplasmic membranes of bacteria. Chlorhexidine acetate has been formulated into topical dressings to protect minor wounds from infection (Bactigras, Smith &

Nephew). Polytracin dressings (polymyxin B, bacitracin zinc, neomycin sulfate) are also available from Galaxy Medicare Ltd. (Orissa, India).

Cadexomer iodine also has been used in wound dressings (Iodosorb Sheet Dressing, Smith & Nephew) and as an ointment or powder (Iodosorb Ointment/Iodosorb Powder, Smith & Nephew). Cadexomer iodine is a biodegradable mixture of cadexomer polysaccharide beads as a carrier for 0.9% iodine. Cadexomer iodine–based products slowly release iodine, unlike povidone-iodine dressings, which deposit their iodine immediately on application to the wound. They have a high rate of fluid absorption for exudative wounds. Dressings with cadexomer iodine should be used cautiously over large surface areas due to the risk of iodine toxicity.

BIOACTIVE DRESSINGS

Dressings composed of materials that originate from living tissue are called *bioactive dressings*. The following are examples of this family of dressings. They may have properties similar to other dressings discussed. Occasionally, companies will combine bioactive products with hydrocolloid or hydrogel dressings and topical agents.

Collagen (Extracellular Matrix Bioscaffold) Dressings.
Bovine collagen can be used as a topical agent: it may

be applied as a powder, gel, pad, or packet form for a variety of applications (see Chapter 4). However, collagen can be applied as a biological dressing that may serve as a scaffold to facilitate wound healing. The organized collagen fibrils serve as a substrate or filamentous network for fibroblast, endothelial, and epithelial cell migration. Research into skin substitutes has focused on the use of artificial dermal scaffolds that better mimic the natural properties of the dermis, in contrast to organized scar tissue secondary to granulation tissue maturation. These products are reported to promote angiogenesis and the chemotactic recruitment of white cells and fibroblasts (see Chapter 2). Prisma (Johnson & Johnson) for example is a *composite* dressing with 55% collagen, 44% oxidized regenerated cellulose, and 1% silver. Prisma is used in the management of chronic ulcers and other open wounds. Biobrane (Smith & Nephew) is a biosynthetic wound dressing constructed of a silicone film and a nylon complex three-dimensional trifilament network to which collagen is chemically bound. Blood and sera will clot in this matrix, firmly adhering the dressing to the wound surface: the moist environment created promotes epithelialization.

Porcine small intestinal submucosa (SIS) has been integrated into an extracellular wound matrix dressing (e.g., Oasis—Healthpoint CO., Cook Biotech Inc., West Lafayette, IN; CollaMend—Bard Medical Division, Genitrix Ltd.; Vet BioSISt, Smith's Medical PM, Waukesha, WI) that provides a three-dimensional collagen scaffold to help "direct" collagen deposition and facilitate the in-growth of cells and capillaries into this matrix for partial or full-thickness wounds. (SIS comprises type I, III, IV, V, VI, and VIII collagen; fibronectin; hyaluronic acid; chondroitin sulfate; and heparin.) It has been used to assist in the repair of hernia and chest wall defects in humans. Acellular urinary bladder matrix or submucosa (UBM or UBS) also has been used as an inductive scaffold for tissue replacement. Acell Vet (Acell Inc., Columbia, MD) has been advocated for a variety of soft tissue and orthopedic procedures. Both SIS and UMB/UBS reportedly also contain growth factors to promote wound healing.

These bioscaffold dressings can be integrated into the healing process; as healing progresses, an additional layer of these materials can be placed over the original dressing without its removal. Loose dressings or hydrolyzed fragments can be removed prior to replacement with a fresh dressing at the time of bandage change.

A study using porcine-derived SIS on exposed bone in dogs failed to demonstrate its effectiveness in promoting wound contraction and epithelialization. A study in horses also failed to demonstrate efficacy.

Equine amnion dressings have been used experimentally as occlusive dressings. They were noted to be effective in promoting contraction and epithelialization in experimental dogs.

> With the presence of other economical dressing alternatives, the routine clinical use of these products is unclear.

Chitosan Dressings.   As previously noted (Chapter 4, Topical Agents), Chitosan is derived from chitin, a natural polysaccharide biopolymer originating from crustacean shells. Partial deacetylation of chitin gives rise to a linear polysaccharide with interspersed D-glucosamine and acetyl-D-glucosamine units. Chitosan has antimicrobial properties and is biodegradable. It may improve the strength of newly formed collagen in granulating wounds and enhance the function of inflammatory cells, cytokines, and fibroblasts. It has been used in a variety of biomedical, nutritional, and cosmetic products. Chito-Seal Topical Hemostasis Pads (Abbott Laboratories, Abbott Park, IL) has been designed to manage actively bleeding wounds: positively charged chitosan molecules attract negatively charged red blood cells and platelets. The HemCon Dressing (HemCon Medical Technologies Inc.) is a commercially available chitosan dressing in the United States.

SPRAY-ON AND LIQUID DRESSINGS

Spray-on and topical dressings are available for providing a protective film on minor abrasive wounds, small nicks or cuts, and sutured incisions. OpSite Spray (Smith & Nephew) is a fast-drying transparent film that is permeable to vapor and air. A variety of over-the-counter liquid bandages are available (Band-Aid, New-Skin, Newphase, Skin Shield, 3M Pet Care, Scientific Angler Spray On, 3-M Nexcare, Invacare, Johnson & Johnson Liquid Bandage) that reportedly form a breathable and flexible seal. Most liquid bandages are cyanoacrylate formulations that polymerize, usually with an activator. They may be useful in protecting incisions or minor nicks and scrapes in areas where contact contamination would be a concern. Alternatively, surgical cyanoacrylate glues can be used over skin sutures or staples to provide an incisional seal.

SILICONE DRESSINGS

Silicone dressings are used primarily to reduce the formation of hypertrophic and keloid scarring in humans. Silicone dressings have been used to reduce exuberant granulation tissue formation in horses. Silicone may promote hydration of scar tissue. It is postulated that the silicone dressing occludes microvessels, gradually decreasing oxygen tension in the tissues, reaching a point of anoxia in which fibroblasts cannot function and undergo apoptosis. There is no information regarding the clinical use of silicone dressings in small animals.

CELLULOSE DRESSINGS

Hydrogel and hydrocolloid dressings may contain carboxymethylcellulose. A woven microfiber cellulose dressing has also been developed with both absorbent and hydrating properties (XCell, Xylos Corp., Langhorne, PA). As a result, it can be used to promote autolytic debridement and absorb discharge from the wound surface. The fine microfiber reduces wound adherence.

Cost Factors

Is special wound preparation required?

Is it easy to apply?

Is it easy to remove?

How frequently must it be changed?

Is a supportive bandage required to maintain dressing?

What is the length of use in relation to the changing wound environment?

Is it readily available?

Is it the best product for the task?

Is this a problematic wound that requires a more innovative approach to facilitate closure?

Is surgical excision/closure of a problematic wound a better alternative at a given stage of open wound management?

Some Practical Considerations

Is a small amount of necrotic tissue present?

- Consider moisture retentive dressings and topical products, including hydrogels, hydrogel dressings, and hydrocolloid dressings

- Use wet-to-dry dressings on a limited basis to facilitate removal of necrotic tissue.

Is infection present?

- Consider dressings and topical agents with antimicrobial properties.

- Early removal of necrotic tissue dramatically reduces bacterial numbers.

Are these moderately exudative and effusive wounds?

- Consider dressings and topical products that facilitate absorption and retention, including alginates and polyurethane foams.

- Is there a healthy granulation bed?

- Consider moisture-retentive dressings and topical products, including semiocclusive and occlusive dressings.

Are these low-moisture or dry wounds?

- Consider moisture retentive dressings.

Note: As wounds respond in a positive fashion to appropriate therapies, dressings can be changed to support the current status of a given wound.

The Secondary Layer

The secondary layer of a bandage is the bulk or absorptive layer. Roll cotton, cast padding, absorptive combination pads, gauze pads, and roll gauze usually comprise this layer of the bandage. The bulk or thickness of this layer will depend on the function of the bandage.

Factors Influencing the Thickness of the Secondary Bandage Layer
- Must it secure the primary dressing layer?
- To what extent does it need to protect or shelter traumatized tissues?
- How great is the volume of wound discharge?
- Is there dead space to be controlled?
- Is it intended to immobilize a given body region?
- Is it necessary to control local bleeding?
- Are there drains or exposed surgical devices that need protection from contamination or patient tampering?

In a wound with a copious discharge, the secondary layer can facilitate the wicking and retention of tissue fluids from the wound surface. Moisture retention in this intermediate layer depends on the volume released from the wound surface, the absorptive or retentive properties of the dressing, and the rate of moisture lost by evaporation through the outer tertiary wrap. For this reason, larger wounds in the early stages of healing (first week) generally require more frequent bandage changes.

Practice Tip

When a large bandage is used to immobilize an area while also managing a wound, the area overlying the wound can be cut out, creating an access window to the wound. The soiled bandage area can be removed and redressed without necessarily removing the entire supportive bandage. The access window is more easily created at the time of bandage application. See Chapter 12, Plate 41 as an example of this technique.

As a healthy granulation bed forms during the second week after injury, the volume of discharge decreases as the capillary bed matures, and the surface area of the wound begins to decrease by wound contraction and epithelialization. Unless a thicker bandage is required for immobilization, the volume of the sec-

ondary bandage layer can be reduced as the amount of discharge progressively declines. As the discharge decreases, moisture retaining or absorptive dressings are better able to contain the fluid for a greater period of time with less spill-over into the secondary bandage layer. Both dressing and bandage changes may be reduced to every 2–4 days in many cases, depending on the products used.

Frequency of Bandage/Dressing Changes in Open Wound Care
- During the first week of open wound management, bandage changes are normally required on a daily basis (one to three times per day depending on the condition of the wound and dressing required).
- During the second week, granulation tissue has formed, and the volume of discharge normally declines. Bandage changes may be extended to every second day in many cases, depending on the severity of the wound and the types of dressings used.
- By the third week, wound contraction and epithelialization usually assume prominent roles in wound closure. As they occur the surface area of the open wound progressively declines. In many cases, the bandage/dressing change interval may be extended to every third or fourth day.
- As noted, a variety of dressings and topical products are available for use as a healthy granulation bed is forming (see Chapter 4). The frequency of bandage changes also is dependent on how often a given wound product requires reapplication based on the manufacturer's suggestions.
- When using moisture-retaining dressings on healthy granulation beds, changes normally are scheduled every 3–5 days. This is a relatively safe time to reassess an otherwise uncomplicated open wound.

Application of the Secondary Layer

As noted in Plate 2, cotton padding is overlapped by 50% to provide an orderly, more uniformly thick supportive layer. On the extremities, materials are applied from a distal to proximal direction. Tape stirrups and padding around pressure points are commonly applied prior to application of the secondary layer. (see Plate 3). Additional absorbent pads may be imbedded in the secondary layer or applied over the wound area before application of the roll cotton. Following one or two revolutions of cotton padding, self-adherent gauze helps stabilize the cotton layer before additional cotton/gauze layers are applied. The final outer cover of gauze provides a suitable substrate for application of the tertiary layer of the bandage. This layered application also provides more uniform compression, improving stability and reducing the risk of applying a bandage too tightly. Thicker secondary layers reduce the risk of circulatory compromise that otherwise may occur if the outer elastic cover is applied with moderate tension.

Baby Diapers?

For large exudative wounds involving the trunk (including the management of peritonitis with the open abdomen technique), diapers may be used as an economical outer absorbent and protective layer. A sterile primary and secondary bandage layer may be followed by integrating the diaper into the outer nonsterile secondary layer of the bandage.

The Tertiary Layer

The outer or tertiary layer serves as a binding or security layer for the contact and absorptive layers of the bandage. There is a wide variety of elastic products on the market, many of which come in an array of colors. Most tertiary wraps are self-adherent as a result of their texture and slightly tacky surface properties (Vetrap, 3M Animal Care Products) (Fig. 5-13). For pets that chew at their bandages, Petflex "No Chew" (Andover Healthcare, Salisbury, MA) is flexible, cohesive bandaging impregnated with a bitter chemical to discourage this behavior. Other products adhere to the contact layer of the secondary bandage layer (usually gauze) with a tenacious adhesive (for example, Elasticon from Johnson & Johnson) (Fig. 5-14). Standard (porous or nonporous) surgical tape (Zonas, Johnson & Johnson) also may be used as a tertiary wrap. Elastic wraps have the advantage of compressing the underlying secondary bandage layer and have better conformation to the contour of the body region. They also provide a pleasing "tailored" appearance to the completed bandage compared to surgical tape alone.

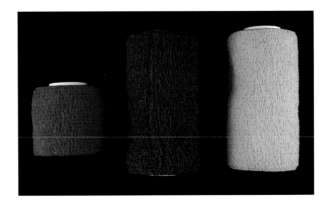

FIG. 5-13 Vetrap (3M). Vetrap adheres to itself but does not adhere to the skin. Vetrap can be autoclaved and used as a temporary sterile tourniquet for lower extremity surgeries.

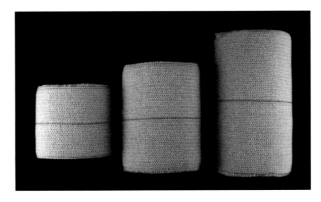

FIG. 5-14 Elasticon 2-inch, 3-inch, and 4-inch widths. Elasticon is a durable, elastic adhesive wrap that is effective for a variety of uses, including as a durable outer bandage wrap; for a variety of sling applications; and as a supplemental adhesive layer to prevent bandage slippage.

Caution

Elastic wraps provide a risk to the patient. Excessive use of elastic tension during application can compromise circulation, especially for bandages involving the extremities. This is more commonly seen in bandages with a relatively thin secondary bandage layer.

Most outer wraps are porous or breathable, allowing a variable amount of moisture to evaporate from the secondary bandage layer. Unfortunately, they also permit wicking to occur, thereby promoting contamination from absorption of fluid into the bandage unless precautionary measures are taken. Occlusive (nonporous) tapes may be advisable for areas in contact with moisture only if the veterinarian remembers that excessive use of this tape will also restrict evaporation from the secondary layer, necessitating more frequent bandage changes from moisture retention. The author generally limits the use of occlusive (nonporous) tape to that portion of a bandage susceptible to fluid contamination (e.g., lower foot): a breathable outer wrap is used for the remaining bandage area.

Elasticon (Johnson & Johnson) and similar materials can be expensive, but the materials are quite durable. They are most useful for bandages and slings that do not require frequent changes. Because of their sticky backing, they will adhere to the skin (see Fig. 5-14).

Vetrap (3M Animal Care Products) and similar products are thinner and more elastic than Elasticon. They do not adhere to the skin. They are more economical to use in those cases requiring more frequent bandage changes.

Standard surgical tape (1 or 2 inch) is economical, but lacks the physical advantages of Elasticon and Vetrap. It is useful for those cases that require frequent (daily) bandage changes.

Vetrap and Elasticon can be effectively used in combination. Vetrap can be used for the bulk of the tertiary wrap; strips of Elasticon can be used to secure the Vetrap to the adjacent skin to prevent bandage slippage.

PREVENTING BANDAGE DISPLACEMENT

Bandages can shift or slip as a result of a number of factors including the contour of the body region bandaged, the lack of a frictional body surface to resist slippage, the normal effects of gravity and body motion, subsequent stretching and loosening of the bandage layers, or forcible removal or partial destruction by the patient. (Cats, for example, are notorious for "flicking" bandages off their extremities using a short, rapid snapping motion of the involved limb.) Resolution of edema, and variable degrees of disuse muscle atrophy also contribute to bandage laxity and displacement over time. Periodic bandage inspection is required by the owner and veterinarian to assure bandages are properly maintained. However, there are techniques that can be used to reduce the likelihood of bandage slippage including *tape stirrups* for extremity bandages (see Plate 3); elastic adhesive tape (Elasticon) to join bandage borders to the adjacent skin (Fig. 5-15); adhesive tape "friction saddles" (trunk) and anchor bands (trunk, tail, limbs) (see Plate 4); spica bandage extensions (limbs) (see Plate 5); and figure 8 or "bandelero" adhesive straps for thoracic bandages. Long

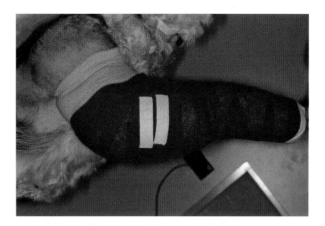

FIG. 5-15 Elasticon can be used to secure the Vetrap-encased bandage to the proximal skin. Elasticon has excellent adherent properties and is one of the most durable tertiary wraps available for bandages, splints, and slings.

fur may be clipped shorter, thereby improving adherence of sticky or adhesive tape materials.

The Double-edged Sword of Aggressive Tape Adhesive

Adhesive bandage materials (Elasticon, Johnson & Johnson, being one of the best) are very effective in securing bandage borders to the skin. Removal of the tape, especially in contact with bare skin, can be difficult and painful to the patient. Adhesive tape solvents (Mueller Tape Remover, etc.) can facilitate its removal. If the tape is adhered to the fur, gently pulling the tape off in the direction of hair growth also facilitates its removal. The underlying fur also may be judiciously trimmed with scissors in problematic areas to facilitate removal as slight traction is applied to the adhesive tape.

Skin staples also may be used to secure dressings and link gauze layers together; they are especially useful for skin graft bandages. Casts and splinting materials can be used to further immobilize body regions, thereby reducing motion and subsequent stretching of bandage layers.

Bandage displacement from chewing can be restricted or eliminated by the judicious use of E-collars, neck braces, body braces, slings, and tape stirrups (see Miscellaneous Protective Devices). Foul-tasting topical agents can be used to discourage licking or chewing of exposed bandages (bitter apple, etc.). Metallic splints and fiberglass casting material also can be applied to the tertiary layer, forming a barrier to chewing.

TIE-OVER DRESSING/ BANDAGE TECHNIQUE

The tie-over dressing/bandage is a method of securing bandages to dependent areas of the body and areas of the trunk, head, or neck where conventional bandage wraps have limited effective use. In humans, the tie-over dressing uses sutures to secure the perimeter of the graft. The sutures are left long and are gathered (twisted) together over the top of a small preformed dressing or bandage. A removable metallic clip is applied to the twist to secure the dressing. Unfortunately, this technique is tedious to execute (Fig. 5-16).

A variation of the conventional tie-over technique, developed by the author, uses a series of 2-0 monofilament suture loops placed in the skin surrounding the wound (or graft area), approximately 2-3 cm from the wound border. A loop (with a 10- to 15-mm profile above the skin surface) is created to facilitate insertion of a strand suture or umbilical tape using forceps or mosquito hemostats.

The dressing or light bandage is applied to the wound surface prior to lacing the suture or umbilical tape between opposing loops in a crisscross or zigzag fashion. A piece of water-resistant paper surgical drape also can be placed over the gauze or bandage to limit bandage topical contamination or "strike-through." As a result, a tie-over dressing immobilizes the immediate wound without restricting regional motion. Bandages are removed and easily replaced in

identical fashion using this technique (Fig. 5-17). Practitioners will find this dressing technique to be simple, economical, and very effective for areas otherwise difficult to bandage. Motivated owners can be instructed to change bandages (in cooperative pets) with minimal difficulty.

PRESSURE POINTS: BANDAGE OPTIONS

See the Chapter 7 discussion of pressure sores. (See also see Plate 9, Pipe Insulation Protection Technique for Elbow Wounds.)

BANDAGE "ACCESS WINDOWS"

When a large bandage is used to immobilize a body region and also protect an open wound, constructing an access window at the time of its initial application can facilitate wound inspection without removal of the entire bandage. With this technique, the bulk of the bandage is applied, leaving an area (access window) over the open wound. With completion of this bandage, a local dressing, secondary padding, and outer cover can be placed in the access window and secured with adhesive tape. Subsequent bandage removals require removal of the local wound bandage only, saving both

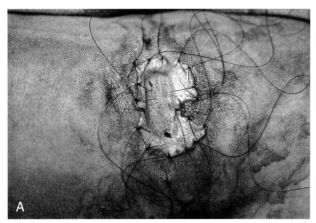 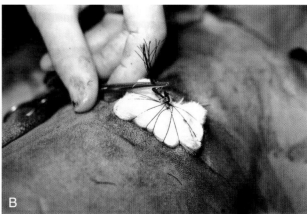

FIG. 5-16 (A) Conventional tie-over dressing. Suture strands that secure the graft are used to secure the dressing into place.
(B) Ointment, a nonadherent dressing, and a layer of gauze cut to the dimensions of the wound bed are applied. Suture strands are twisted and tied. Alternatively, a removal clip can be used if replacement of the bandage is required. A sterilized coin or metallic disc can be inserted into the middle layer for added rigidity.

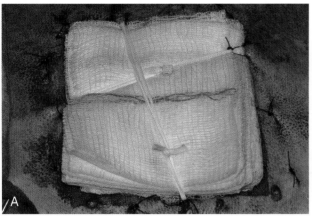 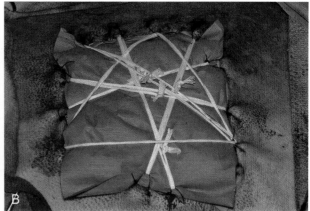

FIG. 5-17 (A) Author's tie-over dressing technique. Suture loops (eyelets) placed around the graft site secure the dressing by lacing suture material or umbilical tape between opposing loops. Loops are created approximately 2–3 cm from the wound borders; loops are 10–15 mm in diameter to permit passage of suture strands or umbilical tape. (B) A piece of sterile paper surgical drape was applied prior to final application of umbilical tape to minimize contamination to the gauze layer.

time and money during open wound care. Alternatively, the surgeon may cut a window in the bandage segment overlying the wound and replace the local dressing and bandage as described at the time of the first change. (See Plate 41.)

BANDAGING TECHNIQUES FOR SKIN GRAFTS

See Chapter 14 for specific details on bandaging skin grafts.

BANDAGING TECHNIQUES FOR SKIN FLAPS

As a general rule, the author avoids applying bandages over most skin flaps. When properly developed, skin flaps have an inherent blood supply. Bandages and splints, unless carefully applied, could compromise vital circulation to the flap

Unlike free grafts, flaps do not require a bandage for their early revascularization and survival. On occasion, a protective bandage and splint are used to protect a flap over a flexion surface (e.g., carpus, tarsus) (Fig. 5-18). The author also has carefully constructed bandages reinforced with splints to protect local flaps and axial pattern flaps placed in areas where excessive motion or trauma could compromise postoperative healing.

Bandages are used in distant direct flaps in which the involved limb is secured beneath a skin flap elevated on the side of the dog and cat. These bandages are important to support the elevated extremity and prevent the patient from displacing the flap from the wound site (see Plates 41 and 42 on distant flap techniques).

SPLINTS, CASTS, REINFORCED BANDAGES

The bandage is the most common method of protecting and supporting the injured area. As previously noted, inappropriately applied bandages can be detrimental to wound healing. Tight bandages can restrict circulation. Loosely fitting bandages, however, may permit regional motion resulting in rubbing and abrasion of the wound surface, especially wounds involving the joints and mobile areas (flank, axilla, neck, etc.). Additional immobilization or rigidity of the bandaged area may be advisable under these circumstances. Half-shell or clamshell fiberglass casts (Scotchcast Plus, 3M), plastic or aluminum Mason metasplints (metal splints by Surecraft, Upton, MA), tongue depressor splints, aluminum bars (aluminum rods, Burns Veterinary Supply, Jericho, NY), and heat-

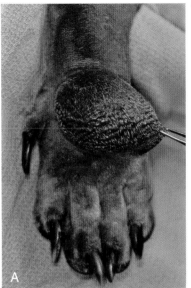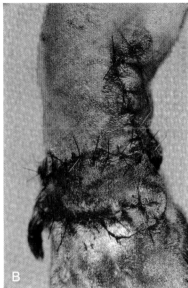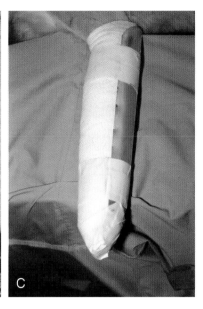

FIG. 5-18 (A) Benign adenoma overlying left carpal area. (B) Excision and closure with a transposition flap. (C) Because the closure was directly over the carpal surface, a metasplint was applied over a protective bandage to minimize motion until suture removal.

malleable plastic (Orthoplast, Johnson & Johnson) are effective for immobilizing lower limb wounds when applied just inside or outside of the tertiary bandage layer.

Splinting in Soft Tissue Wound Care

When external fixation is used for fracture immobilization, excessive padding between the bone and splint reduces its efficacy in immobilizing the fracture site.

In contrast to fracture stabilization, supplemental splinting of soft tissue bandages is primarily used to minimize joint movement and motion of the bandage in relation to the wound surface. As a result, splints can be applied over thicker soft tissue bandages safely and effectively.

External splints can compress the underlying tissues, depending on the thickness of the secondary bandage layer. To reduce the risk of pressure necrosis over bony prominences (olecranon, tarsus, accessory carpal pad), supplemental padding should be place around the base of bony depressions; this padding reduces the pressure cone effect that otherwise can occur between the bony prominence and overlying splint. See Plates 2 and 3.

Schroeder-Thomas splints provide excellent immobilization to the limbs, using aluminum rods or sturdy coat hangers for smaller dogs and cats. The Schroeder-Thomas splint is excellent for immobilizings the elbow, carpus, knee, and tibiotarsal joint and allows the veterinarian to change small bandages without removing the splint (Fig. 5-19 and 5-20). The bars provide protection to these body regions from direct impact. See Plates 6 and 7.

Spica bandages or splints also are effective in immobilizing the upper extremities. The spica bandage envelopes the limb and trunk, restricting motion to the shoulder or hip joint. It can be reinforced with an aluminum bar or a thin plywood silhouette of the affected limb to increase spica rigidity (Figs. 5-21, 5-22.). In the more difficult wound closure areas, including the flank, inguinal, and axillary areas, combined bandaging techniques may be required for achieving optimal healing results. See Plate 5.

MISCELLANEOUS PROTECTIVE DEVICES

Body (Side) Brace

On occasion, a body or side brace fashioned with aluminum rods is useful to prevent dogs from licking or chewing at wounds involving their caudal trunk and hindquarters. An aluminum rod is fashioned into a circular central loop to fit over the head and around

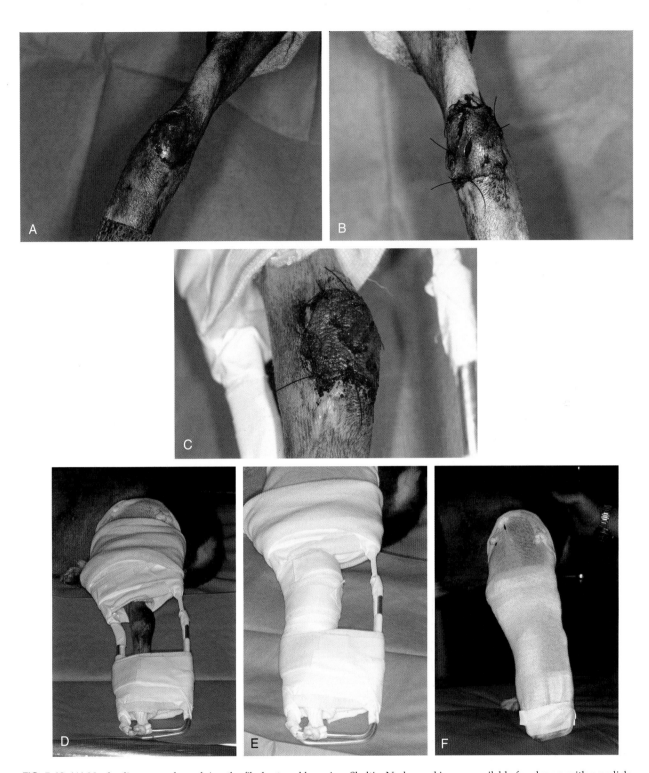

FIG. 5-19 (A) Nonhealing wound overlying the fibular tarsal bone in a Sheltie. No loose skin was available for closure with a pedicle graft.

(B) A mesh graft was applied over the granulation bed. A Schroeder-Thomas splint was used to protect the surgical site from motion and trauma.

(C) The graft on day 5 with 100% viability.

(D) Note that the local bandage overlying the graft can be replaced without removing the splint. Stockinette strips and tape were used to secure the limb to the splint.

(E) Reapplication of the bandage.

(F) A piece of stockinette is secured to the outer ring of the Schroeder-Thomas splint and pulled over the bandaged area for added protection.

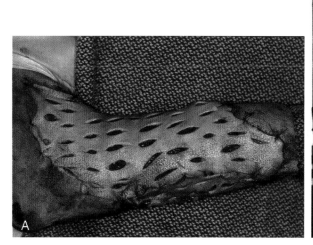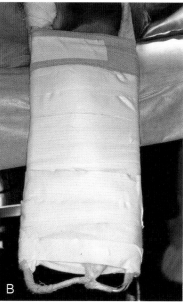

FIG. 5-20 (A) Mesh graft application to the forelimb. Immobilization of the carpus and elbow were considered essential to graft survival in this active golden retriever. (B) A Schroeder-Thomas splint was applied to provide rigid immobilization to the graft.

FIG. 5-21 (A) A spica bandage of the hind limb, encircling the trunk of a cat. This bandage was used to immobilize a difficult wound closure. Note the vacuum drain, using a syringe. Spica bandages are commonly used for grafts that extend into the proximal area of the limbs. This is especially true for cats who have a propensity to remove bandages.

(B) A large flank wound was temporarily covered with a spica bandage. Note the bandage encircles the trunk for added security to prevent the bandage from slipping. Reinforcement material can be incorporated into the bandage if rigid immobilization is required. In this example, a tie-over dressing could have been more effectively used.

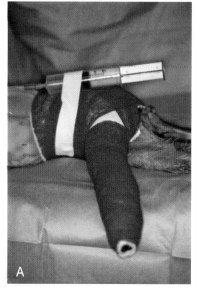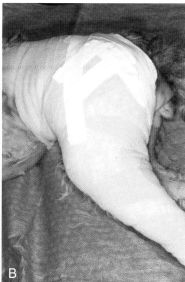

the neck of the dog. Padding is applied to the cervical ring. The remaining left and right aluminum "arms" are bent and positioned along the lateral thorax and abdomen. A second extension piece of aluminum can be added using surgical tape if the arms are too short to complete a dorsal support arch. The aluminum extension contours the dorsal lumbar area and is sufficiently long to allow the lateral bars to rest in the midthoracic and lateral abdominal area. Padding is applied to its surface. Elastic adhesive tape is used to secure the brace to the dog by applying strips between each bar above and below the trunk. Tension on each elastic strip can be adjusted to position the aluminum arms at the midthoracic/abdominal region to inhibit the dog from bending its trunk (Fig 5-23). See Plate 8.

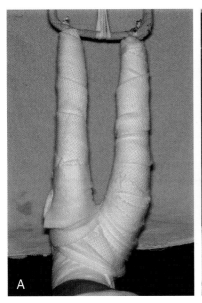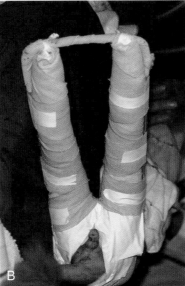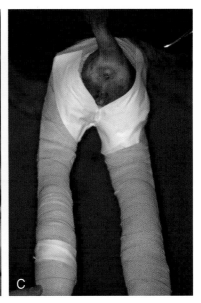

FIG. 5-22 (A) Cat, inner thigh, and inguinal wound (see Fig. 5-9). A full-thickness mesh graft was applied to the large defect. Skin staples were used to secure nonadherent dressings. A tie-over dressing was applied over the nonadherent dressing before application of the spica. The legs were suspended by an aluminum U bar secured to the rear paws with tape stirrups. This set-up was used for subsequent bandage changes, by suspending the bar base, to which the paws were taped.

(B) The spica bandage was complete, followed by the application of each arm of the aluminum bar with Elasticon tape.

(C) Caudal view of the spica splint. Note this spica bandage kept the limbs apart, approximating the width of the pelvis. Waterproof white tape was applied to the bandage around the perineal area to facilitate cleaning around the area. The cat was placed on baby diapers to collect urine and feces. The patient was turned every 2 hours. This device was removed 2 weeks after surgery.

Tape Hobbles

Tape hobbles have been employed to restrict limb abduction and motion of the forelimb or hindlimb. They also can be used to prevent the dog from using his front or hind paws to scratch at a surgical site. The author also has used rear leg hobbles to restrict cats from licking at perineal wounds and urethrostomy incisions. Tape hobbles are applied with the apposing limbs in a normal vertical position in relation to the trunk width. Tape bands are applied below the opposing carpal or tarsal joints. Tape is never applied in a dangerous circular ring pattern around the limbs. Rather, tape ends arc around the limb and the adhesive surfaces are squeezed or sandwiched together. This tape pattern has less likelihood of restricting circulation; swelling is better able to spread or separate the tape-to-tape interface.

Elizabethan Collars

Several commercial Elizabethan collars (Butler Animal Health Supply, Dublin, OH, etc.) are available to veterinarians to prevent dogs and cats from licking or chewing at surgical sites. Alternatively, the plastic collar can protect the head and neck from scratching and rubbing.

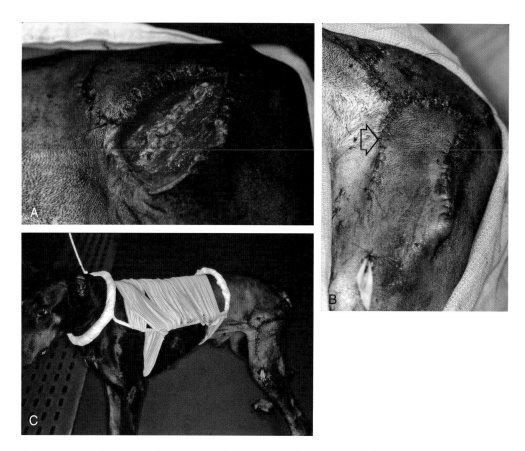

FIG. 5-23 (A) Open wound on the left rear limb. The dog chewed the surgical area apart where a skin tumor was resected. This occurred despite the use of an appropriate sized Elizabethan collar. Infection was treated before closure was attempted. (B) Transposition flap (open arrow) used to close this skin defect. (C) A body brace was fashioned to prevent the patient from repeating his earlier performance.

Note:
Elizabethan collars also can be effectively used to reduce the risk of being bitten by more aggressive dogs and cats.

X-ray film can be fashioned into Elizabethan collars for cats and small dogs. Plastic buckets can be effectively used in a similar fashion for larger dogs. Butler Animal Health Supply also sells a soft, coated fabric variation of the classic Elizabethan collar that may be better tolerated by some feline patients. Veterinarians must remember that dogs are particularly effective at bending plastic collars against cage doors, pushing the collar backward, or chewing the collar borders sufficiently to gain access to their bandage and surgical incisions. When appropriately applied and properly maintained, Elizabethan collars can be very effective in protecting wounds, although the veterinarian must be certain the patient is capable of eating and drinking while wearing one (Fig. 5-24). Owners may need to elevate food and water bowls. In cooperative animals, the collar may be temporarily removed when the patient is fed. Owners are warned that removal of a collar requires direct supervision of their pet; leaving the room even "for a minute" can allow ample time for the patient to damage the surgical site.

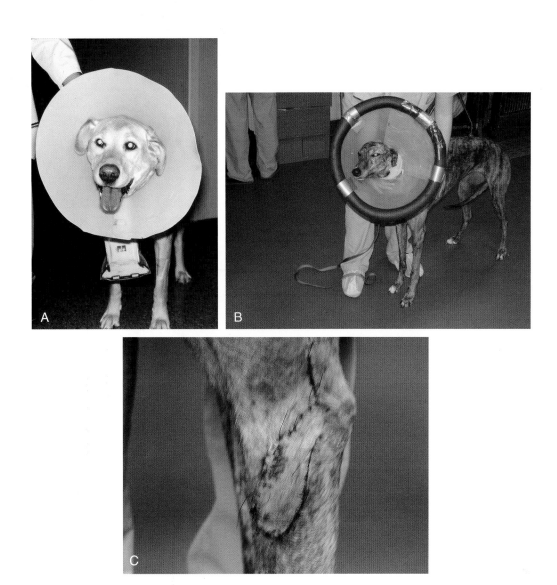

FIG. 5-24 (A) An Elizabethan collar was used to prevent the patient from chewing at a caudal superficial epigastric axial pattern flap used to close an extensive flank defect. Note the reservoir of the closed suction unit attached to the patient's collar.
(B) Pipe insulation used to pad the edge of an Elizabethan collar. A transposition flap was used to close a problematic wound of the left forelimb. Duct tape also can be used to create a softer edge to the collar. (Pipe insulation is best avoided if a patient has a history of chewing and consuming foreign objects. From the author's experience this is a rare occurrence.) (C) Close-up view of the flap, 10 days postoperatively.

Elizabethan Collar Tips:

Selection of the appropriate size is critical to preventing the dog and cat from licking at a surgical area. The edge of an Elizabethan collar can be somewhat sharp, and some dogs occasionally will accidentally rub it on the surgical site. In some cases dogs will learn to use the collar to scratch at an irritated area. This can be detrimental to a flap, graft, or open wound. Pipe insulation (see Chapter 7, Plate 29; Armacell Self-Seal Pipe Insulation, Armacell Engineered Foams, Mebane, NC) can be purchased at most hardware stores and home supply businesses. This versatile material can be applied around the perimeter of the collar. Duct tape can be used to enhance its adherence to the Elizabethan collar border. The soft layer prevents rubbing and is sufficiently light that it does not weigh down the collar excessively. Alternatively, duct tape can be folded lengthwise around the perimeter of the collar, creating a softer, flexible edge to reduce abrasiveness (Fig. 5-24).

Cervical Collars

Cervical collars (Bitenot Collar, Butler Animal Health Supply) provide another option to reduce or prevent patients from licking or chewing at a bandage, wound, or surgical area. The efficacy of cervical collars has had mixed reviews from veterinarians. They normally are considered for those patients in which the Elizabethan collar is ineffective.

Slings

Slings have limited use for most wound closures. They can be employed to restrict motion of a limb when movement could promote wound dehiscence. Examples include axillary, inguinal, and flank wounds closed under tension. The sling should not be applied in a position that could interfere with regional circulation (extreme flexion) or healing of the affected limb. The Velpeau sling can be used for the forelimb. The hind limb sling can be fashioned with a loop of elastic adhesive tape from the lower foot over the lumbar area to prevent weight-bearing (usually for flank wounds closed under tension). For a male dog, the rear limb must be positioned so that the patient does not urinate on his foot or the sling. (A variation of this simple sling is the Robinson Sling; see Robinson and McCoy 1975). If the sling is intended simply to limit a wide range of motion and weight placement on the limb, placement of the limb in extreme flexion is unwarranted. Mild elevation of the limb is capable of restricting motion and preventing weight-bearing without compromising comfort.

Slings must be assessed closely to assure they do not cause swelling to the lower extremity, compromise regional circulation, or irritate the underlying skin. Slings must be kept clean and dry to prevent dermatitis. Similarly, skin folds and flexion creases should be assessed for moisture accumulation and dermatitis. Talcum or medicated powders may be useful in managing these skin fold areas until sling removal. In general, the author rarely uses slings.

Miscellaneous Commercial Protective Devices

A variety of protective devices are available for use in dogs, including elbow pads, protective boots, and covers for external fixators (Dogleggs, www.dogleggs. com; Handicappedpets.com). Wound care dressing holders (Tapeless Wound Care Products; www.tapelesswoundcare.com) are also available to help maintain the position of dressings/bandages. Many of these products can be examined at major veterinary conferences to determine their potential usefulness for a given veterinary practice.

Suggested Readings

Anderson DM, White RAS. 2000. Ischemic bandage injuries: a case series and review of the literature. *Vet Surg* 29:488–498.

Bohling MW. 2007. Open wound care. *NAVC Clinician's Brief* Jan:19–21.

Campbell BG. 2006. Dressings, bandages, and splints for wound management in dogs and cats. *Vet Clin No Am* 36:759–791.

Dean P. 1998. Robinson sling (pelvic limb sling). In: Bojrab MJ, ed. *Current Techniques in Small Animal Surgery*, 4th ed. 1298–1299. Philadelphia: Williams and Wilkins.

DeCamp CE. 2002. External coaptation. In: Slatter DS, ed. *Textbook of Small Animal Surgery*, 3rd ed. 1835–1848. Philadelphia: WB Saunders.

Ducharme-Desjarlais M, Celeste CJ, Lepault E, et al. 2005. Effect of a silicone containing dressing on exuberant granulation tissue formation and wound repair in horses. *Am J Vet Res* 66:1133–1139.

Eaglstein WH, Falanga V. 1997. Chronic wounds. *Surg Clin No Am* 77:689–700.

Fahie MA, Shettko D. 2007. Evidence-based wound management: a systematic review of therapeutic agents to enhance granulation and epithelialization. *Vet Clin No Am* 37:559–577.

Gomez JH, Hanson RR. 2005. Use of dressings and bandages in equine wound management. *Vet Clin No Am* 21(1):91–104.

Gomez JH, Schumacher J, Lauten SD, et al. 2004. Effects of 3 biologic dressings on healing of cutaneous wounds on the limbs of horses. *Can J Vet Res* 68:49–55.

Hodge S, Degner D. 2006. A novel bandaging method. *NAVC Clinicians Brief* Oct.:7–9.

Knecht CD. 1981. *Fundamental Techniques in Veterinary Surgery*. 2nd ed. Philadelphia: WB Saunders.

Krahwinkel DJ, Boothe HW. 2006 Topical and systemic medications for wounds. *Vet Clin No Am* 36:739–757.

Lee AH, Swaim SF, McGuire JA, et al. 1987. Effects of non-adherent dressing materials on the healing of open wounds in dogs. *J Am Vet Med Assoc* 190:416–422.

Lee AH, Swaim SF, Yang ST, et al. 1986. The effects of petrolatum, polyethylene glycol, nitrofurazone, and a hydroactive dressing on open wound healing. *J Am Anim Hosp Assoc* 22:443–451.

Lee AH, Swaim SF, Newton JC, et al. 1987. Wound healing over denuded bone. *J Am Anim Hosp Assoc* 23:75–84.

Lee WR, Tobias KM, Bemis DA, et al. In vitro efficacy of a polyhexamethylene biguanide impregnated gauze dressing against bacteria found in veterinary patients. *Vet Surg* 33(4):404–411.

Morgan PW, Binnington AG, Miller CW, et al. 1994. The effect of occlusive and semi-occlusive dressings on the healing of acute full-thickness skin wounds on the forelimbs of dogs. *Vet Surg* 23:494–502.

Pavletic MM. 1993. Surgery of the skin and management of wounds. In Sherding RG, ed. *The Cat: Diseases and Clinical Management*, 2nd ed. New York: Churchill Livingstone.

Ramsey DT, Pope ER, Wagner-Mann C, et al. 1995. Effects of three occlusive dressing materials on healing of full-thickness skin wounds in dogs. *Am J Vet Res* 56: 941–949.

Robinson GW, McCoy L. 1975. A pelvic limb sling for dogs. In: Bojrab MJ, ed. *Current Techniques in Small Animal Surgery*, 567–569. Philadelphia, PA: Lea & Febiger.

Simpson AM, Beale BS, Radlinsky MA. 2001. Bandaging in dogs and cats: basic principles. *Compend Contin Ed Pract Vet* 23(1):12–16.

Simpson AM, Radlinsky MA, Beale BS. 2001. Bandaging in dogs and cats: external coaptation. *Compend Contin Ed Pract Vet* 23(2):157–163.

Swaim SF. 1990. Bandage and topical agents. *Vet Clin No Am* 20:47–65.

Swaim SF, Gillette RL. 1998. An update on wound medications and dressings. *Compend Contin Ed Pract Vet* 20:1133–1144.

Swaim SF, Henderson R. 1990. *Small Animal Wound Management*, 9–11, 33–40. Philadelphia: Lea & Febiger.

Vermeulen H, Ubbink D, Goossens A, et al. 2006. Dressings and topical agents for surgical wounds healing by secondary intention. *Cochrane Database Syst Rev* 1464–780X2. Available at: http://www.cochrane.org/reviews/en/ab003554.html.

Winkler JT, Swaim SF, Sartin EA, et al. 2002. The effect of a porcine-derived small intestinal submucosa product on wounds with exposed bone in dogs. *Vet Surg* 31: 541–551.

www.dermnetnz.org—Synthetic Wound Dressings

Plate 2   **Basic Bandage Application for Extremities**

DESCRIPTION

Basic bandage application can be uncomplicated if a few general rules are followed.

TECHNIQUE

(A) In this example tape stirrups have been applied prior to the application of standard cast padding (Specialist Cast Padding, BSN Medical, Brierfield, UK). The key to a stronger, more secure bandage is to overlap each revolution by 50% as the material is spiraled up the leg. This process is repeated with every subsequent layer applied. Note that the skin depression around the accessory carpal pad was padded (arrow) prior to application of the roll cotton, preventing a "pressure cone" effect on the accessory carpal bone.

(B) Note that the axillary skin fold can be pressed or flattened with the index finger, thereby allowing the forelimb bandage to cover the lower humeral region more effectively.

(C) In the hind limb, the flank fold is pushed upward, facilitating the more proximal extension of the bandage into the upper thigh region. *Note*: The tape stirrup strips can be separated and folded proximally prior to application of roll gauze, giving added security to keep the bandage from slipping off the foot.

(D) When possible, exposure of the central two toes allows the veterinarian and owner to assess the lower extremity for soft tissue swelling. In the average dog, the index figure can be inserted between the central toes. Excessive swelling would preclude this maneuver. The exposed digits also can be examined more closely for swelling. If swelling is present, immediate bandage removal and inspection of the limb is indicated.

COMMENTS

When building a bandage, cotton cast padding is commonly used as the bulk of the secondary bandage layer. Overlapping by 50% reinforces the strength and thickness of each layer. This is followed by a layer of self-adherent or elastic gauze; this roll gauze is used to compress the cast padding as each subsequent cotton/gauze layer is applied. Bandage thickness is dependent on the purpose of the bandage. As subsequent layers are added and the bandage thickness increases, gauze can be applied with progressively greater tension. An outer tertiary wrap (Vetrap, Elasticon, etc.) completes the bandage.

For greater security, distal extremity bandages are more secure if the bandage is extended proximal to the carpal or tarsal joints. Small, tight bandages are best avoided for lower extremity wounds.

Plate 2

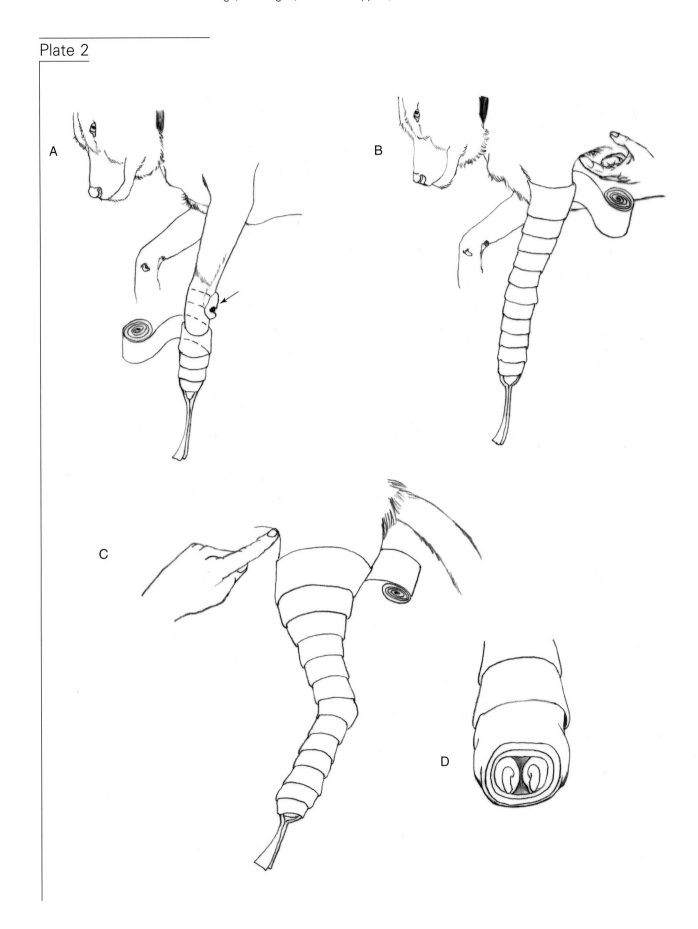

Plate 3	**Tape Stirrups and Padding Dos and Don'ts**

DESCRIPTION

Common safety tips pertaining to tape stirrups and protection of bony prominences are discussed. Tape stirrups help prevent bandages from slipping off the limb and secure bandages to coaptation splints. Stirrups can be used to apply gentle traction to the extremity and may be used to temporarily suspend a limb when changing dressings/bandages.

BANDAGING TECHNIQUES

(A₁, A₂)   Tape stirrups can be placed on the paw in two fashions: (1) over the anterior and posterior surfaces of the paw and (2) over the lateral and medial aspects of the paw. The strips cover the metacarpal and metatarsal surfaces. (*Warning:* Do not apply a caudal tape stirrup over the accessory carpal pad; traction can result in pressure necrosis of the pad. The tape is applied just distal to the lower border of the accessory pad.) Their placement may be determined in part by the condition of the skin. Tape segments can be sandwiched together when traction is required during splint application: these conjoined strips can be secured to the secondary layer of the bandage with tape. Alternatively, each stirrup strip of tape may be separately reflected back and incorporated into the secondary layer of the bandage. There is a particular disadvantage of the lateral-medial application of stirrups: tape traction compresses the toes together and occasionally results in one or more nails compressing into the adjacent toe, causing pain, skin inflammation, local ischemia, and infection that can lead to tissue necrosis. Traction on stirrups placed over the cranial-caudal surface of the paw does not cause this problem.

(B)   Supplemental bands of tape are occasionally used to support tape stirrups.
1. **Encircling bands or tape must be avoided**: under traction, they can shift, creating a tourniquet effect. If left undetected, ischemia and necrosis of the paw can occur.
2. A safer alternative is an open spiral strip that can help secure the stirrup without the risk of creating a tourniquet.

(C, D)   A key point in protecting bony prominences is to pad the depressions around their base. Placement of padding over the surface of a bony prominence actually can enhance the pressure cone effect on the overlying skin, especially if a cast or rigid splint material is applied over these structures. Padding around the prominences better protects the area by distributing direct pressure over its surface, rather than over the bony prominence exclusively. Examples include padding around the point of the elbow, fibular tarsal bone, accessory carpal pad, and first digit. Padding between the toe pads, and metacarpal/metatarsal crease (arrows) can reduce moisture accumulation and secondary dermatitis prior to covering the paw with a protective bandage.

COMMENTS

Tape stirrups are not necessary or practical for every bandage application but can provide added security to prevent a bandage from slipping. A surprising number of complications arise from improperly applied or supervised bandages. Wet bandages secondary to external contamination or progressive moisture accumulation within the bandage can have an adverse effect on the skin. The problems noted in this section, namely skin infections, skin necrosis over bony prominences, necrosis of the accessory carpal pad, necrosis of the paw, and skin necrosis involving the digits have been seen by the author. These problems could have been avoided by careful bandage application and proper maintenance and vigilance by the owner. Proper bandage care should be discussed with the owner; basic handouts on proper bandage and splint care are a useful reference for veterinary clientele.

Plate 3

A₁ A₂ B₁ B₂

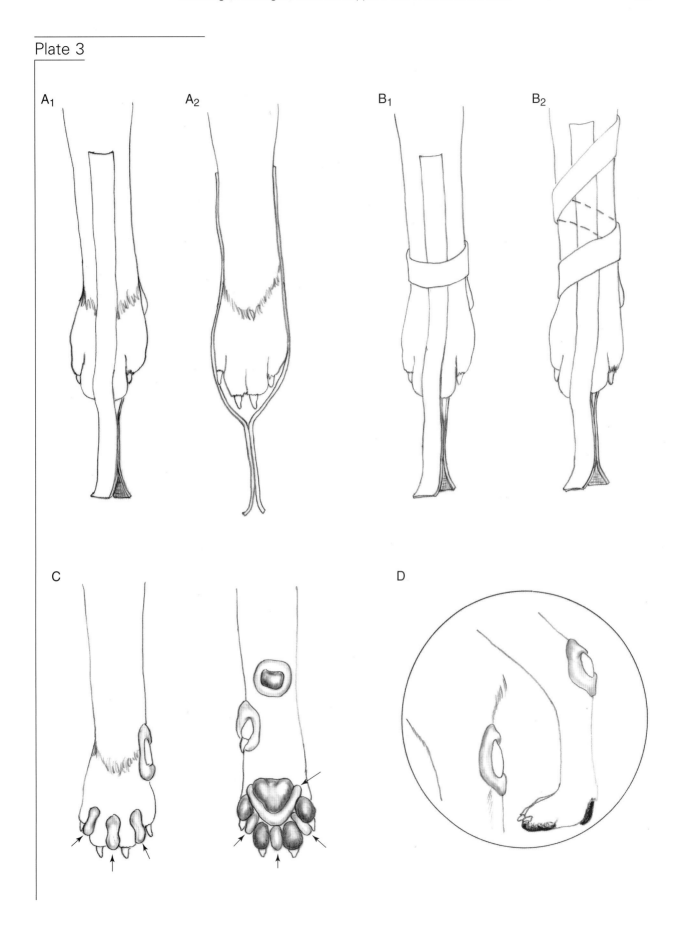

C

D

Plate 4	**Elasticon Bandage Platforms and Saddles**

DESCRIPTION

Securing bandages to the trunk, limbs, and tail can be problematic. The tapered thorax and abdomen result in the tendency for bandages encircling the trunk to slip or shift caudally. Regional bandages of the forelimb and tail, for example, are difficult to maintain as a result of slippage secondary to gravity and motion of the patient. Adhesive Elasticon (Johnson & Johnson) can be used to create a platform for bandage application. The bandage proper overlaps the Elasticon base: subsequent bandage changes are performed without removing the Elasticon until healing is complete.

TECHNIQUE

(A) An Elasticon "saddle" is applied over the back of the dog or cat by running strips parallel or perpendicular to the long axis of the body. In most cases, this elastic adhesive tape is applied to a clean, flat hair coat. The rough surface of Elasticon provides a friction surface to help maintain the bandage in its proper position. The Elasticon is left in place during subsequent bandage changes. (Note: Applying an encircling band of Elasticon to the cranial and caudal borders of the bandage and adjacent skin can further reduce the tendency of the trunk bandage to slide caudally.)

(B) Two Elasticon strips are applied proximal and distal to a forelimb wound prior to application of the bandage.

(C) *Note:* Elasticon is sandwiched to itself when applied to the limbs and tail to reduce the risk of circulatory compromise, rather than being wrapped around the limb in a circular fashion (cross-sectional view). The bandage subsequently overlaps the Elasticon anchors, preventing bandage displacement. The Elasticon is left in place during subsequent bandage changes.

(D) As with the forelimb, this technique can be effectively applied to secure bandages to the tail.

COMMENTS

Elasticon saddles or anchors are simple to apply and effective in keeping most bandages in place. For the forelimb, less bandage material is required when compared to applying a bandage encompassing its entire length. When applied to the fur, removal is relatively simple and pain free by pulling the Elasticon off in the direction of hair growth. Elasticon applied directly to the skin surface is best removed using commercially available medical solvents (see text).

Plate 4

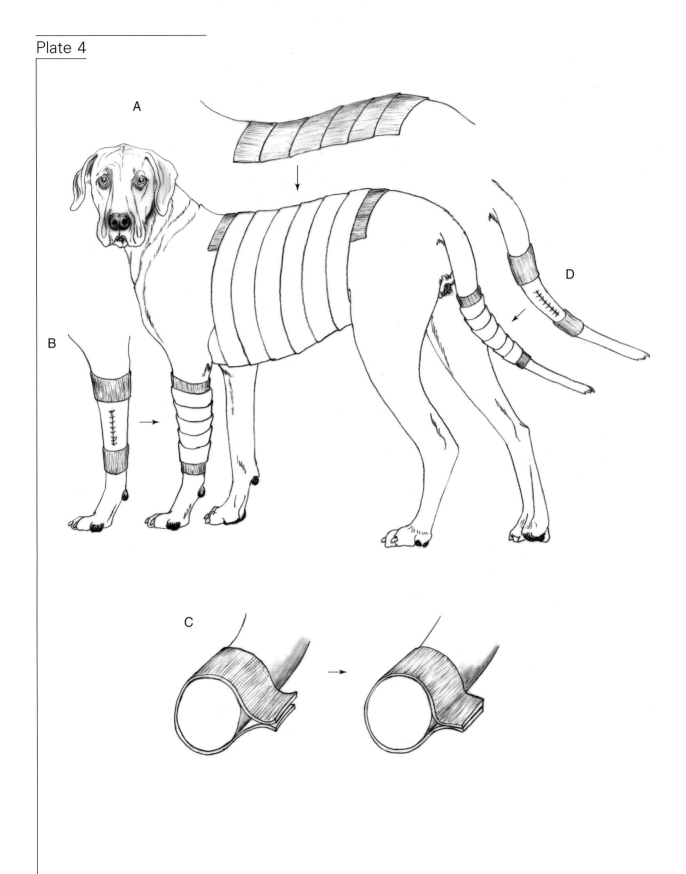

| Plate 5 | **Spica Bandages/Splints** |

DESCRIPTION

Spica (Latin, ear of grain) is used to describe a bandage, splint, or cast that envelopes an extremity and the circumference of the trunk. It is especially useful for immobilizing the upper extremity and restricting motion of the entire limb. In cats the spica technique can effectively prevent the patient from removing bandages of the extremities, a particularly important consideration when skin grafting the limbs.

TECHNIQUE

(A) The bandage is applied by adding alternate layers of cast padding and self-adherent gauze. The thickness of that portion of the bandage overlying the limb is built up so that it better approximates the lateral shoulder silhouette. Layers of the cast padding, roll gauze, and outer wrap are extended around the trunk.

(B) On the forelimb, the spica encircles the trunk behind the opposing leg. On the hindlimb, the bandage encircles the trunk cranial to the opposite leg. Care must be taken to avoid compression of the penis and provide access for normal urination. Elasticon (Johnson & Johnson), Vetrap (3M) or a combination of materials can be used for the tertiary layer. *Note:* Care must be taken to assure the bandage is not abrading the axillary and flank regions of the opposite limb. Keep in mind that these materials can curl and bunch, causing abrasive injuries or cuts to the skin in these areas. Owners should be instructed to watch these areas closely for signs of skin irritation.

(C) Fiberglass strips can be incorporated into the tertiary bandage layer to immobilize the extremity. Alternatively, a rigid aluminum bar can be bent and curved at the top of the arch to conform to the scapular area and curvature of the back. Although rarely used today, 1/4-inch plywood can be used to form a narrow silhouette of the limb for added rigidity. In cats and small dogs, tongue depressors can be overlapped and taped to the outer bandage.

COMMENTS

Spica bandages are a must when grafting the forelimb or hind limb in the cat. This effectively prevents complete removal of the bandage. They are a potential alternative to the Schroeder-Thomas splint for immobilizing and protecting surgical areas susceptible to movement and trauma (for example, the elbow). In some instances, a window can be cut out of the area overlying a surgical site and patched with bandage material and tape to facilitate future bandage changes without removal of the entire spica. Spicas usually require replacement within 2 weeks: bandage materials have a tendency to stretch and loosen from the underlying limb. Muscle atrophy may further contribute to loosening.

Plate 5

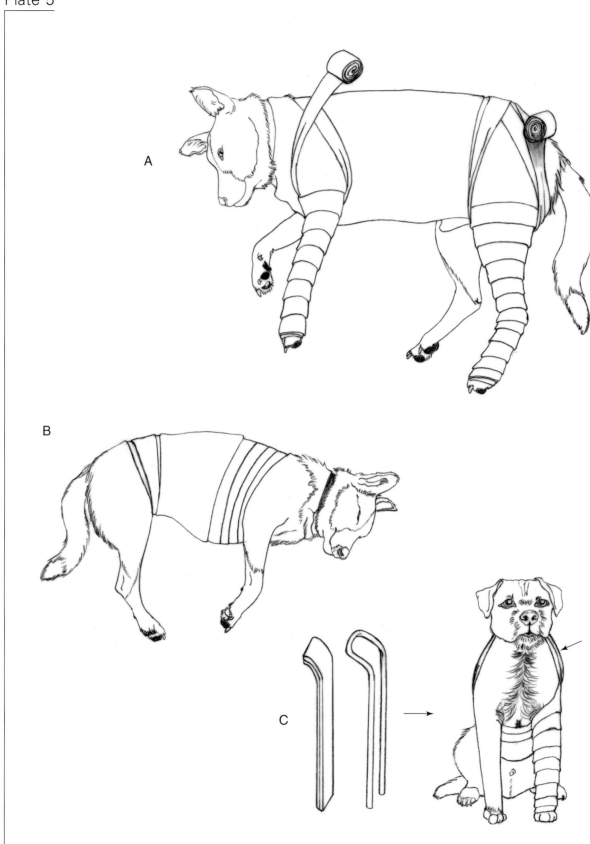

Plate 6	**Schroeder-Thomas Splint**

DESCRIPTION

The Schroeder-Thomas splint is a modification of the Thomas splint used to stabilize fractures in humans. Dr. Erwin F. Schroeder, a former staff member at Angell Memorial Animal Hospital, modified and adapted this splint for fracture repair in small animals. In the 1958 edition of *Canine Surgery* (Lacroix JV, Reiser WH. Fractures. In: Mayer K, Lacroix JV, Hoskins HP, eds. Pp. 636-642. *Canine Surgery*, 4th ed. Santa Barbara: American Veterinary Publications.), the Schroeder-Thomas splint was called "one of the most widely used and adaptable splints for small animals," permitting both traction and fixation of many types of fractures. A variety of angles can be bent into the aluminum bars to facilitate fracture alignment, depending on the nature and location of a fracture.

    Proper design and application of this splint is now a lost art due to the advent of superior internal and external fixation techniques. However, the Schroeder-Thomas splint is occasionally very useful in immobilizing the forelimb and hind limb for problematic wound closures, especially those involving the elbow, fibular tarsal bone, and knee. It also can be used to immobilize grafts applied to the radial and ulna region or tibial region. Commercially available Schroeder-Thomas splints are inferior to manually creating a splint specifically crafted to conform more exactly to the shape of the patient's extremity. Construction of the splint does require more time and patience compared to other bandage and splinting techniques used to protect problematic wound closures in small animals.

SPLINT TECHNIQUE

(A)   The forelimb and hind limb angular circumference are assessed by molding your hands around the upper extremity. This will serve as a general guideline regarding the size and shape of the aluminum ring needed to conform to the upper extremity. (The Thomas ring molds—if they still make them—are not necessary for proper ring formation.) The forelimb ring forms an oval, whereas the hind limb ring is circular in shape.

(B)   The center of an aluminum bar of sufficient rigidity (Burns Veterinary Supply Inc., Guilderland Center, NY) is the starting point for bending the ring. As the ring is symmetrically bent, it is periodically applied to the limb (patient in lateral recumbency) and its shape adjusted accordingly. Allowance must be made for padding the ring, if so desired (see comments). Once the ring is of sufficient size to comfortably slide over the upper extremity, the limbs of the bar are initially bent at approximately a 30-degree angle at the midpoint of the ring. The base of the ring will partially contact the lower thorax and pelvis. The angle can be adjusted so that the limbs or the aluminum bar will support the affected limb, parallel to the lateral silhouette of the trunk. A rubber hammer and vise can be used to slightly bend or cup the lower ring border to better conform to the lower thorax and pelvis if necessary (arrow).

(C, D)   The limbs of the aluminum bar are bent to conform to the elbow, knee, and tarsus as illustrated. Otherwise, the bars remain parallel to each other. The end of each bar is bent at right angles and overlaps with the opposing bar end as illustrated. If the aluminum limbs are too short, a common problem in long-legged patients, a second short segment of aluminum bar is bent to overlap each aluminum limb several inches. Overlapped bar segments are taped together with 1-inch surgical tape. Note: It is important that an index finger can be comfortably inserted between the inner ring and thigh (G) to prevent tissue compression.

Plate 6

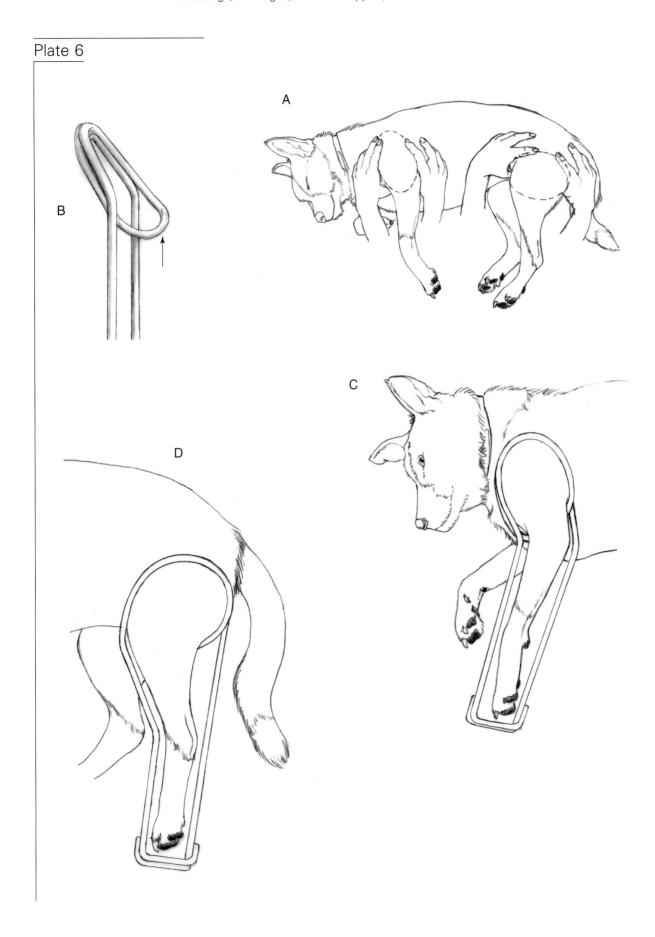

Plate 6

(Continued)

(E) A long tape stirrup is applied to the cranial and caudal aspects of the paw. *Warning:* Do not extend the tape over the accessory carpal pad, as this can lead to pressure necrosis. The tape stirrups are compressed together and split down the middle lengthwise to the level of the central toes.

(F) The stirrups are crisscrossed over the inner bar and tied together in a knot on the central area of the bar. Note that the outer overlapped bar protects the stirrup from erosion when the dog bears weight on the splint (or simply drags it over the floor). The stirrup is important to the proper alignment and security of the limb to the splint.

(G, H) Support bands are positioned to keep the limb cradled between the bars while providing exposure of the wound closure site. Note: An Elasticon band (G) is applied to the caudal portion of the ring to prevent its tendency to rotate forward. Bandage changes can be performed without disturbing the splint and support bands. See Plate 7, a supplement to this plate, Application of Schroeder-Thomas Splint: Security Band Application. A band of Elasticon (Johnson & Johnson) is applied to the caudal-dorsal aspect of the forelimb ring and wrapped around the thorax to neutralize the tendency of the splint to pivot forward over the shoulder.

COMMENTS

See Plate 7 regarding the proper application of the Schroeder-Thomas splint bands. The splint requires the close attention of the clinician and owner to assure no swelling of the toes is noted and that the tape stirrups and bands remain in place. In intact male dogs, it is important to make certain the scrotum and testicles are not accidently trapped between the ring and inner thigh. Because the limb bends to the shape of the bars, there is a tendency to overestimate the length of the splint. Unnecessarily long splints make it difficult for the dog to ambulate. Fortunately, the length can be adjusted by shortening the terminal portion of the splint, as needed.

The rings can be padded by applying surgical tape over the metal prior to application of a layer of cast padding, gauze, and a tertiary wrap (Elasticon or Vetrap). Padding the ring may not necessarily improve patient comfort: the padding can chafe the inner inguinal and axillary skin, whereas the smooth aluminum surface does not rub or irritate the skin. Most patients do not fully bear weight on the Schroeder-Thomas splint and have a tendency to push or drag it.

Plate 6

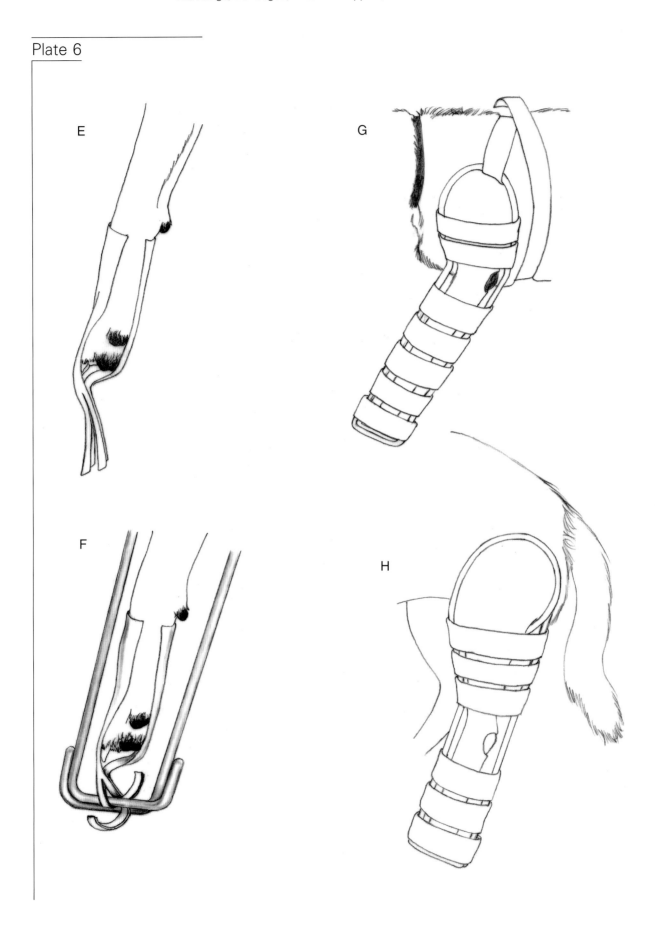

Plate 7   # Schroeder-Thomas Splint: Security Band Application

DESCRIPTION

Many veterinarians unfamiliar with the Schroeder-Thomas splint attempt to secure the limb to the bars with gauze and tape, encircling the splint and leg together. The proper method of applying rings is discussed.

TECHNIQUE

(A) Prior to band application, a layer of white tape is sandwiched or spiraled over the aluminum bars (arrows): this creates a friction surface to assure bands do not slip on the otherwise smooth surface of the aluminum rod. The bands are applied only after securing the paw's tape stirrup to the bottom of the splint (see Plate 6). In this example, the band is folded or looped around the front bar with the end tucked securely medial to the limb. The band is comprised of stockinette (Tex-Care Stockinette, Tex-Care Medical, Burlington, NC; 3M Stockinet, 3M Healthcare, St. Paul, MN). In general, 1 inch is used in small dogs and cats; 2-3 inches in medium sized dogs; 3-4 inches in large breed dogs.
(B) The band completes one revolution around the limb and the front bar.
(C) Under slight tension or traction, the band is rotated around the lateral aspect of the back bar and directed forward to the front bar.
(D) The band is continued around the lateral surface of the front bar and the limb.
(E) Under traction the band rotates around the back bar a few centimeters.
(F) A long strip of surgical tape is used to secure the band.

COMMENTS

Stockinette is the most effective product to create bands for the Schroeder-Thomas splint. Note that this banding technique essentially creates a supportive sling for the leg, elevating the limb somewhat lateral to the bars of the splint. Splints normally will maintain themselves over a 2-week period before adjustment of the stockinette bands is necessary. Weekly examinations of the splint coincide with assessment/management of the surgical area. Band placement is adjusted so that proper dressing and bandage application to the surgical area can be performed. Subsequent bandage changes do not require removal of the splint or the security bands, greatly simplifying wound care.

Upon completion of the splint and bandage application, a strip of wide stockinette can be stretched over the entire Schroeder-Thomas splint as a protective sock. The proximal end of this stockinette sock can be secured to the top of the ring with a few loops of umbilical tape. The bottom of the stockinette can be folded over the end of the splint and taped into place: the tape can be removed and the stockinette sock rolled up to expose the bandage as needed.

Plate 7

A

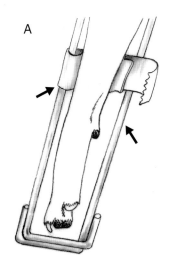

B

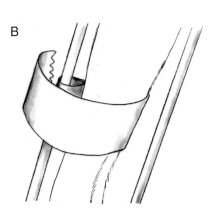

C

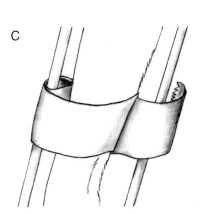

D

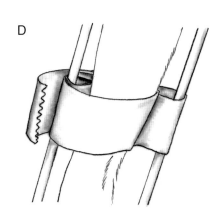

E

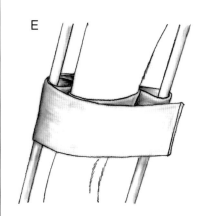

F

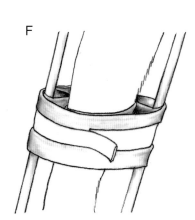

Plate 8   **Body Brace**

DESCRIPTION

The body brace is a simple aluminum bar device designed to prevent the dog from twisting its body to reach a caudal body region. They are most commonly used to prevent a patient from disturbing a surgical area or surgical drain involving the hind limbs and perineum when other protective devices have failed.

TECHNIQUE

(A) An aluminum bar (Burns Veterinary Supply Inc., Guilderland Center, NY) of appropriate rigidity is selected. The diameter of the bar circle must accommodate the passage of the patient's head and neck. As the estimated circle is progressively bent (beginning at the center of the length of the bar), it is periodically passed over the patient's head and neck to ensure it comfortably encircles the lower cervical area. (Keep in mind the ring diameter will require adjustment in size if padding is applied.) The two straight arms are bent backward, at the midpoint of the aluminum ring. The angle of the bar limbs, relative to the circle, is adjusted to assure the ring seats over the cervical region without compressing or irritating the neck. A second "back bar" is bent in a curve to rest over the mid- to lower lumbar area, anterior to the hind limbs.

(B) The body brace is aligned in place prior to taping the two components together. Note the long arms of the bar run along the mid- to upper third of the lateral thoracic and abdominal walls.

(C) Elasticon (Johnson & Johnson) is used to create an adhesive sling support: bands are secured to one bar and run over the back to the opposite bar. This is alternated with bands placed over the lower thorax and abdomen in a similar fashion.

COMMENTS

Although uncommonly required, the body brace is highly effective in preventing dogs from reaching their hind limbs and perineal area. It is normally reserved for those clever dogs adept at removing Elizabethan collars or bending the collar and contorting their body sufficiently to reach the surgical area. The material costs are relatively modest, but it does take about 30 minutes to properly shape and apply the body brace. The cervical ring and top of the back bar can be lightly padded for added comfort and to compensate for small errors in its design. (Padding is not illustrated in this example.) Surgical tape is spiraled around the ring and back bar to create a nonslip surface prior to applying a layer of cast padding, gauze, and outer wrap (Vetrap, 3M).

Plate 8

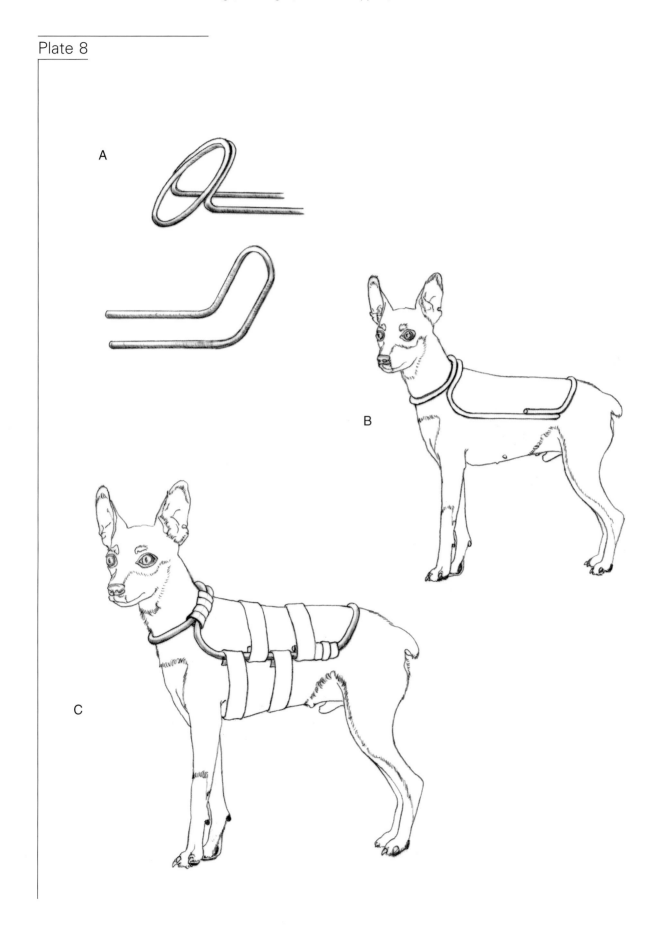

A

B

C

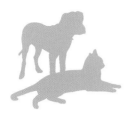

6

Common Complications in Wound Healing

IMPROPER NUTRITIONAL SUPPORT

The majority of our veterinary patients heal in a normal and predictable fashion. As a result of improved health care and nutrition, pets are generally healthier today than at anytime in the past. Despite this, a percentage of pets fall outside this category due to neglect and/or ignorance on the part of the owners. Disease, trauma, and prolonged stress increase the nutritional needs of veterinary patients. A malnourished patient, under these adverse circumstances, is at significant risk for delayed healing with an increased risk of infection.

> The following are common examples of patients that may present malnourished to referral centers:
>
> • Neglected stray animals
> • Animal cruelty/starvation cases
> • Chronic gastrointestinal anomalies/disorders
> • Oral anomalies (major palatal defects, etc.)
> • Advanced neoplasia

The first year of life is particularly critical to the growth and normal development of the dog and cat. Nutritional impairment from congenital defects, disease, or neglect not only restricts growth and development of the patient but also can have serious adverse effects on wound healing. In animals suffering from protein depletion, particularly actively growing animals, impairment of collagen production may delay healing. This has been reported to occur if serum protein concentration falls below 2 g/100 ml. While feeding DL-methionine or cysteine alone can prevent a delay in healing in protein-deficient animals, a balanced nutritious diet is indicated. A plasma protein level of 6.0 g/dl slows healing (normal is 7.0–7.5 g/dl): plasma protein levels below 5.5 g/dl increases the risk of wound disruption by 70%.

Sufficient calories must be provided to help spare body protein from being metabolized to supply amino acids for gluconeogenesis. Glucose is the primary source of energy for fibroblasts and leukocytes and its loss will impair cellular function. Although this breakdown of body protein does yield substrate for wound repair, it places the patient in a harmful state of negative nitrogen balance. In malnourished animals skin and muscle protein is preferentially metabolized. The protein-depleted kitten, puppy, or debilitated geriatric patient is in particular jeopardy of healing complications (Fig. 6-1). It is advisable to delay performing an elective surgical procedure in an undernourished

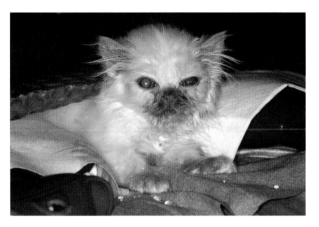

FIG. 6-1 Siamese cat approximately 1 year of age. The patient weighed less than 1 kg. A chronic rhinitis was present as a result of a congenital cleft palate. The poor nutritional status of the patient resulted in serious stunting of growth as noted in the facial features of this adult cat. Any elective surgical procedure should be preceded by a balanced nutritional program to correct the long-standing effects of protein depletion and imbalance.

animal. Prompt enteral or parenteral feeding is particularly important to the seriously ill or injured surgical patient in order to minimize delays in wound healing and reduce the risk of complications during hospitalization. Whether the patient is healthy or malnourished, severe stress, illness, and trauma increase the metabolic demands on the patient and the need for supplemental nutritional support. Urgent or emergency surgical procedures require thoughtful use of surgical materials that will support tissue apposition for prolonged periods of time as a result of a delay in healing. For example, a bowel anastomosis, hernia repair, or routine closure of a laparotomy incision would necessarily require the selection of nonabsorbable (or very slowly absorbed) suture material that would retain tensile strength well beyond the normal range of healing in a healthy patient.

> The following should be considered for prolonged nutritional support for those patients that will not or cannot ingest food to maintain their normal nutritional intake. Selection is based on the specific needs of the patient.
>
> • Esophagostomy tubes
> • Gastrostomy tubes
> • Jejunostomy tubes
> • Pharyngostomy tubes
> • Total or partial parenteral nutrition

Vitamins are essential to proper wound healing. Vitamin C, required for hydroxylation of proline and lysine for collagen synthesis, is normally not required as an exogenous source in the dog and cat. However, supplementation should not be overlooked in severely stressed, debilitated, or traumatized patients with a history of inadequate nutritional support.

Vitamin B_{12} and folate are required for normal protein synthesis, vitamin B_6 is necessary for amino acid metabolism, and iron is required for hemoglobin production and cellular respiration. Excessive vitamin A *labilizes* lysosomes, thereby enhancing inflammation. Vitamin A at high levels can counteract the effects of corticosteroids, which *stabilize* lysosomes. Vitamin E at high levels also stabilizes lysosomes: like cortisone, excessive vitamin E can inhibit wound healing. Vitamin A can counteract the effects of vitamin E, which may or may not be beneficial to a given patient.

Zinc has been reported to be necessary for normal epithelial and fibroblastic proliferation. Absence of trace amounts of zinc slows epithelialization, fibroblast multiplication, and impairs protein synthesis. However, oversupplementation of zinc stabilizes lysosomal and cell membranes and can inhibit macrophage function, thereby reducing phagocytosis. High zinc levels may interfere with collagen cross-linkage. Since small amounts are required for patient health, most balanced diets contain sufficient zinc without the need for additional supplementation.

While the healthy patient normally obtains adequate amounts of these vitamins and elements, the debilitated patient may not be in a position to meet the increased demands of disease, chronic wounds, and previous nutritional inadequacies. In these patients, supplemental water- and fat-soluble vitamins are as essential for a favorable surgical outcome as the caloric and protein supplementation.

MEDICATIONS AND THEIR INFLUENCE ON HEALING

Some medications can interfere with appetite and gastrointestinal function of the patient, thereby reducing the total amount of food ingested and possibly absorbed. Drugs used in veterinary medicine that may have this effect include adrenal corticosteroids, chloramphenicol, sulfonamides, diuretics, salicylates, tetracyclines, and trimethoprim.

Moderate levels of exogenous corticosteroids can have an adverse affect on the early stages of healing, especially administered prior to surgery and over a prolonged period of time. A single dose of corticosteroids will not impair healing. Corticosteroids can reduce vascular permeability; inhibit macrophage migration, fibroplasia, and collagen deposition; and delay angiogenesis. Early suppression of the inflammatory phase of healing delays the subsequent onset of the proliferative and maturation phases of healing. These negative effects are less pronounced if corticosteroids are administered in the latter phases of wound healing. As an immunosuppressant, they have the potential to promote wound infection. If a patient has been on corticosteroids for an extended period of time and requires surgery, nonabsorbable or slowly absorbable suture materials should be considered. Skin sutures or staples should not be removed in 8–10 days: rather, it may be advisable to leave the skin sutures in place for at least 3 weeks as a cautionary measure. An intradermal suture pattern in conjunction with skin sutures or staples also can reduce the risk of dehiscence.

Case Example

At one time, prolonged use of corticosteroids was common in conjunction with laminectomy procedures for patients with thoracolumbar disc disease. There were a few occasions where patients had skin sutures removed 8–10 days postoperatively. As the dogs walked to the owner's vehicle, the skin incision spontaneously separated. Although the patients recovered after resuturing the incisions, this problem could have been avoided.

Leaving sutures in the skin several days beyond the last dose of corticosteroids is a practical option to reduce the risk of wound dehiscence; reinforcing the skin closure with an intradermal pattern provides an added measure of safety.

From the author's experience, leaving sutures in the skin for long periods of time has no adverse effect on the skin, although suture scars may be more pronounced. Epithelial cells will migrate down the suture tract, which may elicit an inflammatory reaction along with the retained suture. In fur-bearing animals, this is normally a minor consideration.

Chemotherapeutic agents in cancer therapy can interfere with B_6, B_{12}, folic acid, ascorbic acid, zinc, and iron metabolism to variable degrees. Prolonged use of these drugs warrants close assessment of the patient's nutritional status and, possibly, nutrient supplementation. Although chemotherapy has the potential to interfere with wound healing, there are no exact wound-healing guidelines pertaining to its use. Again, if a healing delay is of potential concern, use of non- or

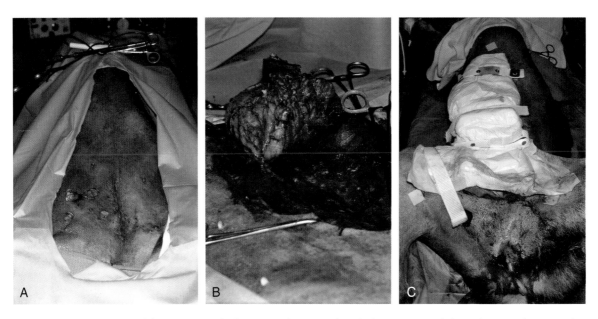

FIG. 6-2 (A) Patient being treated for carcinoma; the biopsy site became infected after initiation of chemotherapy. The patient became profoundly septic. (B) Massive tissue necrosis, secondary to a fulminating infection, necessitated wide excision of necrotic tissue. (C) Initial use of a medicated tie-over dressing secured with skin stretchers (see Chapter 9). The patient died within 24 hours from overwhelming sepsis.

slowly absorbable sutures may be advisable. Like corticosteroids, cytotoxic agents (including cyclophosphamide, methotrexate, and doxorubicin) may exert their greatest negative effect in the early phase of wound healing. Perhaps the greatest concern with drugs that cause immunosuppression is the risk of infection (Fig. 6-2).

Extravasation of chemotherapeutic agents may result in tissue necrosis and wounds that are slow to heal. Doxorubicin, vincristine, and vinblastine are three commonly used drugs known to cause tissue damage that may require surgical debridement and surgical closure of the defect (see Perivascular Injection of Irritating Drugs, below).

HYPOVOLEMIA AND ANEMIA

Dehydration can lead to tissue breakdown, poor appetite, constipation, and renal impairment. Hypovolemia can be particularly devastating to healing by reducing circulation to the wound. Without an adequate blood supply to provide oxygen and nutrients, healing can come to a complete standstill. Surprisingly, anemia must be relatively severe before it has a significant effect on healing as long as blood volume, cardiac output, and the nutrient supply are adequate. Impairment of oxygen delivery has been reported when the hematocrit is below 15%. However, considering blood loss and the dilutional effects associated with intravenous fluid therapy, whole blood transfusion cannot be ruled out based on the initial hematocrit alone.

THE NONHEALING WOUND: GENERAL CONSIDERATIONS

The term *chronic wound* is used to describe wounds that fail to heal in a timely fashion. A variety of factors have the potential to impede key steps in the three phases of wound healing. Successful management requires their identification and elimination.

In otherwise healthy patients, the surgeon has the ability to minimize or eliminate many of the complications noted in wound healing by adhering to the basic surgical principles outline by Halsted and Esmarch (see Chapter 3). Healthy tissue is surprisingly resistant to infection. As previously discussed, the presence of necrotic tissue can have a devastating effect on the wound environment. Dead tissue promotes bacterial infection and delays healing. Surgical closure cannot be performed without completely excising areas of necrotic tissue. Injuries heal more slowly and are more susceptible to infection in the presence of ischemia: minimizing surgical trauma is essential to the promotion of optimal healing.

A necessary component to wound management is proper assessment of the injury and the patient's history to determine whether surgical closure of a wound is the best option. Surgery can bypass the difficulties associated with prolonged management of an open wound. In a debilitated patient, primary closure requires less physiologic effort compared to healing by second intention.

> Neoplasia can be mistaken for a chronic nonhealing wound, abscess, or ulcer. Chronic nonhealing wounds also can result in the development of malignant tumors (e.g., squamous cell carcinoma [Marjolin ulcer] in chronic burn wounds.) If there is any doubt, submit tissue samples for histopathologic examination (Fig. 6-3).

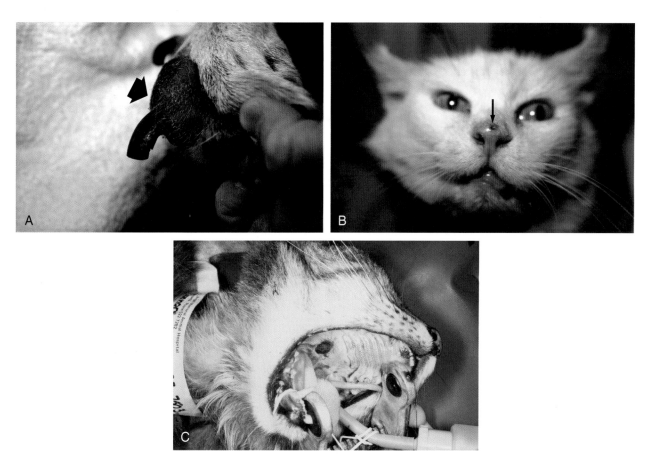

FIG. 6-3 Example of neoplasms mistaken for infection. (A) An acute nail bed infection was later diagnosed as squamous cell carcinoma, with significant bone lysis noted on radiographs.

(B) A cat being treated for a chronic draining abscess beneath the left ear had, in fact, metastatic squamous cell carcinoma to a regional lymph node. The small ulceration on the nose was the primary site of the neoplasm. Squamous epithelium can elicit a foreign body reaction, resulting in abscessation. A secondary bacterial infection, based on culture, masked the underlying cause until biopsies confirmed neoplasia.

(C) This thin geriatric patient was referred for assessment of an ulcer involving the soft palate area. Physical examination detected large, irregular kidneys secondary to renal lymphoma. This case underscores the importance of a complete physical examination.

FAILURE TO HEAL BY SECOND INTENTION

There are a variety of reasons for failure to heal by second intention. Granulation tissue and the processes of wound contraction and epithelialization will be discussed separately.

Problems in Granulation Tissue Formation

A healthy granulation bed is comprised of a well-developed capillary network; fibroblasts, macrophages, and neutrophils; and an extracellular matrix. Granulation tissue develops only from viable vascularized regional tissues. Once formed, the granulation bed affords significant protection from microorganisms that survive on the surface transudate. Its formation is surprisingly rapid in healthy puppies and kittens. In adult animals, early granulation tissue formation may be noted as early as 4–5 days in an uncomplicated open wound. (Chapter 2 details wound healing in the dog and cat.) Granulation tissue serves as a "body putty," filling in gaps within the wound. Collagen deposition increases tensile strength within the area as healing progresses.

In time, capillary channels and fibroplasia subside as collagen content increases in the older wound. In a long-standing open wound, a chronic granulation bed forms, which is poorly suited to healing without appropriate surgical intervention (Fig. 6-4).

> Chronic (collagen laden) granulation tissue is characterized by a dull, pale pink to gray wound bed as a result of a decline in the capillary population. The wound is fibrotic and is an unsuitable wound bed for supporting epithelial cell migration. The collagen dense bed lacks the environment necessary for wound contraction.
>
> If the underlying tissues are healthy, chronic granulation tissue can be excised tangentially: a healthy granulation bed quickly reforms 4–5 days after chronic wound excision (Fig. 6-4).

A healthy granulation bed serves as a vascular scaffold for epithelial cell survival and migration toward the center of the defect. Independently, myofibroblasts within the granulation bed promote wound contraction. Delay in formation of granulation tissue usually is due to a lack of vascularity in the wound bed. Debridement of necrotic tissue, control of local infection, preservation of regional tissue viability, and maintenance of normal cardiovascular output are practical measures to promote a granulation bed.

On occasion, local tissue injury and circulatory compromise may result in a wound area incapable of forming and supporting healthy granulation tissue. A chronic irradiated wound bed is one such example (see Chapter 7). Under these circumstances, local muscle flaps, omental transplantation, or skin flaps (local or axial pattern flaps) may be required since they have an inherent blood supply upon proper elevation and transfer. Muscle flaps and omental flaps are capable of "bringing" new circulation to the area; in turn, the

FIG. 6-4 (A) Dense fibrotic bed involving the antecubital surface of a dog. The pale collagen-laden bed was tangentially excised down to the viable underlying tissues to stimulate formation of a new granulation bed. (B) A healthy vascular granulation bed reformed within 5 days, suitable for closure.

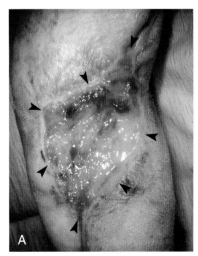
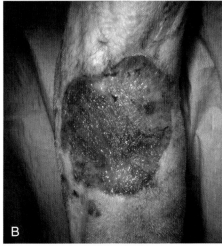

surface of the muscle or omentum can support the survival of a skin graft. However, distant direct flaps and free grafts placed on an ischemic wound cannot survive long term, since their revascularization is dependent on the recipient bed.

Perivascular Injection of Irritating Drugs

Some intravenous drugs are capable of causing extensive tissue trauma and necrosis if accidentally injected into the perivascular tissues (read the drug insert) (Fig. 6-5). The extent of tissue injury is, in part, dependent on the pH, volume, and concentration of the drug. Diluting the offending agent by instilling sterile saline or lactated Ringer's solution into the area is the single best therapeutic measure. Doxirubicin, however, is an exception.

The chemotherapeutic agent doxirubicin is capable of causing massive tissue sloughing; dying cells can release the drug, helping to perpetuate the cycle of tissue destruction. (*Note:* At the time of perivascular injection of doxirubicin, the area should be aseptically prepared for surgery. A skin incision is used to expose the area, allowing for the surgical debridement of the involved tissues, including the infused vein. Skin debridement is kept to a minimum, and open wound management is initiated for several days before closure is attempted.)

The brown recluse spider bite is another example of a toxin capable of destroying tissue and impairing the normal healing process. Debridement of the damaged and necrotic tissue may be advisable to prepare the way for the healing (see Chapter 7).

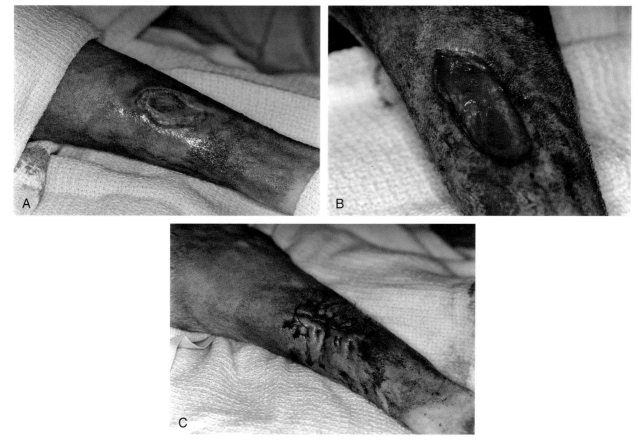

FIG. 6-5 (A) Extravasation of adriamycin, resulting in a nonhealing slough. (B) Excision of necrotic tissue was performed, down to viable tissues. (C) Closure was performed with vertical mattress sutures (3-0 monofilament nylon).

Failure in Wound Contraction

As discussed in Chapter 2, myofibroblasts are responsible for wound contraction. The contractile properties of these cells "pull" the skin toward the center of the defect in a centripetal fashion. Experimentally, square wounds contract more readily than round wounds since the linear borders of skin do not impair skin advancement. By 42 days, wound contraction is nearly complete. Thereafter, the body must rely on epithelialization to close the remaining defect. Wounds on animals less than 1 year of age (especially within the first 6 months of life) demonstrate a remarkably rapid ability to contract.

Keep in mind that wound contraction has a time limitation. As a general rule, the maximal amount of contraction is within 6 weeks of injury. Any remaining defect likely will need to heal by epithelial cell migration after this time. Surgical intervention may be advisable if epithelialization is unlikely to complete this final task.

The two most common factors that halt wound contraction are (1) significant peripheral skin tension (countertension from a lack of loose/elastic skin), which neutralizes myofibroblastic contraction and (2) restrictive fibrosis (within the granulation bed and adjacent skin border), which mechanically impairs skin advancement. A thickened eschar can mechanically "splint" the wound margins and halt contraction. Similarly, rigid adherent hydrocolloid dressings also can impair contraction by preventing the centripetal advancement of the cutaneous margins.

Unless surgical intervention (e.g., flaps, grafts, scar excision, release incisions, cutaneous undermining) is performed, the burden of wound coverage is dependent upon epithelial cell migration alone. Complete epithelialization is not likely to occur in many of the larger defects encountered in small animals.

It also must be kept in mind that excessive contraction and scarring may cause sufficient tissue distortion (e.g., contracture formation) to warrant surgical correction in these situations (see Wound Contracture, below.) Periodic assessment of the patient during the healing process is necessary so that corrective surgery can be performed in a timely fashion.

Wounds that close primarily by wound contraction are far more cosmetically pleasing than defects that heal by epithelial cell migration. Epithelialized scars are thin, hairless, and relatively sensitive to external trauma. Wound contraction literally pulls healthy, fur-bearing skin centripetally, covering the defect. As a result, the cosmetic outcome may be remarkably good.

Failure in Epithelialization

Wound epithelialization is independent of wound contraction. As noted in Chapter 2, cells from the germinal epithelial layer migrate down the dermal edge onto the granulation surface as they extend toward the center of a full-thickness skin defect. Partial-thickness wounds that have viable hair follicles (external root sheaths) are capable of re-epithelializing the exposed dermis. In some situations, deeper hair follicles located in the hypodermis may survive after complete loss of the overlying skin. Small islands of epithelium may be noted as a granulation bed develops during open wound management (see Fig. 2-2).

Epithelial cells require direct contact with a viable vascular tissue bed for survival. Epithelialization occurs optimally in a protective moist environment. Necrotic tissue and dense fibrotic scar tissue are incapable of supporting healthy epithelial coverage without debridement and promotion of a vascularized wound bed. One of the more common factors impairing epithelialization in small animal practice is repeated surface trauma. Improperly applied bandages may abrade the wound surface, preventing normal healing by second intention.

The epithelial layer overlying scar tissue is only a few cell layers thick: this thin layer of coverage is much more susceptible to external trauma compared to normal skin. As a result, epithelialized scars overlying bony prominences and body regions subject to repeated "use and abuse" are susceptible to abrasion and ulceration. Similarly, improperly applied bandages and dressings can abrade migrating epithelial cells from the wound bed during normal body movements. External fixation or immobilization with splints and bandages are occasionally necessary to provide local wound protection for optimal epithelialization.

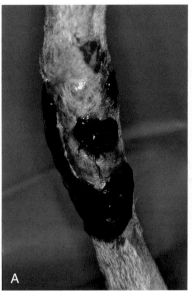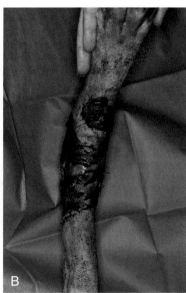

FIG. 6-6 (A) Geriatric German shepherd with nonhealing skin wounds, secondary to vehicular trauma. Contraction and epithelialization failed to close these comparatively small wounds. Multiple topical ointments touted to promote healing failed. Occlusive dressings failed. (B) Closure was accomplished successfully by full-thickness mesh grafting and proper bandage application.

Antecubital wounds are particularly challenging and are quite susceptible to bandage trauma. Flexion of the forelimb places direct bandage pressure over the wound. Rubbing and abrasion to the wound surface occurs during ambulation. Immobilization of the elbow is needed to prevent this problem from occurring.

If second intention closure fails, a local skin flap often can be used to effectively close these small but problematic skin wounds.

The optimal period for an open wound to heal by second intention is finite; repeated interference or insults in the wound-healing process will result in the formation of an indolent ulcer (Fig. 6-6). The use of exogenous growth factors, and more effective topical agents that "stimulate" growth factor production may provide a future role in the closure of many problematic wounds (see Chapter 2, Chapter 4, and Chapter 5). Until then, there are a variety of effective surgical options to close these challenging defects.

Indolent "Pocket" Wounds

On occasion, skin wounds fail to contract and epithelialize despite the presence of a healthy granulation bed surrounded by pliable skin. The surrounding skin remains separated from the underlying muscle fascia despite the formation of granulation tissue on opposing surfaces. The wound forms a pocket or pouch beneath the skin margin. These indolent wounds are most commonly seen in the cat.

Normal wound contraction and epithelialization cannot occur properly because the elevated skin has not attached to the granulation surface overlying the body surface. Healing quickly reaches an impasse. Myofibroblastic contraction is limited to the skin margins, causing the cutaneous surface to curl inward on itself. Similarly, epithelial cells migrate down the inner (granulation-covered) dermal surface. The inguinal, axillary, and flank areas appear to be especially prone to pocket formation. Why the dermal surface and underlying granulation bed fail to heal together remains uncertain. Infection with enzymatic fibrinolysis may destroy this component of the extracellular matrix necessary for fibroblast migration and collagen deposition. Motion between the surfaces also may impair healing of the two granulation surfaces.

Successful closure of indolent wounds is possible using a few basic surgical techniques, depending on the size and location of the defect. Any infection must be addressed with appropriate wound care and topical/systemic antibiotic therapy. Dead space after closure is best controlled with a vacuum drain: evacuation of residual air and fluid by the vacuum will draw the wound surfaces together. The fibrotic epithelialized skin margins are excised. If sufficient skin is present, the skin margins can be sutured together to close the defect. If the underlying dermal collagen surface is impairing skin elasticity, carefully placed *release* incisions can be used to divide the restrictive dermal granulation surface. Incising the restrictive "dermal scar" surface requires a delicate touch, using

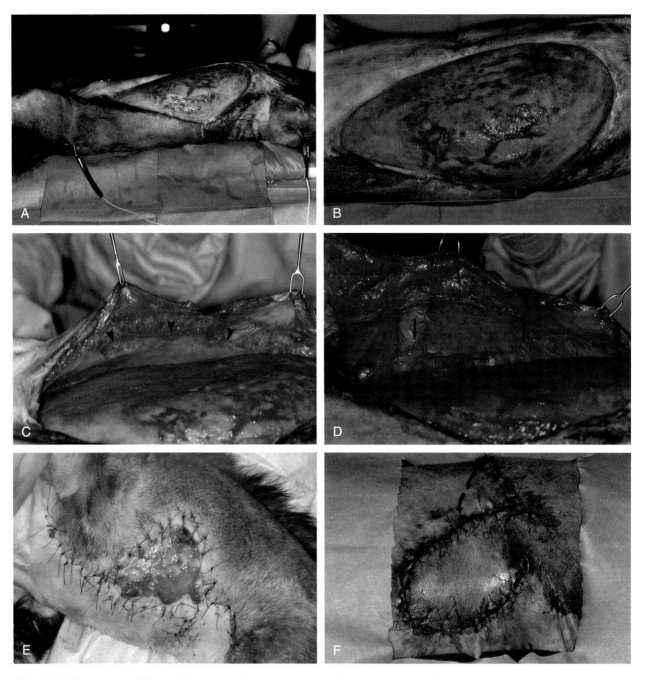

FIG. 6-7 (A) Example of a feline indolent pocket ulcer secondary to a bite wound sustained 6 months previously.

(B) The nonhealing wound involving the ventral thorax and abdomen.

(C) After topical antimicrobial management, 48 hours prior to surgery, the patient was anesthetized. Note the subcutaneous pocket lined by a flat granulation bed.

(D) Release incisions were made in horizontal and vertical directions through the restricting membranous connective tissue layer, with care taken to avoid division of direct cutaneous vessels in the overlying subcutis.

(E) The wound was primarily closed. However, because of excessive tension, a portion of the wound was left open, although skin borders were sutured directly to the granulation bed.

(F) When contraction and epithelialization failed to occur after 1 month, a transposition flap was rotated into position to successfully complete the closure (See Fig. 5-11).

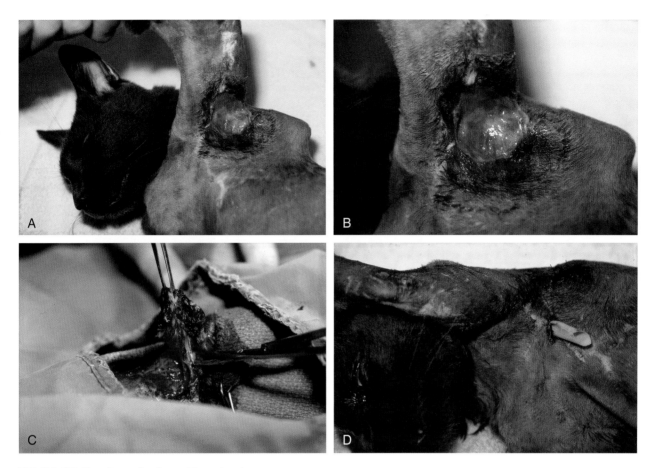

FIG. 6-8 (A) Chronic, nonhealing axillary ulcer in a cat.

(B) Close-up view of this chronic granulation bed.

(C) En bloc excision of the entire wound bed, down to healthy tissue.

(D) The skin margins were carefully undermined: interrupted intradermal sutures were followed by the use of vertical mattress and simple interrupted monofilament 3-0 nylon sutures. The key to successful closure of axillary wounds includes (1) minimal skin tension, (2) use of a two-layer closure to maintain accurate apposition, (3) accurate skin apposition, and (4) cage confinement of the cat to minimize activity for 1 month postoperatively. (Cats often prefer a small box they can crawl into for privacy, thereby reducing their activity level.) Transposition flaps are useful to close more problematic wounds. It is the author's experience that omental flaps are not necessary to close these challenging wounds.

a no. 15 scalpel blade: the granulation surface is lightly incised until the overlying subcutaneous fat is seen. Care is taken to avoid a deeper incision that may compromise circulation to the skin. Successful division of the scar surface will result in widening of the surgical gap as the skin is retracted. A series of parallel and perpendicular grid incisions can be used to improve skin advancement to close the defect. Skin margins must be sutured directly to each other or firmly anchored to the granulation bed to promote wound closure (Fig. 6-7).

Local skin flaps or axial pattern flaps are practical choices when primary closure cannot be achieved by scar release and skin advancement (Fig. 6-8). Skin grafts also are a consideration when skin flaps are not feasible. As discussed in Chapter 10, elastic skin stretchers can be used to prestretch skin in combination with scar release to achieve closure.

In more difficult wounds, omentum (see Plate 128) passed through a slit created in the abdominal wall can be used to manage problematic pocket wounds: the omentum obliterates the cavity and is a supplemental source of circulation to the area. While omentalization of feline axillary wounds has been reported, the author has not found this technique necessary.

SCARRING AND WOUND CONTRACTURE

Formation of scar tissue is a normal response to healing. While scarring is beneficial in some injuries, its formation in other wounds is undesirable. Formation of granulation tissue and deposition of collagen is desirable for many shearing injuries involving the carpal or tarsal joints. Collagen deposition improves joint stability and creates a soft tissue surface promoting closure of the defect. Large skin defects, particularly those involving flexion surfaces (usually of the extremities), may result in restrictive scar formation during second intention healing. The term *wound contracture* implies a loss or restriction of motion and function to an area (e.g., joint), usually as a result of excessive scarring. Muscle atrophy and fibrosis also may contribute to contracture formation. Infection can prolong the inflammatory response and further contribute to scar tissue deposition.

> Large skin wounds involving a flexion surface are most susceptible to contracture formation. From the author's experience, this is most evident when dealing with large skin defects involving the popliteal area.
>
> Patients will naturally hold the involved area in flexion, which decreases pain by reducing the surface area exposed to the environment and reduces movement.
>
> Unfortunately, collagen deposition "connects" the contact surfaces of the wound, resulting in contracture formation. Surgical division of the scar followed by closure of the skin defect usually prevents contracture recurrence. Physical therapy can be useful in accelerating recovery.

Prevention of wound contracture requires early recognition of the developing problem and the proper steps to combat it. In veterinary medicine, early appropriate coverage of open wounds with skin flaps and related Z-plasty techniques or by free grafts, followed by physical therapy, can *prevent* wound contracture. Scar excision, partial myotomies, flap or free graft coverage, and physical therapy may be required once a contracture has developed (Fig. 6-9 and 6-10). Temporary traction or splintage to the area occasionally is used to combat recurrence until healing is complete and physical therapy can be implemented. Physical therapy can be effective in modifying collagen deposition and cross-linkage to improve mobility of the affected region. Early resumption of normal physical activity in a staged fashion generally is the best form of physical therapy for veterinary patients.

INFECTION

Bacterial infection results in the release of toxins and associated inflammatory infiltrates that can result in cell death and vascular thrombosis. Resistance to infection and promotion of healing critically depends upon maintaining adequate circulation to the wound. Delivery of antibiotics also depends on maintaining perfusion to the compromised tissues. Infection can be considered as an imbalance between bacterial population and virulence versus host resistance. The mere presence of organisms is less important than the level of bacterial growth. Bacterial growth greater than 100,000 organisms (10^5) per gram of tissue is necessary to cause wound infection. Although surgeons cannot alter systemic host defense factors in many trauma cases presented, they can play a significant role in adversely affecting local wound properties that can promote infection and deter host defense mechanisms in the wound.

> Quantitative cultures, based on the gram weight of tissue samples submitted, is an experimental gold standard of confirming infection. Clinically, this technique is rarely used or needed. Its use may be limited to particularly problematic wounds, the identified presence of resistant/virulent organisms, and in debilitated-immunocompromised patients.

Although a laceration and puncture wound may have the same degree of tissue injury, the environment of each wound is vastly different. Open wounds rarely are the source of invasive infection. A puncture wound lacking drainage forms a closed, hypoxemic pocket that provides an ideal environment for bacterial proliferation unless steps are taken to prevent

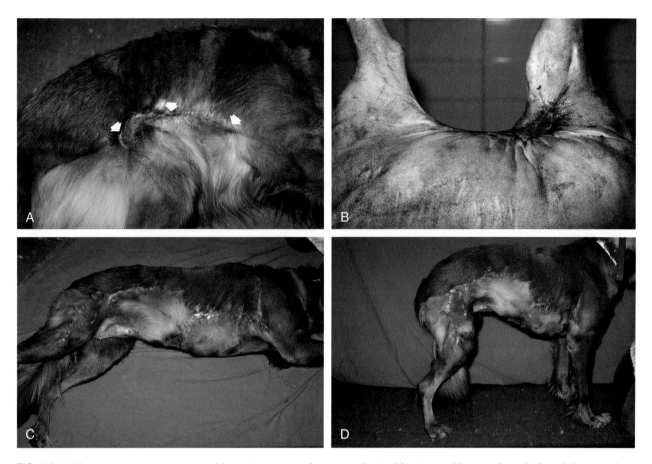

FIG. 6-9 (A) Bowstring contracture in a golden retriever secondary to an electrical heating pad burn to the right lateral thorax and abdomen. Healing was incomplete after 1 year.

(B) The restrictive scar seriously impeded use of the involved limbs.

(C, D) Following surgical removal of the scar tissue, the large defect was closed with a series of skin flaps, including the caudal superficial epigastric axial pattern flap. Note restoration of the range of motion to the right forelimb and hind limb.

infection (open, lavage, debride, establish drainage) (Fig. 6-11). Chronic infections can be more problematic to manage as a result of the prolonged inflammatory response and fibrosis associated with this condition.

Systemic (prophylactic) antibiotics have potential value to blunt the occurrence of infection if tissue levels can be achieved within 4 hours of wounding. After this time, bacterial lodgement will occur: antibiotics at this point generally are ineffective in preventing infection. Cases of cellulitis associated with early bacterial colonization may respond to antibiotics, whereas a purulent discharge or abscess (loculation) requires the wound to be opened for inspection, lavage, debridement, and drainage.

Bacterial Cellulitis: Treat with Antibiotics?

Whether or not to treat bacterial cellulitis with antibiotics is a common clinical question. In the presence of a foreign body, abscess formation will inevitably result following cessation of antibiotic therapy. *Early* cellulitis without foreign bodies may be more responsive to antibiotics than cases of advanced cellulitis, in which edema, inflammation, and fibrosis are noted during examination (palpation, ultrasonography). In the latter case, infection is coalescing into an abscess: warm compresses alone (usually for 12–24 hours) may be considered to facilitate abscess formation. Surgical drainage, bacterial cultures, debridement, lavage, topical therapy, and systemic antibiotics can then effectively resolve the definable abscess.

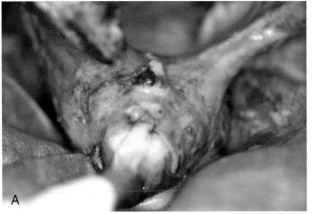

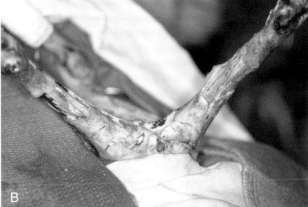

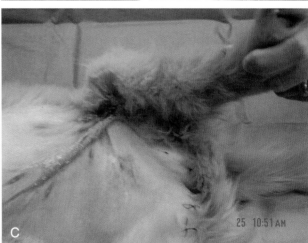

FIG. 6-10 (A) Note contractures behind each knee of a cat, secondary to extensive burns. Contractures were managed by incising the scar, thereby "releasing" the restrictive tissue bands. (B) A no. 15 scalpel blade was used to make "feather light" incisions through the restrictive granulation layer without damaging the underlying musculature. Traction is applied to straighten the leg as the scar bed is incised. A mesh graft was successfully applied to each site. A spica splint was used to keep each limb extended and immobilized (see also Figs. 5-9 and 5-22).
(C) A second example of wound contracture in a gold retriever puppy. The dog fell onto a sump pump motor, burning the left inner thigh on the exposed hot metal. A severe contracture restricted motion of the left hind limb and contributed to severe angular limb deformities that necessitated its amputation.

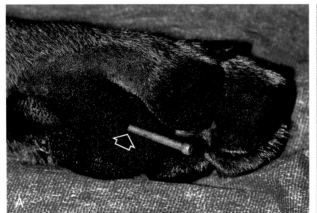

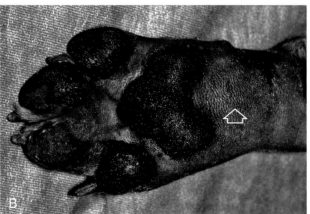

FIG. 6-11 (A) Finishing nail driven deeply through the metacarpal pad (arrow). (B) A severe cellulitis culminated into an abscess proximal to the metacarpal pad (arrow). The area proximal to the metacarpal and metatarsal pads is a common area for abscesses to "point."

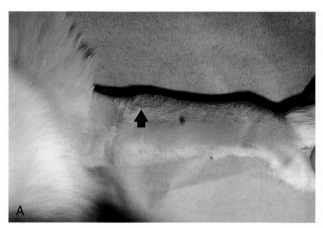 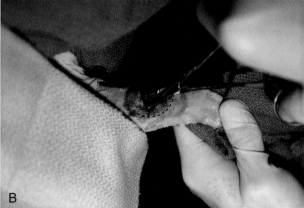

FIG. 6-12 (A) Abscess as a result of a bite wound from another cat. (B) After sterile surgical preparation, a scalpel blade was inserted into the dependent area of the abscess. Pus was evacuated followed by insertion of a hemostat to gently explore and examine the cavity. A few millimeters of skin were excised (dotted line) to enlarge the drainage site.

Abscesses

Abscess formation is common in dogs and cats. Cat abscesses are commonly the result of bite wounds from other cats. The small puncture holes readily seal, and the closed wound pocket is an ideal incubator for bacterial infection. Common examples of infectious microorganisms include *Staphylococcus* spp. (including MRSA—methacillin resistant *Staphylococcus aureus*—commonly pronounced as "mersah"), *Streptococcus* sp, and *Pseudomonas* sp. *Pasteurella* spp is a common oral contaminant in small animals and frequently is responsible for bite wound infections. Uncommonly seen, other infections include norcardiosis, actinomycosis, and atypical mycobacterial infections.

Areas of cellulitis eventually coalesce to form the abscess cavity. Abscesses are drained ventrally once they have "pointed." Warm compresses can facilitate their coalescence. Many of the smaller abscesses in small animals readily respond to this regimen followed by gentle exploration, flushing, debridement, and systemic broad-spectrum antibiotic support for 7 to 10 days (Fig. 6-12). Warm compresses, as discussed below, are useful to promote drainage, maintain cleanliness to the area, improve regional circulation, and promote healing.

Cervical-pharyngeal abscesses in the dog are most commonly seen in the late summer/early fall in New England. They are usually attributed to dogs eating stiff, dry blades of grass, fragments of which perforate the pharyngeal mucosa and migrate into the cranial cervical region. This abscess is characterized by a rapidly forming, firm edematous swelling. (Many patients have a history of chewing wood and grass.) A variation of this condition is the retrobulbar abscess. With retention of this plant material, infection commonly recurs with antibiotic therapy alone. In these cases, the abscess should be opened, explored, debrided, lavaged and drained. (In a low percentage of these cases, the grass fragment can be identified floating in the pus being evacuated from the abscess cavity.) Owners are informed that recurrent abscess formation is likely if any foreign debris remains (Fig. 6-13).

Larger abscess cavities can be packed open for 2 or 3 days with moistened medicated cotton gauze packs, changed two or three times daily over a 3- to 5-day period. Partial drying of the pack facilitates the absorption of the discharge and helps to strip out necrotic tissue adhered to the cotton fibers (Fig. 6-13). Other

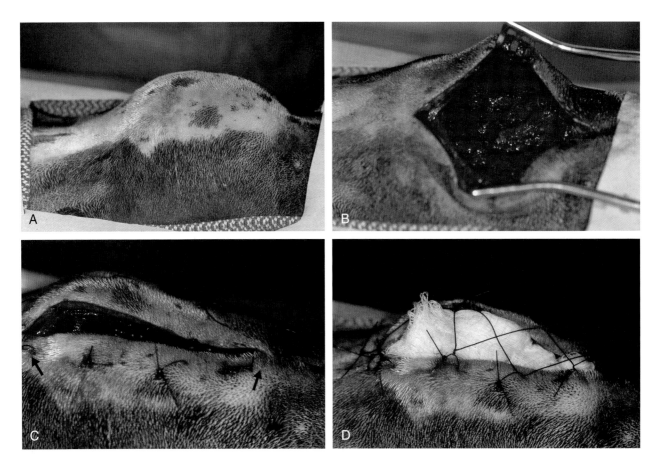

FIG. 6-13 (A) Deep ventral cervical abscess from a migrating fragment of grass. In New England, cervical abscesses are most commonly seen in the late summer and early fall. The dry grass tips are stiffer, facilitating oral mucosal penetration and perforation.
(B) The abscess cavity was explored, lavaged, and suctioned. Surgical debridement also was performed.
(C) The cranial and caudal wound borders were partially closed, and this was followed by the placement of suture loops around the periphery of the wound (arrows).
(D) Tie-over dressing. A medicated wet dressing was inserted into the cavity and secured by lacing suture material through opposing loops. Wet-to-dry dressings were used to mechanically debride the cavity for 48 hours. Thereafter, sutures were placed through opposing loops to loosely approximate wound edges. It is important to count the number of gauze sponges used to pack wound cavities in order to prevent their accidental retention into the healing wound.

useful packing materials include alginate dressings and absorptive foam pads after surgical exploration-debridement. Thereafter, periodic warm compresses (three times daily for 10–15 minutes) are followed by the application of a topical antimicrobial agent to protect the developing granulation bed from desiccation until second intention healing is complete. In some deeper body abscesses, closed vacuum drains can be effectively employed to remove pus and inflam-

matory tissue fluids for several days, but only after necrotic tissue and any foreign debris have been removed to help ensure their more effective use (See Fig. 4-7).

Culture and sensitivity testing and Gram stains usually are not warranted for the smaller abscesses seen in small animal practice: deep abscesses, recurrent infections, persistent or recurrent draining tracts, and potentially life-threatening infections do

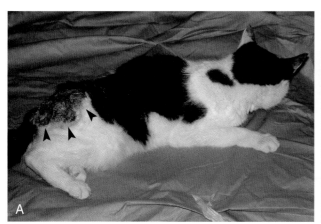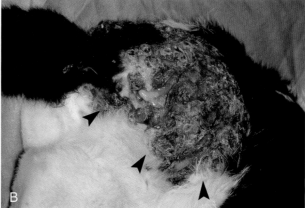

FIG. 6-14 (A) Diffuse suppurative abscesses involving the skin and subcutis of a domestic short hair. (B) Close-up view revealed multiple small abscesses coalescing and interconnecting through numerous tracts. Histopathologic analysis and aerobic and anaerobic cultures were submitted revealing *Nocardia asteroides*. The patient was negative for feline infectious peritonitis, toxoplasmosis, and feline leukemia virus.

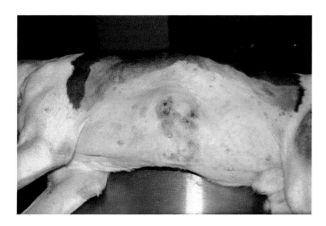

FIG. 6-15 Multiple draining tracts entering the thoracic wall of a walker hound (hunting dog). Diagnosis was actinomycosis secondary to imbedded wood fragments.

warrant these additional diagnostic techniques. These clinical observations should alert the practitioner that the condition is not a "minor" local infection, but one that warrants a detailed clinical work-up, examination, and, if necessary, surgical exploration (Fig. 6-14 and 6-15). Aerobic and possibly anaerobic cultures should be submitted for bacterial analysis under these circumstances. The most effective method of obtaining an accurate culture from an infected pocket is by taking a sample of the abscess wall for culture. Deep aspiration of the cavity is preferable in order to obtain a representative culture. Cultures obtained from the purulent drainage are more likely to contain bacterial contaminants rather than the primary organism responsible for infection.

Fungal infections can mimic bacterial infections, and culture and biopsy samples should be taken when this condition is suspected. Fungal infections have a regional incidence pattern in the United States (Fig. 6-16). A detailed patient history should include the pet's travel history.

Fungal Infections
- Blastomycosis
- Coccidioidomycosis
- Histoplasmosis
- Mycetomas
- Phaeohyphomycosis
- Pythiosis
- Sporotrichosis
- Zygomycosis

As discussed, neoplasia with an ongoing infection can be diagnosed with the submission of appropriate biopsy samples. Immunosuppression by various chemotherapeutic agents or underlying disease (e.g., feline leukemia, feline infectious peritonitis) may explain an animal's susceptibility to infection and poor healing, and these possibilities should be investigated. Autoimmune disorders and immune-mediated vasculitis can present as a cellulitis with progressive necrosis. Appropriate diagnostic tests (antinuclear antibody [ANA], direct antiglobulin test, Coombs test) should be performed (Fig. 6-17).

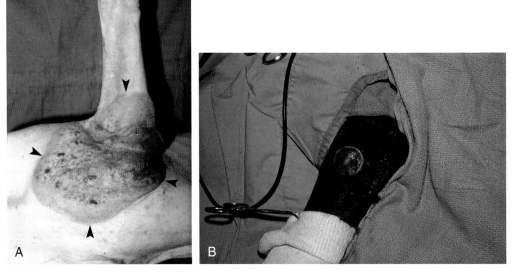

FIG. 6-16 (A) Large granulomatous mass with multiple draining tracts involving the axilla and inner brachium of a malamute. Histopathologic analysis of biopsy samples revealed phycomycosis. Deep, wide excision and closure with a thoracodorsal axial pattern flap was curative. (From Pavletic MM, MacIntire D. 1982. Phycomycosis of the axilla and inner brachium in a dog: surgical excision and reconstruction with a thoracodorsal axial pattern flap. *J Am Vet Med Assoc* 180:1197.)

(B) Expanding, ulcerated mass overlying the lateral aspect of the left elbow. Histopathologic analysis revealed cutaneous histoplasmosis; thoracic radiographs were within normal limits in this young Labrador retriever. Surgical excision was curative.

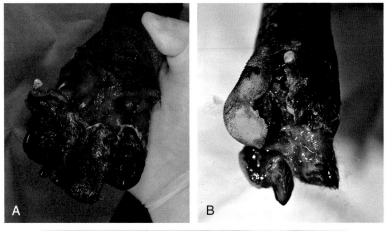

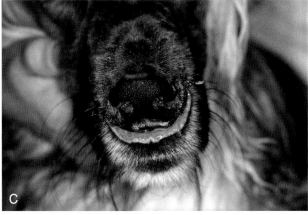

FIG. 6-17 (A, B) Two case examples of immune-mediated vasculitis resulting in loss of digits to the hind limbs. Both patients were positive on the Coombs test and for the presence of antinuclear antibodies. (See foot pad salvage techniques in Chapter 18.) (C) Infarction and mummification of the entire cartilaginous external nose secondary to immune-mediated vasculitis.

DRAINING TRACTS

Persistent or intermittent sinus tracts have been seen with the presence of necrotic tissue that cannot be expelled by the body; osteomyelitis and bone sequestra; bone fragments harboring bacteria; bacterial or fungal organisms resistant to the current treatment regimen; and foreign bodies (grass fragments, wood, grass awns, porcupine quills [see Chapter 7], etc.). These tracts also occur in conjunction with tooth fragments retained in the patient (especially between the radius and ulna); surgical foreign bodies such as implants or braided nonabsorbable suture material (silk, Vetafil, cotton, polyester, etc.; Fig. 6-18A,B); and neoplastic conditions (with or without the presence of microorganisms) that mimic infection or foreign bodies. A sinus tract is essentially a fibrotic tunnel lined by granulation tissue, allowing accumulated discharge from around the offending object to exit via the skin surface. Occasionally the inciting cause may extrude spontaneously with resolution of the sinus

tract infection. In most cases, surgery is required to locate and remove the retained material.

> Although uncommon today, braided nonabsorbable suture materials used in ovariohysterectomies have the potential of initiating a draining tract. Tracts involving the ovarian pedicle normally drain through the sublumbar area; the uterine pedicle may form tracts exiting the caudal abdominal area. Surgical correction requires removal of all suture material fragments.

Radiographs occasionally reveal radiopaque objects amenable to removal. Contrast studies (fistulogram or sinogram) occasionally are useful in highlighting foreign bodies, determining the magnitude of the tract(s), and examining their relationship with regional anatomy (Fig. 6-18C). Ultrasonography may be useful in select cases. Although cannulation and injection of

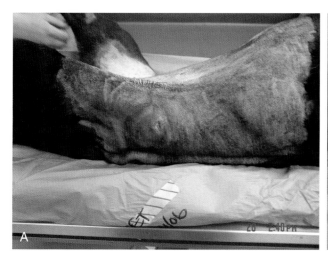
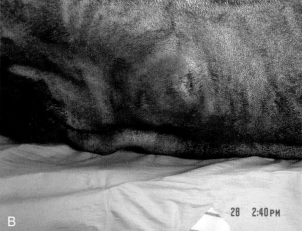
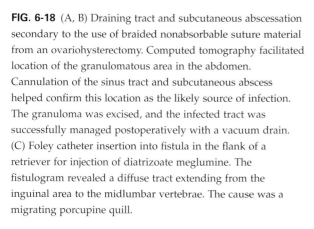
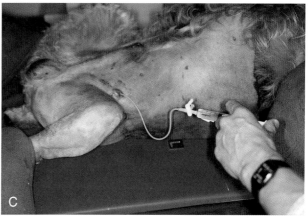

FIG. 6-18 (A, B) Draining tract and subcutaneous abscessation secondary to the use of braided nonabsorbable suture material from an ovariohysterectomy. Computed tomography facilitated location of the granulomatous area in the abdomen. Cannulation of the sinus tract and subcutaneous abscess helped confirm this location as the likely source of infection. The granuloma was excised, and the infected tract was successfully managed postoperatively with a vacuum drain. (C) Foley catheter insertion into fistula in the flank of a retriever for injection of diatrizoate meglumine. The fistulogram revealed a diffuse tract extending from the inguinal area to the midlumbar vertebrae. The cause was a migrating porcupine quill.

dyes such as sterilized methylene blue can stain the tracts, facilitating their removal, the author has not considered this technique useful or necessary (Fig. 6-19). Deep wound biopsy cultures should be obtained for aerobic and anaerobic microorganisms. Fungal cultures also should be considered based on geographic location and historic exposure.

Definitions to Remember

Sinus: A canal or passage leading to an abscess.

Fistula: An abnormal tubelike passage from a normal cavity or tube to a free surface or to another cavity. They may be the result of a congenital anomaly, trauma, infection, or other inflammatory processes.

Foreign bodies can be elusive by migrating through tissue planes or they can be hidden by layers of scar tissue and necrotic debris (Fig. 6-20). The most direct approach is to cannulate the tract and dissect around the tract while minimizing spillage of its contaminated contents into the neighboring tissues. Dissection is extended down to the base or origin of the sinus tract and the entire area excised. Upon completion of the surgical procedure, the excised tissue is open and examined, culture samples are taken, and the tissue submitted for histopathologic examination.

Many surgical implants have the potential to develop draining tracts, secondary to tissue irritation, foreign body reaction, and/or secondary infection.

The accidental retention of Penrose drains or fragments of the drain will initiate a foreign body reaction and formation of a sinus tract. Radiographs normally will highlight these radiopaque drains. Their removal is normally curative (Fig. 6-21).

Dermal Sinuses

A pilonidal sinus (dermoid sinus) is a congenital defect in which ectodermal cells fail to cleanly separate from the neural tissue during embryogenesis. As a result, an epithelial tube forms below the skin surface to variable depths; in extreme cases it can extend to the dura mater. Because the sinus tract is lined by cutaneous epithelium, hair and epithelial debris will accumulate in the tract and elicit a foreign body reaction. Bacteria can secondarily infect the sinus tract, compounding the problem. Although rare, for those cases in which the sinus attaches to the dura mater, a septic meningitis and the onset of neurologic signs may be noted.

Rhodesian ridgebacks most commonly present with this condition, and it is considered a simple recessive mode of inheritance (Fig. 6-22). However, the

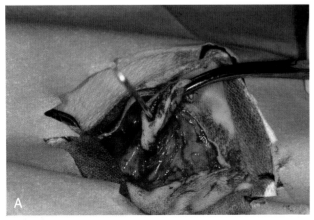
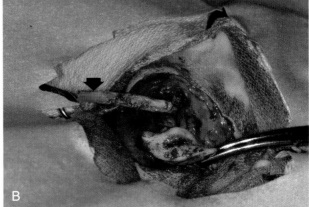

FIG. 6-19 (A) Case example of plant material causing a draining tract. Chronic draining tract caudal to the left mandible. A fistulogram demonstrated a linear object medial to the digastricus muscle. A metallic probe was inserted into the tract, serving as a guide during surgical dissection. (B) The tract led to a small cavity containing several fragments of plant material. The owner later reported the cat had a habit of chewing on a broom used for sweeping ashes from the fireplace. Surgeons must look closely for more than one foreign body, as this case demonstrated.

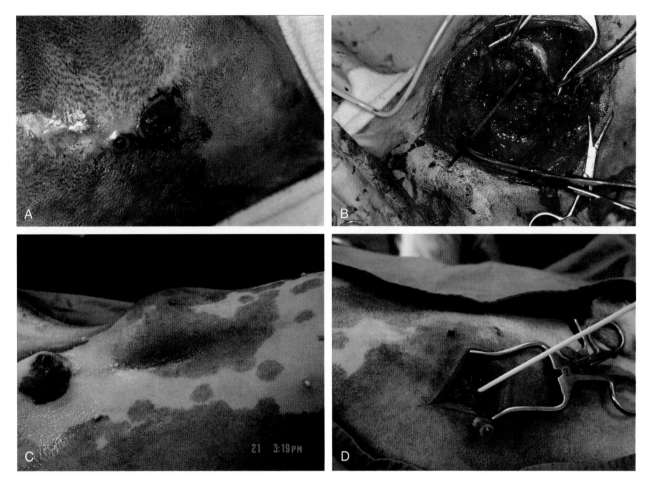

FIG. 6-20 Two case examples of migrating teriyaki sticks. (A) Chronic draining tract overlying the sternal area in a boxer. Previous attempts to locate the source of the infection failed to locate the cause.

(B) Careful dissection of the draining tract uncovered a "teriyaki" bamboo stick of the sort the owner frequently used for barbecuing. The migrating stick was firmly lodged in thoracic cavity muscle and fascia adjacent to the sternum. The bamboo shaft likely migrated through the esophagus. The author has removed similar sticks from the abdominal cavity and retroperitoneal space that migrated through the gastric wall, resulting in abscess formation.

(C) Lower abdominal wall abscess. Ultrasonography noted a 5-cm linear foreign body.

(D) Insertion of a hypodermic needle to locate the depth of the abscess cavity after surgical preparation of the area. The needle is left in place, serving as a guide for surgical incision. The white pointer denotes the outer abscess wall.

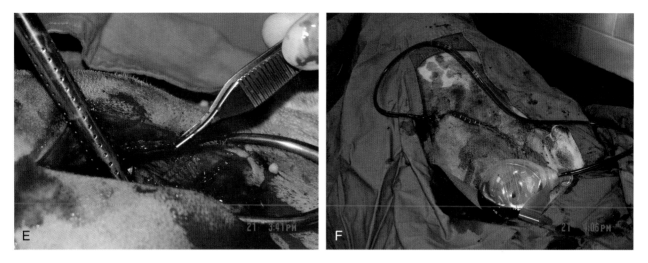

FIG. 6-20 *Continued* (E) The abscess pocket was suctioned; digital palpation located the teriyaki stick segment, and forceps were used to remove this foreign body.

(F) After flushing and suctioning the abscess cavity, the wound was closed, using a vacuum drain. The patient healed uneventfully.

Note: The author strongly advises owners to immediately dispose of teriyaki sticks by placing them in a secure refuse container. Dogs love to chew on the sticks, which absorb the flavor of the meat and marinade. Teriyaki sticks can perforate the gastrointestinal tract or esophagus and migrate to a variety of body regions. Please see suggested readings: Hunt et al. 2004, Pennick and Mitchell 2003, and Walmsley et al. 2009.

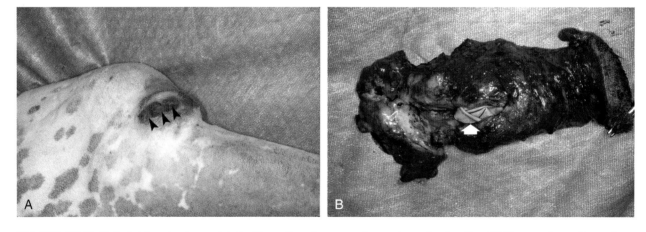

FIG. 6-21 (A) Multiple fistulous tracts associated with an elbow hygroma of several months duration. (B) Preoperative radiographs taken to assess the underlying bone demonstrated a radiopaque Penrose drain retained in the granulomatous mass (arrow). Excision of the large granuloma and drain (from a previous surgical attempt to manage the elbow hygroma) was curative.

condition also has been reported in other dog breeds, including the boxer, chow chow, English bulldog, shih tzu, Siberian husky, and springer spaniel. (The author has removed one pilonidal sinus from the dorsum of the head of a black Labrador retriever, with the winding tract terminating at the level of the occipital crest.) The mode of inheritance in these breeds is unknown. In Rhodesian ridgebacks, the sinus opening is usually found along the spinal column and normally opens in the midst of a whorl of hair. Palpation of the subcutaneous tissues between the thumb and index finger often reveals a cordlike structure extending into the deeper tissues.

Radiographs can be taken to assess the underlying spinal column. Contrast studies have been suggested to outline the extent of the tract, although filling of the cavity with a contrast medium can be problematic due to the accumulation of discharge and tissue debris. If neurologic signs are present, CT and MRI are advisable to assess the extent of the condition prior to surgery.

Surgical excision is the best course of managing a pilonidal sinus. The area should be liberally clipped to compensate for the occasionally irregular course of the tract. A circular skin incision is made around the sinus opening; skin incisions can be used to simplify exposure of the deeper aspects of the sinus tract. Most pilonidal sinuses tend to taper as dissection progresses into the deeper tissues (Fig. 6-22). Insertion of a feline urinary catheter or metallic probe can orient the surgeon during this process. Self-retaining retractors improve visualization of the deeper portions of the tract. If the sinus extends to the dura mater, a small dorsal laminectomy may be needed to assure that complete removal of the sinus is accomplished. A culture of the deeper portion of the sinus tract is advisable in the face of infection; broad-spectrum antibiotic therapy can be initiated pending the final culture results.

In general, it has been the author's experience that removal of most pilonidal sinuses is not difficult surgery, but complete removal of the entire tract is critical for a successful outcome.

Nasal Dermoid Sinus Cyst

Nasal dermoid sinus cysts (NDSCs) are uncommon congenital lesions similar to the embryologic origin of the pilonidal sinus. NDSC is recognized in golden retrievers. During embryologic development, the meninges in the frontal bones protrude through the foramen cecum. This canal normally closes, but persists in NDSC cases. As a result, a sinus opening can be found in the dorsal midline of the skull, caudal to the external nares. The sinus passes through an incomplete suture line in the nasal septum. In the young adult golden retriever with NDSC, a sebaceous discharge may be noted caudal to the nasal planum. Surgical removal is indicated, with the assistance of a probe or catheter to facilitate dissection of the entire tract. Communication with the meninges has been reported in humans; although meningitis has been reported in humans, it has not been reported in the dog to date.

USE OF TOURNIQUETS FOR LOWER EXTREMITY PROCEDURES

A tourniquet is useful in creating a bloodless field for exploration of draining tracts for foreign bodies in the limbs of small animal patients. However, tourniquets should be avoided in traumatized limbs or limbs with vascular injury or circulatory compromise. Pneumatic tourniquets are the best available method of applying uniform pressure to a wide area. Venous blood is expelled prior to tourniquet application by elevating the affected limb for 5 minutes.

An Esmarch bandage or elastic wrap can be used as a short-term tourniquet by applying it from the digits proximally without excessive tension (or tissue compression). An Esmarch bandage can be used alone or in conjunction with a pneumatic cuff. Exsanguination should not be done in the presence of local suppuration, deep venous thrombosis, or neoplasia. A thin layer of cotton padding may be applied before wrapping the limbs for more uniform pressure distribution. The elastic wrap is removed upon inflation of the pneumatic cuff. The cuff is positioned at the point of maximal limb circumference where the bulk of the muscle protects underlying nerves and vessels from compression over bone.

Tourniquets are not without risk. Muscle ischemia, nerve palsies, and tissue necrosis may result from improper application or prolonged usage of tourniquets. When using a pneumatic cuff, pressure should be kept to the minimum required to provide a bloodless field; pressures greater than 300 mm Hg should be avoided. While a properly applied tourniquet can be applied for up to 3 hours, the surgeon should minimize its usage. Some recommend releasing the tourniquet 10 minutes for every hour of inflation, although the benefits of this maneuver are questionable. Fortunately, most cases of tract exploration involving the extremities can be performed within 30 to 45 minutes.

Vetrap (3M Corp.) can be autoclaved and used effectively as a short-term tourniquet to obtain a

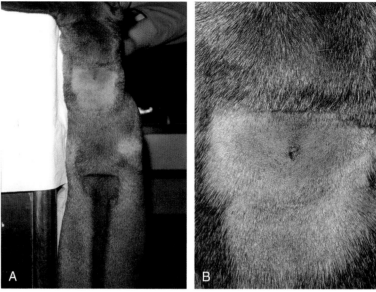

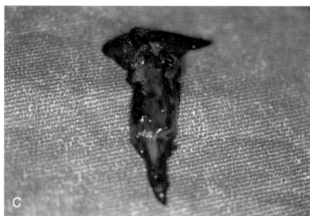

FIG. 6-22 (A) Pilonidal sinus in a Rhodesian ridgeback. (B) Close-up view of the tract. (C) The tract was cannulated with a tom-cat catheter to outline the tract. A circular incision was made around the sinus tract; skin incisions can be used to improve exposure. The entire sinus "cylinder" progressively tapered and ended dorsal to the vertebral surface. Epithelium, hair, and tissue debris are commonly observed when the tract is dissected open.

relatively bloodless surgical field. After wrapping the limb, beginning at the toes and working proximally, scissors can be used to cut the Vetrap and expose the surgical area for exploration. Care must be taken to avoid excessive elastic tension during application and minimize the time of application, as discussed above.

SEROMAS

Seromas are pockets in which serum accumulates, usually as a result of trauma. Seroma formation is most commonly associated with surgery, especially in areas where considerable dissection has been performed, leaving a dead space or pocket where serum can accumulate. Capillary leakage and lymphatic injury secondary to inflammation result in fluid accumulation. Traumatic surgical technique, harsh wound-cleansing techniques, the presence of foreign debris and irritants,

and areas subject to constant movement also contribute to seroma formation. Small seromas beneath the skin are of no major consequence and resolve in time. Larger seromas on many occasions will require drainage (in Chapter 4, see the sections Passive Drains and Active Drains). Postoperative seroma of an abdominal incision may be difficult to distinguish from a hernia. Careful aspiration can help confirm a seroma; removal of the fluid can facilitate palpation of the abdominal incision for any hernia ring or herniated tissue in the area.

Microscopic examination of fluid from a seroma normally shows a variable number of red blood cells and very few white blood cells. They are easily distinguished from infection, where the neutrophil population clearly predominates.

Treatment and Prevention

A single aspiration is generally insufficient for treatment of large seromas. On occasion, the application of a firm compression bandage after aspiration may help to control dead space to promote healing of the separated tissue planes. Intermittent seroma drainage by aspiration every few days is occasionally successful (usually over a 2-week period): however, rapid fluid reformation (usually within 24 hours) after initial aspiration is a clear indication that drain insertion is required to definitively manage the serum pocket. Prior to any attempt at aspiration, the area must have a basic surgical preparation before introducing a sterile hypodermic needle. An 18-gauge hypodermic needle and 35- to 60-cc syringe may be used to aspirate the serum pocket; the addition of a three-way stopcock will facilitate evacuation of the syringe. Butterfly catheters are useful for aspiration in restless patients, since the tube extension reduces the risk of needle displacement during movement. Larger-gauge needles or a trocar (14- to 6-gauge) can facilitate drainage but would require a lidocaine block at the point of insertion. Serum may be allowed to escape passively from the dependently placed trocar (facilitated by the manual compression of the serum pocket) or by application of a syringe and three-way stopcock or vacuum pump. A compression bandage may be applied to help prevent reformation. There is minimal risk of infection after seroma aspiration provided that strict aseptic technique is maintained.

Aspiration is a simple method of managing seromas, but is frequently unsuccessful. Rapid reformation (less than 24 hours) after aspiration is an indicator that a drain is required. (This should be clearly stated to the owner prior to using this technique.) Aspiration with a syringe can be frustrated by the bevel of the hypodermic needle contacting soft tissue as the fluid pocket collapses during aspiration. The needle will require repositioning within the fluid pocket to continue serum removal. Owners that travel a distance to your practice may prefer the more reliable drain.

Nearly all seromas respond well to the use of a Penrose or vacuum drain system, depending on the size and location of the seroma. Vacuum drains are preferred for large seromas; Penrose drains (1/4-inch) are useful for smaller seromas. Depending on the patient, sedation/lidocaine block or general anesthesia can be used to insert a surgical drain as a day case or on an outpatient basis.

Drains are most commonly required both to prevent and treat seromas. A Penrose drain is retained for 2 to 5 days in most cases. When applicable, a compression bandage is useful to protect the drain from contamination, restrict movement, and collapse the dead space. Alternatively, closed suction units can be highly effective in removing fluid and obliterating dead space instead of Penrose drains. As noted in Chapter 4, syringes (35, 60 cc) can be adapted as closed suction reservoirs for smaller seromas, but are considered inferior to the commercially available vacuum drain system. Compression bandages, Penrose drains, or close suction units should be employed any time the surgeon feels that the accumulation of fluid is likely in an area where dead space is present.

Buried "tacking" sutures also can be employed to discourage seroma formation in small, sterile, dead space areas. However, large areas of dead space may be impossible to tack down completely. Excessive use of buried sutures may promote wound infection and cannot be advocated for routine use in contaminated wounds. Buried sutures also may result in the formation of smaller seroma pockets that may not communicate with one another for simple drainage.

HEMATOMAS

Hematomas usually are the result of external trauma or hemorrhage secondary to incomplete hemostasis after completion of a surgical procedure. Small hematomas normally require no specific treatment. Large hematomas, however, are capable of pushing tissue planes apart and creating pressure beneath the suture line. Large clots can take considerable time to resorb and delay the normal healing of the tissues displaced by their presence. When feasible, the surgical area should opened, the hematoma evacuated, and the area suctioned and lavaged. Bleeders should be identified and ligated; small bleeders may respond to electrocautery. A vacuum drain can be inserted into the dead space prior to closure of the surgical incision.

EXPOSED BONE

Exposed bone is most commonly associated with shearing and avulsion injuries to the lower extremities. The metacarpal and metatarsal surfaces are especially prone to injury when the foot of the dog is trapped beneath the tire of a moving vehicle. The foot is compressed and ground into the pavement, avulsing skin and grinding soft tissue and bone. Avulsion of skin over bone surfaces lacking muscle immediately

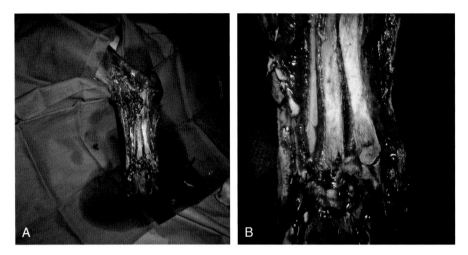

FIG. 6-23 (A) Severe shearing injury to the lower portion of a canine hind limb. (B) A close-up view revealed 50% of the metatarsal bones were sheared off, leaving multiple joints exposed. Despite the severity of this injury, the leg was potentially salvageable. However, the owner's financial restrictions required hind limb amputation.

exposes the periosteum or cortex to the external environment (Fig. 6-23).

In the dog and cat, most exposed viable bone will be covered by granulation tissue, arising from the viable periosteum, the exposed viable medullary cavity, or by "creeping coverage" from granulation tissue arising from viable soft tissue adjacent to the bone surfaces. Tissue between exposed metatarsal and metacarpal bones frequently is the source of granulation tissue coverage after road pavement shearing injuries. In many of these cases, the periosteum and bone below the wound surface are viable despite the significant loss of the outer "half" of their circumference. Because portions of the periosteum and the cortical and medullary bone are destroyed in these injuries, there is a potential for osteomyelitis or sequestrum formation. However, most cases encountered in the dog and cat do not require the removal or "decortication" of exposed bone (Fig. 6-24).

Surgical promotion of a granulation bed over exposed bone can be accomplished by drilling a series of small holes with a 1/16-inch Steinmann pin or drill bit into the vascular medullary canal of the bone. These channels facilitate capillary bud formation from the vascular medullary tissues to promote granulation tissue formation over the exposed cortical surface. A blood clot may form over the bone, providing an extracellular matrix for the ingrowth of fibroblasts and capillary buds. The resultant granulation bed can, in turn, support a free graft. Caution must be exercised, however, when using this technique for metatarsal and metacarpal bones due to the risk of fracturing bones already weakened by trauma.

Most lower extremity shearing wounds seen in practice can heal by second intention; skin grafts can be considered for the more extensive injuries. Joint instability of the tarsal joint, secondary to loss of collateral ligamentous support, may require wire stabilization using cortical screws to serve as anchors for (20- to 22-gauge) stainless steel orthopedic wire placed in a figure 8 pattern. Over time, collagen deposition can stabilize the joint, usually by the time the wire fractures due to cyclic stress within weeks after placement. Alternatively, prolonged splint support can be used to stabilize an unstable joint. Failure in obtaining sufficient stability may necessitate arthrodesis once skin closure is complete.

Despite the rather gruesome appearance of lower extremity shearing wounds, most heal satisfactorily by second intention using the basic wound management principles previously discussed. The rate of infection is remarkably low, and the wound size is exaggerated by the soft tissue swelling that normally accompanies these wounds.

After debridement and lavage, partial approximation of portions of the wound, without excessive tension, will reduce the magnitude of the defect. This can shorten the time required for second intention healing. Drainage is preserved through the open portions of the wound.

Serial applications of medicated dressings can provide a protective medium to support granulation tissue formation, wound contraction, and epithelialization. In turn, fibroblasts will provide the collagen needed to stabilize the exposed joint(s).

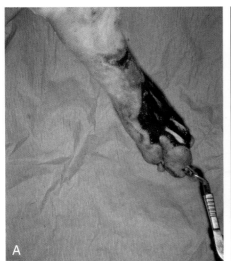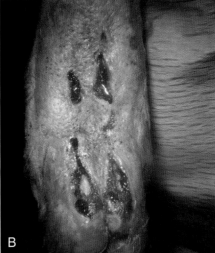

FIG. 6-24 (A) Healing shearing wound overlying the metatarsal surface. Metatarsal bones and first phalanges were exposed. Over the next 4 weeks, a healthy granulation bed formed from viable soft tissue surfaces. Granulation tissue slowly covered the exposed bone. (B) A skin graft was applied to the granulation bed. Slits were created in the graft over areas of exposed bone. Note that bone coverage by granulation tissue is nearly complete, with final wound coverage over the bony surface by second intention healing.

Devitalized bone that is protruding above the wound is not likely to be covered by granulation tissue (Fig. 6-25). This exposed, desiccated bone, which is not integral to the surgical salvage of the extremity, should be excised below the surface of the granulation bed with bone rongeurs or bone-cutting instruments (Fig. 6-26).

WOUND DEHISCENCE

Wound dehiscence, or the disruption of apposed surfaces of a wound, is the result of several factors, either alone or in combination. The following are the most common causes noted by the author:

1. Wound closure under excessive tension, with suture cut-out, secondary to ischemic necrosis.

2. Suture placement too close to incisional border with cut-out (collagenase activity within 5-mm cutaneous zone bordering skin incision).

3. Improper suture material selection (size, tensile strength, suture pattern, placement, rate of resorption/ degradation).

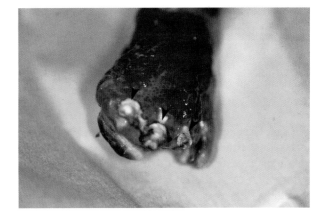

FIG. 6-25 Massive skin loss to the rear paw of a cat. A healthy granulation bed has formed although the exposed third phalanges were nonviable. The exposed bone was resected below the granulation surface, and a full-thickness mesh graft was used to close the wound.

4. Closure of severely compromised skin, with subsequent necrosis.

5. Suture placement, compromising cutaneous circulation.

6. Moisture accumulation contributing to tissue overhydration, maceration.

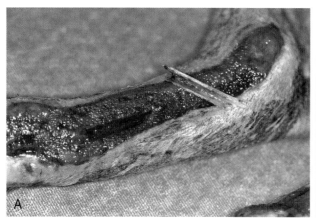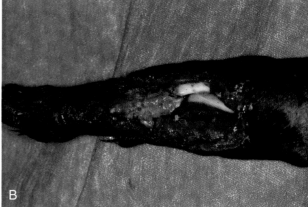

FIG. 6-26 (A) Devitalized metatarsal fragment: granulation tissue typically will not fully cover necrotic bone; in this case the loosened fragment was removed with forceps. (B) Devitalized radius, ulna, and carpus secondary to extensive bite wound trauma. Granulation tissue will circumvent completely devitalized bone.

7. Underlying pocket of infection, necrosis, foreign body, neoplasia.

8. Lack of postoperative protection/support from motion, licking, external trauma.

9. Premature suture removal.

10. Delayed healing precipitated by corticosteroids and other agents.

11. Suture placement in scar tissue, which has poor suture-holding ability.

12. Underlying healing disorder or delay in healing, excluding the above causes, suspected.

Critical evaluation of the separated wound can assist the surgeon in determining the most likely cause(s) of dehiscence. Incisional gaps with absent sutures suggests the premature removal of sutures, usually by the patient. Presence of the sutures often demonstrates suture cut-out from one side of the incision, with an irregular right-angle tear from the suture hole to the incision. An intact suture with the presence of an incisional gap usually is associated with stretching or deformation of suture material (from incisional tension, or sutures deliberately placed loosely) (Fig. 6-27). Often a veterinarian may place sutures loosely when edema of the skin is evident or anticipated. When swelling subsides, the incisions retract, leaving an incisional gap. Unfortunately, many surgical instructors at teaching institutions overemphasize loose suture placement to offset anticipated swelling. It is the author's opinion that surgical instructors should emphasize a traumatic surgical technique that

minimizes postoperative swelling, thus enabling the surgeon to place sutures that more effectively appose and immobilize the incision.

Suture cut-out can occur from placement too close to the incision. Because collagenase activity remains high within 5 mm of the skin incision, sutures placed near or within this zone are more likely to cut through the weakened dermal collagen weave, especially in the presence of motion and incisional tension. Larger suture bites are less likely to pull out. Cutting needles have the cutting edge within the curvature of the needle. Under tension, with placement in susceptible skin, the suture is more likely to cut along the V-shaped cut created by the suture, in the direction of the incision. Today, most surgeons use reverse cutting needles (cutting edge on the outer curvature of the needle) almost exclusively, since the flat edge of the needle hole facing the incision line is more resistant to tissue tear.

It is useful to select an elastic suture material that can stretch to a limited degree to accommodate possible tissue swelling, but of sufficient size and strength to prevent permanent stretch deformation. Suture material size and selection should be tailored to the skin thickness, durability, location, and the anticipated postoperative incisional forces that require neutralization. All surgeons have a preferred suture material for skin closure. This preference may be based on the materials with which they were trained and the surgeon's familiarity with the handling (physical) properties of the product. While many of us prefer monofilament nylon and polypropylene for closure, other materials may be quite acceptable for many of the wounds encountered. In more difficult wound closures, complete familiarity with the physical prop-

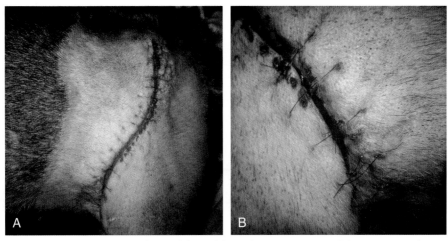

FIG. 6-27 (A) Closure of a long laceration along the caudal shoulder and upper extremity. Dehiscence is evident several days after surgery. (B) A close-up view reveals no sutures cut out. Rather. the 3-0 monofilament nylon has stretched as a result of patient activity. Sutures also were placed loosely for anticipated postoperative swelling. Intradermal sutures, the addition of vertical mattress sutures, the use of 2-0 monofilament material, restricted activity, and other methods to offset incisional tension could have prevented this case of dehiscence.

erties of a given suture material is essential for more consistent success in wound closure.

Closure of an incision under moderate tension increases the likelihood of dehiscence. Closure under tension, with the addition of motion, can further promote suture serration of the skin and cut-out. Although mechanical creep and stress relaxation of skin can, almost miraculously, reduce incisional tension within hours after closure, a veterinarian cannot rely on this natural dermal collagen phenomenon as a reliable "bail out" for all difficult closures. Techniques to offset skin tension should be considered (see Chapter 9) in concert with immobilization of the area to promote uncomplicated healing.

Delays in healing from inflammation, trauma, or malnutrition, for example, will further increase the likelihood of dehiscence. Suture placement, pattern, and selection are particularly important under these circumstances. It is not always clear at the time of traumatic wound closure whether the onset of necrosis was the result of "dying skin" or additional ischemia precipitated by tight suture placement. Large areas of skin necrosis would suggest preceding trauma was primarily responsible for necrosis. In areas with ample regional skin, aggressive debridement could prevent dehiscence by removal of compromised or potentially compromised tissues. Necrosis limited to the suture site would be compatible with suture compromise to the skin (Fig. 6-28).

Underlying pockets of infection, necrotic tissue, or foreign bodies will result in persistent wound drainage at the expense of incisional closure until the underlying causes are alleviated. Future continuous discharge and prolonged moisture exposure can hydrate or soften the skin, enhancing the likelihood of suture cut-out. As a result, failure in abiding by basic wound management principles can have a negative, cascading effect on wound healing and closure until the problems are recognized and remedied.

Finally, proper bandage and external support can be critically important in preventing dehiscence in areas subject to motion or weight bearing. Care is used to avoid circulatory compromise during bandage application along with proper bandage care.

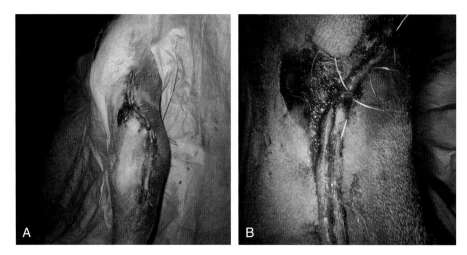

FIG. 6-28 (A) Closure of a laceration over the right stifle area, secondary to vehicular trauma. Early dehiscence noted approximately 48 hours later.

(B) Horizontal mattress sutures were placed too snugly, aggravating tissue swelling as a result of circulatory compromise. Early tissue necrosis also is evident in this view. A vertical mattress tension suture pattern, in combination with alternating simple interrupted sutures, would have been a better choice for stabilizing the incisional border. In cases of moderate trauma and swelling, delayed closure may be a better choice of wound management. Resolution of swelling and hemorrhage would improve the likelihood of subsequent successful skin closure.

Suggested Readings

Amalsadvala T, Swaim SF. 2006. Management of hard-to-heal wounds. *Vet Clin No Am* 36:693–711.

Atkinson JB, Kosi M, Srikanth MS, et al. 1992. Growth hormone reverses impaired wound healing in protein-malnourished rats treated with corticosteroids. *J Pediatric Surg* 27:1026–1028.

Beardsley SL, Schrader SC. 1995. Treatment of dogs with wounds of the limbs caused by shearing forces: 98 cases (1975–1993). *J Am Vet Med Assoc* 207:1071–1075.

Blass CE, Moore RW. 1984. The tourniquet in surgery: a review. *Vet Surg* 13:111–114.

Bradley DM, Swaim SF, Stuart SW. 1998. An animal model for research on wound healing over exposed bone. *Vet Comp Orthop Traumatol* 11:131–135.

Brockman DJ, Pardo AD, Conzemius MG, et al. 1996. Omentum-enhanced reconstruction of chronic nonhealing wounds in cats: techniques and clinical use. *Vet Surg* 25:99–104.

Carlson MA. 1997. Acute wound failure. *Surg Clin No Am* 77:607–636.

Clark GN. 2001. Bone perforation to enhance wound healing over exposed bone with shearing injuries. *J Am Anim Hosp Assoc* 37(3):215–217.

Delany HM, Demetrius AA, Teh E, et al. 1990. Effect of early postoperative nutritional support on skin wound and colon anastomosis healing. *J Parenter Enter Nutri* 14:357–361.

Hong A-H, Khanna C. 2003. Chemotherapy of neoplasia. In: Slatter D, ed. *Textbook of Small Animal Surgery*, 23–52. Philadelphia: WB Saunders Co.

Hunt GB, Worth A, Marchevsky A. 2004. Migration of wooden skewer foreign bodies from the gastrointestinal tract in eight dogs. *J Sm Anim Pract* 45:362–367.

Hunt TK, Dunphy JE. 1979. *Fundamentals of Wound Management*. New York: Appleton and Lange.

Hunt TK, Williams H. 1997. Wound healing and wound infection. *Surg Clin No Am* 77:587–606.

Johnston DE. 1990. Care of accidental wounds. *Vet Clin No Am* 20:27–46.

Johnston DE. 1990. Wound healing in skin. *Vet Clin No Am* 20:1–25.

Jyung RW, Mustoe TA, Busby WN, et al. 1994. Increased wound-breaking strength induced by insulin-like growth factor I in combination with insulin-like growth factor binding proteins-1. *Surgery* 115:233–239.

Lavy UI. 1972. The effective oral supplementation of zinc sulfate on primary wound healing in rats. *Brit J Surg* 59:194–196.

Lee AH, Swaim SF, Newton JC, et al. 1987. Wound healing over denuded bone. *J Am Anim Hosp Assoc* 23(1):75–84.

Nwomeh B, Yager DR, Kelman CL. 1998. Physiology of the chronic wound. *Clin Plast Surg* 25(3):341–356.

Pavletic MM. 1995. *Bite Wound Management in Small Animals*. The Professional Library Series. Denver: American Animal Hospital Association.

Pavletic MM. 2005. Preventing wound dehiscence: tension-relieving and closure options. *Stand Care* 7(10):7–10.

Peacock EE. 1984. *Wound Repair*, 3rd ed. Philadelphia: WB Saunders.

Pennick D, Mitchell SL. 2003. Ultrasonographic detection of ingested and perforating wooden foreign bodies in four dogs. *J Am Vet Med Assoc* 223:206–209.

Robson MC. 1997. Wound infection. *Surg Clin No Am* 77:637–650.

Rudolph R, Noe JM. 1983. *Chronic Problem Wounds*. Boston: Little, Brown and Co.

Stanley BJ. 2007. Nonhealing wounds. *Clinician's Brief* 5(5): 67–71.

Swaim SF, Angarano DW. 1990. Chronic problem wounds of dog limbs. *Clin Dermatol* 8(3/4):175–186.

Swaim SF, Henderson RA. 1997. *Small Animal Wound Management*, 2nd ed. Baltimore: Williams and Wilkins.

Temple WJ, Voitk AJ, Snelling CFT, et al. 1975. Effect of nutrition, diet and suture material on long term wound healing. *Ann Surg* 182:93–97.

Walmsley GL, Scurrell E, Summers BA, et al. 2009. Foreign body induced neuritis masquerading as a canine brachial plexus nerve sheath tumour. *Vet Comp Orthop Traumatol* 5:427–429.

White RAS. 2003. Surgical treatment of specific skin disorders. In: Slatter DH, ed. *Textbook of Small Animal Surgery*, 3rd ed., 339–355. Philadelphia: WB Saunders.

White, RAS. 2006. Management of specific skin wounds. *Vet Clin No Am* 36:895–912.

White RAS, Williams JM. 1995. Intracapsular prostatic omentalization: a new technique for management of prostate abscess. *Vet Surg* 24:390–395.

Wusteman M, Hayes A, Stirling D, Elia M. 1994. Changes in protein distribution in the rat during prolonged "systemic injury." *J Surg Res* 56:331–337.

Wykes PM. 1982. Cutaneous sinus tracts of the dog. *Compend Contin Educ Pract Vet* 4(4):293–296.

Zaizen Y, Ford EG, Costin G, et al. 1990. Stimulation of wound bursting strength during protein malnutrition. *J Surg Research* 49:333–336.

Zaloga GP, Bortenschlager L, Black KW, et al. 1992. Immediate postoperative enteral feeding decreases weight loss and improves wound healing after abdominal surgery in rats. *Crit Care Med* 20:115–118.

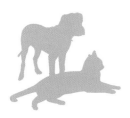

Management of Specific Wounds

BITE WOUNDS

Introduction

Bite wounds are among the most serious injuries seen in small animal practice, and account for 10% to 15% of all veterinary trauma cases. The canine teeth arc designed for tissue penetration, the incisors for grasping, and the molars/premolars for shearing tissue. The curved canine teeth of large dogs are capable of deep penetration, whereas the smaller, straighter canine teeth of domestic cats can penetrate directly into tissues, leaving a relatively small cutaneous hole. The jaws of larger dogs in particular can generate tremendous crushing (up to 450 psi) and shearing forces, and the canine teeth can tear and lacerate the skin, hypodermis, and underlying musculature.

A struggling victim may promote additional tissue injury while attempting to wrest free of its attacker. Small dogs and cats are at special risk since most portions of their body can be completely grasped by a large dog (Fig. 7-1). In one study, male dogs weighing less than 10 kg presented with more severe multiple bite wounds. (Miniature pinchers, Pekinese, and small terrier breeds were overrepresented.) Many of these victims are lifted and violently shaken by the attacker. Direct and indirect trauma to internal organs frequently occurs. The kidneys in small animals are particularly susceptible to bite wounds over the back. In addition, bone fractures, joint injuries, and spinal trauma also may occur.

The untrained observer can mistakenly dismiss the gravity of the bite wounds since the only obvious injuries may be a few puncture wounds confined to the skin. Wounds may be covered by a thick hair coat and go unrecognized. The skin and underlying issues can be lacerated, stretched, crushed and avulsed. Circulatory compromise from the division of vessels and compromise to collateral vascular channels can result in massive tissue necrosis. It may take several days before the severity of tissue loss becomes evident. All bites are considered contaminated wounds: the presence of bacteria in the face of vascular compromise can precipitate massive infection.

Wild Animals and Bite Wounds

Bite wounds from black bears (*Ursus americanus*) and the grizzly bear *(Ursus arctos horribilis)* are infrequent, but are most commonly seen in hunting dogs or unsupervised dogs where these bear species are most prevalent. Although bears frequently attack the head and neck area, hunting dogs may be bitten in the trunk and pelvic regions, most likely when the bear lunges at a retreating dog. Tissue trauma can be massive. Coyote *(Canis iatrans)* attacks on dogs and cats have been reported throughout the United States as a result of their expanding range. Wolves *(Canis* spp.) are less prevalent and are limited to selective areas of the northern United States. Attacks from other large carnivores, including mountain lions *(Felis concolor),* alligators *(Alligator mississippiensis),* and crocodiles *(Crocodylus acutus)* are far less prevalent due to their comparatively small populations and limited range. Of particular concern are bite wounds from wild

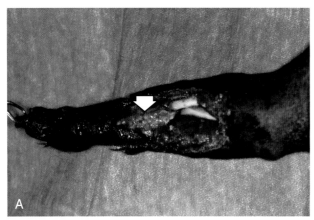
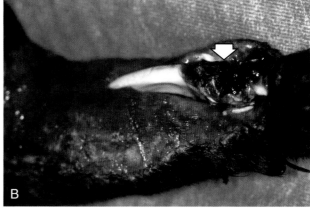

FIG. 7-1 (A, B) Medial and lateral view of extensive tissue necrosis to the left forelimb of a Scottie. A neighborhood pit bull attacked the dog and refused to let go of the patient's limb. Due to extensive skin, muscle, and bone necrosis, with destruction of the carpal joint (arrows), amputation was performed.

animals, including raccoons, skunks, and bats, in which rabies is an endemic problem, (see Rabies and the Transmission of Infectious Diseases below).

Initial Patient Assessment

A complete physical exam is required. A history of the attack may help in locating the body region(s) bitten. Latex gloves must be worn during the examination and management of open wounds.

> A complete medical history should include the patient's medical history and current rabies vaccination status.

The patient's head should be restrained or muzzled during examination to protect the practitioner from injury. The hair coat must be parted and skin areas visualized. Small spots of dried blood and matted hair frequently overlie puncture wounds. Careful palpa-

tion and observation may demonstrate muscle tears or hernias.

> Keep in mind that Elizabethan collars also can be useful in shielding veterinary personnel from being bitten, especially in the less aggressive canine and feline patients.

Care must be taken to minimize pain to the patient and avoid manipulating unstable fractures or spinal injuries. Analgesics or sedation may be used in an otherwise stable patient. (A neurologic examination would be advisable prior to using medications that could obscure these injuries.)

Blood loss, shock, respiratory distress (including laryngeal wounds, tracheal injuries, pneumomediastinum, pneumothorax, hemothorax, flail chest) are emergency situations that frequently require the clinician's immediate attention before completing the examination (Fig. 7-2 and 7-3). The prognosis of the patient, definitive course(s) of action required, and potential complications in managing the patient are essential to the owner's decision regarding whether or not to proceed with treatment in the seriously injured

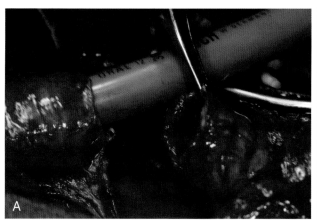
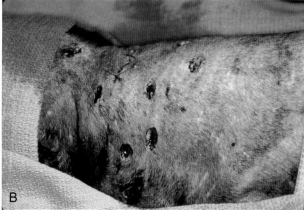

FIG. 7-2 (A) Massive cervical trauma to the trachea and cervical muscles as a result of a dog fight. The patient was administered oxygen prior to anesthesia. The cervical area was prepared for surgery. Anesthetic induction was immediately followed by a cervical incision, with placement of a sterile endotracheal tube into the lacerated trachea. The gas anesthetic machine was connected to this tube. Once the patient was stable, the technician passed a sterile endotracheal tube through the larynx. The surgeon then guided the tube past the tracheal tear.

(B) Surgical repair included tracheal anastomosis, thorough debridement of necrotic muscle, copious lavage, and delayed primary closure. Small puncture wounds were uncapped and locally assessed using a pair of mosquito hemostats as tissue retractors. These wounds were left open to heal by second intention. However, complete excision of small puncture wounds can permit primary closure.

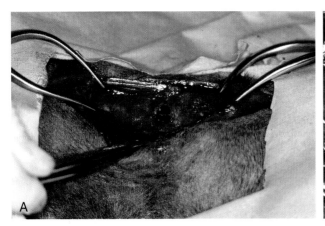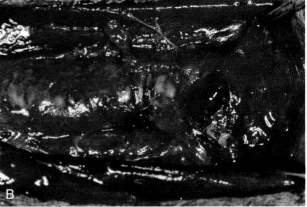

FIG. 7-3 (A) Puncture to the cervical trachea as a result of a dog bite: intraoperative view. A canine tooth created the opening that enabled air to pass into the cervical tissues, impairing the ability of the patient to breath. Manual compression of the skin over the puncture site halted the air excursion until anesthesia and intubation could be accomplished. (B) Closure was accomplished by conservative debridement of the wound borders followed by placement of 3-0 polydioxanone sutures.

pet. In the interim, basic life-support procedural guidelines include the following areas of emergency resuscitation: (1) airway, (2) breathing, (3) cardiac function, and (4) hemorrhage control. Intravenous fluid support and whole blood would be indicated in the presence of extensive tissue trauma and blood loss. Details on emergency management can be obtained in standard textbooks. A complete blood count, serum chemistry profile, and urinalysis can serve as baseline data for the seriously injured patient.

> Treatment of hemorrhage requires (1) recognition of the condition, (2) control of further blood loss, and (3) intravenous fluid support to treat the patient's hypovolemia.
>
> In many cases, blood loss is not the result of an obvious spurting artery. Internal hemorrhage can be difficult to quantitate. Individual bite wounds may result in little hemorrhage; collectively, multiple bite wounds can result in a sizeable loss of blood.

Systemic Effects

Multiple and severe bite wounds can initiate a systemic inflammatory response syndrome (SIRS). What

normally is a regional response to injury becomes an exaggerated systemic inflammatory response secondary to extensive tissue trauma. Resection of necrotic tissue and aggressive management of infection is critical to the prevention and management of this condition. Acute respiratory distress syndrome (ARDS) may be noted as a sequela to SIRS.

Bite Wound Management

All penetrating bite wounds are ideally explored under anesthesia. If the patient is in critical condition, exploration, debridement, and definitive repair may be necessarily delayed until the patient can be stabilized. However, basic wound management can be instituted in the interim. The procedures for short-term treatment before definitive exploration are described below.

Temporary Bite Wound Care in the Critical Patient

The following steps should be taken for the initial management of bite wounds in the critical-care patient in which general anesthesia cannot be administered.

1. Minimize further contamination of open wounds prior to preparing the wound for

surgery. Cover the open wound with sterile gauze sponges; sterile water-soluble gel or saline is applied to the gauze before application.

2. Liberally clip hair around each puncture wound.

3. Gently cleanse the skin around each wound with warm sterile saline and a surgical preparation solution.

4. Inject small amounts of lidocaine with a 25-gauge hypodermic needle into and around the bite wound punctures. Trim off any tattered borders. Insert a pair of sterile hemostats and inspect the underlying tissues.

5. Perform liberal pressure lavage of the puncture site using an 18-gauge needle and 35-cc syringe with warm sterile saline. The wound should be opened sufficiently to permit fluid to flow out freely. A three-way stopcock valve connected to sterile intravenous tubing can be used to facilitate refilling the syringe. A dilute povidone-iodine (1%:1 part solution/9 parts sterile saline) or chlorhexidine (0.05%:1 part solution/40 parts sterile saline) solution can be made by adding these stock solutions to the lavage receptacle. The access site must be sufficiently large to allow the lavage solution to exit the area.

6. Apply a topical antimicrobial ointment and dressing over the open wound.

7. Systemic broad-spectrum antibiotics may be administered if deemed necessary (see below).

The primary goal of this short-term therapy is to reduce the amount of contamination present and reduce the possibility of further contamination from organisms in the hospital environment (nosocomial infection).

Once stabilized, the patient can be anesthetized for wound exploration if necessary. (See the next section.) On occasion, critically injured patients with serious underlying injuries cannot be stabilized to the desired degree. Under these circumstances surgical intervention would be necessary since these wounds are the primary cause of the patients deterioration (bowel rupture, sepsis, etc.). Such a serious endeavor requires the coordinated efforts of the emergency clinician, anesthesiologist/anesthetist, and the surgeon.

Definitive Management: Bite Wound Exploration

The following steps summarize the approach for the definitive management of bite wounds.

1. General anesthesia.

2. Open wounds should be temporarily covered or packed with sterile gauze sponges moistened with saline; a water-miscible lubricant can be applied to the sponges in place of saline in order to protect individual wounds from contamination associated with preparing the area for surgery.

3. The bite wound area should be clipped *liberally*. In particular, the thoracic and abdominal area should be completely clipped and prepared for surgery in the event the exploration requires conversion to a thoracotomy or exploratory laparotomy. The surgical area then is prepared and draped for aseptic surgery.

4. Puncture wounds are "uncapped" using a scalpel blade by excising the puncture-wound borders, thereby creating a 1.0-cm-plus circular opening. Sterile mosquito hemostats are inserted into the opening and spread to expose the underlying hypodermis, fascial tissues, and muscle. Wounds with little or no underlying tissue damage may be left open to drain and heal by second intention or may be closed with one or two skin sutures after lavaging the wound.

5. If significant tissue damage is suspected, a skin incision is made over the puncture site; tissue retractors are inserted to permit exploration and debridement of traumatized tissues. Adjacent puncture wounds may be connected with a single incision to facilitate exploration (Fig. 7-4). Care must be taken not to inadvertently divide direct cutaneous arteries, especially those vessels supplying skin already compromised by bite wound trauma.

6. Any hair or foreign debris is removed. Shredded or necrotic muscle, fat, and fascia are excised. A more aggressive

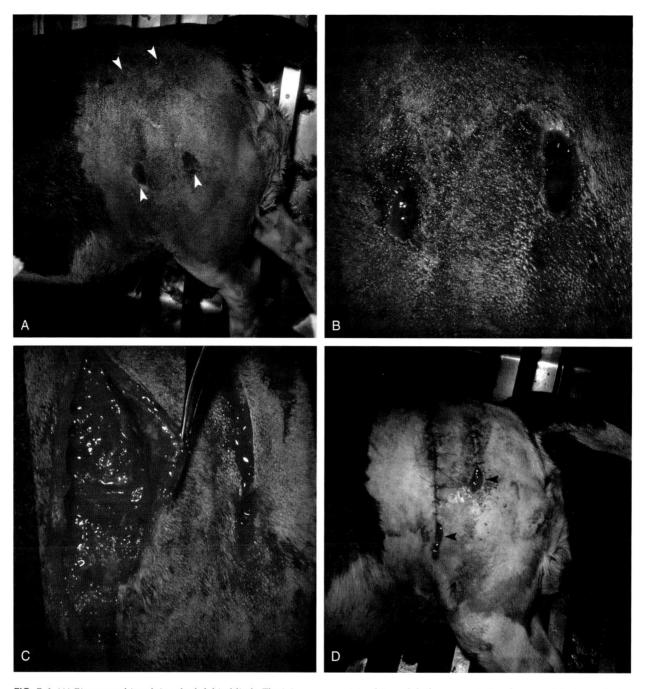

FIG. 7-4 (A) Bite wound involving the left hind limb. The injury was sustained 1 week before presentation for a persistent purulent discharge. Arrows denote the four canine puncture wounds.

(B) A close-up view of the puncture wounds. The comparatively benign appearance of these injuries masks the more serious underlying tissue destruction.

(C) Two parallel incisions were made between the respective left and right canine puncture wounds, demonstrating a layer of necrotic subcutaneous fat. This tissue was excised and the wound lavaged.

(D) Partial closure was performed; the lower 2 cm (arrows) were left open for drainage. The narrow tracts were poorly suited to drain insertion.

debridement can be performed for those tissues of questionable viability that are not essential to normal function. As noted, additional care is warranted when exploring bite wounds over the thorax. Retraction of muscle and fascia may unseal penetrating thoracic wounds. Sucking sounds may emanate from the area as air enters the thoracic cavity, necessitating assisted ventilation, aspiration of the thorax, or temporary insertion of a thoracostomy tube.

7. Debridement ideally is accomplished in one stage, especially in critical areas (thoracic cavity and abdominal cavity involvement) where the presence of necrotic tissues can promote life-threatening sepsis. In less critical areas, such as the extremities, a more conservative daily or staged debridement (open-wound management followed by delayed primary closure, secondary closure, healing by second intention) is indicated for tissues of questionable viability, where important muscle groups and the limited availability of skin could compromise salvage of the limb.

8. Skin viability may be difficult to determine on initial presentation. Necrosis may not be evident for 5 to 7 days after injury. The loose skin available over the cervical area and trunk permits more aggressive debridement of skin of questionable viability. However, a more conservative "wait and reassess" approach is indicated for compromised skin of the lower extremities. With the limited amount of loose skin available for closure, unnecessarily wide debridement will increase the likelihood that reconstructive surgery will be required to close the resultant defect.

9. Wound drainage is necessary in areas where dead space is present, especially after wide debridement of contaminated bite wounds. Closed vacuum drains or Penrose drains may be considered (see Chapter 4).

10. Open wound management is advisable in the presence of infection and tissues of questionable viability (see Chapter 3).

"Uncapping" the Puncture Wound

A simple method of assessing a puncture wound is by lifting the puncture site with forceps and excising the area with a scalpel blade, thereby creating a 10- to 15-mm opening to inspect the underlying tissues. A mosquito hemostat can be inserted and spread open, serving as a tissue retractor or speculum to examine the subcutaneous tissues and underlying muscles. If the subcutaneous fat is undisturbed, the wound is considered minor. If the fat has been separated and fragmented, the underlying muscle is examined. Lavage and suctioning facilitate visualization of the tissues by removal of tissue fragments and debris.

If tissue damage is minor, the wound can be lavaged and apposed with one or two skin sutures; if there are any doubts, the wound may be left open to maintain postoperative drainage and open wound care.

If more significant tissue trauma is noted or suspected, a scalpel blade is used to incise over the area for wound inspection, debridement, lavage, and repair. Adjacent punctures can be connected through a single incision.

Prolonged wound drainage is common after extensive muscle trauma and formation of dead space. It is not unusual to retain use of drains for several days under these circumstances. Closed suction units (as discussed in Chapter 4) limit the risk of ascending infection and can be used to prevent air entry into the wound cavity. Subcutaneous emphysema associated with sucking wounds of the flank and axilla may be prevented with vacuum drains. Similarly, they can provide wound drainage overlying the thorax or thoracic inlet where air entry (with the use of Penrose drains) may result in pneumothorax. Vacuum drains can be used effectively for the drainage of abdominal wall wounds and the abdominal cavity simultaneously (as needed).

Regional Considerations

Head and Neck

The head and neck areas are most commonly attacked by predators. Small dogs and cats can sustain skull fractures from larger predators (Fig. 7-5). Injury to eyes and ears are occasionally noted. Bite wounds involving the pinna are common; occasionally, the ear canal will sustain punctures, lacerations, or avulsion injuries

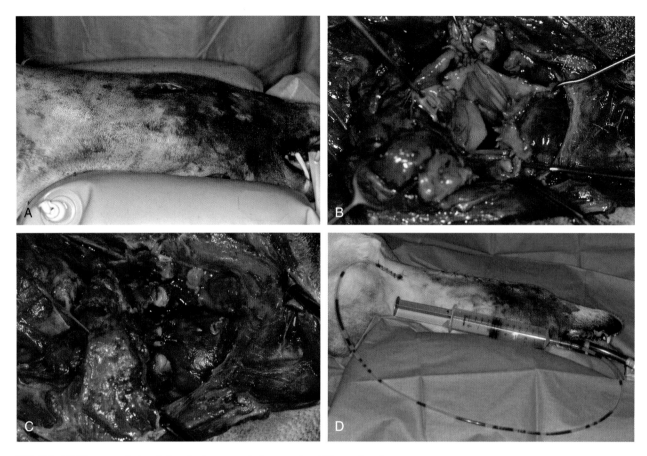

FIG. 7-5 (A) Bite wounds involving the larynx and pharynx should be explored.

(B) Pharyngeal tears permit extensive tissue exposure to saliva and oral contaminants.

(C, D) Debridement, closure of the pharyngeal laceration, and repair of the damaged hyoid apparatus was followed by wound lavage and closure over a closed suction unit. Skin hooks are invaluable in elevating the borders of the pharyngeal mucosa, facilitating suture apposition of this surface.

(at the junction of the vertical and horizontal ear canal, or canal avulsion at the external acoustic meatus). Cervical wounds must be closely assessed for injuries to the trachea, larynx, esophagus, pharynx, major vessels, and salivary glands, in particular. The spinal column is most susceptible to trauma in small dogs and cats. Skin and muscle are most prone to injury. A tracheostomy may be necessary when upper respiratory distress is evident. Traumatic division of the trachea may require a prompt cervical incision upon anesthetic induction for proper intubation before tracheal repair can be instituted. Alternatively, an endotracheal tube can be temporarily inserted into the tracheal tear to stabilize the patient until proper placement can be instituted intraoperatively (Fig. 7-2). Puncture or laceration of the rigid trachea also can result from penetrating canine teeth without tearing of the overlying skin (Fig. 7-3).

Extremities

The comparatively narrow diameter of the extremities make them particularly susceptible to extensive bite wound trauma (crushing, laceration), especially in the smaller patients. Circulatory compromise to the skin, muscle, and bone can result in massive necrosis, necessitating limb amputation in many cases. Overlooked puncture wounds involving the elbow, carpal, knee, and tarsal joints may result in problematic infections. A complete neurologic examination of the involved limb and close assessment of circulation is in order in the days following bite wound care. Fracture repair and stabilization normally is performed at the time of bite wound exploration. However, in the face of extensive swelling and circulatory compromise, a delay in fracture repair may be advisable: surgical trauma could further compromise circulation to the lower extremity and precipitate loss of the limb. As discussed, when debriding extremity wounds, a more conservative approach is in order when tissue viability is equivocal. (See Orthopedic Injuries and Spinal Trauma, below).

> Retention of fractured teeth is rarely seen in small animals. The dense interosseous ligament between the radius and ulna is the most common region where the tip of a canine tooth can be broken off. Its retention will result in a draining tract. Radiographs will easily identify the denser tooth fragment in contrast to the adjacent bone (Fig. 7-6).

Thoracic Trauma

Small patients are more susceptible to thoracic wall trauma, although the canine teeth in larger dogs are capable of penetrating the intercostal area of most dogs. Open wounds at the thoracic inlet can result in pneumomediastinum; direct open wounds involving the thoracic wall can result in fatal pneumothorax. On occasion, flaps of tissue may overlap and seal the thoracic wall defect, limiting the severity of the pneumothorax until surgical repair can be performed.

Both pneumothorax and hemothorax should be immediately suspected in patients presenting with respiratory distress. Pyothorax may be noted in patients with older bite wounds (Fig. 7-7). Hyperresonance would suggest pneumothorax, whereas dull areas of percussion would suggest fluid accumulation in the dependent areas of the thoracic cavity. In relatively calm and stable patients, a lateral thoracic radiograph may be obtained to confirm each condition. Thoracocentesis can be used to initially alleviate respiratory

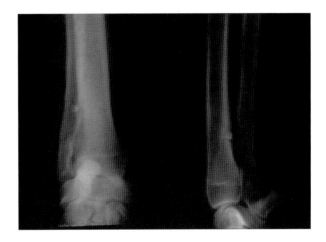

FIG. 7-6 Radiographs of the distal forelimb in a dog, demonstrating retention of the tip of a canine tooth in the interosseous ligament between the radius and ulna. The tooth fragment and associated draining tract were removed. The greater density of the retained canine helps to distinguish it from the adjacent bone. (Radiographs courtesy of Dr. Paul Gambardella.)

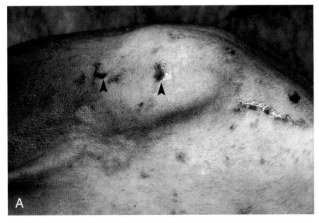
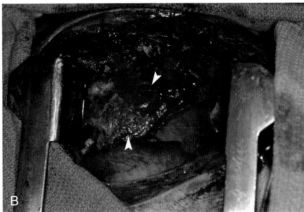

FIG. 7-7 (A) Bite wounds (arrows) overlying the sternum 4 days prior to presentation. The dog presented with respiratory distress as a result of pyothorax. Necrotic sternal bone was excised followed by a thoracotomy. (B) A restrictive pleuritis (arrows) was noted as a result of fibrin deposition and early fibrous connective tissue. Decortication of this layer with gauze pads was followed by closure after placement of a thoracostomy tube for continuous closed suction postoperatively.

distress and confirm the presence of air or fluid. The diameter of a bronchus noted on radiographs can serve as a relative guideline for estimation of the size of the thoracostomy tube that may be required. Immediate placement of a thoracostomy tube may be preferable when tension pneumothorax or significant hemothorax is diagnosed at presentation. The tube can be connected to a continuous thoracic suction unit in more serious cases. Drainage may be continued for 48 hours after cessation of air leakage. Significant, unabated leaks beyond the initial 72-hour period may require surgical (re)intervention. Similarly, brisk continuous hemorrhage following initial evacuation of blood in the thoracic cavity would justify prompt surgical intervention.

The hypodermic needle or, preferably, butterfly catheter, attached to a three-way stopcock and 35- to 60-cc syringe, can be used for thoracocentesis. The needle is angled slightly with the bevel toward the patient to reduce the risk of lung laceration. Plastic intravenous catheters also may be used to reduce the risk of lung laceration.

- If the patient is in lateral recumbency, air is drawn from the central third of the midthorax.

- If the patient is standing, air is withdrawn from the upper third of the midthorax.

- If the patient is standing or in lateral recumbency, fluid is removed from the lower third of the thorax, between the third and eighth ribs. Care is required to prevent advancement of the needle into the pericardium.

Open skin wounds can be temporarily stapled or sutured to limit air entry prior to surgery. Alternatively, a bandage containing a heavy layer of ointment can be cupped over the wound temporarily. Bite wounds entering the thoracic cavity are best explored, due to the significant risk of tissue necrosis and pyothorax present in these cases. Surgical staplers (TA, Covidien/USSC/Kendall) are useful in removing traumatized pulmonary tissue.

Fractured ribs with significant displacement can be repaired at the time of exploration. Sharp, pointed edges can be trimmed with rongeurs to reduce the risk of lung laceration. Cases of flail chest can be stabilized in a similar fashion with fine wire or nonabsorbable suture to realign the fracture segments. Holes can be drilled approximately 1 cm from the fracture ends.

Stainless steel orthopedic wire (22-gauge) is commonly used to realign the rib segments; overtightening should be avoided in this soft bone. In most cases of flail chest, preoperative external stabilization of the area is usually unnecessary.

Bite wounds involving the caudal thoracic and cranial abdominal areas are capable of tearing the underlying diaphragm: the pars costalis and pars sternalis are relatively superficial at the area of the xiphoid and caudal thoracic cage. Rents in the diaphragm may not be visible on initial thoracic radiographs; additional radiographs are indicated if deterioration of clinical signs warrants reevaluation of the patient. The diaphragm should always be inspected during exploratory laparotomy.

Abdominal Trauma

The larger canine teeth are capable of deep penetration through the soft and compressible abdominal wall into the peritoneal cavity, especially in smaller patients. It is important to note that the skin and abdominal wall may appear to be intact, although internal organs can be crushed. The kidneys, bowel, mesenteric vasculature, spleen, and liver can be traumatized by direct contact with the canine teeth or indirectly as a result of the stretching and tearing of tissues if the patient is shaken during the attack. Ultrasonography may be used to assess the integrity of the internal organs; abdominal radiographs can be used to assess the abdomen and determine the presence of free air and fluid. An intravenous pyelogram may be used to assess traumatized kidneys based on these findings.

Internal hemorrhage can have an insidious onset and can be easily overlooked in the trauma patient. A fist-sized hematoma may vary from 300 to 500 ml of blood. Retroperitoneal hemorrhage may not be apparent on physical examination. For example, half the patient's blood volume (40 ml/kg body weight) must be present to cause overt abdominal distention. If 20% to 25% of the blood volume is lost or sequestered over a 10-minute period, profound hypovolemic shock will occur.

It is also worthy to note that small volumes of blood loss from multiple small bite wounds and contusions cumulatively can result in a significant loss of red cells.

A midline celiotomy is advisable when teeth have penetrated or crushed the abdominal cavity (as occasionally noted in small dogs and cats). Superficial bite

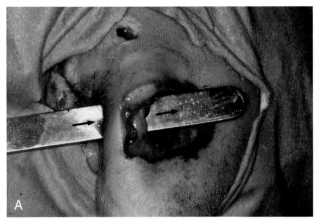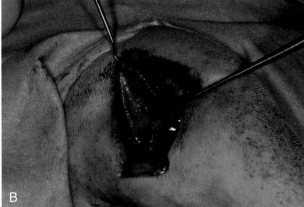

FIG. 7-8 (A) Bite wounds to the perineum completely severed the rectum from the anocutaneous junction; as noted by passage of a spay hook handle from the anus into the bite wound. (B) Skin hooks were used to manipulate the rectum. Polydiaxonone 3-0 sutures were used to repair this laceration. Skin wounds were only partially closed. It is best not to attempt primary skin closure with grossly contaminated rectal wounds.

wounds limited to the outer abdominal wall can be managed as discussed above. However, the abdomen should be prepared for possible exploratory surgery in the event that more significant trauma is noted during surgery.

Orthopedic Injuries and Spinal Trauma

As discussed, smaller dogs and cats are more susceptible to injury as a result of *direct trauma* (crushing, penetration) or *indirect trauma* (violent shaking of the victim with wounds created distant to the point of direct contact). Most fractures can be stabilized at the time of bite wound management. External fixators may be particularly useful in fracture stabilization, thereby reducing the risk of internal fixation in proximity to a contaminated bite wound. As noted, surgery should be delayed in those cases where circulatory compromise to the lower extremity is of concern. Resolution of tissue swelling normally follows improvement in circulation and lymphatic drainage. A modified Robert Jones bandage or supportive splints may be used to stabilize the fracture while managing the bite wounds.

A complete neurologic examination is essential to diagnosing spinal trauma. Radiographs and supplemental diagnostic imaging are used to confirm vertebral fracture/luxations. Depending on the nature of the injury and the severity of clinical signs, external stabilization, internal stabilization, and/or decompression of the spinal cord may be necessary.

Infection and Bite Wounds

The polymicrobial flora of the oral cavity can inoculate wounds with aerobic and anaerobic bacteria. Bite wounds resulting in perforation of the gastrointestinal tract can result in the spillage of additional bacterial contaminants (Fig. 7-8.) In human studies, aerobic infections are more common than anaerobic infections alone. (Bite wounds have a 5% to 10% risk of infection in humans; nonbite lacerations have an infection rate of 5% by contrast.) However, with the presence of anaerobic bacteria, the severity of the infection is often increased. *Pasteurella* spp. are gram-negative nonmotile pleomorphic coccobacilli that are commonly isolated from the oral cavity of dogs and cats. In one report, up to 50% of canine and 90% of feline bite wound infections in humans were the result of *Pasteurella* spp. Management of *Pasteurella* infections in humans can be problematic, especially in older, debilitated patients; individuals with orthopedic implants and internal prosthetic devices; and persons with a compromised immune system.

> The risk of infection is affected by several factors, including
>
> - Overall health of the patient
> - Body region bitten
> - Severity of tissue trauma
> - Bacterial inoculum and virulence
> - Delays in proper medical management

In the face of this acute tissue trauma, the selection and use of antibiotics remains somewhat controversial. Over the last decade, the prophylactic use of antibiotics has been demonstrated to be of limited clinical efficacy in preventing infection. Prophylactic use of antibiotics is of proven value only for carefully selected high-risk procedures when properly administered before surgery. Antibiotics are normally administered after bite injuries, and several hours may transpire before administration and effective blood levels are achieved. In general, 3 hours is considered the maximum acceptable delay in administration of antibiotics in bite wound management. To avoid the several-hour delay to achieve an adequate serum level associated with oral antibiotics, intravenous administration is advisable for seriously injured patients and is 4 to 12 times faster than intramuscular administration for developing an effective tissue-fluid concentration at the wound.

Bacteriocidal antibiotics are best employed in bite wounds. Cephalosporins, ampicillin, and penicillin rapidly enter the wound (within 1 hour). In contrast, erythromycin and gentamicin take 2–4 hours for wound concentrations to match serum concentrations, whereas tetracycline and clindamycin never reach wound levels equivalent to serum levels. Cephalosporins are generally effective against *Pasteurella* spp. and a variety of other microorganisms. Amoxicillin or clavulanate potassium can be useful against *Pasteurella multocida* resistant to penicillins and β-lactamase *Staphylococcus* spp. Fluoroquinolones are useful for resistant gram-positive and gram-negative infection. In the presence of gram-negative organisms, an aminoglycoside such as gentamicin should be considered. Antibiotics are *not* a substitute for the appropriate surgical management of bite wounds.

In the presence of infection, wound cultures (aerobic, anaerobic) are advisable in order to select the most appropriate antibiotic(s), especially in the septic patient. Culturing the acute uninfected bite wound is useless in determining the potential infection organisms. Culture samples should be submitted from deep within the wound by aspiration or incision, drainage, and exploration of the area. Aspiration of lymph nodes or areas of cellulitis also can be employed to obtain accurate culture samples. More superficial wound cultures are more likely to include contaminants that will lead to misleading results. The most accurate source for culturing infected wounds is from tissue samples from the abscess wall.

Although uncommonly performed in practice, Gram stains may be useful in determining the type of organisms present and the most appropriate initial antibiotic selection prior to obtaining definitive culture and sensitivity results.

Rabies and the Transmission of Infectious Diseases

Of the infectious diseases transmitted by bite wounds, rabies is the single greatest concern because of the human health implications of this viral disease.

It has been recommended that unvaccinated pets bitten by a wild mammal (unavailable for testing) should be euthanized. If the owner refuses, the pet must be isolated for 6 months and vaccinated 1 month before release.

Vaccinated pets should be revaccinated immediately, confined by the owner, and monitored carefully for 45 days. For specific details, the veterinarian should consult with local and state authorities to ensure that regulations are precisely followed.

Cats can transmit feline leukemia virus and feline immunodeficiency virus through bites. Assessment of transmission can be evaluated by serologic testing 6 months after the injury. These two diseases can result in nonhealing wounds.

BURNS

Veterinarians see few burns compared to human physicians. Most burns seen by the author are not life-threatening but are referred for definitive closure of the wound.

Types of Burns Seen in Veterinary Practice

1. Fire/flame burns
2. Scalds
3. Electrical heating pads
4. Hot air dryers
5. Heating lamps
6. Exothermic (chemically activated) heat packs
7. Electrical cords
8. Faulty electrocautery units
9. Wood-burning stoves
10. Household radiators
11. Stove tops
12. Automobile mufflers
13. Solar (actinic) radiation
14. Chemical burns
15. Radiation burns
16. Automobile muffler burns

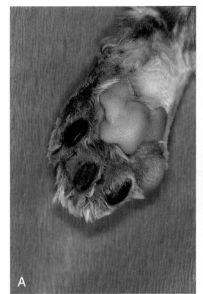
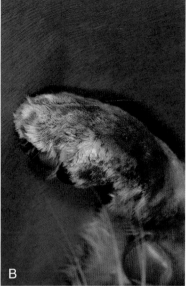
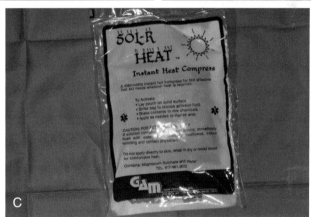

FIG. 7-9 (A, B) Contact burns involving a foot of a feline patient recovering from anesthesia. (C) Unfortunately, chemically activated heat packs were placed in direct contact with the foot, resulting in full-thickness skin necrosis. Hot water bottles and other supplemental heat sources should be well covered with towels to prevent burns from occurring.

Ironically, the most common thermal injuries seen by the author are caused by veterinarians using various heat sources to warm the patient (Fig. 7-9). Electrical heating pads in particular can generate considerable heat: prolonged contact in combination with local tissue retention of heat can produce full-thickness burns of considerable dimension (Fig. 7-10). Less commonly seen are faulty ground plates used with electrocautery units, resulting in contact burns (Fig.7-11).

Burn Classification

The severity of the burn is evaluated by the degree or depth of the injury, as well as the percentage of the surface area involved. A full-thickness burn site usually has three concentric zones of tissue injury: a central zone of coagulative necrosis, a middle zone of vascular stasis with compromised tissue perfusion, and an outer zone of hyperemia. Progressive circulatory compromise can result in necrosis extending into the middle zone, in an outward direction.

Superficial burns (first degree) are burns confined to the outermost epidermis. The skin can appear erythematous and is hyperesthetic to the touch. Properly managed, healing can be rapid and complete within a week after injury. Partial-thickness burns (second degree) involve a variable depth of the dermis. Burns confined to the more superficial layer normally have a favorable outcome when properly managed, with healing noted 3 weeks after injury. Deep dermal burn healing, however, is more problematic, especially when involving large surface areas. Systemic effects may be noted under these circumstances. Healing can be prolonged since the epidermis and a majority of compound hair follicles, residing in the dermis, are destroyed.

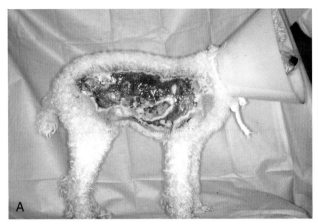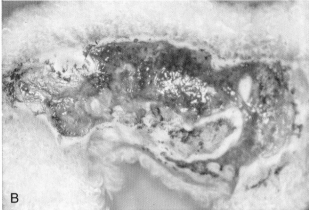

FIG. 7-10 (A) Electrical heating pad burn in a poodle. (B) Close assessment of the wound suggested that sufficient loose skin was present for closure by wound contraction and epithelialization. (From Parritz DL, Pavletic MM. 1992. Physical and chemical injuries: heat stroke, hypothermia, burns and frostbite. In: Murtaugh R, Kaplan P, eds. *Veterinary Emergency and Critical Care Medicine.* St. Louis, MO: Mosby Year Book.)

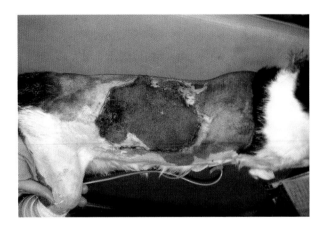

FIG. 7-11 Improperly grounded electrocautery units can result in contact burns, as noted in this patient. The eschar was excised and the wound was closed primarily.

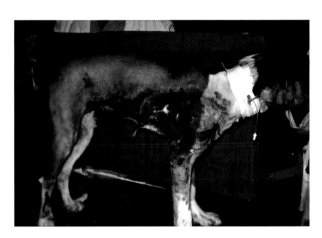

FIG. 7-12 Muffler burn in a dog. Animals can tumble beneath a car on impact, coming in contact with the hot muffler. Animals also may suffer from deep abrasions when dragged beneath the car for a distance.

Full-thickness burns involve the complete destruction of the epidermis, dermis, and possibly underlying hypodermal tissues (Fig. 7-12 and 7-13). In large areas involving major surface areas of the body, systemic signs may be noted. Closure of the lost skin may require plastic surgery for the larger wounds. Full-thickness burns involving greater than 20% of the total body surface area can result in a cascading series of pathophysiologic changes that require considerable medical management in addition to the challenges associated with the surgical management and closure of the wounds.

Burn Classification Based on Depth of Injury

- Superficial (first degree): Limited to the epidermis.
- Partial-thickness (second degree): Epidermis and a variable portion of the dermis.
- Full-thickness (third degree): Complete involvement of the entire skin thickness,
- Fourth-degree burns are those that extend to the deeper tissues, including muscle and bone.

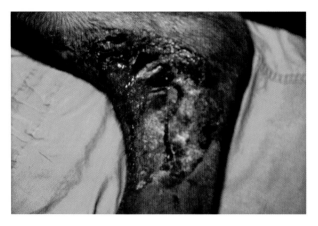

FIG. 7-13 Thermal injury in a dog struck by an automobile. The burn was sustained by friction/abrasion on the road pavement. This wound had a central third-degree burn (note burn eschar) with more peripheral second- and first-degree burns. (From Parritz DL, Pavletic MM. 1992. Physical and chemical injuries: heat stroke, hypothermia, burns and frostbite. In Murtaugh R, Kaplan P, eds. *Veterinary Emergency and Critical Care Medicine.* St. Louis, MO: Mosby Year Book.)

Estimating the Surface Area of the Burn

An estimation of the size of the burn can be somewhat subjective in animals that have comparatively greater amounts of loose elastic skin covering their body (as compared with humans). A basic estimation of the surface area can be determined by employing the "rule of nines" formula commonly used in humans. Accurate assessment of the depth of the burn, however, can be problematic in the first several days after sustaining a thermal injury.

Rule of Nines: Surface Areas Estimates Based on Body Region

Each forelimb: 9%

Each hind limb: 18%

Head and neck: 09%

Dorsal half of the trunk: 18%

Ventral half of the trunk: 18%

Although conversion charts and surface area formulas are available (see Table 7-1), a working estimate can be determined using the rule of nines. Patient management is primarily directed at the patient's needs and response during the course of therapy. This estimate will serve as the initial point for fluid therapy in patients with probable full-thickness burns over greater than 20% of their body surface area.

Speaking to the Client

After evaluating a patient with extensive burns, it is critically important to discuss the care required and costs associated with managing the pet. The cost of managing these patients can easily run into thousands of dollars.

When a major surface area of the patient is involved with probable full-thickness burns, euthanasia becomes a realistic option. When in doubt, consult with a board-certified surgeon familiar with these injuries.

Burn Pathophysiology

The pathophysiology of major thermal injuries can create serious metabolic derangements beyond the margins of the wound. Among the potential problems associated with partial- and full-thickness burns involving a wide surface area (greater than 20%) are: hypovolemic burn shock; sequestration of fluid in the extravascular extracellular space; red cell destruction; myocardial depression (negative inotropy), arrhythmias, and high output cardiac failure; postburn pneumonitis, acute respiratory insufficiency, and pneumonia; immunosuppression with impaired function of leukocytes, macrophages, and T cells; reticuloendothelial cells; fluid and electrolyte derangements; acid-based imbalance; disseminated intravascular coagulation and thromboembolism; hepatic and renal failure; adrenal insufficiency; increased gastrointestinal mucosal permeability with disruption of the intestinal barrier; and gastrointestinal ulceration or Curling's ulcers; burn sepsis; hypermetabolism; nonhealing wounds, contracture, and Margolin's ulcer (squamous cell carcinoma); scarring; and poor cosmetic results.

Experimentally, dogs that sustain 50% scald burns without intravenous fluid support demonstrate a sharp decline of cardiac output and an abrupt rise in hematocrit value from a loss of plasma volume. Although the body can institute compensatory mechanisms to improve cardiac output, early aggressive intravenous fluid replacement therapy is essential to correct the abnormalities noted.

TABLE 7-1
Body weight-to-surface area conversion.

Body Weight		Surface Area*	
Kilograms	Pounds	Square Centimeters	Square Meters
2	4.4	1600	0.16
4	8.8	2500	0.25
6	13.2	3800	0.33
8	17.6	4000	0.40
10	22.0	4600	0.46
12	26.6	5200	0.52
14	30.9	5800	0.58
16	35.3	6400	0.64
18	39.7	6900	0.69
20	44.1	7400	0.74
22	48.5	7900	0.79
24	52.9	8300	0.83
26	57.3	8800	0.88
28	61.7	9000	0.92
30	66.1	9700	0.97
32	70.6	10,100	1.01
34	75.0	10,500	1.05
36	79.4	10,900	1.09
38	83.8	11,300	1.13
40	88.2	11,700	1.17
42	92.6	12,100	1.21
44	97.0	12,500	1.25
46	101.4	12,800	1.28
48	105.6	13,200	1.32
50	110.0	13,500	1.35
52	114.4	13,900	1.39
54	118.8	14,300	1.43
56	123.2	14,700	1.47
58	127.6	15,000	1.50
60	132.0	15,300	1.53
62	136.4	15,700	1.57
64	140.8	16,000	1.60
66	145.2	16,300	1.63
68	149.6	16,600	1.66
70	154.0	17,000	1.70

* Calculated from the following equation: Area (in meters)^2 = 0.1 × Wt.2/3 (in kilograms).
Modified from Davis LE. Thermal burns. In: Swaim SF, ed. 1980. *Surgery of Traumatized Skin: Management and Reconstruction,* 222. Philadelphia, PA: WB Saunders.

Clinical Observations

A number of referral burn patients who have sustained burns estimated to be somewhat greater than 20% of their body surface area have been noted to be surprisingly stable (oftentimes days after injury) despite the fact they received little or no fluid therapy.

This may have to do with the fact that most dogs and cats have loose, elastic skin, resulting in a tendency for clinicians to overestimate the burn surface area.

Appropriate medical therapy should be instituted to ensure the patient is in the best possible health for the wound care/surgical procedures required to close the cutaneous defects.

Fluid Therapy for Major Thermal Injuries

After sustaining a serious burn, capillary permeability increases rapidly, not only at the burn site itself, but also throughout the body, resulting in a free exchange of all noncellular elements of the blood within the extravascular space. The loss of plasma, electrolytes, and plasma proteins (less than 350,000 Daltons) occurs at a rate of 4 to 4.5 ml/kg/h during fluid administration of seriously burned humans. This extracellular fluid (edema) is sequestrated from the vascular compartment proportional to the severity of the burn. The dramatic loss of plasma volume results in a notable rise in hematocrit, despite the fact that red cells have been destroyed, and their life span is reduced to 30% of estimated normal value. The loss of fluid combined with polymerization of plasma protein increases blood viscosity. However, capillary integrity does improve 18 to 24 hours after the burn. Adequate fluid replacement at this time results in early restoration of cardiac output. After 24 hours, colloids may be useful in expanding plasma volume as capillary permeability declines.

The fluid loss of burn patients is essentially iso-osmolar; isotonic fluids are used as the basic replacement solution. Hypertonic saline also has been used to a lesser degree. During the first 24 hours, lactated Ringer's solution is commonly used for volume expansion. To maintain normal renal function, fluid administration should be adjusted to maintain a urine output of 1 ml/kg/h. In the first 24 postburn hours, fluid input may be as much as 3 to 4 times urine output (3 to 4 ml/kg/h) because of the increased capillary permeability. An initial shock dose of 80–90 ml/kg intravenously may be indicated during the first hour of critical presentation.

Fluid Resuscitation Formulas

Burn formulas (Parkland and modified Brooke formulas) have been developed as a general guideline for initial treatment of human patients sustaining major burns. These formulas combine both maintenance and replacement volumes based on the weight of the patient and surface area burned. The Parkland formula, commonly employed in humans, uses the percentage of surface area burned to estimate fluid needs: 4 ml/kg body weight × percentage of burn area. Half of this volume is given within the first 8 hours after injury. One quarter of this volume is given during the second 8-hour period, followed by the remaining quarter in the last 8 hours. Delayed presentation of the patient would require a more aggressive approach. Colloid, plasma, or 5% albumin can be administered in this last 8-hour period if urine output remains below normal value. Although this formula has been adapted to small animals, treatment must be tailored to the individual needs of the patient. Central venous pressure monitoring may be useful in assessing the rate of fluid administration.

All formulas are potentially imprecise. Treatment is based on the patient's response to treatment, monitoring by

Vital signs

Mental status

Serial blood work

Blood gas analysis

Central venous pressure

Urine output and analysis

Adjustments in the rate of fluid administration are based on the serial measurements of these parameters.

When capillary permeability returns to near normal levels after 24 hours, less Ringer's intravenous fluid support is required for intravascular volume expansion and urine output. With evaporative loss of water through a large burn surface area, 5% dextrose in water is additionally used to offset this deficit in the second 24-hour period: 1–2 ml/kg × percentage of burn per day. If needed, colloid or plasma at 0.3–0.5 ml/kg per percentage of burn or 0.5% albumin at 1 g/kg/d has been used in persons during this time period. They also have potential use in the veterinary patient. Body weight; urine output; and blood analysis of hematocrit, serum protein and albumin, electrolytes, blood urea nitrogen (BUN) and creatinine, blood glucose, blood gas determination; and serum/urine osmolality are closely monitored to determine the adequacy of fluid administration. BUN, hematocrit, total protein, and blood glucose samples can be repeated throughout the day until chemistry profile results are obtained. Blood chemistry units that are common in many veterinary hospitals can be used for more frequent testing if necessary.

After 48 hours, mobilization of burn wound edema occurs and the body weight gradually returns to preburn levels over the following days. Less intravenous fluid support is required as the patient begins eating and drinking during this resorptive phase, although evaporative water loss must be assessed during this period. Continued analysis of blood and urine samples are necessary. Fluid therapy is judiciously tailored to maintain serum values in a low normal range as edema fluid is mobilized. Urine output is closely monitored. It is desirable to maintain serum protein between 3.5 and 6.5 gm/dl and a hematocrit above 25% to prevent hypoxia during the patient's hypermetabolic state. Anemia may become apparent in this stage, necessitating packed red cells or whole blood transfusions.

Common Fluid and Electrolyte Problems

Hypernatremia

Hypernatremia is the most common electrolyte abnormality encountered in human burn patients, and it is a result of unreplaced evaporative water loss from the burn surface. It can be noted in dogs under similar circumstances. The clinical response to this fluid deficit is loss of weight and blood volume. There is a rise in serum sodium and chloride above 145 mEq/l and 110 mEq/l, respectively. There is a concomitant rise in BUN as well as serum and urine osmolalities. Osmotic diuresis can cause similar signs in uncontrolled hyperalimentation regimens and sepsis. Serum sodium levels rising to 170–180 mEq/l leads to delirium, convulsions, and death.

Electrolyte-free fluids (5% dextrose in water; D5W) or hypotonic solutions are used to re-expand the extracellular fluid loss and correct this abnormality.

Hyponatremia

Hyponatremia, or water intoxication, is most prevalent in children who receive large volumes of electrolyte-free (D5W) or hypotonic solution during resuscitation. Dogs allowed to consume large amounts of water before proper fluid resuscitation may also manifest this condition. Convulsions ensue when serum sodium and chloride levels plummet below 130 mEq/l and 80 mEq/l, respectively. Serum and urine osmolalities decrease and an increase in urine output with low specific gravity can be seen. This problem can be corrected by restriction of free water and sodium replacement (3% to 5% solution) administered slowly over 6–12 hours.

Hyperkalemia

A modest degree of hyperkalemia is a common result of hemolysis and tissue necrosis in the first 48 hours in burned animals. Acidosis can enhance potassium elevation. Renal failure can cause a dramatic rise in serum potassium levels. Adrenocortical insufficiency in humans can promote hyperkalemia. Electrocardiograms can reflect the severity of hyperkalemia. Therapy for hyperkalemia is directed at protecting the heart from potassium's depressive action on the conducting system and toward reducing those levels, while correcting the underlying cause(s). Serious cardiac conduction toxicity can be reversed with the judicious administration of calcium. Serum potassium can be decreased by sodium bicarbonate or glucose and insulin to promote the shift of potassium from the extracellular space. Peritoneal dialysis, hemodialysis, and cation-exchange resins have been used in severe cases of hyperkalemia in humans.

Potassium levels are ideally maintained at 3.5–4.5 mEq/l. Intravenous administration of fluids low in potassium, including 0.9% saline or lactated Ringer's, should be used.

Hypokalemia

After 48 hours, renal excretion of potassium is accelerated and may result in hypokalemia unless supplementation is instituted. Potassium (15–20 mEq/l) may be added to commercial replacement solutions (4–5 mEq/l) to maintain serum potassium in the normal range. Supplementation should be increased to 80 mEq/l if serum potassium falls below 2.5 mEq/l as long as renal function is maintained and an electrocardiogram is monitored for signs of potassium toxicity (mild hyperkalemia: peaked T waves, widening QRS, decreased P wave; moderate hyperkalemia: amplitude prolonged P-R; severe hyperkalemia: ventricular fibrillation, asystole). A safe rate of potassium administration is 0.5 mEq/kg/h.

A second method to maintain adequate potassium levels is that of alternating commercial replacement fluids (containing 4–5 mEq/l potassium) with maintenance fluids (containing 13–35 mEq/l) on an equal basis.

Acidosis

Acidosis is most commonly seen in the early postburn period. Metabolic acidosis is the result of poor tissue perfusion but may be compounded by respiratory acidosis secondary to smoke inhalation or pulmonary disease. Patients attempt to compensate with an increased respiratory rate to reduce pCO_2. Blood and urine pH may drop below 7.35 and 5.5, respectively.

Treatment consists of improving tissue perfusion, maintaining adequate oxygen saturation, and the judicious use of sodium bicarbonate, if necessary, based on a blood gas analysis and base-deficit calculations.

Overload Syndrome

Administration of crystalloids and colloids in excess of volume losses results in overexpansion of extracellular fluid spaces. One should be suspicious of fluid overload if urinary output approaches intravenous fluid administration. In animals, rales on thoracic auscultation and the appearance of pulmonary edema on radiographs are most commonly noted. Peripheral edema unrelated to the burn injury, a decreased urine specific gravity, and an elevated serum sodium level should alert the clinician to this complication. Treatment consists of decreasing volume replacement, diuretics, and closely monitoring serum electrolytes.

Oliguria

The most frequent causes of oliguria is hypovolemia from inadequate fluid resuscitation in relation to fluid losses from evaporative water loss, diarrhea, hemorrhage, and increased capillary permeability. Acute tubular necrosis due to myoglobin casts in the kidney or administration of nephrotoxic drugs can result in complete renal failure.

Increased fluid volume replacement can reverse prerenal oliguria by improving renal blood flow and restoring vascular volume. Additional medical management directed at improving renal perfusion may be necessary, including the judicious use of intravenous dopamine. Mannitol or furosemide can be instituted. Failure to respond suggests acute renal tubular necrosis. Acute renal shutdown necessitates intensive monitoring and dialysis to maintain the patient until renal function (if possible) can improve. Acute renal tubular necrosis in face of major thermal injuries is particularly foreboding in the veterinary patient.

Anemia

Assuming patients have a normal hematocrit in the preburn period, anemia in severely burned patients is the result of direct red cell destruction and a significant reduction of the life span of red cells. Following successful fluid resuscitation, the artificially high hematocrit noted in the early postburn period will decline after 48 hours. Hemolysis from sepsis, internal bleeding, and related complications can enhance the anemia. Whole blood or packed cell replacement should be instituted to maintain a hematocrit above 25%. Supplemental oxygen is advisable in seriously burned patients due to increased oxygen consumption in their hypermetabolic states. Conditions contributing to red cell destruction or a fall in production require correction.

Nutritional Support

In view of the hypermetabolic state of the severely burned patient and the expenditure of energy from evaporative heat loss through the burn wound, efforts must be initiated to keep the patient in a state of positive nitrogen balance. Nutritious high-calorie, high-protein diets can be introduced provided that renal and liver function is adequate. A balanced diet can be offered in increasing amounts after 48 hours. Vitamin supplements can be added to the nutritionally balanced diet. Keeping the room temperature at 31 °C can reduce the caloric expenditure of the patient. Patients who are able to display a healthy appetite are introduced to greater amounts of food up to 2–2.5 times maintenance requirements, depending upon the severity of the burn. Weighing patients is useful to determine how they are responding, keeping in mind that resorption of extravascular extracellular fluid after 48 hours will account for initial weight reduction to a preburn weight.

Assessment of the Thermal Injury

Following initial patient stabilization, the primary goal in the management of all burn patients is early wound closure. Burn depth and regional involvement must be determined in order to develop a proper medical/surgical plan.

Early assessment of burn depth can be difficult. Pinching of the skin to assess burn depth by the fissure created is inaccurate in the early hours after injury unless the wound is obviously deep. Advanced full-thickness thermal necrosis is distinguishable as a thickened, leathery, brown-black eschar (Fig. 7-13). In some cases full-thickness burns are a bloodless "pearl" white. A fissure or separation at the interface between viable and nonviable tissue commonly forms within 7–10 days after full-thickness thermal injury. Superficial burns may appear as reddened, inflamed skin with a thin scab or crust formed on the surface. Partial-thickness (second degree) burns, however, may be indistinguishable grossly from full-thickness (third-degree) burns in the initial days until separation of viable and nonviable tissue occurs. Unsinged hair may be plucked effortlessly from deep partial thickness and full-thickness burns (Fig. 7-14). Adding to the confusion is the fact that progressive circulatory compromise from thrombosis may result in further tissue loss within the first 72 hours after injury. Depending on the

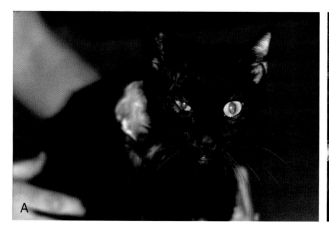
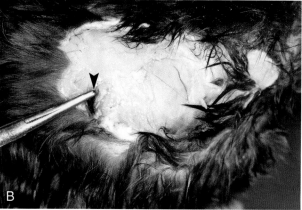

FIG. 7-14 (A, B) Hair easily plucks out of the third-degree scald injury on the shoulder of this cat.

heat source and its application, the veterinarian may see a halo effect of first- and second-degree burns surrounding a third-degree burn.

> ## Partial or Full Thickness?
>
> With the presence of a burn eschar, it is not possible to determine immediately the amount of dermis damaged or destroyed. During conservative management, the necrotic surface may delaminate over several days, allowing assessment of the surviving tissues.
>
> At the time of surgical debridement, a scalpel blade can be used to partially incise through a portion of the eschar, giving a cross-sectional view of the skin edge. In the case of partial-thickness burns, viability can be observed in the lower dermal segment. The thicker skin overlying the dorsum of the trunk and cervical areas is easier to visualize.

As noted in Chapter 1, the poorly developed capillary loops of the superficial plexus explains the general lack of blister formation with thermal injuries.

Extreme burns can result in destruction of tissues below the skin (fourth-degree burns). A detailed physical examination is required to assess other regional structures, including the eyes, ears, oral cavity, respiratory tract, urogenital tract, anus, and footpads. However, patients may be subject to multiple forms of trauma simultaneously: neurologic injuries, fractures, and other internal injuries should not be overlooked.

Burn Wound Infection

Sepsis presents the greatest threat to the seriously burned patient. Protection from sepsis includes containment and control of bacteria colonizing the burn wound, prevention of the accumulation of purulent discharge on the burn wound, prevention of secondary contamination, avoidance of additional tissue trauma, promotion of an environment conducive to healing, and removing all nonviable tissue as early as possible. In the case of large areas of necrotic skin, the author firmly believes in early surgical excision of the necrotic eschar. Early eschar removal does more to control infection and promote a viable vascular bed suitable for closure than any other treatment modality. This is reserved only for areas of distinguishable full-thickness skin necrosis. Superficial- and partial-thickness burns are not routinely excised: topical

management is instituted to control infection, promote separation of the nonviable surface, and promote epithelialization of the denuded areas.

Extensive burns generate extensive costs. Materials, supplies, medication, surgery, and hospitalization easily can result in bills up to several thousand dollars. Owners must be prepared for the financial and emotional commitment they will face in seriously burned animals. In some cases euthanasia is a humane and logical alternative.

Initial Wound Management

After excessive hair is carefully clipped from the burn area, the wound is examined to help determine its depth and extent. Because skin has low thermal conductance and releases retained heat slowly, thermal damage can continue after the initial injury. Application of chilled saline or water to the burn wound within 2 hours after injury can decrease the duration of thermal retention and reduce the depth of tissue injury. The optimal liquid temperature is 3°C–17°C, and the burned area should be cooled by immersion or compresses for at least 30 minutes. (Unfortunately, most cases are not presented promptly).

Avoid packing areas in ice and be aware that prolonged cold may further injure compromised tissues. Discretion must be employed when cold fluid is applied over a broad burn area in order to avoid hypothermia in a shocky patient. Topical cool water with a spray nozzle also is useful in removing caustic agents from the skin surface.

Analgesics are an integral part of burn wound management. Sedatives or general anesthesia also may be required during procedures in which pain may be inflicted. Good systemic analgesics include the following: oxymorphone at 0.02–0.06 mg/kg IV every 4 hours (dogs); butorphenol 0.05–0.20 mg/kg IV every 6 to 12 hours (dogs, cats); and morphine sulfate 0.20–0.50 mg/kg SQ, IM every 4 hours (dogs). Consultation with an anesthesiologist is advisable not only to discuss optional analgesics and dosages but also to select the most appropriate anesthetic protocols for surgery.

Topical Agents

Detergents, peroxides, and harsh antimicrobials should not be applied to burns. Additional tissue trauma and circulatory compromise can convert a partial-thickness burn to a full-thickness loss. Copious lavage with sterile isotonic solutions followed by a broad-spectrum antimicrobial ointment is satisfactory for small superficial and partial-thickness thermal injuries. Until the veterinarian can clearly delineate between partial-thickness and full-thickness thermal injuries, this initial conservative approach is appropriate.

Topical agents can be applied beneath a bulky, sterile, protective bandage. This is most effective when dealing with the lower extremities in order to protect the wound from contamination and external trauma. Extensive burns involving multiple regions are more difficult to cover. In many cases, topical agents may be applied more easily without a bandage. "Open therapy" by buttering burn ointment on the areas with a sterile glove or applicator can be performed two or three times daily. Areas can be gently dabbed or rinsed with warm isotonic solutions to remove debris prior to reapplication of the ointment. Serial debridement also may be performed as necrotic tissue separates.

A variety of nonirritating topical antimicrobial agents are available on the market. Selection is of minor importance in small thermal injuries. In large thermal wounds, a broad-spectrum ointment that is easily applied and rinsed is desirable. Furthermore, the ointment should be nonpainful, nonirritating, minimally absorbed systemically, and nontoxic. Of the agents commonly available, including polymyxin-bacitracin, furacin, povidone-iodine, gentamicin, mafenide (Sulfamylon), and silver sulfadiazine (Silvadene); only silver sulfadiazine fulfills most of these criteria. This water-miscible ointment is sold in jars or small tubes (see Chapter 4).

Escharotomy

A burn eschar that embraces the circumference of the trunk or extremity can form a biologic tourniquet that impairs blood and lymphatic flow. In the thoracic area, respiration can be impaired. Although a rare event in veterinary medicine, an escharotomy (eschar-relaxing incision) is indicated. Escharotomy incisions can be used to facilitate the penetration of enzymatic debriding agents (see Chapter 4).

Debridement

Debridement, the removal of devitalized tissue, is a key component to management of partial-thickness and full-thickness burn areas. Conservative mechanical debridement (e.g., wet-to-dry dressings), aggressive surgical debridement, and enzymatic debridement are commonly employed to remove necrotic tissue. Removal of dead tissue is essential to the control of

sepsis and the promotion of a viable vascular bed suitable for surgical closure.

Conservative Debridement

Conservative debridement in veterinary medicine includes the use of enzymatic debriding agents, the application of wetting agents to the injured area by immersion into water or isotonic solutions (hydrotherapy), and the application of wet dressings. All three methods can be used to facilitate softening and separation of necrotic tissue from the surrounding and underlying viable tissues.

Stainless steel surgery buckets can be sterilized and used effectively for the cat and smaller dog (Fig. 7-15). Small containers also can be covered with sterile plastic liners. The patient is immersed in warm sterile saline for 15–30 minutes once or twice daily. Following soaks, loose necrotic tissue is removed with thumb forceps and scissors. Floating the affected area improves visualization of strands of attached necrotic tissue for removal. Hydrotherapy is most difficult and time consuming in large dogs. After dabbing water from the patient's body, silver sulfadiazine ointment is applied prior to returning the patient to a heated cage. The cage must be cleaned with antiseptic agents periodically to prevent wound contamination from urine and feces.

Wet-to-wet dressings are an alternative to immersion hydrotherapy. They are best used for extremities or local areas of the trunk. Periodic application of sterile saline or lactated Ringer's solution using a syringe is necessary to offset moisture evaporation

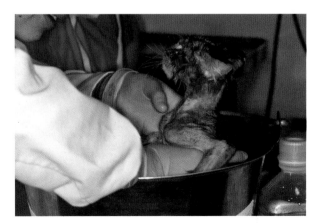

FIG. 7-15 Kitten with extensive burns. The patient was immersed in warm saline placed in a sterilized stainless steel bucket. This facilitated softening dried, necrotic skin adhered to the wounds. Forceps and scissors were used to trim off the tissue in a serial fashion.

from the bandage surface. Alternatively, a plastic perforated catheter can be incorporated into the secondary or absorptive layer of the bandage for easier fluid infusion with a syringe. (See Chapter 5.) Bandages are left on the wound for several hours. Antimicrobial agents can be included in the wetting agent employed. Wounds can be debrided during bandage changes as required.

Conservative debridement is used by the author when aggressive surgical debridement is difficult or inadvisable. This includes the removal of small areas of necrotic tissue adherent to tendons, ligaments, or underlying body structures where no clear delineation of a fascial plane can be employed for accurate excision. When necrotic tissue is largely removed and infection is under control, other topical dressings and agents also may be considered (see Chapter 4).

Aggressive Debridement

Aggressive debridement or "wound excision" is the removal of the entire burn. Large areas of full-thickness skin necrosis impede granulation bed formation and dramatically increase the risk of infection. Several days or weeks may pass before spontaneous separation of the necrotic tissue can occur with more con-

servative treatment. Under these circumstances, surgical excision using general anesthesia has the potential to eliminate the necrotic wound in a single stage. Grafting knives can facilitate tangential excision of the nonviable tissue at the level of the hypodermis (Fig. 7-16). A healthy granulation bed , suitable for flap or graft closure, rapidly forms within 5–7 days. Electrocautery, vascular clips, and ligatures are essential for hemostasis.

Wound Closure Options

Once a viable vascular wound bed is free of necrotic tissue and infection, there are several options for closure. Superficial- and partial-thickness burns frequently re-epithelialize within 3 weeks with supportive care. Deep dermal partial-thickness burns take longer. Full-thickness skin defects may heal by contraction and epithelialization from the bordering skin. Extensive burns usually require closure with skin grafts or skin flaps, depending upon the extent and location of the wound(s).

While allografts and xenografts have been used for temporary coverage of thermal injuries in humans, autogenous free grafts are required for permanent cov-

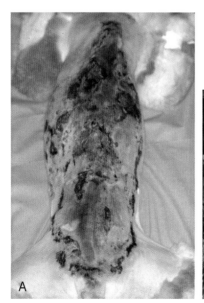
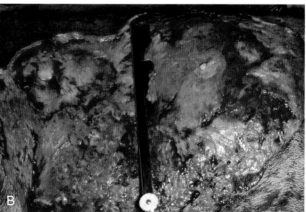

FIG. 7-16 (A) Extensive thermal wound in a dog. The burn eschar contained numerous abscesses. (B) A graft knife facilitated excision of the necrotic skin and hypodermis. A healthy granulation bed formed within 1 week, which was suitable for wound closure using a combination of axial pattern flaps, skin advancement, and punch grafts (See Fig. 2-3). (From Pavletic MM. 1990. Massive trunk wound caused by thermal trauma. *Vet Med Report* 2:159).

erage of large full-thickness thermal wounds. Partial-thickness grafts harvested with a dermatome and meshed with a 3:1 ratio is considered the best free-grafting technique for resurfacing large wounds. On occasion, axial pattern flaps can be used alone or in combination with free grafts and/or skin advancement techniques.

Excessive scarring and wound contracture are serious complications in the burned patient, often occurring when preventative medical/surgical intervention was not instituted for serious wounds. Areas subject to constant motion, such as flexion surfaces, are most susceptible to wound contracture development if major cutaneous losses occur. Splints, braces, and other devices have been employed to minimize these complications in humans. Z-plasty, pedicle grafts, and free grafts with scar division may be necessary to prevent and treat contractures. Prevention of contracture is obviously preferable to their treatment after formation.

Cosmetic results depend upon the extent of the burn. In contrast to the human, hair growth is an essential component to the cosmetic outcome of the veterinary patient. Superficial and minor partial-thickness burns may heal and retain a majority of their hair follicles for regrowth of the hair coat. Deeper burns result in a greater loss of dermis and hair follicles. Complete surgical coverage with skin flaps and full-thickness grafts can provide an adequate hair coat, whereas split-thickness grafts provide fewer follicles and are less durable than full-thickness skin coverage. On occasion, wound contraction, combined with the overlapping of hair, can reduce the visibility of the burn scar with a satisfactory cosmetic outcome. It is important to discuss cosmetic results with owners who may have unrealistic expectations.

In summary, surgical management of burns is primarily limited to full-thickness skin wounds, especially when the wound involves a significant area of the patient. Once defined, large burn eschars are best treated by surgical excision; a healthy granulation bed is expected within 5 to 7 days after careful and thorough debridement of the dead skin. Topical silver sulfadiazine, with nonadherent dressings, is commonly employed to protect the wound and reduce the bacterial population until split-thickness mesh grafts, axial pattern flaps, or skin undermining and advancement can be employed for wound closure.

INHALATION INJURIES

Smoke contains several toxic gases including CO, SO_4, NO_2, aldehydes, H_2SO_4, HCl, benzene, halogens, and hydrogen cyanide. Many of these compounds combined with inhaled particulate matter (superheated soot) can reach the pulmonary tissue, causing serious damage. Bronchial spasm, laryngeal spasm, pulmonary edema, mucosal edema, loss of ciliary function, and compromised pulmonary surfactant will aggravate hypoxia associated with a smoke-filled room. Hot, dry air has a low specific heat, and respiratory injuries are confined to the upper respiratory tract. Live steam, with a high specific heat, is capable of causing atelectasis, severe pulmonary edema, and alveolar damage.

> Dogs and cats trapped in burning buildings often have a strong smoke odor. The hair coat may have soot particles. Pets close to flames may have singed hair. These clinical findings should alert the clinician to closely assess the patient for smoke and heat-related pulmonary injury.

Pulmonary parenchymal dysfunction from severe smoke inhalation is frequently fatal in humans. Hypoxemia refractory to oxygen therapy, with the presence of bronchospasm/pulmonary edema, requires aggressive treatment to save the patient. High mortality rates (60%–70%) are associated with humans who develop pulmonary edema within 72 hours after injury.

Clinical Signs

Overt clinical signs in dogs suffering from smoke inhalation include coughing, gagging, and respiratory distress. Occasionally, ataxia, foaming at the mouth, rubbing at the eyes, and nasal bleeding are noted.

Overt clinical signs in affected cats suffering from smoke inhalation include dyspnea, vocalization, open mouth breathing, lethargy, wheezing, gagging, nasal mucoid discharge, third eyelid protrusion, and foaming at the mouth.

Loss of consciousness may be indicative of hypoxia and possible brain injury.

In two case reviews in the dog and cat (Drobaz), most patients with nonthreatening smoke inhalation clinically improved within 24 hours: severe cases worsened within this time frame.

With major inhalation injuries, an adequate airway must be established. Intubation and ventilatory support with positive-pressure ventilation is indicated in severe cases. Temporary tracheostomy should be considered for problematic patients; ventilatory support also can be used in conjunction with the tracheostomy tube. In mild cases of smoke inhalation and direct thermal injury, oxygen therapy alone may suffice. Nebulization of saline and coupage may facilitate clearance of respiratory secretions. In most cases, the tissue injury associated with mild direct thermal injury resolves within 5 days. Serial thoracic radiographs are useful in assessing changes in the respiratory tract. Bronchoscopy can be used to assess the severity of injury. It may be advisable to transfer the more serious patients to a veterinary emergency referral center that is better equipped to handle these challenging cases.

Carbon monoxide poisoning is suspected if the mucous membranes and blood are cherry red. Carbon monoxide blocks the oxygen-carrying capacity of hemoglobin. Blood oxygen levels may be low despite normal levels of dissolved oxygen in the bloodstream. Carbon monoxide poisoning requires 100% oxygen therapy to rapidly reduce the level of carboxyhemoglobin. Mild cases may benefit from an oxygen cage alone. In humans, the half-life carboxyhemoglobin is 4 hours breathing room air, whereas this is dramatically reduced to 45–60 minutes with oxygen administration by mask or nasal tube. If accessible, hyperbaric oxygen can reduce the half-life of carboxyhemoglobin to 30 minutes or less. Carboxyhemoglobin can be measured to assess the severity of carbon monoxide poisoning and progress in treatment of the patient. Local human hospitals may be required for precise measurements in problematic patients.

As previously stated, additional caution is necessary during the administration of intravenous fluids. Efficacy with short-term (12–24 hours) use of corticosteroids is questionable: prolonged use can compound the immunosuppression already seen with concomitant major thermal injuries. Diuretics (furosemide) may decrease intravascular volume without significant benefits in the treatment of pulmonary edema. Bronchodilators (albuterol) and expectorants may be beneficial. Prophylactic antibiotics are ineffective and may select out resistant organisms. Their use should be based on airway culture. Many respiratory infections in animals are noted to be caused by gram-negative bacteria. Because respiratory equipment is a potential source of bacterial infection, care must be taken to ensure that sterile tubes and uncontaminated equipment are used.

CHEMICAL BURNS

Many caustic agents are available for home and industrial use. On occasion these chemicals cause "burns" to animals accidentally or from their malicious application to pets (Fig. 7-17). The extent of the injury depends upon the chemical, its concentration, dura-

tion of contact and penetration, and its particular mechanism of action. Chemical agents damage the skin by oxidation or reduction, dehydration, protein denaturation, corrosion, or vesication. Drain cleaners and oven cleaners may contain caustic soda, causing tissue corrosion. Phenolic disinfectants also may exert a corrosive effect on tissues. Sulfuric acid and hydrochloric acid may be found in cleaning compounds and exert a dehydrating effect on tissues. Hypochlorite, potassium permanganate, and chromic acid are oxidizing agents and cause protein coagulation. In contrast, picric acid, tannic acid, acetic acid, formic acid, and hydrofluoric acid cause protein denaturation. Halogenated hydrocarbons, gasoline, ethylene oxide, and catharides are vesicants, liberating tissue amines (histamine and serotonin) and creating vesicles or blisters from tissue contact. Some solvents used for painting (turpentine, mineral spirits), furniture strippers, and concentrated flea dip solutions are examples of household chemical agents also capable of causing superficial and partial-thickness skin injuries with prolonged contact.

In general, caustic agents can be divided into strong acids and strong alkalis. Most of these agents destroy skin by coagulation necrosis. Vascular thrombosis may be noted with prolonged exposure to stronger agents. Strong alkalis in particular are capable of causing deep-tissue destruction by colliquation, extraction of water, and precipitation of protein (Fig. 7-18). An alkali-albuminate bond may form and redissolve in excess water. Alkalis form soluble soaps and protein complexes within the tissues, which facilitate the passage of hydroxyl ions into deeper layers. In contrast, hydrogen ions from acids are not complexed.

The medical history may reveal the nature of the injury, the chemical concentration, and duration of contact. However, most cases of caustic burns noted by the author are the result of malicious attacks in which the agent in question is unknown. Inhalation of vapors or consumption of the material should be determined by physical examination, thoracic radiographs, and oral/laryngeal/pharyngeal examination. Eyes should be examined very closely.

Management of Chemical Burns

Most chemical burns encountered should be lavaged with large volumes of water. Eyes are best lavaged copiously with sterile saline when available. Under experimental conditions, the results of chemical burn treatment required returning skin pH to normal and varied between acid and alkali burns. While lavage of 30% acid burns for 2 hours returned the skin to normal

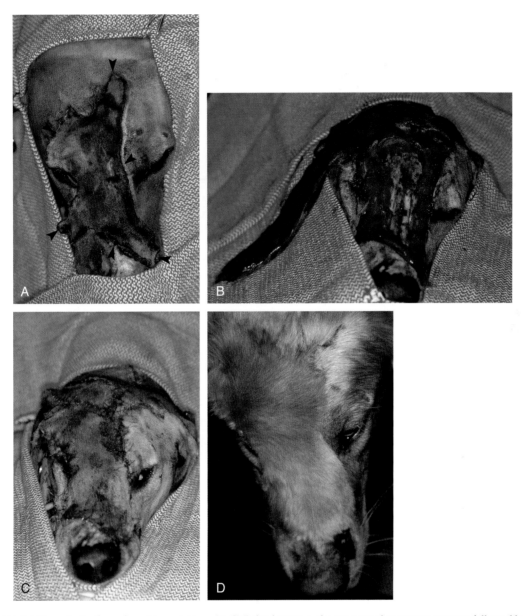

FIG. 7-17 (A) Acid burn to the face of a golden retriever. (B, C) Debridement and open wound management were followed by closure with a local transposition flap.

(D) Close-up view after early hair growth. (From Pavletic MM. 1993. Pedicle grafts. In: Slatter DH, ed. *Textbook of Small Animal Surgery*, 2nd ed. Philadelphia, PA: WB Saunders.)

pH, it took over 12 hours of lavage to reestablish normal pH following a burn with 50% sodium hydroxide. Deep chemical burns, especially alkali compounds, may require deep surgical excision if the contact has been prolonged.

Neutralizing agents are occasionally useful in limiting the extent of injury. They are not a substitute for copious lavage and should never be applied to undiluted chemical. If used, they can be applied to the wound in the form of gauze sponges loosely wrapped over the area for 20 minutes. This may be repeated if necessary. Table 7-2 summarizes several chemical compounds and their neutralizing agents.

Removal of fur facilitates close examination of the skin surfaces. Management of superficial and partial-thickness chemical burns, excluding the potential systemic effects of absorption, is similar to thermal burns. Once defined, deeper necrosis involving the skin and underlying tissues is best managed by excision and closure, unless the minor size, depth, and location of

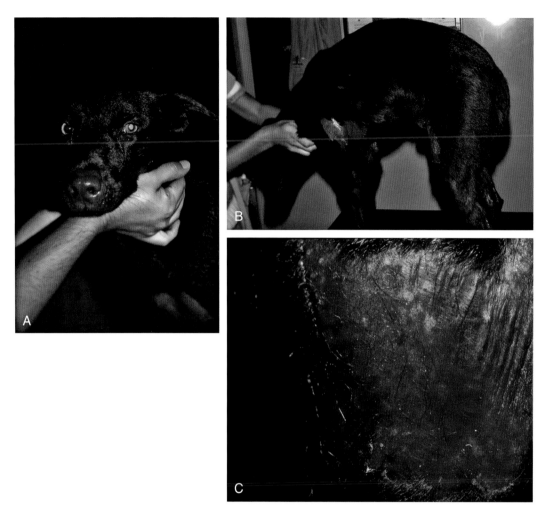

FIG. 7-18 (A, B) Patient that fell into a caustic soda pit at a petrochemical plant. Extensive chemical burns were present. The patient was bathed extensively with a water spray to remove any residual caustic soda. (C) Close-up view of the patient demonstrating coagulation of the dermis. The patient went into acute renal failure despite aggressive medical therapy and was euthanized.

the wound warrants spontaneous separation and healing by second intention.

ELECTRICAL INJURIES

Electricity can cause electrothermal burns due to arcing of the current between the source and the conductor or when the arc crosses a flexor surface, causing flame burns when the arc ignites materials adjacent to it. It can cause deep thermal burns, with cellular and vascular destruction of tissue in the path of the current; and crushlike injuries occurring secondary to massive cellular, ischemic, and muscular damage. The severity of the electrical injury is dependent upon the type of circuit, voltage, amperage, duration of contact, pathway of the current, tissue resistance, and the tissue's spatial relationship with the current. Electrical injuries are classified as low-voltage (<1000 V) or high-voltage (>1000 V). Most dogs and cats present with low-voltage (alternating household current in the United States) injuries. High-voltage injuries are rarely seen but are often fatal: wild birds, cats, and animals capable of climbing poles occasionally contact high-tension power lines, usually causing instant death.

TABLE 7-2
Injurious chemical agents.[*][+]

Agent	Clinical Presentation	Mechanism of Systemic Toxicity	Immediate Cleansing	Neutralization
Common Acids				
Sulfuric, nitric, hydrochloric, trichloracetic	Yellow, brown grey or black eschar	Vapor	Water and soap	$Mg(OH)_2$ or $NaHCO_3$ solution
Hydrofluoric	Erythema with central necrosis	None	Water	Calcium gluconate (10%) subcutaneously
Oxalic	Chalky white indolent ulcers	Ingestion only	Water	Calcium gluconate (10%)
Phenol (carbolic) and analogs	Painless, white or brown skin burn	Skin absorption	Water	Ethyl alcohol (10%) or glycerol
Chromic	Ulceration, blisters	Vapor	Water	Sodium hyposulfite
Hypochlorous (Clorox)	Second-degree	None	Water	Sodium thiosulfate (1%)
Other Acids				
Tungstic, picric, tannic, cresylic, formic, (cavity fluid)	Hard eschar	Skin absorption	Water	Cover with oil
Lyes				
$NaOH$, KOH, $Ba(OH)_3$, $Ba_2(OH)_3$, $LiOH$	Bullous erythema; slimy or slick eschar	Ingestion only	Water	Weak (0.5%–5.0%) acetic acid; lemon juice
Ammonia (NH_4OH)	Bullous erythema; slimy or slick eschar	Vapor	Water	Weak (0.5%–5.0%) acetic acid, lemon juice
Lime	Bullous erythema; slimy or slick eschar	Ingestion only	Brush off lime in water	Weak (0.5%–5.0%) acetic acid; lemon juice
Alkyl mercury salts	Erythema, blisters	Skin absorption from blisters	Water and remove blisters	Copious irrigation
Sodium metal	Painful deep burns	None	Cover with oil	None, except excision
Vesicants				
Mustard gas	Painful bullae	Vapor	Water; open vesicles during copious lavage	British antilewisite (BAL)
Tear gas	Erythema, ulcers	Vapor	Water	No specific agent
Phosphorus	Erythema to third-degree burn	Tissue absorption	Water; cold water packs	Copper sulfate ($CuSO_4$) for identification only
Ethylene oxide (ETO)	Erythema to third-degree burn	None	Allow to vaporize; then water lavage	No specific agent

[*]For complete discussion of chemicals and antidotes see Jelenko C. 1974. Chemicals that burn. J *Trauma* 14:65–73.
[+]A complete listing and description of injurious chemical agents may be found in the *Fire Protection Guide on Hazardous Materials,* 7th ed. National Fire Protection Association, 470 Atlantic Avenue, Boston, MA 02210.

Aqueous electrolyte solutions are relatively good electrical conductors with electrical current carried by mobile ions rather than free electrons. The frictional interaction of colliding molecules generates heat. An electrical current generates heat as it passes through body tissues. The rate of heating tissues depends upon the current intensity, the electrical and thermal properties of the tissues, and the spatial relationship of the tissue with the current. Tissues have different electrical conductivities and dissipate heat at different rates. In tissues electrically parallel relative to the source of the current, heat generation occurs at a rate directly proportional to tissue conductivity. In tissues that are electrically in series, heat generation is inversely proportional to tissue conductivity. In experimental models, muscle generates the highest temperatures; on cessation of the current, the muscle can heat other adjacent tissues, including bone. Convective transport of heat through blood is critical for rapid cooling. Tissue injury is severe where the current density is greatest—at the point of contact. Electrical contact with a small surface area results in a concentration of energy that causes coagulation necrosis. As a result, injuries to the tissue deep to the contact burn can be extensive. Electrical contact with a broad surface area of the body decreases the current density with dissipation of the energy. No burns may be noted in these cases, although fatal ventricular fibrillation may occur. More recent studies indicate the local electrical field can be of sufficient magnitude to cause electrical breakdown of cell membranes. Muscle destruction may be caused in part by *electroporation*, in which electrical current causes the formation of enlarged pores in the lipid cell membrane: this results in cellular rupture. Muscle and nerve cells appear to be more vulnerable to electrical breakdown.

Electrical current follows the path of least resistance, particularly with low-voltage sources. Skin resistance is lowered, however, when the surface is wet. Neurovascular channels offer the least resistance followed by muscle, skin, and bone. Nerves and vessels are particularly sensitive to electrical injury whereas bone is least sensitive to injury. Studies suggest that all tissues beneath the skin function as a single conductor (or resistor). Tissue damage is the result of converting electrical current to heat. Current intensity is greater in small cross-sectional areas such as the extremities, whereas large areas dissipate current over a wider area. Small vessels undergo thrombosis, whereas large vessels may maintain blood flow despite the occasional formation of mural thrombi. Small nutrient vessels in skeletal muscle are particularly sensitive to thrombosis, resulting in deep muscle necrosis in selected cases. Production of thromboxane A, a vasoactive prostanoid that causes vasoconstriction, thrombosis, and ischemia, enhances tissue necrosis.

The majority of small animal electrical injuries in the United States are associated with low-voltage household alternating current (60 Hz) within the frequency range known to cause striated muscle tetanization and nervous tissue paralysis. The heart and respiratory centers are more sensitive to alternating current than direct current. Low-amperage 60-Hz current passing through the head of the dog and cat produce convulsions and respiratory paralysis. Low-voltage current is capable of causing fatal ventricular fibrillation, whereas high voltage (>1000 V) can produce respiratory and cardiac arrest. Ventricular rhythm may resume in those cases when the high-voltage current is removed. Cardiopulmonary resuscitation may be necessary once the patient is separated from the electrical source.

Resultant low-voltage oral burns commonly involve the commissure of the lips, gums, tongue, and palate in small animals (Fig. 7-19). A centroneurogenic-mediated increase in peripheral vascular resistance has been implicated as the cause of the fulminating pulmonary edema occasionally seen with oral electrical burns in young dogs and cats that bite live electrical cords. Pulmonary edema would appear to be a greater problem in dogs. Aggressive treatment with oxygen, diuretics, and corticosteroids is indicated (see below).

As noted, high-voltage current injuries are uncommon in pets and are usually fatal. The contact or entry point is usually depressed, charred, and leathery, whereas the exit wound at the ground point may be explosive. Electrical current also can arc to an adjacent area if immediate grounding does not take place. Among the organs injured in association with high-voltage electrical passage through the body of humans are the esophagus, pancreas, gall bladder, small intestine, colon, skeleton, and lungs; depending upon the point of contact, course of the current through the body, and the point of exit. Immediate and delayed spinal cord injuries have been reported in humans from vascular and thermal damage. Such injuries may be temporary or permanent.

Necrosis of small intestine, secondary to low-voltage injury has not been reported in animals, but has been reported in humans. This may be explained by current passage down the anterior mesenteric artery, with heat dissipation in the terminal arteriolar branches causing bowel infarction. Paralytic ileus may also be noted. Despite the fact that this injury has not been noted in small animals, the veterinarian should be alert to vomiting and abdominal pain that may suggest bowel injury to animals known to have been injured by electrical current.

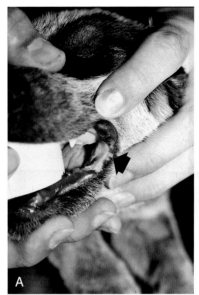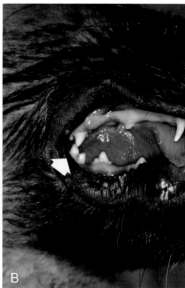

FIG. 7-19 (A) Electrical cord burn involving the oral commissure. Note the pale, bloodless wound. (B) Other electrical burns can appear brown to black, with possible local hemorrhage.

Management of Electrical Wounds

Typically, the owner will report seeing their pet bite an electrical cord or encountering their pet in a state of tetany with the cord in its mouth. After disconnecting the cord from the electrical outlet, many dogs will resume breathing. On occasion, owners will report that they resuscitated their dog or cat by breathing through the pet's nose. Intravenous fluid therapy must be performed with caution, since many dogs and cats will develop pulmonary edema, as discussed above. Close auscultation of the patient for moist rales is indicative of edema which can be confirmed with thoracic radiographs.

In the presence of life-threatening pulmonary edema, oxygen therapy and the intravenous administration of a fast-acting diuretic, such as furosemide (Lasix, Butler, Dublin OH), are indicated. Corticosteroids may be useful. Analgesics (morphine, etc.) are useful to reduce pain and patient anxiety. Morphine can have a sympatholytic and vasodilatory effect; bronchodilators (aminophylline) also may improve respiration and cause vasodilation. In refractory cases, sodium nitroprusside has been cautiously administered. Readers are directed to standard medical textbooks for further information.

As noted, most electrical burns from household current occur in and around the oral cavity. The burns are pale yellow, tan, or gray and are usually slow to slough and heal (Fig. 7-19). Many of the mild injuries slough and heal within 3 weeks without the need for surgical debridement. Oronasal fistula development in dogs and cats requires closure with mucosal flaps, labial advancement flaps, or skin flaps (Fig. 7-20). Damage to the adjacent dental arcade in young dogs and cats can result in deviation of teeth, possibly necessitating their extraction.

Like other major thermal injuries, large areas of necrosis warrant debridement and eventual closure as the severity of the wound becomes more apparent. In humans, fasciotomy has been required for injured muscle groups in order to prevent development of the compartmental syndrome secondary to high-voltage electricity.

RADIATION INJURIES

Radiation is a general term for any form of radiant energy emission from roentgen ray tubes, radioactive elements, luminous bodies, or fluorescent substances. Burns from solar (actinic) radiation are not a common problem in veterinary medicine; however, in regions where solar intensity is the greatest, body areas lacking hair and pigmentation are susceptible to actinic injury (Fig. 7-21). The majority of the discussion in this section, however, is devoted to complications associated with radiotherapy. Radiation injury concerns the veterinary surgeon from two perspectives: first, its influence on healing in association with surgery and second, management of nonhealing radiation ulcers.

Radiation particles are composed of one of three particles: alpha particles, beta particles, and gamma

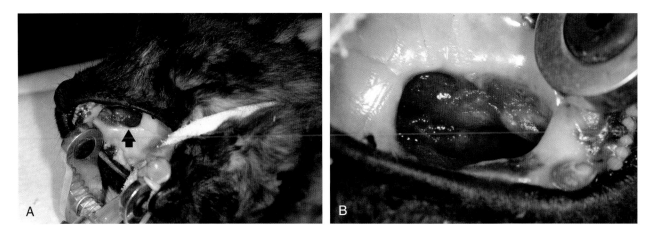

FIG. 7-20 (A) Oronasal fistula in a cat secondary to biting an electrical cord. (B) Full-thickness necrosis of the hard palate is evident. Closure was accomplished with a labial advancement flap (see Plate 99).

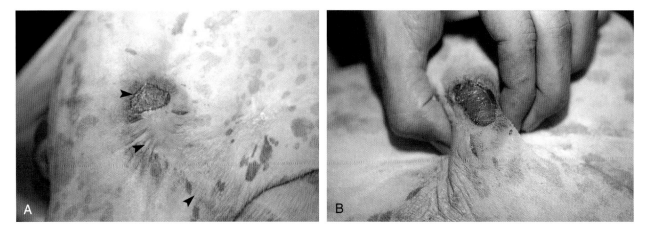

FIG. 7-21 (A, B) Repeated blistering and ulceration of an epithelialized scar in a field trial dog from prolonged solar exposure (actinic radiation). The scar was the result of the dog falling out of a moving pickup truck several months before presentation. Scar excision and advancement of hair-bearing peripheral skin was curative. Tissue was submitted for histopathologic examination to assure squamous cell carcinoma was not present.

particles. Alpha (helium nuclei) particles emitted by radium implants have limited penetrating ability. Beta particles (negatively charged electrons) can penetrate tissue 1–2 cm; its use in radiation therapy generally is limited to skin cancer and other superficial lesions. Gamma particles are capable of deep tissue penetration and are the major form of therapeutic radiation for cancer. Orthovoltage radiotherapy is delivered by X-ray–producing units, capable of a power range of 250–500 kV. Photons at this energy level are concentrated in the skin and superficial tissues. Orthovoltage

may be useful for superficial neoplasms. If used for more invasive tumors, use of excessive doses can result in a greater likelihood of significant skin damage. Orthovoltage is uncommonly used today in favor of megavoltage therapies.

Megavoltage radiotherapy is delivered by radioisotope teletherapy or linear accelerator units in the form of high-energy X-rays, gamma rays, or electrons. Photons provided by megavoltage units have an energy range of 1–35 million volts. High-energy photons are capable of deeper penetration and a skin-sparing effect. Neutron radiotherapy involves neutron bombardment of tissues but is not commonly used these days in veterinary medicine.

The success of radiation therapy resides in applying lethal doses to cancer cells, while subjecting normal tissues to sublethal levels. Unfortunately, because higher doses of radiation may be required to achieve cancer control, there is an increased likelihood of damage to normal tissues, including tissue necrosis, extensive fibrosis, and compromise to local tissue circulation.

Changes occur in irradiated tissue that can have early or delayed effects on healing. The acute reactions to skin or mucosa are erythema and desquamation. Acute radiodermatitis has been classified into four degrees: a first-degree reaction is cutaneous reddening; a second-degree reaction is characterized by a dry desquamation resulting from a loss of the outer epidermis; a third-degree reaction is characterized by moist desquamation resulting from destruction of the basal epidermal layer; and a fourth-degree burn is characterized by complete skin necrosis (Fig. 7-22). These changes are dose related. Severe erythema shortly after radiation therapy indicates a more serious burn injury. Other changes observed following radiation therapy include hair loss and alterations in skin pigmentation, depending upon the radiation dose, area irradiated, and individual sensitivity. Hair-covered skin is less sensitive compared to hairless skin. Surviving germinal cells repopulate areas when epithelial cells are destroyed. Severe radiation damage can result in acute ulceration with a loss of germinal cells required for epithelial repopulation.

Acute skin reactions generally heal within 10–14 days after cessation of therapy, except in the more severe injuries. Most cases of simple radiation dermatitis can be managed with a variety of basic topical agents. Surgeons, however, are concerned with the management of the more severe wounds, particularly in chronic ulceration where healing is problematic.

Late or chronic changes noted in previously irradiated skin include thinning and flattening of the epidermis, a decline in adnexal structures, and obliteration of rete pegs. Grossly, the skin may demonstrate dryness, thinning, induration and loss of pliability from fibrosis, and increased pigmentation with a reduction of hair growth (Fig. 7-23).

The most significant late change is a progressive decline in circulation over time. Chronic obliterative endarteritis is noted, characterized by endothelial proliferation, subintimal fibrosis, and gradual reduction in lumen diameter. Perivascular infiltrate also is present. The ischemia that ensues will impede healing to a variable degree. If incising into a previously irradiated field is unavoidable, the surgeon should avoid or minimize surgical maneuvers that may further compromise tissue. Precautions are essential to prevent contamination during surgery, since ischemic tissues are more susceptible to infection. Open wounds have a particularly difficult time healing by second intention, since neovascularization, wound contraction (myofibroblastic activity), fibroplasia, and epithelialization are impaired. A loss of fibroblasts and their stem cells also impair formation of blood vessels. The low capillary content and collagen-laden wound bed present form an unstable base for migrating epithelial

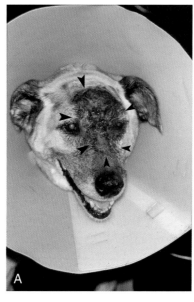 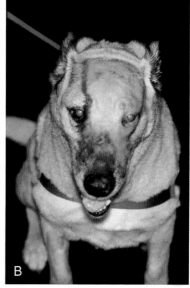

FIG. 7-22 (A) Erythema and moist desquamation after completion of orthovoltage therapy for the treatment of a nasal carcinoma. (B) The patient 10 days later. Moist crust patches have disappeared, the result of reepithelialization from germinal epithelial cells of the epidermis and cutaneous adnexa.

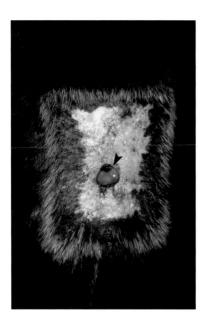

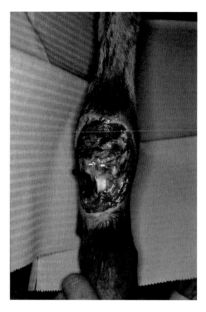

FIG. 7-23 Chronic ulcer several months after completion of radiotherapy (arrow). Note the sparse hair growth, nonpigmented hair at the periphery of the radiation field, and the dry, flaky epithelial surface.

FIG. 7-24 Necrosis of skin, muscle, and tendon overlying the carpus as a result of radiation therapy. Necrotic tissue, infection, and impaired regional circulation create a major challenge to the veterinary plastic surgeon who attempts to close this wound.

cells. Any epithelialized surface formed is more susceptible to trauma. Split-thickness grafts and direct distant flaps cannot be sustained on wound beds characterized by these chronic changes (Fig. 7-24).

In general, an uncomplicated closed surgical wound can safely receive radiotherapy as early as 1 week postoperatively. Similarly, elective surgery can be performed 4–8 weeks after radiation therapy is discontinued because inflammation secondary to irradiation is subsiding and circulation is still satisfactory. As time passes, however, tissue looses vascularity to a degree proportional to the radiation source, size of the area irradiated, fractionation of the total dose, and length of time during which the total dose was administered.

Management of Radiation Wounds

Radiation ulcers can develop 10–20 years after exposure in humans. In small animals, ulceration is more likely to occur within weeks to months after therapy. Treatment includes debridement of necrotic tissue, control of infection, and early wound closure. If the wound can be excised down to healthy vascular tissue, skin grafts can survive. However, skin grafts are unlikely to survive on an incompletely excised, chronic,

irradiated wound bed. It must be noted that more powerful radiotherapy units can damage deeper tissues, making complete excision down to viable vascular tissue difficult or impossible. Tissue excised should be submitted for histopathologic examination to assure neoplasia has not recurred. Additionally, neoplasms can develop as a result of irradiation or chronic inflammation such as Margolin's ulcers (squamous cell carcinoma) in nonhealing burn wounds.

Skin flaps, myocutaneous flaps, muscle flaps, and omentum may be used to close chronic ulcers. Properly created flaps have their own inherent circulation and do not require circulation provided by the wound bed, as long as their vascular pedicle is maintained. Local skin flaps can be attempted in order to close smaller debrided ulcers, although the veterinarian must consider that the regional skin also may have been affected by the previous radiation treatment. Local flap failure is more likely than flaps created outside the general region irradiated. Axial pattern flaps may be ideally suited due to their excellent circulation and length compared to flaps based upon the subdermal plexus alone. Muscle flaps can contribute circulation to ischemic areas and provide a vascular surface for free graft coverage. Myocutaneous flaps can provide simultaneous wound coverage while providing a muscle surface to supply circulation to ischemic areas. Omentum can be mobilized and passed through a small abdominal access incision, delivering this vascular tissue to poorly vascularized ulcers within its reach. Improvement in regional circulation will enable the surgeon to apply a graft to the viable omental surface, if needed.

> Ischemic radiation ulcers normally do not support free grafts. Local flaps may not be possible if the skin peripheral to the ulcer also was exposed to the radiation field. Distant direct flaps will likely fail, since division of the pedicle(s) relies on revascularization of the transferred flap from the recipient bed. As a result, any tissue flaps require an intact vascular pedicle to support their long-term survival in areas with marginal circulatory support.

FROSTBITE

Frostbite is the freezing of, or effect of freezing on, a part of the body. Contact with metal and other materials that rapidly conduct cold, including water, gasoline, and other industrial chemicals, can rapidly accelerate the freezing process. The thermal conductivity of water, for example, is 32 times greater than still air. Cold air alone, however, is not nearly as dangerous a freezing factor as the combination of chilling air and wind. Animals who lose their insulation properties are susceptible to hypothermia and frostbite as peripheral circulation is diverted to maintain body core temperature. Accidental or inappropriate use of liquid nitrogen and nitrous oxide during cryosurgical procedures can result in serious injury to adjacent healthy tissues as well. In all, the type and duration of cold contact are the two most important factors in determining frostbite.

High-altitude locations with lower oxygen content in the air can increase the likelihood of cold injury in animals and persons unaccustomed to it. Exertion and labored breathing in this environment accelerate heat loss through the lungs. Inadequate caloric intake can reduce the ability of the animal to generate heat. The heat production capacity of the body and the ability to conserve heat are two of the most important factors in the prevention of cold injuries. Frostbite can occur in above-freezing temperatures from prolonged immersion in animals who lack the insulation and protective physiologic mechanisms other species possess for adverse conditions.

Several mechanisms have been proposed to explain tissue injury and death after exposure to cold. Extracellular ice crystal formation may damage cells. Rapid freezing can result in fatal intracellular ice crystal for-

mation. Endothelial cell injury may precipitate thrombosis. Arteriolar vasospasm combined with shunting of blood from arterioles to venules directs oxygen, nutrients, and warmth from the frozen tissue in an effort to preserve central core temperature. Ischemia–reperfusion injury likely plays a significant roll in the loss of tissue. As blood viscosity increases, sludging and thrombosis also may occur. Unless the source of cold is removed, tissues continue to freeze, and the depth of the damage increases with prolongation of contact.

Frostbite Assessment

Frostbite in small animals is not particularly common in the United States. In veterinary practice, it is usually diagnosed in retrospect. Animals are most susceptible to frostbite during bitterly cold days with high winds. Animals lacking shelter and protection from the elements combined with a prolonged exposure period may suffer frostbite to the toes, tips of the ears, scrotum, tip of the tail, preputial orifice, flank skin, or other cutaneous surfaces lacking an adequate protective hair coat. Unless examined by an astute owner or clinician immediately, the injury will remain undiagnosed and untreated until tissue separation becomes evident days later.

Upon initial manual examination, superficial frostbite is classically characterized by soft and resilient tissues underlying the outer layer of rigid tissue. Deep frostbite is characterized by firm or stiff tissue beneath the outer rigid tissue layer. Unless the injury is obviously minor, the severity of the frostbite injury cannot be determined initially. Frostbite classification is made retrospectively: first-degree results in cutaneous erythema after warming; second-degree, in cutaneous blistering patchy skin; third-degree, in skin necrosis; and fourth-degree, in soft tissue loss or gangrene of the extremity. Mild and severe cases of frostbite may be indistinguishable for several days. Conservative therapy is advisable until the severity of the injury is clearly defined (Fig. 7-25).

Management of Frostbite

If there is no chance that the tissues will later refreeze, the affected area(s) should be rewarmed. Immersion of the affected area in a receptacle of sufficient volume to maintain a uniform temperature of 104°F–108°F (40°C–42°C) for approximately 20 minutes or until rewarming is judged complete is ideal. Tissues should never be rubbed or massaged. Soft, dry protective bandages are indicated in small animals. Restriction of activity is required when the feet are involved.

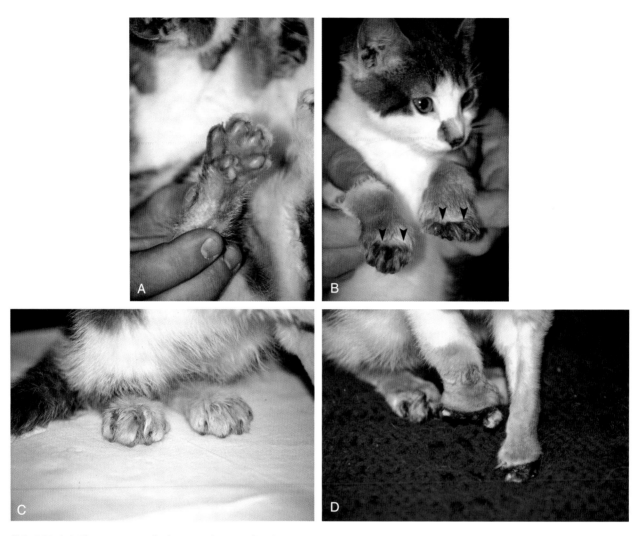

FIG. 7-25 (A) Close-up view of a kitten with severe frostbite to its paws as a result of being trapped in a freezer for several hours. Extensive edema is noted. The patient reportedly climbed into the refrigerator when the owner's children left the door open. Direct contact with the cold metallic shelving enhanced the freezing process.

(B, C) Within days, a clear demarcation of viable and nonviable tissue was noted: digits on all four paws subsequently sloughed.

(D) Necrotic tissue was trimmed; portions of the skin wounds were sutured. Other areas healed by second intention. The patient did well as a house cat despite these unfortunate circumstances. A similar injury in larger dogs would be considered catastrophic.

Maintaining hydration and a balanced diet are essential. Analgesics may be indicated. Topical antiseptics and judicious debridement of necrotic tissue or ruptured blisters is advisable. Systemic antibiotics are indicated for cases where sepsis is noted.

Rapid rewarming causes vasodilation, capillary extravasation, and vascular stasis. Treatment for persistent vasospasm at one time regularly included heparin or low-molecular-weight dextrans. However, no beneficial effect has been consistently demonstrated. Chemical sympathectomy with the use of alpha-blocking agents has shown promise when treatment has been instituted between 2 and 10 days after injury in humans. Nonsteroidal anti-inflammatory drugs may have some benefit in blocking inflammatory products of cyclooxygenases, prostaglandin F2-α, and thromboxane A_2, thereby reducing platelet aggregation and thrombosis. The methylxanthine derivative pentoxifylline alone or in combination with aloe vera cream has shown promise in a rabbit ear model. A rat foot model demonstrated less tissue necrosis when pentoxifylline and aspirin were used in combination. Controlled clinical trials are required to confirm these previous reports and the treatments' efficacy in small animals.

As noted, because of the low incidence of frostbite in small animals and the initial lack of its recognition by most owners, the veterinarian is usually contacted only after signs of necrosis become evident. Surgical debridement or amputation of the affected area may be necessary if natural separation has not occurred.

PROJECTILE INJURIES

Gunshot wounds to pets and wildlife are not uncommon in rural and inner city areas of the United States. Most veterinarians have limited knowledge of the subject of ballistics and the treatment of projectile injuries. This section reviews the basic concepts of this surprisingly complex subject, known as *projectile injuries.*

Ballistics is the science of motion of a projectile during its travel through the barrel of a firearm (interior ballistics), its subsequent path through the air (exterior ballistics), and its final path into the target (terminal ballistics). The seriousness of bullet wounds often is considered to be limited to those tissues in the direct path of the projectile. However, under some circumstances, the wounding potential of projectiles can occur beyond the pathway of a projectile.

Missiles are any projectiles, including bullets, pellets, fragments from grenades, and explosive shells. A cartridge (round) is composed of four basic components: primer, case, powder, and bullet. The primer, located at the base of a centerfire or rimfire cartridge, usually contains the compounds lead styphnate, barium nitrate, and antimony sulfide. Small arms cartridges are classified as *centerfire* or *rimfire*, depending on the location of the primer. In centerfire cartridges, there are two types of primers: Boxer and Berden. American centerfire cartridges are Boxer primers. When struck, the primer at the cartridge base explodes and ignites the powder charge (propellant) in the casing as the flame passes through the flash hole(s) (Fig. 7-26). Black powder, a mixture of charcoal, sulfur, and potassium nitrate was the propellant used until the end of the 19th century. Modern weapons use smokeless powder, comprised of a single- or double-base nitrocellulose. Burning of the propellant within the confines of the casing releases gas to propel the bullet. Pyrodex, a synthetic black powder, has replaced the orignal black powder for older black powder

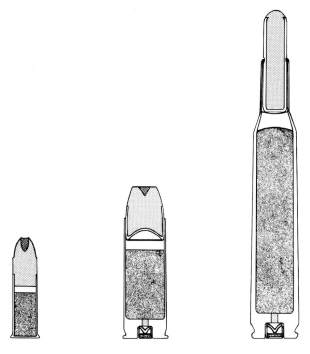

FIG. 7-26 Cross-section of three cartridges (rounds) demonstrating the components of a cartridge: primer, case, powder, and bullet. The example includes (left) a .22 caliber hollow-point rimfire cartridge, (center) a .38 caliber partially jacketed centerfire handgun cartridge, and (right) a .30 caliber partially jacketed centerfire hunting rifle cartridge. The priming mixture in the .22 rimfire is located at the rim base of the cartridge case, unlike the centrally located primer in the centerfire cartridges. (From 1981 Winchester Sporting Arms and Ammunition Catalog, Olin Corp., Winchester Group, New Haven, CT. Modified with permission.)

weapons and replicas. Spiral grooves cut in the interior bore or barrel (rifling) impart rotation or spin along the bullet's longitudinal axis, thus stabilizing its flight in a gyroscopic fashion. The metal between the "twist" or length of a complete revolution of rifling varies by manufacturer. The grooves are called *lands.*

The three basic theories that have been used to explain the wounding capacity of projectiles in the medical literature include the momentum theory, kinetic energy theory, and the power theory. None takes into account all factors that influence bullet destructiveness. The kinetic energy theory, however, is the most popular and is considered the most accurate in describing the potential lethal effects of projectiles.

$$\frac{\text{Mass} \times \text{Velocity}^2}{2g \text{ [where accleration of gravity } (32.16 \, \text{ft}/\text{s}^2)]}$$

The formula demonstrates an important fact pertaining to the kinetic energy of a given projectile: doubling the missile mass increases the energy of the projectile by a factor of 2, but doubling the velocity quadruples the kinetic energy. Lighter bullets can be driven at greater velocities and maintain a commensurately lower chamber pressure than can larger projectiles, with a lower recoil or rifle "kick." Moreover, a smaller projectile traveling at a high velocity has a flatter trajectory for greater accuracy. The mass, shape, design, and composition of a bullet also will influence its function and capacity to inflict trauma.

Projectile Caliber and Design

Bullet caliber generally is considered the diameter of the slug or weapon bore (from land to land) measured in millimeters or thousandths of an inch (2 digits, hundredths; 3 digits, thousandths). However, caliber may be given in terms of bullet, land, or groove diameter. Unfortunately, caliber specification using the U.S. system is neither accurate nor consistent. Although U.S. ammunition has been measured in fractions of an inch in the past, many presently employ metric terminology, including the 5.56mm M-16 and 7.62 NATO. For historic reasons, some cartridges corresponding to caliber .30 rifles show cartridge designations made of two figures: the first referring to the caliber and the second to the year of introduction or the original powder charge. For example, a cartridge designated .30-06 means a .30 caliber bullet introduced in the year 1906. This is a common cartridge employed in the M-1 and other rifles. A .30-30 and .30-40 designation indicates the caliber and the number of grains of gun powder (30gr, 40gr) in the cartridge. Occasionally, the second number indicates the muzzle velocity of the projectile (250 to 3000 ft/s). Some of the caliber .30 designations include the name of the manufacturer or person who developed the cartridge (.30 Remington, .30-30 Winchester, .30-40 Krag, .30-06 Springfield, etc.). U.S. cartridges that originally used black powder are designated by caliber, powder charge, and bullet weight (for example, .45-70-405). Some manufacturers refer to bullet caliber and cartridge length. In all, literally thousands of handgun and rifle cartridges have been developed over the years, with nomenclatures that are modified and formulated by manufacturers.

It is important to note that bullets of the same caliber can vary according to their weight, velocity, design, shape, composition, and accordingly, potential wounding capacity. Most military rifle bullets throughout the world weigh between 40 and 200 grains, including the .223 caliber (5.56mm) M-16 cartridge with a slug weight of 55 grains. Hunting bullets range from 50 to 350 grains, depending on their intended use. Shotguns are measured according to their gauge and are capable of firing pellets of variable diameters.

Low-velocity projectiles travel less than 1000 ft/s, medium-velocity projectiles between 1000 and 2000 ft/s, and high-velocity projectiles faster than 2000 ft/s. However, 2500 ft/s and above generally is selected as the designated speed for high-velocity projectiles. Most handguns fire bullets in the low- to medium-velocity range, whereas most rifles fire bullets in the medium- to high-velocity range. The projectile design and composition also will influence how rapidly the bullet loses its velocity and the wounding capability upon impact. High-velocity bullets are of two basic designs: full patch (military) and expanding (hunting). In 1908 the Hague Convention (and the subsequent 1949 Geneva Convention), recognizing the horrendous wounding potential of expanding (deforming) bullets, advocated the use of fully jacketed (full patch) bullets in warfare (Fig. 7-27). The outer jacket, composed of metals with a higher melting point than the lead alloy core (copper, cupronickel, brass, soft steel), restricts bullet deformation during passage through the barrel, lead residue fouling of the barrel, and deformation on impact with the target. Most bullets are composed of 90% lead with 10% antimony or tin employed as a hardener. However, some are composed of zinc, magnesium, clay, wood, plastic, rubber, or wax, depending on their intended purpose. Fully jacketed bullets have greater penetration into the target than partial or nonjacketed bullets which flatten or "mushroom" to a variable degree on impact, thus increasing their resistance during penetration and passage(Fig. 7-28).

The conically shaped tract formed by mushrooming hollow-point, or soft lead-tipped, partially jacketed hunting projectiles can form wounds up to 40 times the volume of a military bullet of similar weight and velocity, although the full-patch projectile also is capable of causing sizable tracts due to flight instability and occasional fragmentation achieved at very high velocities.

As noted, bullets can be modified in various fashions to enhance deformation by exposing a variable portion of the soft lead alloy at the tip (partially jacketed bullet), by designing bullets with an exposed hollow tip, or by flattening the bullet and scoring two crossed grooves on its surface (improperly termed *dum-dums*). Other bullet designs are on the market that promote deformation upon impact. A hollow point soft-tip bullet can expand twofold to threefold. A partial jacket may be included to protect the soft lead

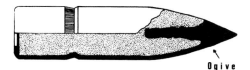

SPORTING-Expanding

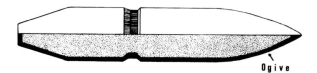

MILITARY - Full Jacket
(Boat-tail)

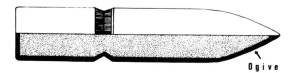

MILITARY RIFLE

FIG. 7-27 Cross-section of the sporting or hunting bullet and military fully jacketed (full-patch) spitzer bullets. Note the exposed soft-lead tip in the hunting bullet, which promotes expansion (mushrooming) and fragmentation on impact. Fully jacketed bullets have the lead core encased in an outer metallic sheath to minimize expansion on impact; however, many military bullets have been known to fragment on impact at high velocity. The boat-tail design has a minor influence on the bullet's velocity. (From DeMuth WE. 1966. Bullet velocity and design as determinants of wounding capability: An experimental study. *J Trauma* 6:222. Modified with permission.)

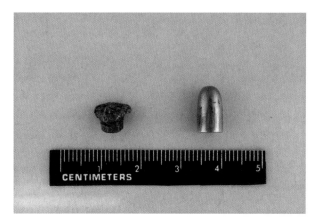

FIG. 7-28 Illustration of bullet performance on impact with bone. The bullet on the left is an unjacketed .22 handgun bullet that traversed the abdomen of a cat before striking the wing of the ilium. The bullet on the right is a .25 caliber fully jacketed bullet that fractured a lumbar vertebra. Note the lack of deformation compared with the soft-lead .22 slug. (Pavletic MM. 1986. Gunshot wounds in veterinary medicine: projectiles ballistics—part I. *Compend Contin Ed Pract Vet* 8:47.)

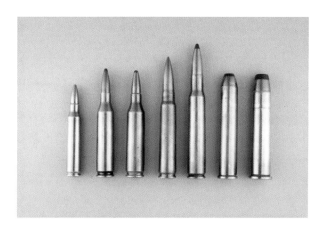

FIG. 7-29 Various rifle rounds (from left to right): 5.56 mm full-patch M-16; .243 Winchester hunting; 6.0 mm hunting; .30 military, armor piercing; .30-06 Springfield hunting; .444 Marlin hunting; .45-70 Government hunting. The partial copper jacket of the sport or hunting bullet provides controlled expansion of the exposed lead core on impact. (Pavletic MM. 1986. Gunshot wounds in veterinary medicine: projectiles ballistics—part I. *Compend Contin Ed Pract Vet* 8:47.)

from deformation and fouling during its passage through the barrel and to provide controlled expansion and penetration in the target. Rapid deceleration and instability of the expanding bullet as it passes through the target may promote bullet fragmentation and enhance tissue destruction (Fig. 7-29 and 7-30). Some bullets are not jacketed, but have an outer metallic plating (copper, copper-zinc) and lubricant as exemplified by the common .22 caliber rimfire cartridge (Fig. 7-31). These thin "protective veneers" do not restrict bullet collapse on impact. Air-powered projectiles, shotguns, and exploding bullets have a few unique features that are worthy of discussion separately. Bullets may have circumferential indentations, called *cannelures*, in which a lubricant is inserted to improve passage through the barrel. A cannelure may be present to allow the casing to crimp onto the bullet and seal the propellant.

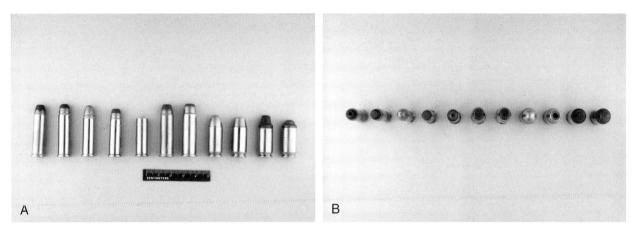

FIG. 7-30 (A) Side and (B) top views of various handgun rounds (from left to right): .357 Magnum, partial jacket, hollow point; .357 Magnum, partial jacket; .38 Special unjacketed; .38 Special partial jacket; .38 caliber wad cutter (flat face); .41 Magnum partial jacket; .44 Remington Magnum; .45 caliber full-patch military; .45 copper jacketed hollow point; .45 caliber unjacketed; .45 caliber unjacketed. Each bullet varies in weight, velocity, and performance on impact. Bullets with an exposed lead core, especially with a hollow point, would be expected to deform on impact compared with a full-patch bullet. The full-patch bullet would be expected to have greater penetration, other factors being equal. (Pavletic MM. 1986. Gunshot wounds in veterinary medicine: projectiles ballistics—part I. *Compend Contin Ed Pract Vet* 8:47.)

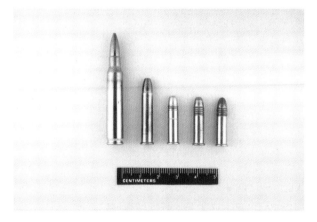

FIG. 7-31 These .22 cartridges demonstrate the various sizes and designs of these rounds (left to right): 5.56 mm (.223), 55 grain, full-patch centerfire M-16; .22 Magnum jacketed rimfire; .22 Winchester long rifle high power, 29 grain hollow point; 22 Remington long rifle, high velocity, 36 grain hollow point; .22 long rifle with uncoated lead bullet. The .22 Winchester and .22 Remington have a metallic coating that has little influence on minimizing bullet deformation. The decorative coating is reported to shun dirt, grit, and lint. A waxy coating or priming on the rimfire long rifle illustrated lubricates the bullet and minimizes fouling of the gun barrel. Note that the .22 designation does not indicate the projectile's weight, composition, design, or velocity, only its diameter. (Pavletic MM. 1986. Gunshot wounds in veterinary medicine: projectiles ballistics—part I. *Compend Contin Ed Pract Vet* 8:47.)

Air-Powered Projectiles

Air-powered rifles, developed in 16th-century Germany, use compressed air to drive the projectile in place of gases released by exploding powder. Today, air rifles, air guns, and air pistols are used for target shooting and small-game hunting. The air gun is distinguished from the air rifle in that the gun is a smooth-bored barrel, whereas the rifle has a rifled barrel. Air pistols may have a smooth or rifled barrel. Standard calibers for air arms in the United States include .177, .22, and .20 (5 mm). The basic types of air gun ammunition are the BB and "air rifle" shot. These plated balls are steel of .175 caliber. The most common missile employed in the air rifle is the waisted diabolo pellet, possessing an hourglass shape. The diabolo pellet weighs an average of 8.2 grains in .177 caliber and 15.0 grains in .22 caliber. The Sheridan rifle employs a .20 or 5 mm pointed conical bullet weighing 15.3 grains with a hollow base that expands to seal the bore and engage the rifling (Fig. 7-32). Because of their extremely light weight, these pellets rapidly lose velocity and become nearly harmless at 100 yards.

All modern air rifles operate on one of three gas-compressing systems: the pneumatic system, the spring-air system, or the gas-compression system. Despite their modest size, velocity, and poor aerodynamic design, air-driven pellets are capable of causing serious injuries and fatalities at close range. Indeed, many air pistols and rifles have muzzle velocities comparable to the low-velocity bullets propelled by gunpowder. The skin has the ability to absorb a considerable amount of energy and will limit the penetration of low-velocity projectiles. It is not uncommon to find air pellets or BBs on radiographs, residing in the hypodermal and adjacent muscle/fascia.

Shotguns

Shotguns, by design and function, differ from handguns and rifles. Shotguns are smooth-bored long-barreled guns designed to fire a shot charge consisting of a large number of small spheres that form a pattern depending on the distance and "choke" of the barrel. Although there are handgun and rifle cartridges that fire bird shot, the comparatively low number of these small pellets limits their effective use to small varmints.

The shotgun shell is composed of a paper or plastic casing, fused into a metallic cup or base that contains a centerfire primer. Brass or steel casings occasionally are employed outside North America. In the bottom of the shell casing, the powder charge is located adjacent to the primer. Wads of plastic, felt, paper, or cork are used to compartmentalize the powder and shot charge: the wadding also plays a role as a compressor or shock absorber to improve shot dispersion. The shot charge is in turn sealed within the casing by a thin wad or by crimping the end of the shell casing (Fig. 7-33). Upon discharge, the shot and wadding materials in front of the propellant are pushed forward. At close range, this wadding may enter the body, along with the advancing shot charge or deer slug.

In the United States and other countries the caliber of shotguns is expressed in *gauge* or *bore*. This unit of measurement is derived from the early 19th-century method of measuring the weight of one cannon ball in pounds; the caliber of a shotgun is a comparison with lead balls of the same diameter contained in 1 lb of lead for a specific gauge. A 12-gauge shotgun, for example, has a caliber corresponding to the diameter of a lead ball, 12 of which are equivalent to 1 lb. Shotgun gauges in common use are the 10 (.775 inch), 12 (.73 inch), 16 (.670 inch), 20 (.615 inch), and 28 (.550 inch). Another common shotgun is the .410, a number that designates a caliber of 410 thousandths of an inch.

Shot charges spread from the muzzle in a conelike fashion. The pattern is influenced by the shotgun's

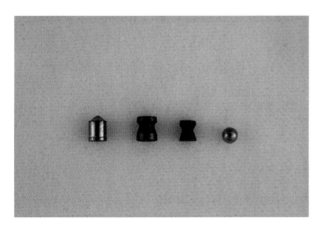

FIG. 7-32 Side view of air-powered projectiles (from left to right): .20 (5 mm) Sheridan pellet; .22 diabolo pellet; .177 diabolo pellet; .175 BB copper-plated steel sphere. Each pellet has a hollow base. Sheridan pellets are harder than the conventional diabolo pellet. These projectiles are commonly encountered as incidental findings subcutaneously or in a muscle during radiographic examination. At close range, these projectiles are capable of seriously wounding or killing small animals. (Pavletic MM. 1986. Gunshot wounds in veterinary medicine: projectiles ballistics—part I. *Compend Contin Ed Pract Vet* 8:47.)

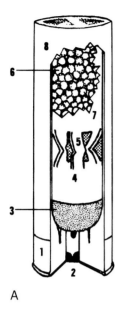 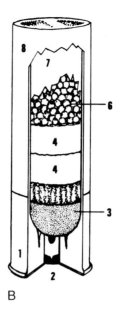 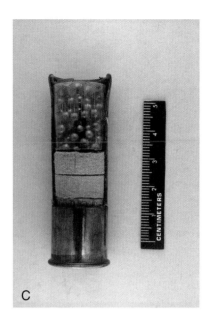

A   B   C

FIG. 7-33 (A) Cross-section of shotgun shell: (1) metal head, (2) primer, (3) gunpowder propellant, (4) plastic wad and (5) plastic baffle, (6) shot, (7) plastic collar, (8) outer plastic hull.

(B) Cross-section of shotgun shell with (4) cardboard wadding. The other numbers correspond to the descriptions in (A). (Diagram redrawn from 1981 Winchester Sporting Arms and Ammunition Catalog).

(C) Cross-sectional view of a shotgun shell. A portion of the casing was removed to show its contents. Compare this shell to (B).

choke or constriction at the barrel end. Choke variations include full-choke (maximal constriction or tighter cluster pattern over a greater distance), modified choke, improved cylinder, and skeet-bore or cylinder-bore (little or no constriction with a wide pattern for hunting at close range). In the game field, 30 to 40 yards is the effective range for most shotguns. Within 20 yards the dense pattern is too destructive, whereas beyond 40 yards the wide dispersion of shot and the loss of velocity limits its effectiveness.

Various gauge shotguns are capable of firing a variety of pellet or shot sizes (Fig. 7-34). Occasionally, shotguns are used for hunting large animals by shooting buckshot or single slug loads. Foster "deer" slugs, most commonly used in North America, compare favorably with high-powered rifles at ranges of 100 yards, but perform poorly past that range due to their mass and design, resulting in rapid dissipation of energy (Fig. 7-35). Although uncommonly used, shotgun shells designed to fire metallic arrowlike darts, called flechettes, have been employed primarily as a military weapon.

Charges fired from shotguns of all types have a muzzle velocity between 1100 and 1350 ft/s, although rifle slugs may reach a velocity of 1850 ft/s. Strikes to an animal in which the shot pattern is contained within a 12-inch diameter will have a velocity of 1000 to 1350 ft/s (Fig. 7-36). Considering that a single pellet or shot imparts a striking force of 9.56 ft-pounds at a muzzle velocity of 1295 ft/s and the combined force of 235 pellets at point blank range delivers 2247 ft-pounds, there is a formidable comparison to the muzzle energy of the 1250 ft-pounds of an M-16 rifle. Buckshot and slugs, by virtue of their greater mass, maintain their velocity more effectively at longer ranges. Considering that large shot can have a weight comparable to a .22 bullet, with a velocity over 1000 ft/s, the combined wounding potential of the larger shot is evident.

The use of shotguns as weapons against dogs is not uncommon. The variety of loads, pellet sizes, and their wounding capability in relation to the distance from the muzzle adds a number of additional factors for the veterinarian to consider when confronted with such injuries.

COMPARATIVE SHOT SIZES

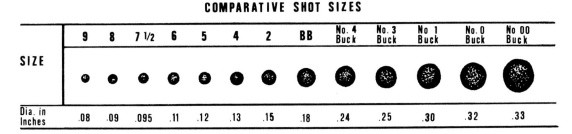

SIZE	9	8	7 1/2	6	5	4	2	BB	No. 4 Buck	No. 3 Buck	No 1 Buck	No. 0 Buck	No 00 Buck
	●	●	●	●	●	●	●	●	●	●	●	●	●
Dia. in Inches	.08	.09	.095	.11	.12	.13	.15	.18	.24	.25	.30	.32	.33

FIG. 7-34 Comparative sizes of shot fired from shotguns. (From 1980 Browning Catalog, Browning, Morgan, UT. Modified with permission).

1   **2**   **3**   **4**

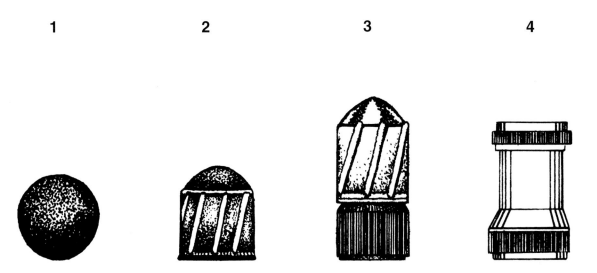

FIG. 7-35 Single projectiles (enlarged) used in shotguns throughout the world: (1) pumpkin ball, (2) rifle slug, (3) Brenneke slug, and (4) Balle Blondeau. (From DeMuth WE. 1979. The mechanism of shotgun wounds. *J Trauma* 11:219. Redrawn with permission).

Sherman and Parrish classified shotgun wounds into three basic types based on the pattern of distribution, depth of penetration, and range. Type I injuries, reflecting a relatively long distance between animal and shooter, are wounds in which the subcutaneous tissue and deep fascia are penetrated; type II injuries, produced at closer range, perforate structures beneath the deep fascia; and type III wounds, inflicted at point blank range (less than 3 yards), produce an extensive central zone of tissue destruction with a small peripheral halo of pellet holes. Extensive tissue destruction at close range is due to the high velocity and wider total surface area formed by the pellet group in flight as compared to a single projectile. Thus, at very close ranges, the shotgun is one of the most destructive weapons available (Fig. 7-37 and 7-38).

Exploding Bullets

Although presently illegal to purchase and very difficult to attain, exploding bullets were available in the 1980s for defense purposes to the public and law enforcement sectors. Exploding bullets initially were developed by the British in the early 1800s to penetrate barriers and ignite enemy powder caissons. They were subsequently employed in limited quantities during the American Civil War for antipersonnel use. There

SHOT PATTERN AT VARYING DISTANCES

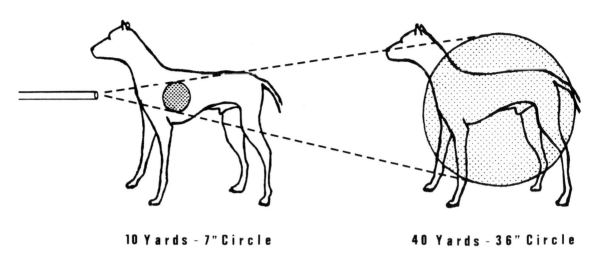

10 Yards - 7" Circle   **40 Yards - 36" Circle**

FIG. 7-36 Shot pattern at varying distances (Drawing modified from Bell, MJ. 1981. The management of shotgun wounds. *J Trauma* 11:522.)

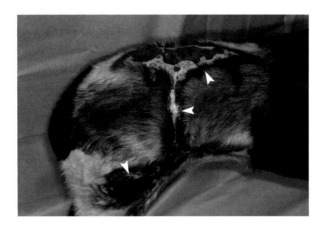

FIG. 7-37 Shotgun (type I) injury to the flanks caudal lumbar area and hind limbs (No. 6 birdshot). The dog presented several weeks after injury: considerable skin loss had occurred. Healing by second intention was nearly complete. The shotgun blast occurred at the level of the deep circumflex iliac artery and vein. Destruction of these major direct cutaneous vessels and regional collateral circulation was the major factor involved in the skin loss.

are several variations of exploding bullets. Bullets have been designed to split or fragment on impact. Alternatively, bullets containing an explosive charge were designed to explode on impact. These latter projectiles can be somewhat troublesome if they fail to

detonate on impact with the patient: rough handling of the projectile during retrieval can result in their explosion. Undetonated bullets retained in the animal present a potential hazard to the patient and the surgeon attempting to remove them. Exploding bullets generally are semijacketed hollow point bullets filled with an explosive powder charge covered by a single lead shot and a percussion cap (or simply a primer anvil) covered by a wax coat. Deceleration of the bullet on impact ignites the percussion cap or primer, resulting in the explosion of the powder charge. From a historical perspective, the .22 bullet that struck President Reagan contained an aluminum canister in its nose filled with the explosive lead azide that is detonated by impact or high heat. Bullet deformation and the release of projectile fragments on impact reportedly increases the local tissue destruction compared to a regular bullet of similar size. However, this contention has been questioned by some authorities.

Interior and Exterior Ballistics

Modern bullets are fired from barrels that contain helical grooves (rifling) that serve to spin the projectile on its longitudinal axis to stabilize its flight. Rifling improves the flight characteristics of a bullet in much the same way the helical fletching of an arrow serves to improve its flight. Despite rifling, projectiles

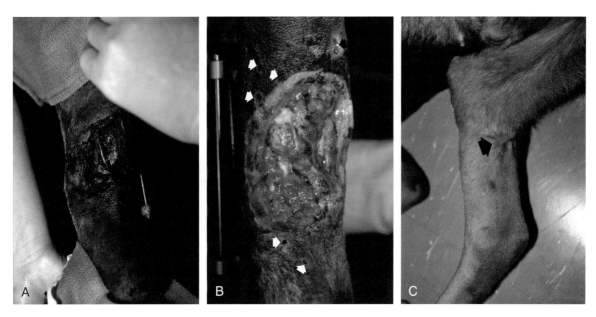

FIG. 7-38 (A) Massive soft tissue injury and a comminuted tibial fracture were the result of a (type III) shotgun injury. Some pellet entry wounds are still evident. Maggots were present, but manually removed during the initial debridement procedure. (B) Serial debridement was performed on a daily basis. (C) The wound healed by second intention. However, the external fixation was later replaced by internal fixation with a bone plate and cancellous bone graft (successfully).

traveling at a high velocity can become unstable in flight. A bullet can deviate from its longitudinal axis: it can yaw or tumble prior to or after impact with a body region, thereby increasing its profile in contact with tissues, resulting in greater tissue trauma. Flight instability enhances the likelihood of greater tissue destruction and promotes bullet fragmentation.

From an "offensive" standpoint, the ideal projectile has the following characteristics: (1) good ballistic shape (needlelike design); (2) high sectional density (ratio of projectile mass to area of presentation); (3) high velocity; and (4) the capability of deep penetration with a controlled expansion.

Terminal Ballistics

The seriousness of bullet wounds is often considered only in relation to those structures in the path of the bullet. Although this generally is true for low-velocity projectiles and stab wounds, it does not account for the severity of injuries associated with some high-velocity missile injuries. Bullets damage tissue in three ways: tissue laceration and crushing, shock waves, and cavitation. Both low- and high-velocity projectiles create permanent tracts as they pass through tissues. Expanding bullets increase the tissue damage of a projectile

by creating a larger wound cavity and enhancing energy absorption by the tissue. The tissue trauma from low-velocity projectiles primarily is restricted to the crushing and laceration of tissues at the permanent tract. By comparison, high-velocity projectiles can expend considerable energy to adjacent tissues in the form of shock waves and cavitation. Cavitation, a temporary cavity (5- to 30-microsecond duration) up to 30 times the diameter of the projectile, is most evident as a projectile's velocity markedly increases (Fig. 7-39). Following the temporary lateral and cranial expansion of the surrounding tissues, a negative pressure forms with a sucking effect that has the potential of drawing debris and contaminants into the wound. The stretching and compression of tissues as a result of cavitation can enhance the magnitude of tissue destruction, especially if circulatory compromise occurs secondary to vascular disruption or thrombosis: fractured bones, torn vessels, bowel ruptures, and contusions of the heart and lungs may occur without direct contact from high velocity projectiles.

A projectile may penetrate or perforate various tissues or structures, depending on its impact velocity, mass, design, and composition of the target struck. A penetrating wound has an entry point with no exit, whereas a perforating wound has an entry and exit (through-and-through) without the projectile's reten-

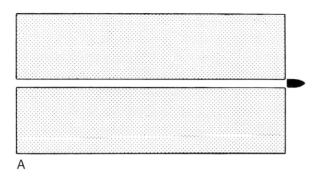

A

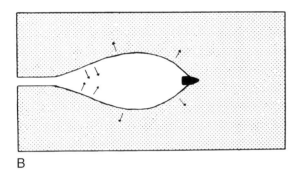

B

FIG. 7-39 (A) Note low velocity, no cavitation, and small entrance and exit. (B) Greater cavitation is noted as velocity increases. Note that the size of the exit wound is influenced by (1) target thickness or depth, (2) tissue density, (3) projectile velocity and composition, and (4) the amount of kinetic energy expended as the projectile(s) exit the target area. (From Swan KG, Swan RC. 1980. *Gunshot Wounds*. Littleton, MA: PSG Publishing. Modified with permission.)

tion in a specified structure or region. To avoid confusion, it is best to restrict the terms *penetrating* and *perforating* to the anatomical structure in question. Projectiles that exit the body make it more difficult to determine the weapon involved. Projectiles retained in the patient without impacting bone are more likely to be lower-velocity projectiles.

Besides velocity and mass, three factors are responsible for the greater destructiveness of projectiles, especially in higher velocity weapons: tumbling prior to impact, which permits a variety of positional contacts with the tissues; flight instability, apart from tumbling, thus adding an additional motion of the projectile; and secondary projectiles formed by missile fragmentation and bone shattering (Fig. 7-40).

The entry wound usually is smaller than the exit wound because bullet tumbling, distortion, fragmentation, and secondary projectile formation increases the bullet's destructiveness in a conelike fashion as it passes through the body. This general rule on wound size, however, is misleading. If the gun muzzle is placed very close to the target when fired, expanding gases are released that accentuate the size of the entry wound, and powder burns also would be noted. The magnitude of the temporary cavity is proportional to the energy imparted by the projectile during target penetration, with the missile's energy decreasing exponentially with the distance penetrated. Smaller projectiles may dissipate their energy more rapidly than larger projectiles with equal energy. A projectile that has expended a majority of its energy in the center of the target may exit without the gaping exit wound expected.

The specific gravity of the tissues struck also will influence the wounds produced. Tissues with greater

TUMBLING

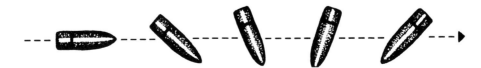

FIG. 7-40 Schematic diagram illustrating tumbling (forward rotation around the center of the mass). This unstable flight pattern increases the projectile's surface presentation to the target, enhancing tissue damage. (From Swan KG, Swan RC. 1980. *Gunshot Wounds*. Littleton, MA, PSG Publishing. Modified with permission).

density, such as bone, are affected more adversely than are soft tissue structures. The retentive forces that combat the disruptive forces of the projectile also vary with the tissue struck. Skin and lung have elastic properties that better accommodate the energy insult which helps maintain the organ's integrity. Liver and muscle have a similar specific gravity and absorb energy from a high-velocity projectile in similar fashion. However, the temporary cavity and permanent tract formed in the liver are greater in magnitude compared to skeletal muscle because the liver parenchyma is less cohesive and resilient. Cavitation in pulmonary tissue is comparatively minor due to the elastic fibers within the spongy network of their parenchyma.

At high velocities, cavitation has also been recorded in bone. The explosive effect on the bone drives splinters of bone ahead of the projectile, increasing the magnitude of soft tissue damage and possibly the exit wound. Greater fragmentation will occur where cortical bone predominates. Thus, long bones composed of large amounts of cortical bone have greater density as compared to flat bones, such as the ribs, with a greater proportion of cancellous bone. High-velocity rounds are more likely to cause massive tissue destruction when bone is struck. Paradoxically, any high-velocity rounds can pass through soft tissue structures and exit the body without resulting in massive tissue necrosis. This can be explained primarily by the fact that a considerable proportion of the projectile's kinetic energy (mass, velocity) is not "deposited in" or "captured by" the body.

High-velocity projectile injuries to the abdomen of anesthetized cats have demonstrated that the abdomen swells immediately and collapses, followed by a second expansion of less intensity, but with a prolonged duration. Damage to the abdominal contents can occur with the first expansion, but the explosive injury noted develops during the second expansion. Intestinal gas expands, resulting in multiple bowel perforations. The explosive shock wave displaces viscera, tears the mesentery, and can rupture blood vessels away from the permanent tract. The extent of soft tissue necrosis associated with high-velocity projectiles is variable and can be difficult to assess. Muscle tissue is extremely resilient, and damage may occur only a few centimeters from the muscle tract. The tissue destruction occasionally noted hours to days later in some high-velocity injuries, most likely is attributable to progressive vascular compromise to the tissues involved. Cavitation and the associated shock wave apparently result in blunt contusion of the associated tissues. The volume of necrosis is influenced by the severity of the vascular compromise. Vessels need not be struck directly by a high-velocity projectile.

Stretching and tearing of the vessels can occur, resulting in hemorrhage or thrombosis of the damaged vessel. The resulting damage has been likened to a crushing-type injury. However, the large arteries, such as the canine femoral artery, are more resistant to indirect trauma. Circulatory insult and tissue necrosis increases the likelihood of infection. Various studies using the thigh muscles of goats and dogs for high-velocity projectile studies have demonstrated the surprising resilience of wound healing in the face of moderate trauma, as long as the circulation to the area remains predominantly intact. From clinical experience in humans, it is known that the extent of devitalization is affected by time.

Many researchers contend that bullet fragmentation better explains the size and severity of high-velocity projectile wounds. Bullet fragmentation and the dispersion of secondary projectiles causing muscle tearing enhances the absorption of the projectile's energy by the target and is more likely responsible for the magnitude of the large conical-shaped tracts formed by hunting bullets. In these cases, radiographs can help define the boundaries of the wounded tissue for debridement by the location of metallic fragments deposited in the area. Fragmentation of projectiles, in association with bone impact and fragmentation, best explains the massive trauma noted with high-velocity rounds and the more powerful handguns.

The severity of tissue injury by a given projectile in large part is determined by the total kinetic energy absorbed by the patient. For example, a jacketed, high-velocity bullet that perforates an upper extremity and exits intact without a significant loss in velocity would cause substantially less tissue injury compared to a bullet that deforms and rapidly decelerates in the same tissue. If this projectile is completely retained, the area has absorbed the damaging energy of the round. Thus, tissue trauma is better understood in terms of how rapidly and completely the energy is lost (absorbed by the body) and the tissues in which the energy is dissipated. As noted, certain body tissues that are elastic and maintain their architectural integrity better sustain projectile trauma.

Gunshot Wound Infection

All gunshot wounds are contaminated. Low- and high-velocity projectiles are capable of driving or dragging topical debris (dirt, hair, etc.) into the permanent tract. Bacteria also are driven into the wound. As noted, the negative pressure formed during formation of the temporary cavity associated with high-velocity projectiles also is capable of "sucking" contaminants into the wound to a variable degree. The notion that projectiles, especially high-velocity projectiles, are sterile due to heat generated during passage of the bullet through the barrel and air is a fallacy. The risk of infection is more likely in the case of high-velocity projectile injuries where extensive tissue damage and circulatory embarrassment in the region are more likely. In general, the incidence of infection associated with low-velocity rounds limited to skin, muscle, and fascia is remarkably low.

Diagnosis and Management Considerations

In many cases, the owner is unaware of their pet being shot; clearly, pets that are allowed to roam unsupervised are at greatest risk of being shot. Without a history, skin wounds may be mistaken for bite wounds or vehicular trauma. There are occasions in which the owner, a witness, or police officer may provide specific information pertaining to the weapon. Knowledge of the weapon can help the veterinarian determine the potential tissue damage and appropriate surgical management of the injuries.

Most gunshot wounds to dogs and cats in a city are due to low-velocity handguns (Figs. 7-41 and 7-42). High-velocity gunshot wounds from hunting rifles are seen more commonly in rural areas. Data from Angell Memorial Animal Hospital indicated that shotgun wounds occurred in urban, suburban, and rural areas. Radiographs of the patient are useful to determine the presence and location of retained bullets or fragments.

Low-velocity projectile injuries cause comparatively less tissue destruction, except to those tissues in their path (Fig. 7-43 and 7-44). Such wounds confined

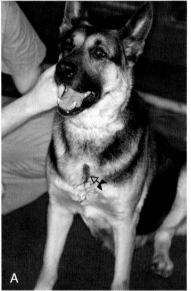
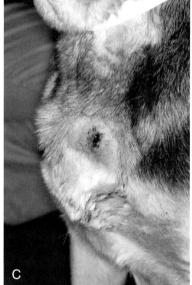
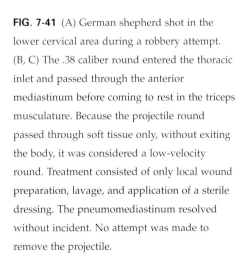
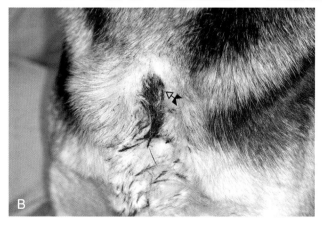

FIG. 7-41 (A) German shepherd shot in the lower cervical area during a robbery attempt. (B, C) The .38 caliber round entered the thoracic inlet and passed through the anterior mediastinum before coming to rest in the triceps musculature. Because the projectile round passed through soft tissue only, without exiting the body, it was considered a low-velocity round. Treatment consisted of only local wound preparation, lavage, and application of a sterile dressing. The pneumomediastinum resolved without incident. No attempt was made to remove the projectile.

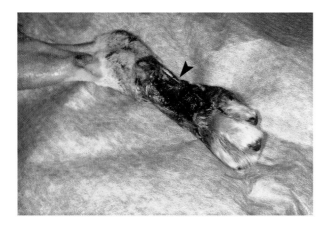

FIG. 7-42 Example of a .44 magnum handgun round to the foot of a German shepherd. The dog was shot by the owner's former boyfriend during a heated argument. The considerable power of the .44 magnum is evident. The paw was suspended by remnants of two metatarsal bones and soft tissue. The limb required amputation.

to the skin and underlying muscle generally are treated by local debridement of the entry and exit wound (if present), local wound lavage, and the application of a sterile dressing. Systemic antibiotics may be advisable in selected cases. Bullets that are easily and safely accessible can be removed. They generally are not pursued unless they involve a joint or vital structure. Attempts to probe and explore the wound simply to find a bullet should be discouraged to reduce the likelihood of further tissue damage and infection. Occasionally, however, bullet retrieval may be required for legal purposes.

High-velocity projectiles, because of their greater kinetic energy, may require wound exploration and debridement due to the greater tissue destruction present. This is most evident when bone is struck, allowing the effect of the projectile's kinetic energy to be more fully expressed. Many of these cases may require considerable debridement, orthopedic repair, and a variable amount of open wound management.

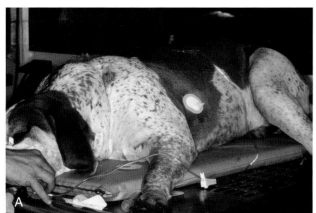

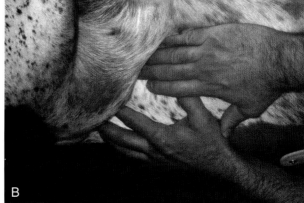

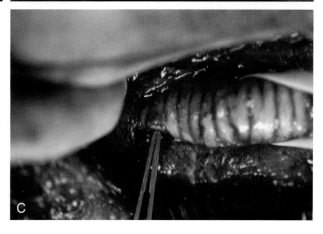

FIG. 7-43 (A) Cervical gunshot wound with extensive subcutaneous emphysema.
(B) Compression of the skin easily displaces the extensive pocket of air.
(C) Tangential perforation of the trachea by the handgun round. This area was minimally debrided and sutured closed. Within 24 hours, over half the air was resorbed; by 48 hours most of the subcutaneous air was gone. (A large-gauge needle and vacuum pump can remove a portion of the air that has accumulated in patients with extensive subcutaneous emphysema. With closure of the air leak, the ability of the patient to resorb the air can be dramatic.) (From Pavletic MM. 1996. Gunshot wound management. *Compend Contin Edu Pract Vet* 18:1285-1299.)

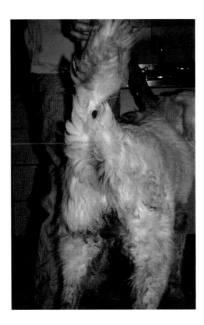

FIG. 7-44 Great Pyrenees with a urethral tear dorsal to the scrotum. A second hole was noted in the tail. What initially appeared to be two gunshot wounds was actually one. The dog was shot from the rear with his tail between his legs. The hole in the patient's tail lined up with the cutaneous hole above the scrotum.

The amount of kinetic energy lost by a bullet depends on four factors: (1) the kinetic energy possessed by the bullet on impact; (2) deviation of the longitudinal path of the bullet (yaw, tumble) enhancing projectile retardation; (3) loss of kinetic energy by loss of bullet mass and shape during passage through tissues; (4) the tissues' density, elasticity, and inherent integrity. High-velocity hunting bullets, with an exposed soft lead tip or hollow point, can deform and fragment readily secondary to flight instability and tissue retardation, especially when bone is struck. A direct hit on dense cortical bone will cause a catastrophic deceleration of the bullet and its fragmentation. Bullet fragments and shards of bone are driven into the adjacent soft tissues (Fig. 7-45 and 7-46). Disruption and pulpification of tissues combined with circulatory compromise results in massively destructive wounds. Skin, muscle, and fascia are sufficiently elastic to absorb a portion of this energy while maintaining their integrity, although cavitation is a major disruptive force during passage of a high-velocity projectile through tissues. Passage of a high-velocity round through the soft tissue of the upper thigh, for example, may not result in a wound that necessarily will require wide debridement: treatment may be more conservative than that suggested by the literature.

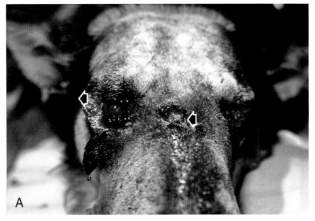
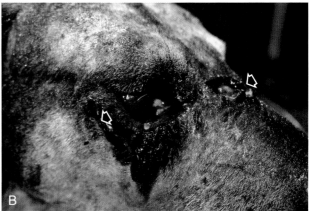

FIG. 7-45 (A) High-velocity rifle round to the head of a German shepherd farm dog. Arrows denote the pathway of the projectile. Massive bone and soft tissue destruction were evident. (B) Lateral view demonstrates the large exit wound through the bony orbit with destruction of the right eye. A long incision was made connecting the entry/exit wounds, and bone fragments and necrotic soft tissue excised. The cosmetic and functional results were comparable to a patient subjected to eye enucleation.

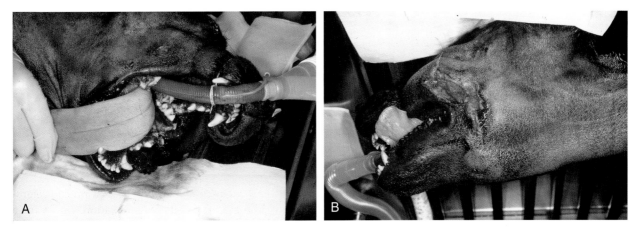

FIG. 7-46 (A) Extensive trauma secondary to a high-velocity rifle round. The entry wound was on the left side of the face of this Labrador. Note the extensive trauma to the mandible. (B) The large irregular exit wound is noted on the right. There were fine fragments of the projectile associated with the bilateral mandibular fractures. The majority of the high-velocity round exited the patient, despite impact with this dense bone.

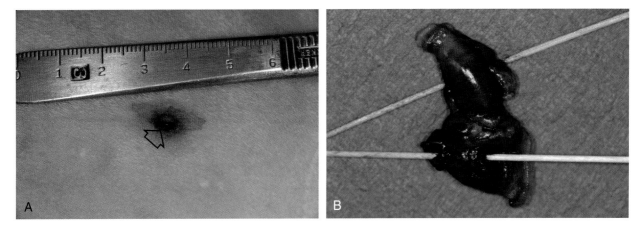

FIG. 7-47 (A) Air-powered B-B gun injury to a Siamese cat. Note the small, seemingly innocuous-appearing entry wound. The patient presented as depressed with abdominal pain. Abdominal radiographs demonstrated the retained projectile. (B) Laparotomy revealed the bowel wall was perforated in two places (highlighted by probes) prompting intestinal resection and anastomosis. Prompt surgical intervention prevented development of peritonitis. However, veterinarians should be aware that retained air-powered projectiles are a common incidental finding.

With few exceptions, gunshot wounds to the brain and abdominal cavity require surgical exploration in the human. This approach can be justified in the small animal as well, although data are lacking regarding the successful management of gunshot wounds to the brain, primarily because of their grim outcome in most cases. Because abdominal gunshot wounds carry a high incidence of bowel injury and peritonitis, exploratory laparotomy is advisable (Fig. 7-47 and 7-48). Thoracic gunshot wounds in the human are second in fatalities only to bullet wounds to the brain. Paradoxically, many of the cases in the human and the dog may be treated by conservative management. A chest tube may be required to treat a hemothorax and pneumothorax, but a thoracotomy is often unnecessary unless the esophagus has been penetrated or perforated,

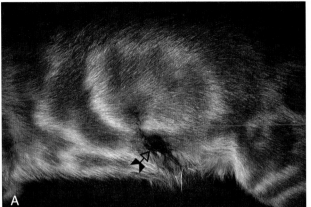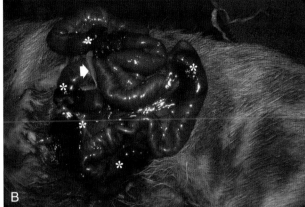

FIG. 7-48 (A) A .22 Rimfire round to the lower abdomen of a cat. The bullet lodged against the wing of the ilium. The owner's boyfriend accidentally shot the cat with his handgun. (B) The owner elected to euthanatize the cat. The abdomen was opened on postmortem revealing multiple bowel perforations (asterisks) with the presence of tapeworm segments throughout the abdominal cavity (arrow). Exploration is mandatory for projectile wounds to the abdomen.

the heart was struck, a major tear in the tracheobronchial tree has occurred, or hemorrhage and air leakage into the thoracic cavity remains unchecked. Gunshot wounds to the neck in humans are explored routinely by many surgeons due to the risk of esophageal injury and the presence of vital vessels. However, it is controversial whether mandatory cervical exploration is justifiable in small animals, depending on the severity of the wound and the neurological status of the animal.

If the bullet cannot be located, it has either exited the body or has passed into another area of the body. The body compartment above and below the area shot should be radiographed in these situations. A bullet passing through the thorax into the abdomen will, at the very least, require an exploratory laparotomy, although a bullet passing in the opposite direction does not automatically mandate a thoracotomy. Bullets have been known to migrate and embolize if they gain access to the circulatory system. Major vascular obstruction may lead to serious consequences. Similarly, bullets have been known to enter the tracheobronchial tree only to be coughed up and swallowed by humans (Fig. 7-49).

A Few Tips

- If a projectile enters and exits a soft tissue area, it may not be possible to determine low versus high velocity by examination of the entry and exit wounds.

- If a projectile enters soft tissue and is retained in the tissues, it is most likely a low-velocity projectile.

- If a projectile impacts dense bony structures and exits the body, the projectile is likely a high-velocity round.

- Keep in mind that high-velocity rounds decelerate over a distance and can impact a target with a significantly lower velocity.

Arrow Wounds

The bow and arrow has been an effective weapon for centuries. Despite its primitive origins, the bow and arrow is a highly lethal weapon in the hands of an

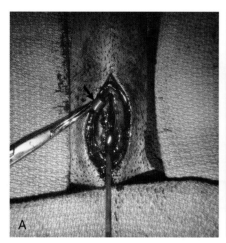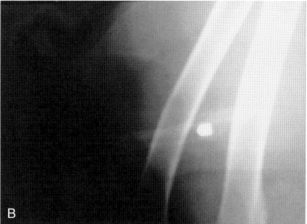

FIG. 7-49 (A) An unusual case of a migrating projectile. A Sheridan pellet was retrieved via urethrotomy at the level of the os penis. The dog presented with an acute urinary tract obstruction during a walk with the observant owner.

(B) Radiographs detected the pellet. Close examination of the lateral abdominal wall revealed a healed entry scar. The dog had apparently been shot some weeks before, with the pellet entering the urinary bladder. Its abrupt passage into the urethra caused the immediate urinary obstruction.

experienced archer. Arrows lack the knockdown power and destructive capacity of high-velocity rifles. Rather, arrows rely on striking a vital area (lungs, heart, major vessels, liver, etc.), resulting in fatal hemorrhage. If an arrow weighing 450 grains has a velocity of 250 ft/s, it generates only 26 ft-pounds of kinetic energy, considerably smaller than that generated by rifles.

Bows are measured by their draw weight, which is the number of pounds required to pull the drawstring to a full draw (full length of the arrow). In order to reduce the effort required to draw the bowstring of a conventional longbow or recurve bow, compound bows were developed in 1967 that employ a series of pulleys, elliptical wheels, and cables. Improvements in the compound bow can reduce draw weights from 50% to 86%. Some states limit compound bows to those with a reduction of no greater than 65%.

A variation of the longbow is the crossbow. A weapon approximately 2000 years old, it gained popularity in the Middle Ages. The crossbow fires a bolt or quarrel approximately half the length (14–18 inches) of the average longbow arrow. A crossbow can have a draw weight from 125 to 200 pounds. One crossbow has been developed with a draw weight of 300 pounds, whereas the upper draw weight of a longbow is around 70 pounds. A 125-pound draw crossbow produces the same energy as a 60-pound draw compound bow. A compound bow can fire a bolt with velocities of over 250 ft/s with an amazingly flat trajectory and short-range accuracy. Crossbows have been criticized as silent, accurate, and highly lethal weapons that could be used to advantage by poachers. However, studies have indicated they are not silent and can be a difficult weapon to master. Furthermore, rifles, especially of a lower caliber with a sound suppressor, are a preferred weapon for illegal hunters, compared to a single-shot crossbow. Crossbows are required by law to have a safety to prevent discharge of the bolt from jarring or dropping. Many states restrict the ownership and use of crossbows for hunting.

Arrows vary in length, weight, shaft composition, fetching, nock style, and arrow point (head). Arrow shafts are commonly composed of cedar, aluminum, or carbon fiber. Composite arrows of aluminum-carbon fiber or wood-fiberglass also have been introduced. Shaft length, width, and weight can be varied depending on the game hunted and bow employed (Fig. 7-50).

Arrow fetching is the guidance system of the arrow, imparting twist or rotation to the shaft to stabilize its flight, similar to the rifling previously discussed. Turkey feathers once were the material of choice for fetching, but have been progressively replaced by plastic because of its durability and greater availability (Fig. 7-51). The arrow nock adjacent to the fetching is the portion of the arrow that is notched to engage the

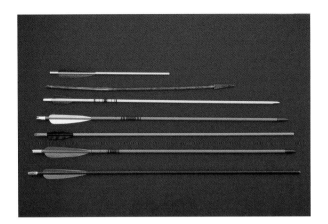

FIG. 7-50 Arrows of various designs and materials. Note the short (aluminum) quarrel of the crossbow (top) and 1800s North Dakota Sioux Indian arrow, second from top (the feathered fetching has long since deteriorated). The remaining arrows are composed of wood, fiberglass, and aluminum. The bow-fishing arrow was composed of heavier fiberglass for greater penetration through water.

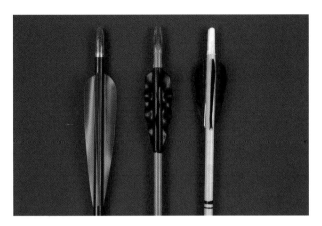

FIG. 7-51 Fetching departs spin on the arrow to improve flight stability. The left and middle arrows have plastic fletching; the right arrow has turkey feather fletching.

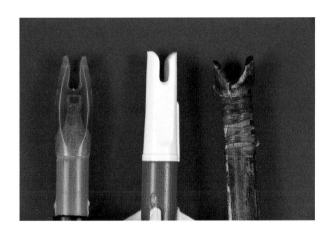

FIG. 7-52 The arrow nock. Right is an example of the Sioux arrow.

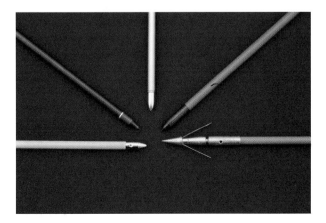

FIG. 7-53 Field points and arrowhead for bow fishing. Field points have a round silhouette that lacks cutting blades. Note the bow-fishing arrow has a metallic barb to capture the fish upon penetration.

"serving" area of the bowstring. The nock design varies according to the personal preference and requirements of the archer (Fig. 7-52).

The head or point is the engaging end of the arrow and varies in shape, design, and weight. The arrowheads made by the early American Indians were chipped into points using flint, obsidian and other hard rock, antler, and bone. Indians later created metal points from scraps of iron. Some primitive tribes use wooden tips formed by tapering the shaft that lacks fetching.

Modern arrowheads are exclusively metal, and are broadly classified as field points and hunting points (broadheads). Field points lack cutting blades, but have a pointed or dull tip for small game or target practice (Fig. 7-53). In contrast, broadheads generally have two to four balanced cutting blades for larger game. There are a wide variety of broadhead designs. Many arrow shafts have threaded tips that allow the hunter to change hunting heads. Some of the older arrows have a tapered shaft with the head applied with adhesives and crimping. Broadheads are usually razor sharp for maximum penetration and laceration. Broadheads are usually designed to slide past bone (ribs) to assure a clean strike to a vital spot. Broadheads are of three general types. Fixed-blade broadheads are fixed to the shaft and sharpened manually. Modular broadheads contain a center column or ferrule holding three to four replaceable blades. Mechanical broadheads are designed to have recessed blades that fly open on impact: in a closed position, they have excellent ballistic properties. Barbed heads are illegal for hunting game (except for bow fishing) since the head will not work out of a wounded animal that receives a nonfatal shot (Fig. 7-54).

Arrow wounds in humans and companion animals are uncommon in the United States compared to gunshot wounds. Few cases are reported in the human and veterinary medical literature. Many cases go unreported.

Management of Arrow Wounds

Most arrows are not barbed and may be able to be removed without great difficulty. Target arrows have a smooth field point equal to the diameter of the shaft and should slide out unimpeded. Broadheads with their rotating cutting edges can "corkscrew" deep into the body, making removal more difficult. Their razor-sharp cutting edges have the potential to lacerate tissue when withdrawn. If the arrow is lodged near a vital area or vessel (based on radiographs and examination), surgical exploration and removal are advisable. There are reported instances when vital organs (e.g., heart) have been penetrated with a foreign object, which paradoxically plugs the hole created and prevents fatal hemorrhage by its presence. Surgical exploration and removal is obviously the safest option in this situation.

From the surgical standpoint, retention of the arrow would allow the clinician to determine the depth and location of the arrow wound prior to exploration (Fig. 7-55). Owners may have removed the arrow before the animal is brought to the clinic. In the field, removal can be attempted if the arrow is lodged in a nonvital area to facilitate transport of the animal. Alternatively, the

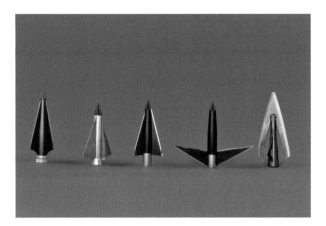

FIG. 7-54 Broadheads vary in shape, design, weight, and number of blades (usually two, three, or four). Broadheads are frequently threaded and screwed onto the arrow shaft. The broadhead, third from the left, has three blades that open in a tripod fashion (fourth from left) upon penetration in order to enhance its cutting surface area.

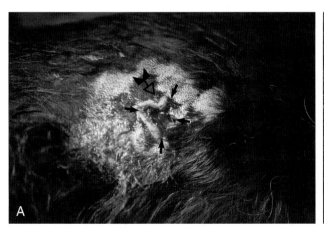
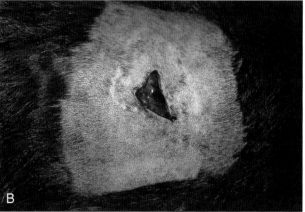

FIG. 7-55 (A) Arrow wound over the lumbar area. Trajectory of the arrow suggested the patient was shot by a hunter from an elevated position. Note the "cross" wound (arrows) created by a four-blade broadhead hunting arrow (symmetrically placed blades). Management consisted of local wound debridement, lavage, and a sterile dressing. Because of the large lacerations created, it was possible to close the skin wounds with establishment of separate ventral drainage.
(B) Lumbar arrow wound: the triangular cut was created by a broadhead arrow with three blades.

exposed shaft can be cut off to prevent accidental jarring of the arrow. The animal should be immobilized to prevent additional injury with a retained arrow during transport. In the emergency clinic, bolt cutters can be used to divide the exposed shaft. Sedatives, analgesics, and/or general anesthesia should be used when manipulating the patient.

Radiographs and a complete examination are followed by surgical preparation of the area, exploration, and extraction of the arrow. If the arrow has perforated a structure, and the broadhead is accessible, it can be unscrewed from the threaded shaft or cut off with bolt cutters to prevent further trauma as the shaft is withdrawn.

Wide aggressive surgical debridement is not indicated for most arrow wounds. Wound lavage and establishing adequate drainage are important. Exploration is necessary when major organs or structures are involved. Like other penetrating/perforating abdominal wounds, laparotomy is indicated (Fig. 7-56 and 7-57).

Legal Considerations

In today's litigious society, veterinarians can find themselves involved in lawsuits, primarily to present testimony as to the physical findings of a given case. Forensic evidence of a shooting may be requested by owners, game wardens, and attorneys. Veterinarians must be able to document such evidence or request assistance from an experienced pathologist. Basic protocols and responsibilities involved with handling forensic evidence must be followed, or legal cases will be contested easily. Detailed records should include notes of conversations.

A complete set of quality radiographs and color photographs of the entire animal should be taken to illustrate the general position of the injuries. This will help orient those reviewing the case. Close photographs of individual injuries should include an area 15 cm around the wounds. A metric ruler should be included in the photographs to indicate scale. The photographs are labeled with the date, case number, and examiner's initials. Projectiles should be photographed in situ before their removal. Flexible plastic probes are best used to highlight the course of a projectile. Care must be taken to avoid scratching projectiles with metallic instruments that could distort rifling marks.

When feasible, an experienced, board-certified veterinary pathologist should perform the detailed postmortem examination. Consultation with the pathologist and knowledgeable law enforcement offi-

cials is advisable to assure evidence is obtained, handled, and transferred properly to assure legal aspects of the case are properly maintained. Other preexisting medical or physical conditions may have affected the circumstances of the animal's demise.

Tissue samples are taken to confirm the presence of any suspected diseases, determine the age of a wound, and help distinguish entry from exit wounds. Tissue samples occasionally are taken for more detailed testing and analysis by law-enforcement officials.

Information commonly requested in court relates to the number and location of wounds, features of the wounds and related tissue areas, course of the projectiles, angle of fire, projectiles and foreign debris recovered, cause and time of death, and details pertaining to the handling and disposition of specimens collected. Entry wounds are closely inspected to determine the proximity of the weapon to the animal. A 15-cm square around entrance wounds should be removed, pinned to a piece of rigid material, and then frozen for analysis to determine the presence of propellant and projectile residue. This tissue specimen should not be washed or placed in formalin.

Careful examination and collection of tissues surrounding the path of a projectile are useful in determining whether game has been illegally killed by a gun during restricted bow-hunting seasons. Some hunters insert a broadhead arrow into a gunshot wound to mask the nature of the weapon. Flesh along the path of the bullet can be collected to recover particles of lead released by frangible projectiles. Lead residue can be identified by atomic absorption spectrophotometry in tissue surrounding the tract. Tissue samples taken from a separate, uninvolved body region of the carcass serve as a control. Examination of gastric contents can also help the pathologist determine the circumstances of the incident.

The *lands* (elevated borders) and *grooves* of a rifled barrel embed marks on jacketed and nonjacketed bullets. Occasionally, the lead core separates from the outer jacket. Retrieval of the jacket is of great importance because the rifling marks are scored on its outer surface. The bullet should be washed with water and alcohol and then allowed to air dry. The washing removes blood and tissue fragments. The bullet can be marked on its base (bottom) to ensure that it can be identified later. Close-up photographs of the bullet may help ensure its identification.

Projectiles can be wrapped in facial tissues and placed in vials or containers that can be sealed with tape. Some pathologists place projectiles in sealed envelopes. The body region from which each projectile was retrieved must be clearly identified and each

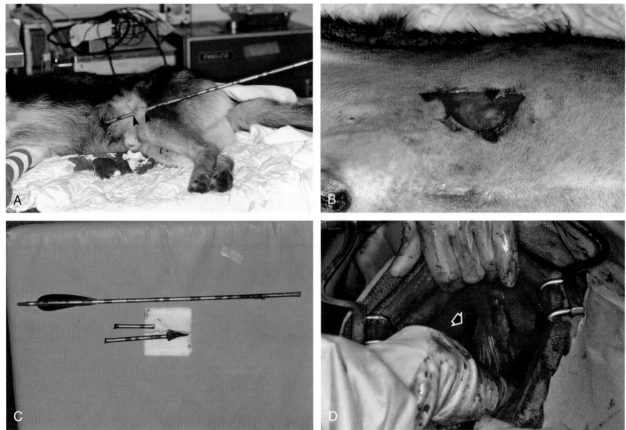

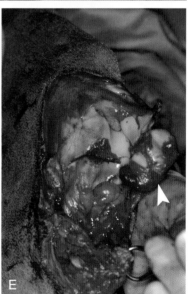

FIG. 7-56 (A) A broadhead arrow wound entering the abdominal cavity of a dog. The arrow initially perforated the stifle area before penetrating the abdomen. A neighbor admitted to shooting the dog for "self defense." However, entry of the arrow from a caudal, lateral direction would suggest the dog was not in an offensive position when struck.

(B) Note the triangular entry wound to the abdomen created by the three blades of the broadhead arrow.

(C) Under anesthesia, the arrow was cut with bolt cutters and removed just prior to the laparotomy.

(D) The arrow penetrated deep into the thoracic cavity (intraoperative view) cutting the liver and diaphragm (arrow).

(E) Exploration of the knee. Note the patellar tendon was severed (grasped with forceps) from its attachment to the patella (arrow).

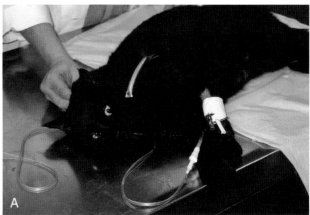

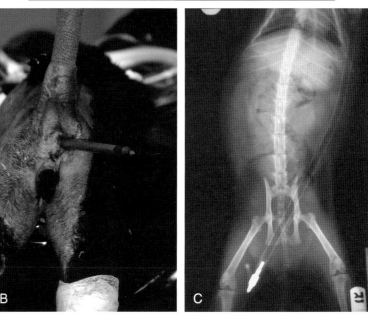

FIG. 7-57 (A) Field point arrow wound. The arrow traversed the thoracic and abdominal cavities. (B) The arrow exited the anus. (C) Radiograph of the patient with the arrow. Despite the gruesome nature of the wound, the patient recovered completely following exploratory surgery and repair. Field points pierce tissue, but lack the cutting blades of broadheads (hunting arrows). If no vital structures are impacted, soft tissue trauma is relatively minor. (Slides courtesy of Gary Spodnick, DVM, DACVS.)

projectile must be placed in a separate, marked container. The container is identified with the date, time, case number, and owner's name, and it is initialed by those present at the necropsy. An indelible marker should be used on the container or on a nonremovable label. The projectiles should be secured from tampering or access by other individuals. Projectiles are turned over only to a qualified law-enforcement officer. Any persons receiving the specimens must add the time and date of the transfer and their initials to the container.

Attention to the legal issues discussed in this section will help clinicians avoid the embarrassing errors and pitfalls associated with inappropriate case preparation in a court of law.

Arrows can have latent fingerprints on the shaft, unless blurred by passage through body tissues,

contact with the entrance environment, or manipulation by individuals. Depending upon the exact nature of the case, arrows can be removed without touching the shaft and placed in a secure area for presentation to law-enforcement officials.

Under no circumstances should the projectile be transferred to the owner, thereby reducing the credibility of the evidence gathered.

IMPALEMENT INJURIES

Impalement by definition is to pierce or transfix with a sharp object. In dogs and cats, this is most commonly the result of running or falling onto a sharp object. Dogs in particular are more susceptible to oropharyngeal and esophageal impalement wounds when chasing or carrying sticks. There are two common scenarios. (1) Dogs occasionally run after a stick or piece of wood tossed by the owner: as the object tumbles or momentarily imbeds into the ground the dog grabs the end in its mouth. The momentum of the dog drives the stick through their oropharynx, in many cases deep into the cervical tissues (Fig. 7-58). (2) Dogs occasionally run with a stick or piece of wood in their mouth: if the end of the stick strikes the ground while the dog is running, the dog again impales their oropharynx.

Dogs occasionally run into a stationary pointed object, resulting in an impalement wound usually involving the head, neck, or anterior thorax (Fig. 7-59). Dogs can impale their trunk by chasing and overrunning a tumbling stick tossed by the owner. One end of the stick contacts the ground while the vertical end of the stick impales the pet (Fig. 7-60). Rarely, dogs and cats impale themselves by falling from an elevated position, striking fencing or other objects upon impact.

Impalement injuries, especially those involving sticks, should be explored to assure that no plant material (bark, wood splinters, leaf fragments, pine needles) is retained in the body. Such retained material normally results in abscess formation and draining tracts. Smooth surfaced objects (finished lumber, metal, plastic) are less problematic. Deeper cervical wounds should be explored through a ventral midline cervical approach. More superficial oropharyngeal wounds can be explored and repaired with an oral approach.

It is an advantage for the surgeon to have the impalement object left in place: exploration can be focused on the exact path and optimal approach to its removal. This also facilitates lavage, debridement, tissue repair, and postoperative drainage. If the object has been removed, examination of the object by the surgeon combined with the owner's description of the wound can help determine the relative depth and direction of the impalement tract. Radiographs and ultrasonography of the involved region(s) can be useful in determining the best surgical approach to problematic impalement wounds. Endoscopic examination also may be useful in assessing the location of an esophageal tear. Magnetic resonance imaging has been suggested for better defining the location of problematic esophageal injuries, although most tears should be visible by surgical exploration of the cervical area. Radiographic evidence of cervical emphysema is a frequent finding with acute penetrating oropharyngeal and esophageal impalement. Repair of esophageal tears can be challenging, depending on the size and location of the tear. Most oral impalement wounds necessarily require debridement and closure of the mucosal wound to prevent oral contaminants from gaining access to the underlying tissues.

Overlooking retained sticks or delays in treatment of oropharyngeal/cervical esophageal tears can result in life-threatening infection and extension into the anterior mediastinum. Prompt intervention can dramatically reduce this risk.

Cervical exploration includes careful inspection for retained plant material and debris. Following closure of the oropharyngeal/esophageal defect, copious

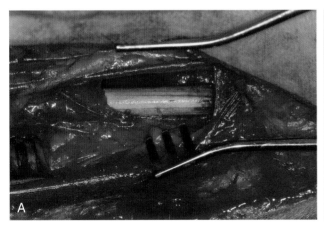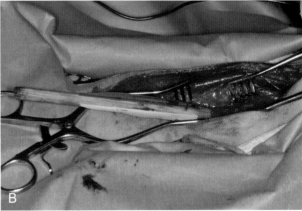

FIG. 7-58 (A). This canine patient chased an arrow in flight. When the arrow struck the ground the dog grabbed the nock end of the arrow. His body momentum drove the arrow through his oropharynx deep into the cervical tissues. (B) A ventral cervical incision was used to remove the arrow and inspect the wound tract. The oropharyngeal tear was sutured. The cervical wound was lavaged and closed with a vacuum drain. The patient made a complete recovery.

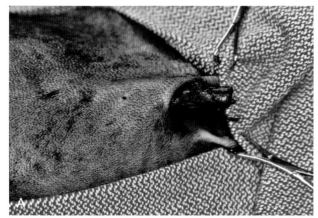
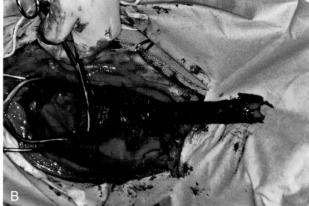
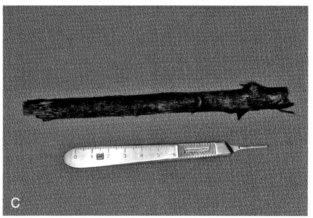

FIG. 7-59 (A) Thoracic impalement on a stick. The dog staggered back to the owner after running into the neighboring woods. The stick entered the thoracic inlet to the level of the diaphragm. (B, C) The stick was left in place to facilitate exploration of the entire wound. A thoracotomy also was performed to ensure no fragments of bark or wood splinters remained. The patient made a complete recovery.

lavage and suction of the area is indicated. A closed vacuum drain can be very effective in controlling dead space and assessing the fluid volume/composition retained in the reservoir after completion of surgery. Most dogs do not require a gastrostomy tube, depending on the assessment of the esophageal repair. Broad spectrum antibiotic administration is advisable.

PRESSURE SORES

Pressure sores (decubital ulcers) are considered a sign of poor nursing care. They are caused by prolonged compression of the skin over bony prominences, resulting in progressive ischemia. Pressure sores do not occur in healthy ambulatory animals who are properly housed. Animals incapable or unwilling to change body positions are prone to pressure sore for-

mation, unless close attention is given to their prevention.

Sick, debilitated, and paralyzed dogs are most susceptible to their formation. Weight loss, protein depletion, and poor nutritional support increases the likelihood of their development. Loss of subcutaneous fat and muscle mass enhances the silhouette of bony prominences including the greater trochanter, ischial tuberosity, acromion, lateral tibial condyle, lateral humeral epicondyle, tuber coxae, olecranon and calcaneal tuber, lateral malleolus, lateral surface of the fifth digit, and the sternum. Denervated skin may be more prone to trophic ulcer development.

Casts and splints are capable of causing pressure sores by compression of the skin overlying a bony prominence. Most commonly, this involves the accessory carpal pad (Fig. 7-61). Prevention is directed at proper padding around the bony prominences to avoid a pressure cone effect to the area.

Large dogs are more prone to pressure sore formation due to their greater weight (Fig. 7-62). Debilitated greyhounds and other breeds with thin skin and a sparse hair coat may be prone to pressure sore formation. The skin overlying the greater trochanter is the most common site for their development. Ischial tuberosity pressure sores are more common in smaller paraplegic dogs who have a tendency to sit up on their perineal region for prolonged periods of time on unpadded surfaces. Cats rarely develop pressure sores due to their small size and less frequent spinal cord injuries.

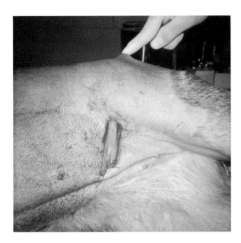

FIG. 7-60 Impalement on a piece of wood. The dog overran the piece of lumber, tossed by the owner, with the stick penetrating the left flank area. Sticks and twigs are more likely to leave fragments of plant material behind and warrant closer inspection than finished lumber, metal, or plastic. The author has removed bark, wood slivers, pine needles, and leaf fragments, all associated with stick-impalement injuries.

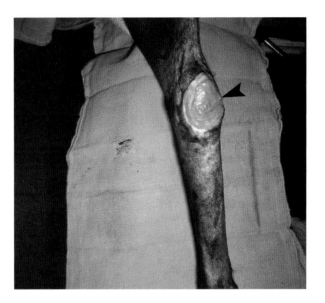

FIG. 7-62 Pressure sore (grade II) over the elbow of a large Labrador retriever. The dog developed the wound during its hospitalization for a serious illness. Closure required the application of a skin flap.

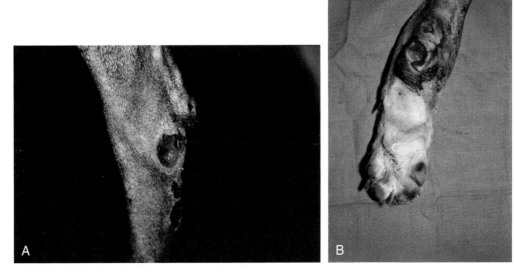

FIG. 7-61 Pressure sores associated with improper casting/padding. (A) Ulcer overlying the calcaneus. (B) Sloughing of the accessory carpal pad.

Nursing care is more difficult for larger dogs. Unfortunately, if they cannot be lifted from their cage, they may be inappropriately dragged out of the cage for treatments and cleaning. The fragile skin overlying the bony prominences then is stretched and abraded against the floor surface. Moisture accumulation on the skin from sweating, environmental moisture, urine, and feces can promote tissue maceration and infection. A dense hair coat affords some natural (padding) protection but may promote moisture retention, mask early stages of pressure sore formation, and delay institution of additional preventative measures.

Prevention

Prevention of pressure sores requires an educated and devoted nursing staff, veterinarian, and owner. The following management steps should be implemented.

1. Provide proper nutritional and fluid support.

2. Keep the patient's skin clean and dry.

3. Change the patient's body position every 2 hours (left lateral, sternal, right lateral).

4. Keep the patient on padded surfaces (artificial washable fleece pads placed over easily cleaned support pads) placed on elevated grates or racks to separate the dog from urine and feces; water or air mattresses; disposable absorbent foam egg crate sheets (convoluted foam pads, Allegiance Health Care Corp., Wilsonville, OR); or coated or closed cell foam pads (Dubicrest Padding 4700, Alpha Protech, Tulsa, OK).

5. Assess skin overlying bony prominences daily for erythema, the first sign of pressure sore development.

6. Avoid dragging over or dropping the patient on hard surfaces. If the patient cannot be lifted, slide the dog on a rug or fleece pad to prevent cutaneous abrasion.

7. Place weak or paralyzed dogs in a sling support for 2–4 hours daily to reduce pressure on lateral bony prominences.

8. Periodically, use hydrotherapy to keep the patient clean while improving muscle tone and circulation to the skin. The patient must be dried appropriately after each session.

Properly maintained, a closed collection system can prevent urine scalding and skin maceration in patients incapable of urinating voluntarily. The perineal area can be clipped of hair to facilitate cleansing in the event of fecal incontinence. Water mattresses are useful as long as they support the weight of the dog. Covers should be applied over the mattresses to protect them from punctures and to facilitate cleaning. Unfortunately, many dogs will bite, chew, and scratch mattresses and foam pads. Because replacement can be costly, one option is to have the owner purchase pads, which they later can take home with them when the dog is discharged from the hospital. Many dogs will not cooperate with periodic attempts to change body position unless barriers (cardboard boxes, pads, etc.) are used to restrict their movements. Providing large patients with appropriate nursing care is time consuming and expensive. However, the cost of pressure sore treatment far outweighs the cost of prevention.

Pressure Sore Classification

Pressure sore gradation is done according to the depth of injury to tissues overlying bony prominences (grades I to IV) (Fig. 7-63). Table 7-3 summarizes this classification.

Management of Pressure Sores

Permanently debilitated or paralyzed dogs prone to pressure sore formation also are prone to redevelopment of them after successful closure. Patients who regain ambulation have the greatest likelihood of maintaining permanent closure. Until patients reach this point, continuous preventative medicine is required to protect the area from reulceration. Several options are available for management of pressure sores; selection of the appropriate technique depends upon the severity of the lesion.

1. Open wound management—healing by second intention

2. Delayed primary closure

3. Secondary closure

4. Excision of the bony prominence in combination with (2) or (3)

5. Muscle flap coverage of the bony prominence in combination with (2), (3), or (4)

6. Skin flap coverage in combination with (2), (3), (4), or (5)

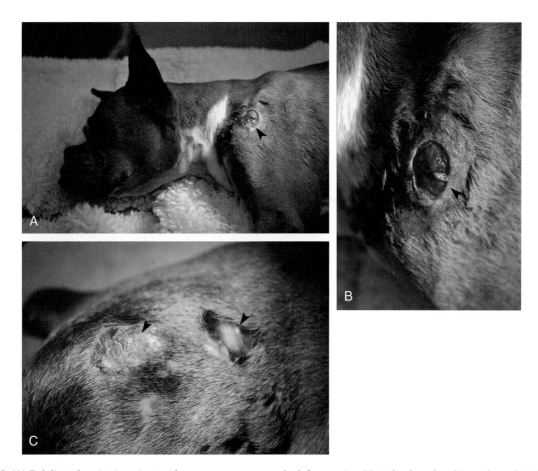

FIG. 7-63 (A) Debilitated geriatric patient with a pressure sore over the left acromion. Note the dog placed on a sheepskin. (B) A closer view indicates a grade II pressure sore (arrow). (C) Two pressure sores also were noted over the wing of the ilium (grade II) and greater trochanter (grade I progressing to a grade II) (arrows).

TABLE 7-3
Pressure sore classification.

Grade I	Erythema; superficial to partial thickness skin loss.
Grade II	Full-thickness skin loss with variable involvement of subcutis.
Grade III	Ulceration extends to deep fascia overlying the bony prominences.
Grade IV	Ulceration extends to bone. Osteomyelitis or joint infection may be present.

Grade I and grade II pressure sores may be amenable to second intention healing, unless they are persistent or recurrent ulcers. In many cases, grade II pressure sores are better closed by wound excision and primary closure, delayed primary closure, or secondary closure (Fig. 7-64). Grade III, grade IV, or recurrent pressure sores may require open wound management to control infection followed by excision of a portion of the bony prominence. A local muscle flap may be used to add padding between the bone and skin. Muscle flaps can contribute circulation to diseased bone and help control chronic infection. The outer muscle surface in turn provides a stable vascular bed for skin flaps or cutaneous advancement.

Healing by second intention may not provide a durable surface to prevent reinjury. Skin closure techniques that place the incision line directly over the bony prominence increase the likelihood of dehiscence unless additional wound protection is provided. Skin flaps (including local flaps and axial pattern flaps) can provide a layer of subcutaneous tissue to cushion the

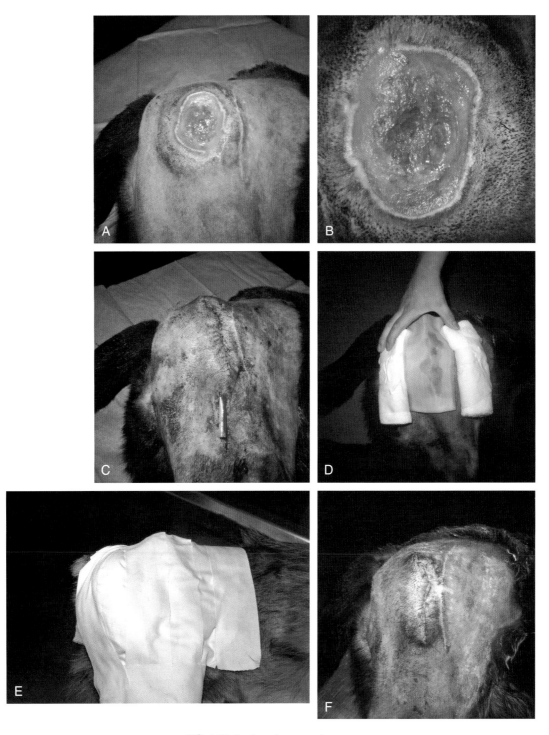

FIG. 7-64 *See legend on opposite page.*

skin over the bony prominence. Moreover, rotational flaps can provide full-thickness skin coverage while placing the suture line peripheral to the bony prominence. Even then, postoperative protective measures must be instituted to avoid trauma and ischemia to the flap until the animal becomes ambulatory.

> Pressure sores over the elbow can be particularly challenging, especially in thin-skinned breeds such as the greyhound.
>
> In many cases, local flaps can be used to close the defect, the simplest being the use of bipedicle advancement flaps (release incisions). The thoracodorsal axial pattern flap is considered only for the most problematic skin defects overlying the elbow area. See Plate 9.

Postoperative Care

Preventative measures, as described in the previous section, must be continued. In addition, bandages are advised in order to protect the healing wound from moisture, microorganisms, and compression and shearing forces that promote ischemic necrosis and dehiscence. Soft, thick, "doughnut rings" fashioned from roll gauze have been used to protect the trochanteric area and lateral prominence of the limbs. The ring encircles the circumference of the bony prominence and protects it from contact with hard surfaces when the dog is placed in lateral recumbency. However, they can be difficult to properly maintain. Their use is controversial since the doughnut ring can create a "halo" compression over the skin surrounding the bony prominence and compromise the cutaneous circulation required to promote healing to the injured area. Doughnut rings require close observation when used. Another option is the use of parallel pads made from gauze rolls. These pads can provide protection without the complete skin encirclement of doughnut rings. Spray adhesive used for plastic surgical drapes can be applied around the neighboring skin followed by the application of surgical tape (Fig. 7-64).

Soft foam pads, spicas, and tie-over dressings may be used to protect bony prominences on the lateral surface of the trunk and limbs. Schroeder-Thomas splints may be useful to manage pressure sores overlying the olecranon and calcaneal tuber after surgical closure. The author has developed a simple foam padding system to protect the elbow region while allowing the dog to ambulate normally (see Plate 9).

Once healing is completed and sutures removed, splints and protective bandages may be removed on a trial basis, although proper nursing care is continued for as long as the dog is not ambulatory.

HYGROMA

An elbow hygroma is a serous subcutaneous fluid pocket overlying the olecranon in large to giant breed dogs (great Danes, Irish wolfhounds, St. Bernards, and

---

FIG. 7-64 (A) Chronic pressure sore over the greater trochanter. The dog developed the wound previously during hospitalization for the repair of pelvic fractures.

(B) Complete excision of the pressure sore was performed. Electrocautery and ligatures were required to control the considerable hemorrhage that occurred during this procedure.

(C) Skin borders were undermined, advanced, and opposed with a subcuticular suture pattern, followed by skin sutures (vertical mattress and simple interrupted suture patterns). A Penrose drain was used to control dead space.

(D) A nonadherent dressing was applied over the incision. Two 6-inch soft gauze rolls were placed in parallel fashion cranial and caudal to the incision. Spray adhesive, used for the application of plastic surgical drapes, was used to stick the gauze sponges into position.

(E) Spray adhesive was used to provide additional adhesive power to the surgical tape placed over the area.

(F) The wound 14 days later. The ability of the patient to freely move and ambulate is critical to the treatment and prevention of recurrence of pressure sores.

Newfoundlands), usually less than 2 years of age. Hygromas form as a result of repeated blunt trauma from the patient striking and compressing the skin against hard floor surfaces. The skin and subcutis in turn is compressed against this bony prominence (Fig. 7-65) Although rare, hygromas have been reported overlying the carpus, nuchal crest, os calcis, and tuber ischium.

Most hygromas are painless fluctuations. Some hygromas remain relatively small and change little in size. Over time, hygromas can enlarge and ulcerate as the overlying skin thins and stretches over the fluid pocket. Ulcerated hygromas frequently become infected. Poor aseptic technique from attempted fluid aspiration can result in abscess formation; this problem may be compounded by futile attempts at prevention by injecting corticosteroids into the hygroma pocket. Both techniques are not advisable.

Conservative prevention and management are essentially the same: soft padded bedding (see bedding options for pressure sores above) and protective elbow pads (protective dog leggings, HandicappedPets.com; www.dogleggs.com). This would be the initial treatment of choice for small hygromas. Larger, persistent hygromas are likely surgical candidates. Similarly, large, ulcerated, and infected hygromas normally require more aggressive surgical intervention.

Penrose Drain Technique

Large, uncomplicated hygromas are managed with the prolonged use of Penrose drains. (See Fig. 7-65.)

1. Liberally clip the elbow area.
2. Use sterile surgical preparation and draping.
3. Make a stab incision in the proximal and distal borders of the hygroma.
4. Drain the fluid and inspect the interior of the hygroma.
5. Remove fibrinous debris with forceps and sharp scissors.

Direct one 1/4-inch or two 1/4-inch Penrose drains through both stab incisions.

6. 3–4 centimeters of the drain length should extend from each drain hole and is secured to the skin with 2-0 monofilament sutures at each end of the hygroma.
7. Apply a nonadherent dressing and topical antimicrobial ointment over the area,

followed by a firm, bulky protective bandage. Apply ample padding over the elbow.
8. Inspect the bandage every 4–5 days. The bandage overlying the drain site requires local removal and replacement due to accumulated discharge from the drain sites.
9. Continue this procedure for 3–4 weeks. The drains are removed at the time of the last bandage change. Thereafter, elbow pads and soft bedding are advisable to prevent recurrence.

The Penrose drain provides continuous wound drainage while the compressive wrap helps to compress the dermal surface to the opposing side of the hygroma. Collagen will connect the surfaces together, obliterating the hygroma dead space (Fig. 7-65).

Surgical Resection

Problematic hygromas less commonly present with ulcerated skin, draining tracts, and an ongoing bacterial infection. Considerable scarring may be noted in the area. Under these circumstances, surgical resection of the ulcerated skin and underlying fibrotic scar should be considered. This surgical procedure runs the risk of wound dehiscence if skin closure is performed under tension. A Schroeder-Thomas splint or rigid spica bandage may be needed for 2–3 weeks to prevent elbow flexion during the healing process. An incision lateral to the olecranon is best used to dissect the underlying diseased tissues from beneath the skin. (An incision directly over the olecranon has a higher probability of dehiscence.) Surgical efforts must be directed at preserving healthy elbow callus and as much skin coverage as possible. Failure to do so will likely result in wound dehiscence. Postoperatively, wound drainage (vacuum drains or Penrose drains) and protective bandaging are essential to control dead space and minimize motion until suture removal. Closure of smaller skin defects overlying the olecranon may be achieved with the assistance of lateral/medial release incisons. In extreme cases, wide skin resection will require reconstructive surgery, usually with the thoracodorsal axial pattern flap. It is strongly recommended that the veterinarian consult with a board-certified surgeon before undertaking surgical removal of problematic hygromas. It is worth remembering that large elbow wounds are among the most difficult defects to close successfully.

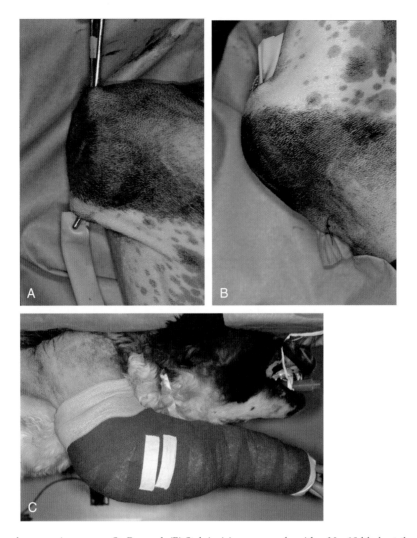

FIG. 7-65 (A) Elbow hygroma in a young St. Bernard. (B) Stab incisions are made with a No. 10 blade at the proximal and distal ends of the swelling. Hemostats can be used as a tissue retractor to examine the cavity. Insertion of two 1/4-inch Penrose drains. Sutures are used to secure both ends of the drains. (C) Application of a bulky compression bandage. The bandage extends down to the paw to prevent distal limb edema.

SNAKEBITE

Although relatively uncommon, snakebites are occasionally seen in the United States primarily in those areas populated with poisonous snakes. An estimated 15,000 domestic animals are bitten by snakes annually in the United States. There are two main families of venomous snakes.

- Elapidae: Elapids include coral snakes, cobras, mambas, kraits, and the tiger snake. Coral snakes can be found in the southeastern areas of the United States.

- Vipers: Rattlesnakes, copperheads, and cottonmouths (water moccasins) are found in various areas throughout the United States. Copperheads have a relatively low order of toxicity. Toxicity can vary between species. Rattlesnakes account for 80% of the poisonous snakebite wounds in North America.

In North America, 90% of snake bites occur between April and October. Toxicity is increased in young or very large snakes during the springtime.

Toxins in elapids are neurotoxic and hemolytic in nature; viper toxins cause local tissue damage (necrogenic) and may initiate systemic bleeding/coagulation (vasculotoxic). Diamondback rattlesnake venom may contain a myocardial depressant factor that can result in cardiac dysrhythmias. Fang marks are a distinguishing feature of vipers; nonvenomous snake bites are characterized by a series of small punctures that reflect the curvature of the mouth. Almost one in four bites of vipers are "dry," with little or no envenomation of the dog or cat. Coral snakes have short fangs and a small mouth, leaving a characteristic convex row of pinpoint puncture wounds.

Unless witnessed by the owner, snakebites can be difficult to diagnose. Typically, viper bites cause local swelling, pain, erythema, petechiae, or ecchymoses, and later cyanosis with subsequent tissue necrosis. Close inspection may reveal fang marks. Most dogs are bitten in the head and facial area and less commonly the paws. Facial swelling may be pronounced, and the patient's airway is closely monitored in the event a tracheotomy is needed. In severe cases tissue around the fang marks may darken and ooze dark blood. Swelling may worsen over the first 24–48 hours, and the damaged tissues may form a hematoma. Copperhead bites, from the author's limited experience, primarily result in regional tissue swelling to the dog, but lack the severity of local and systemic changes noted in the more toxic rattlesnake and water moccasin envenomation (Fig. 7-66).

Elapid venom may have a delayed onset of 1–7.5 hours. Signs include salivation, vomiting, apprehensive behavior, followed by convulsions, quadriplegia, and respiratory paralysis. Fortunately, documented coral snake envenomation is rare.

Baseline blood work (complete blood count, profile) and a urinalysis should be submitted on presentation. A coagulation profile is also advisable. Hemoconcentration, leukocytosis, echinocytosis ("burred" red blood cells may be noted 24–48 hours after envenomation), hypokalemia, elevated creatine kinase, hematuria, and myoglobinuria, may be noted. Prolongation of activated clotting time (ACT), prothrombin time (PT), partial thromboplastin time (PTT), and increased fibrin degradation products (FDPs) also may be noted.

Therapeutic goals include prevention of hypotension (monitor blood pressure, electrocardiograms) and neutralization of the local and systemic effects of the venom. Crystaloids (lactated Ringer's solution, or 0.9% saline) comprise the bulk of intravenous fluid support, with the use of colloids and plasma as needed. Urine output is closely monitored.

Antivenin (polyvalent Crotalidae) can be administered to critical patients. One to three vials is typically given to dogs: there is no specific dosage. Antivenin administration is based on patient response in humans. One canine study involving eastern diamondback rat-

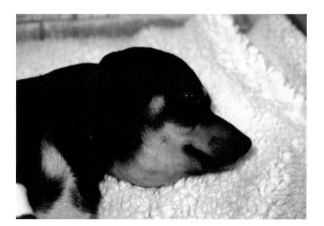

FIG. 7-66 Louisiana dog that sustained a copperhead bite: note the facial swelling. No tissue loss was noted: copperhead venom has a relatively low order of toxicity compared to rattlesnakes. Supportive fluid therapy resulted in complete recovery.

tlesnake poisoning found an 80% survival when anti-venin was administered within 30 minutes of envenomation. The survival rate dropped to 62% if given 4 hours after envenomation. Antivenin is administered slowly intravenously; it can cause an anaphylactic reaction. Unfortunately, antivenin is expensive (up to $300.00 per vial) and has limited availability. (Fort Dodge Veterinary Supplies carries antivenin for veterinary use; Wyeth-Ayerst Laboratories, Philadelphia, PA, carries antivenin for humans.) In emergencies, veterinarians can contact human medical facilities to obtain antivenin. Pain control (opiates), corticosteroids, and antibiotics (cephalosporins) are advisable.

Most patients recover from viper envenomation. Tissue necrosis can be significant and will require standard wound care. Reconstructive surgery may be required for the larger tissue defects (Fig. 7-67).

BROWN RECLUSE SPIDER BITES

Although there are a number of poisonous insects in the United States, only the brown recluse has surgical significance due to its potential to cause tissue necrosis. The brown recluse (*Loxosceles reclusa*) venom contains a variety of enzymes (sphingomyelinase-D, hyaluronidase, esterase, alkaline phosphatase, 5′ ribonucleotide phosphorylase, necrotizing enzymes, and several proteins/polypeptides) capable of causing circular areas of skin necrosis that are slow to heal (referred to as loxoscelism or dermonecrotic arachnidism). Potency varies between species of this spider: the Arizona recluse (*L. rufscens*), desert recluse (*L. deserta)*, and Mediterranean recluse (*L. arizonica*) spider envenomations are less potent.

The characteristic coloration of the bite wound in humans (central red area inflammation; white middle ring ischemia; and outer blue ring thrombosis) may be noted 3–8 hours after envenomation. Systemic signs that may be noted from the bite include hemolytic anemia, thrombocytopenia, hematuria, pyrexia, and myalgia. The hair coat of fur-bearing animals effectively conceals the bite wound; owners note the problem only when a circular necrotic patch of skin becomes evident. Lesions may be 1–25 cm in diameter. The diagnosis of dermonecrotic arachnidism is normally a "default" diagnosis only when other causes are ruled out. Methacillin-resistant staphylococcal infections (MRSA) in humans can mimic recluse lesions.

Brown recluse spiders prefer dry undisturbed areas, including woodpiles, sheds, garages, closets, and cellars. They favor cardboard and paper piles, but can be found in shoes, dressers, behind baseboards, and near furnaces. They have a wide distribution, from the southern Midwest to the Gulf of Mexico. They are rarely found west of the Rocky Mountains.

Recluse spiders are a variable brown to a deep yellow, and usually have a violin-like marking on the dorsal side of the cephalothorax, with the neck of the violin extending caudally. They vary from 6 to 20 mm (1/4 to 3/4 inch). Multiple websites have photographs of this spider to facilitate identification.

The known presence of recluse spiders, possible exposure of the pet to an area frequented by this arachnid, and any supporting clinical signs would reinforce this "after-the-fact" diagnosis. Bite wounds in humans can result in significant medical complications; this does not appear to be the case in small animals. In humans, wounds can be slow to slough and subsequently heal. There are a variety of treatments advocated for treatment of verified *acute* brown recluse bites in humans; this is not the case in veterinary patients. Areas of necrotic tissue and any slow healing wound usually can be excised and closed in veterinary patients with little difficulty.

PORCUPINE QUILLS

Porcupine quill injuries are normally noted in dogs, the majority of wounds being in the facial area. Occasionally, some owners will attempt to remove quills with pliers, but most will seek out veterinary assistance, especially when multiple quills are embedded in their pet.

Quills vary from 2–10 cm in length. Heavy sedation or general anesthesia is advisable since quill extraction can be painful. The fur should be parted to visualize embedded quills; fingers are carefully run through the fur to identify the exposed point of shorter or more deeply embedded quills. Needle holders can be used to grasp and remove each quill. Lightly embedded quills can be extracted with a firm tug, whereas deeply embedded quills can be extracted with quarter turns of the wrist. A No. 11 scalpel blade can be aligned along the surface of problematic quills to create a small cutaneous stab incision to facilitate their removal. Few quill sites become infected after their removal; systemic antibiotics may be administered along with analgesics when the patient is discharged from the hospital.

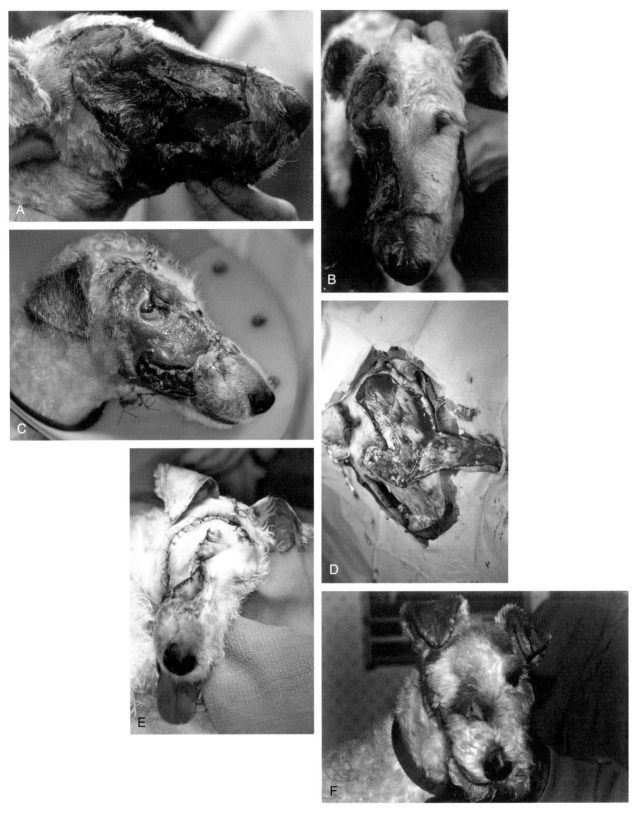

FIG. 7-67 *See legend on opposite page.*

FIG. 7-67 (A, B) Rattlesnake bite to a 6-year-old wired haired fox terrier. The dog was bitten rostral to the right eye. The dog received antivenin (Antivenin Crotalidae Polyvalent, Wyeth-Ayerst Laboratories, Philadelphia, PA) and supportive therapy. Within 4 hours after envenomation, the local skin darkened with serous exudation from the area. Photograph of the necrotic wound at 2 weeks.

(C) The wound at 6 weeks. Debridement and open wound management resulted in a healthy granulation bed.

(D) Enucleation was performed, followed by elevation of a transposition flap.

(E) Completion of the surgical procedure. The small remaining area will heal by second intention.

(F) The patient, 14 weeks after injury. (From Kostolich M. 1990. Reconstructive surgery of a rattlesnake bite. *Canine Pract* 15:15–19. Case slides courtesy of Marilyn Kostolich, DVM, DACVS.)

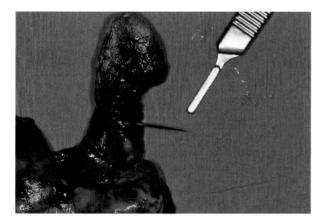

FIG. 7-68 Porcupine quill in the left cranial lung lobe resulting in pneumothorax. A detailed history revealed the dog encountered a porcupine some months before presentation for pneumothorax.

> Contrary to popular folklore, cutting a quill does not cause the quill to deflate, facilitating its removal.

The frictional surface of quills can facilitate their migration deep into the body. A porcupine quill was removed from a canine brain abscess on postmortem examination of a patient at Angell Memorial Animal Hospital: the quill had migrated through one of the formina of the skull. The author has also removed quills from the lungs of dogs that have presented with spontaneous pneumothorax and lung abscessation

(Fig. 7-68). A careful and complete examination of the entire dog is advisable.

Suggested Readings

Bite Wounds

August JR. 1988. Dog and cat bites. *J Am Vet Med Assoc* 193:1394–1398.

Cowell AK, Penwick RC. 1989. Dog bite wounds: a study of 93 cases. *Compend Contin Educ Pract Vet* 11:313–320.

Davidson EB. 1998. Managing bite wounds in dogs and cats. Part II. *Compend Contin Educ Pract Vet* 20:974–991.

Kolata RJ, Kraut NH, Hohnston DE. 1974. Patterns of trauma in urban dogs and cats: a study of 1000 cases. *J Am Vet Med Assoc* 164:499–502.

McKiernan BC, Adams WM, Huse DC. 1984. Thoracic bite wounds and associated internal injury in 11 dogs and 1 cat. *J Am Vet Med Assoc* 184:959–964.

Neal TM, Key JC. 1976. Principles of treatment of dog bite wounds. *J Am Anim Hosp Assoc* 12:657–660.

Pavletic MM. 1990. Bite Wounds. In: *2nd International Veterinary Emergency and Critical Care Symposium*. Lakewood, CO: AAHA.

Pavletic MM. 1995. *Bite Wound Management in Small Animals*. AAHA Professional Library Series. Denver: American Animal Hospital Association.

Shahar R, Shamir M, Johnston D. 1997. A technique for management of bite wounds of the thoracic wall in small dogs. *Vet Surg* 26:45–50.

Shamir MH, Leisner S, Klement E, et al. 2002. Dog bite wounds in dogs and cats: a retrospective study of 196 cases. *J Vet Med* 49:107–112.

Swaim SF. 1980. *Surgery of Traumatized Skin: Management and Reconstruction in the Dog and Cat*. Philadelphia, PA: WB Saunders.

Talan DA, Citron DM, Abrahamian FM, et al. 1999. Bacteriologic analysis of infected dog and cat bites *N Engl J Med* 340:85–92.

Thermal, Chemical, Radiation Burns

Baxter CR. 1970. Present concepts in the management of major electrical injury. *Surg Clin No Am* 50:1401–1418.

Bedenice D. 2007. Smoke inhalation. In: Cote E, ed. *Clinical Veterinary Advisor*, 1011–1012. St. Louis, MO: Mosby.

Bostwick SA. 1987. Comprehensive rehabilitation after burn injury. *Surg Clin No Am* 67:159–166.

Coyne BE, Bednarski RM, Bilbrey SA. 1993. Thermoelectric burns from improper grounding of electrocautery units: two case reports. *J Am Anim Hosp Assoc* 29:7–9.

Demling RH. 1983. Improved survival after massive burns. *J Trauma* 23(3):179–184.

Demling RH. 1987. Fluid replacement in burn patients. *Surg Clin No Am* 67:15–30.

Demling RH, Buerstatte RPH, Perea A. 1980. Management of hot tar burns. *J Trauma* 20:242.

Dernell WS, Wheaton, LG. 1995. Surgical management of radiation injury—Part I. *Compend Cont Educ Pract Vet* 17:181–187.

Dernell WS, Wheaton, LG. 1995. Surgical management of radiation injury—Part II. *Compend Cont Educ Vet* 17:499–510.

Dhupa N, Pavletic MM. 1997. Burns. In: Morgan R, ed. *Handbook of Small Animal Practice*, 3rd ed. Philadelphia, PA: WB Saunders.

Dow KD, Bucholtz JD, Iwamoto R, et al. 1997. *Nursing Care in Radiation Oncology*. Philadelphia, PA: WB Saunders.

Drobaz KJ, et al. 1999. Smoke exposure in dogs: 27 cases (1988–1997). *J Am Vet Med Assoc* 215:1306–1311.

Drobaz KJ, et al. 1999. Smoke exposure in cats: 22 cases (1986–1997). *J Am Vet Med Assoc* 215:1312–1316.

Harris D, King GK, Bergman PJ. 1997. Radiation therapy toxicities. *Vet Clin No Am* 27:37–46.

Heimbach DM. 1987. Early burn excision and grafting. *Surg Clin No Am* 67:93–107.

Hummel RP. 1982. *Clinical Burn Therapy*. Boston: John Wright PSG.

Johnston DE. 1985. Burns, electrical, chemical and cold injuries. In: Slatter DH, ed. *Textbook of Small Animal Surgery*. Philadelphia, PA: WB Saunders.

Kolata RJ, Burrows CF. 1981. The clinical features of injury by chewing electrical cords in dogs and cats. *J Am Anim Hosp Assoc* 17:219–222.

Ladue TA. 2007. Radiation therapy: adverse reactions. In: Cote E, ed. *Clinical Veterinary Advisor, 940–943*. St. Louis, MO: Mosby.

Lee RC, Kolodney MS. 1987. Electrical injury mechanisms: dynamics of the thermal response. *Plast Reconstr Surg* 80:663–671.

Lee RC, Kolodney MS. 1987. Electrical injury mechanisms: electrical breakdown of cell membranes. *Plast Reconstr Surg* 80:672–679.

Luce EA. 1984. The irradiated wound. *Surg Clin No Am* 64:821–829.

Luce EA, Gottlieb SE. 1984. "True" high tension electrical injuries. *Ann Plast Surg* 12:321–326.

Monafo WW, Freedman B. 1987. Topical therapy in burns. *Surg Clin No Am* 67:133–145.

O'Toole TE. 2007. Burns. In: Cote E., ed., *Clinical Veterinary Advisor*, 164–166. St Louis, MO: Mosby.

Pasulka PS, Wachtel TL. 1987. Nutritional considerations for the burned patient. *Surg Clin No Am* 67:109–131.

Pavletic MM. 1990. Management of thermal injuries. In: *2nd International Veterinary Emergency and Critical Care Symposium*. San Antonio, TX.

Pope ER. 2003. Burns: thermal, electrical, chemical and cold injuries. In: Slatter DH, ed. *Textbook of Small Animal Surgery*, 3rd ed., 356–372. Philadelphia, PA: WB Saunders.

Reedy LM, Clubb FJ. 1991. Microwave burns in a toy poodle: a case report. *J Am Anim Hosp Assoc* 27:497–500.

Reinsch JF, Puckett CL. 1984. Management of radiation wounds. *Surg Clin No Am* 64:795–802.

Rudolph R, Noe JM. 1983. *Chronic Problem Wounds*. Boston: Little, Brown and Co.

Thrall DE. 1982. Radiation therapy in the dog: principles, indications, and complications. *Compend Cont Educ Pract Vet* 4:652–660.

Frostbite

Bejerke HS, Tevar A. 2006. Frostbite. www.emedicine.com

Carpenter HM, Hurley IA, Hardenbergh E, et al. 1971. Vascular injury due to cold: effects of rapid rewarming. *Arch Pathol* 92:153–161.

Hummel RP. 1982. *Clinical Burn Therapy*. Boston: John Wright PSG.

Johnston DE. 1985. Burns, electrical, chemical and cold injuries. In: Slatter DH, ed. *Textbook of Small Animal Surgery*, 516–533. Philadelphia, PA: WB Saunders.

Lapp NL, Juergens JL. 1965. Frostbite. *Mayo Clin Proc* 40:932.

Lathrop T. 1975. *Hypothermia: Killer of the Unprepared*. Portland, OR: The Mazamas.

Martinez A, Golding MR, Sawyer PN, et al. 1966. The specific arterial lesions in mild and severe frostbite: effect of sympathectomy. *J Cardiovasc Surg* 7:495–503.

McCauley RL, Hing DN, Robson MC, et al. 1983. Frostbite injuries. A rational approach based on the pathophysiology. *J Trauma* 23:143–147.

Pope ER. 2003. Burns: thermal, electrical, chemical, and cold injuries. In Slatter, DH, ed. *Textbook of Small Animal Surgery*, 3rd ed., 356–372. Philadelphia, PA: WB Saunders.

Washburn B. 1975. *Frostbite*. Boston: Museum of Science.

Wellehan JFX. 2003. Frostbite in birds: pathophysiology and treatment. *Compend Contin Ed Pract Vet* 25:775–780.

Projectile Injuries

Barnes EC. 1997. *Cartridges of the World*, 8th ed. Northbrook, IL: DBI Books.

Combs R. 1987. *Crossbows*. Northbrook, IL: DBI Books.

DiMaio VJM. 1993. *Gunshot Wounds*. Boca Raton, FL: CRC Press.

Dodd GD, Budzik RF. 1990. Identification of retained firearm projectiles on plain radiographs. *AJR* 154:471–475.

Fackler ML. 1996. Gunshot wound review. *Ann Emerg Med* 28:194–203.

Ferguson T. 1991. *Modern Law Enforcement Weapons and Tactics*, 2nd ed. Northbrook, IL: DBI Books.

Heard, BJ. 1997. *Handbook of Firearms and Ballistics*. New York: John Wiley and Sons.

James MR. 1992. *The Bowhunter's Handbook*. Iowa, WI: DBI Books.

Kettner F, Kirberger RM. 2006. Aortic foreign body (airgun pellet) embolism in a cat. *J Sm Anim Pract* 47:221–225.

Pavletic MM. 1985. A review of 121 gunshot wounds in the dog and cat. *Vet Surg* 14:61–62.

Pavletic MM. 1986. Gunshot wounds in veterinary medicine: projectile ballistics—Part I. *Compend Contin Ed Pract Vet* 8:47–60.

Pavletic MM. 1986. Gunshot wounds in veterinary medicine: projectile ballistics—Part II. *Compen Contin Ed Pract Vet* 8:125–134.

Pavletic MM. 1996. Gunshot wound management. *Compend Cont Educ Pract Vet* 18:1285–1299.

Pavletic MM, Trout N. 2006. Bullet, bite and burn wounds. *Vet Clin No Am* 36(4):873–893.

Wallentine D. 1988. *Making Indian Bows and Arrows ... The Old Way*. Liberty, UT: Eagle's View Publishing Co.

Impalement Injuries

Doran IP, Wright CA, Moore AH. 2008. Acute oropharyngeal and esophageal stick injury in forty-one dogs. *Vet Surg* 37:781–785.

Griffiths LG, et al. 2000. Oropharyngeal penetrating injuries in 50 dogs: a retrospective study. *Vet Surg* 29:383–388.

Pressure Sores

Brunner LS, Suddarth DS. 1986. *Manual of Nursing Practice*, 4th ed. Philadelphia, PA: JB Lippincott.

Daniel RK, Hall EJ, MacLeod MK. 1979. Pressure sores—a reappraisal. *Ann Plast Surg* 3:53–63.

Griffith BH. 1979. Pressure sores. In: Grabb WC, Smith JW, eds. *Plastic Surgery*. Boston: Little, Brown & Co.

Nwomeh B, Yager DR, Kelman CL. 1998. Physiology of the chronic wound. *Clin Plast Surg* 25(3):341–356.

Swaim SF, Hanson RR, Coates JR. 1996. Pressure wounds in animals. *Compend Cont Educ Pract Vet* 18:203–218.

Swaim SF, Henderson RA. 1997. *Small Animal Wound Management*, 2nd ed. Baltimore: Williams and Wilkins.

Swaim SF, Lee AH, Henderson RA. 1989. Mobility vs immobility in the healing of open wounds. *J Am Anim Hosp Asoc* 25:91–96.

Hygroma

Johnston DE. 1975. Hygroma of the elbow in dogs. *J Am Vet Med Assoc* 167:213–219.

White RAS. 2006. Management of specific skin wounds. *Vet Clin No Am* 36:905–907.

Snakebite

Hackett TB, et al. 2002. Clinical findings associated with prairie rattlesnake bites in dogs: 100 cases (1989–1998). *J Am Vet Med Assoc* 220:1675–1680.

Hudelson S, Hudelson P. 1995. Pathophysiology of snake envenomization and evaluation of treatments: Parts I,II, & III. *Compend Contin Ed Pract Vet* 17:889–897, 1035–1040, 1385–1396.

Kostolich M. 1990. Reconstructive surgery of a snake bite wound. *Canine Pract* 15:15–19.

Paul A, Rozanski E. 2007. Snakebite. In: Cote, E, ed. *Clinical Veterinary Advisor*, 1012–1014. St. Louis, MO: Mosby.

Peterson ME. 2001. Snake bite: pit vipers and coral snakes. In: Peterson ME, Talcott PA, eds. *Small Animal Toxicology*, 695–720. Philadelphia, PA: WB Saunders.

Waldron DR, Zimmerman-Pope N. 2002. Superficial skin wounds. In: Slatter D, ed. *Textbook of Small Animal Surgery*, 267–268. Philadelphia, PA: WB Saunders.

Willey JR, Schaer M. 2005. Eastern diamond rattlesnake (*Crotalus adamanteus*) envenomation of dogs: 31 cases (1982–2002). *J Am Anim Hosp Assoc* 41:22–33.

Spider Bite/Brown Recluse

Amalsadvala T, Swaim SF. 2006. Management of hard-to-heal wounds. *Vet Clin No Am* 36(4):704.

Dunayer, EK. 2007. Spider envenomation. In: Cote E, ed. *Clinical Veterinary Advisor*, 1020–1021. St. Louis, MO: Mosby.

Roder JD. 2004. Spiders. In: Plumlee KH, ed. *Clinical Veterinary Toxicology*, 111–113. St. Louis, MO: Mosby.

Porcupine Quills

Pavletic MM. 2002. Penetrating wounds. In: Wingfield WE, Raffe MR, eds. *The Veterinary ICU Book*, 966. Jackson Hole: Teton Newmedia.

Grahn BH, Szentimrey D, Pharr JW, et al. 1995. Ocular and orbital porcupine quills in 50 dogs: a retrospective study. *Can Vet J* 36:488–493.

| Plate 9 | **Pipe Insulation Protective Device: Elbow** |

DESCRIPTION

Pipe insulation is used by plumbers and homeowners to insulate water pipes. There are a few varieties available at hardware stores. Black plastic foam pipe insulation (Armacell Self-Seal pipe insulation available at Home Depot) is a soft, light, flexible foam, with a linear split to facilitate its application around a pipe. The split edges have a self-adherent glue, allowing the insulation to completely encase a pipe upon application. Pipe insulation comes in economical 6-foot lengths to cover copper pipes of 1/2-inch, 3/4-inch, and 1-inch diameters. In medium to large dogs, 3/4-inch and 1-inch sizes are the most appropriate. The author designed this technique to protect incisions overlying the olecranon and lateral epicondylar areas in dogs, usually for the management/closure of pressure sores.

TECHNIQUE

(A) Cut two pieces of Pipe insulation. Measure the shorter internal piece below the flexion surface of the antecubital area to the metacarpal-phalangeal joints. The outer segment extends from the metacarpal-phalangeal joints and overlaps the entire elbow surface proximally.

(B) In medium to large dogs, apply strips of 2-inch surgical tape (Zonas, Johnson & Johnson) to the limb in a linear fashion. On patients with longer hair coats, remove the fur. The parallel strips of tape begin below the flexion surface of the antecubital area, down to the metacarpal-phalangeal joints. Avoid placing tape over the accessory carpal pad. This layer of tape forms a friction surface for application of the pipe insulation.

(C) The inner segment of pipe insulation is cupped around the extremity. In this example, the open split of the insulation is positioned over the anterior surface of the forelimb. (The thin plastic strip is removed from the insulation adhesive that covers the split border of the insulation.) Use strips of Elasticon (Johnson & Johnson) to secure the pipe insulation to the exposed white tape overlying the anterior aspect of the limb. Contact of the Elasticon to the white tape prevents the pipe insulation from slipping. Cut the longer (outer) piece of pipe insulation to comfortably overlap the entire olecranon, extending approximately 2–3 inches (5–8 cm) proximally. (In this illustration, this outer pipe insulation layer is transparent, allowing us to see the short pipe segment secured with bands of Elasticon.) Secure the insulation to the exposed surgical tape in a fashion similar to that of the first layer. Avoid excess tape application over the carpus to maintain limb mobility.

(D) To change wound dressings, temporarily fold down the proximal end of the foam insulation, which forms an "overlapping shield" for the elbow, to change dressings. Once released, the foam springs back to its original position. The overlapping foam insulation provides a "slot" to maintain the position of a thin protective dressing/bandage layer. A non-adherent dressing, topical ointment, a light layer of cast padding and a gauze wrap is normally used to cover the wound. *Do NOT apply a tight bandage that will rub on the elbow during ambulation and elbow flexion. It is important NOT to use a thick bandage that could create a "pressure cone effect" on the elbow, thereby defeating the purpose of the bandage.* The owner can change this simple bandage daily over the first 7-10 days and every 2 days thereafter.

Plate 9

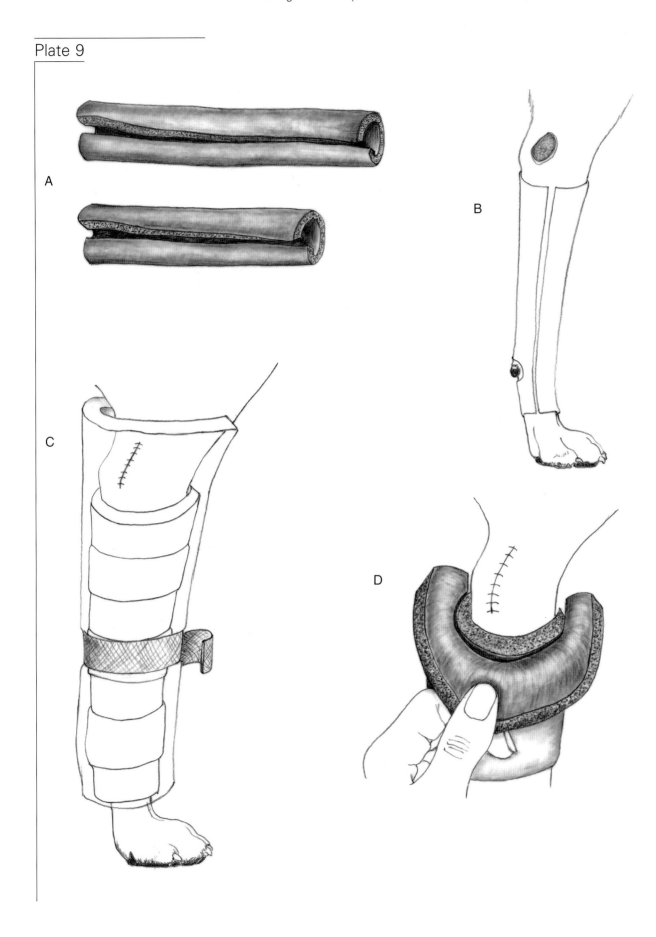

Plate 9

(Continued)

COMMENTS

With a cost around $1 per foot, pipe insulation is both cheap and economical to apply. The pipe insulation bandage is light and flexible, enabling the dog to use the leg unimpeded. The author prefers to use this protective device when wound closure is achieved without excessive incisional tension, or to protect a healing wound.

The overlapping layers of the foam insulation effectively elevate the olecranon and lateral epicondyle from directly contacting hard flooring. A third, shorter layer can be applied to the outer layer of pipe insulation if additional protection is considered necessary. Soft bedding also is recommended. Owners are advised to keep the patient's activity level to a minimum.

Normally, Pipe Insulation Protection for the Elbow (PIPE) will maintain itself for 3 weeks, at which time the entire protective wrap is replaced, as the adhesive tape applied to the skin surface loosens. Moreover, the foam cells tend to compress with continuous pressure application by the third week. Depending on the healing process, the author normally uses this device for 6–9 weeks. Owners must keep the insulation and skin free of moisture to reduce the likelihood of dermatitis. The black foam can temporarily stain the skin, but most of this residue can be washed off with surgical soap and tap water.

For more problematic closures, a reinforced spica bandage (Plate 5) or a Schroeder-Thomas splint (Plates 6 and 7) can be considered if immobilization of the elbow joint is deemed necessary. Most dogs, however, have difficulty ambulating with these latter forms of elbow protection.

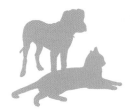

8

Regional Considerations

THE CANINE AND FELINE PROFILES

Description

In dogs the thinnest skin is located along the ventral body surface, the medial surface of the limbs and inner pinna. Thicker skin is located along the dorsum. The most pliable skin regions include the axilla, flank, and dorsum of the neck. The hair coat is thicker over the back and sides of the body, with thinner hair growth located inside the ears, on the inner surfaces of the flanks, along the ventral abdomen, and beneath the tail. Optimal cosmetic results are achieved by selecting closure techniques that match skin thickness and hair growth pattern (hair length, color, and growth direction). By using skin adjacent to a defect, one is more likely able to achieve these goals. However, large defects frequently warrant skin coverage from a distant source. In this situation, closure and restoration of function should be accomplished by the simplest techniques that minimize stress and discomfort to the patient, rather than by techniques selected primarily for achieving the optimum cosmetic result.

> Over the years, the author has found that clients have not complained about hair growth variations since the results are far more pleasing than the wound or disease process that has been corrected. Owners recognize normal variations in their pet's hair coat and generally accept these variations when the facts are explained prior to the procedure.

Both the dog and cat have pliable and elastic skin over most areas of the body, except for extremely obese individuals. Skin laxity varies in each body region along with skin thickness and hair growth. Variations naturally occur between species, breeds, and individual animals.

> Pronounced obesity in dogs and cats will dramatically reduce skin laxity. As a result, wound closure can be problematic in these patients, unlike their normal-weight counterparts.

These cutaneous variations also make universal rules pertaining to flap size and regional applicability difficult. For example, a caudal superficial epigastric axial pattern flap in long-bodied dogs with short legs, such as dachshunds, is capable of extending to the foot, whereas the same flap employing identical anatomic guidelines may not extend beyond the knee in a dog with long extremities, such as an Irish wolfhound. In the cat, this same flap normally can extend to the metatarsal region. Clearly, careful preoperative measurements are required to determine wound coverage.

> The elastic properties of skin vary based on the species, breed, individual, and body location. These elastic properties can be manipulated in some cases for the closure of problematic wounds by using skin-stretching techniques discussed in Chapter 9.

Although dog and cat breeds generally conform to most of the flap techniques discussed, one clinical exception is the greyhound. The author has found that the thin, delicate skin of the greyhound is more prone to dehiscence and partial flap necrosis compared to other breeds. This likely is the scenario for similar breeds such as the whippet and Italian greyhound. Care must be taken to use meticulous surgical technique, avoid unnecessary tissue manipulation, minimize the size (especially length) of skin flap dimensions (when feasible), and keep skin tension to a minimum during wound closure.

Certain skin regions are closely attached to the underlying bone, muscle, and fascia. These areas include the skin over the dorsum of the muzzle, the caudolateral aspect of the upper thigh (overlying the biceps femoris, semitendinous/semimembranous muscles), and the skin overlying portions of the superficial pectoral muscle. Undermining skin in these regions is more difficult; care must be taken to avoid injury to the subdermal plexus when elevating the skin free from the underlying structures. In some cases, it may be advisable to retain the epimysium of the underlying muscle with the skin used for pedicle grafts. From a clinical perspective, the author has noted that skin around the caudal thigh and perineum are not particularly amenable to local flap development. Subdermal plexus flaps developed in these regions are more prone to partial necrosis compared to similar flaps created in other body regions. This is most likely attributable to regional variation in cutaneous circulation.

Ample loose skin is located over the dorsal and lateral aspects of the neck and trunk. Even moderate-sized skin defects are frequently amenable to primary closure. Second intention healing can take advantage of neighboring loose elastic skin for optimal wound contraction. When skin is required for coverage of large wounds involving the extremities, the trunk is the obvious source of donor skin in the form of axial pattern flaps, free grafts, and the less-frequently used distant flap techniques. Wounds involving the most distant areas of the body, including the rostral facial area, tail, distal extremities, and ears are naturally more difficult to close due to the paucity of loose skin and their greater distance from potential donor areas. As skin loss approaches 180 degrees of the circumference of an extremity, some form of skin flap or free-grafting technique will be necessary.

Large defects involving the ventral thorax (sternal region), dorsal pelvic, and inguinal area are similarly troublesome, although somewhat more amenable to closure due to their proximity to the loose skin of the lateral thorax and abdomen. The axilla, flank, and inguinal areas present closure difficulties in association with patient ambulation unless restriction of activity is achieved by cage rest or limb immobilization. Similarly, wounds involving joints may require postoperative immobilization to prevent wound dehiscence. Special care must be taken to assess range of motion during closure of defects involving the limbs, eyelids, and oral cavity to avoid distortion of anatomic structures and compromise to normal function.

Skin loss of the distal extremities need not be great to create wound-closure difficulties. Wounds less than 90 degrees of the circumference have potential to heal by second intention. As wounds approach 180 degrees, closure will require a skin graft or possibly skin flap.

Assessment of true wound size is exaggerated by edema. The surgeon should defer closure decisions until improvement in circulation is followed by resolution of tissue swelling. Tissue edema can make open wounds appear approximately 25% greater than their true size: skin margins retract and dermal fluid accumulation pushes collagen fibers apart.

Plates 10A and 10B **Surgical Technique Menu**

DESCRIPTION

Based on the anatomic region, the following techniques have potential application for closure of major skin, mucosal, and epithelial defects. Selection of the technique(s) depends upon the size of the defect, the regional skin tension, regional and distant cutaneous circulation, and the practicalities and individual limitations of the technique(s) selected. Other techniques, however, may be employed in selected cases based on the individual surgeon's preference and needs of the patient. Open wound management is not on the technique menu, although it remains as a viable option for wound closure using the guidelines previously described. The reader is directed to the respective sections illustrating these surgical techniques.

1. Tension-Relieving Techniques (Chapter 9)
   A. Undermining
   B. Relaxing/release incisions
   C. Multiple relaxing incisions
   D. Subcuticular suture patterns
   E. Walking sutures
   F. Z-plasty
   G. W-plasty
   H. V-Y advancement
   I. Stents
   J. Skin stretchers
   K. Hidden dermal release incision

2. Skin-Stretching Techniques (Chapter 10)
   A. Skin expanders
   B. Presuturing technique
   C. Skin stretchers: open wound management
   D. Skin stretchers: preoperative use

3. Local Flaps (Chapter 11)
   A. Single pedicle advancement flap
   B. Bipedicle advancement flap
   C. Rotational flap
   D. Transposition flap
   E. Interpolation flap
   F. Forelimb fold flap

4. Axial Pattern Flaps (Chapter 13)
   A. Omocervical
   B. Thoracodorsal
   C. Deep circumflex iliac (dorsal branch)
   D. Deep circumflex iliac (ventral branch)
   E. Deep circumflex iliac (ventral branch)
      (Flank fold flap (hindlimb)
   F. Caudal superficial epigastric
   G. Cranial superficial epigastric
   H. Brachial
   I. Genicular
   J. Reverse saphenous

Plates 10A and 10B

    K. Caudal auricular
    L. Lateral caudal (tail)
    M. Superficial temporal

5. Free Grafts (Chapter 14)
    A. Punch/pinch grafts
    B. Strip grafts
    C. Stamp grafts
    D. Sheet grafts
    E. Mesh graft—mesh graft expansion unit
    F. Mesh graft—hand mesh

6. Distant Flaps (Chapter 12)
    A. Direct flap
    B. Indirect flap

7. Myocutaneous Flaps and Muscle Flaps (Chapter 16)
    A. Latissimus dorsi myocutaneous flap
    B. Cutaneous trunci myocutaneous flap
    C. Latissimus dorsi muscle flap
    D. External abdominal oblique muscle flap
    E. Caudal sartorius muscle flap
    F. Cranial sartorius muscle flap
    G. Temporalis muscle flap
    H. Transversus abdominis muscle flap
    I. Semitendinosus muscle flap
    J. Flexor carpi ulnaris muscle flap

8. Facial Reconstruction (Chapter 15)
    A. Labial avulsion closure techniques
    B. Triangular excision/closure—lip
    C. Rectangular excision/closure—lip
    D. Labial advancement—upper lip
    E. Labial advancement—lower lip
    F. Buccal rotation technique—lip and cheek
    G. Labial lift-up technique
    H. Labial pull-down technique
    I. Skin substitution for oral mucosa
    J. Labial/buccal reconstruction with skin flaps
    K. Cleft lip repair
    L. Rostral labial pivot flap
    M. Oral commissure advancement
    N. Brachycephalic facial fold resection
    O. Cheilopexy technique

9. Oral Reconstruction Surgical Techniques (Chapter 17)
    A. Oral mucosal flaps
    B. Palatoplasty: bipedicle advancement
    C. Mucoperiosteal flap technique

Plates 10A and 10B

(Continued)

    D. Palatine (artery) mucosal flap
    E. Soft palate and pharyngeal mucosal flaps
    F. Full-thickness labial advancement flap
    G. Cartilage graft technique
    H. Angularis oris mucosal flap

10. Nasal Reconstruction Techniques (Chapter 20)
    A. Septal resection technique
    B. Septal coverage: cutaneous advancement flap
    C. Bilateral sulcus flap
    D. Alar fold flap
    E. Musculofascial island labial flap
    F. Cantilever suture technique
    G. Labial mucosal inversion technique

11. Foot Pad Reconstruction (Chapter 18)
    A. Digital pad transfer
    B. Metatarsal/metacarpal pad transfer
    C. Whole pad grafting
    D. Segmental pad graft
    E. Digital flap technique—interdigital defects
    F. Digital flap technique—digit 2, 5 defects
    G. Fusion podoplasty

12. Major Eyelid Reconstruction (Chapter 19)
    A. "Lip-to-lid procedure"
    B. Mucosal graft/transposition flap reconstruction
    C. Third eyelid reconstruction of lower eyelid

13. Preputial Reconstructive Surgery (Chapter 22)
    A. Preputial ostium enlargement
    B. Preputial ostium reduction
    C. Preputial advancement technique
    D. Phallopexy
    E. Urethral reconstruction for subanal hypospadias
    F. Preputial urethrostomy technique

14. Miscellaneous Reconstructive Surgical Techniques (Chapter 23)
    A. Omental Flaps
    B. Scrotal Flaps
    C. Caudectomy for tail fold intertrigo
    D. Episioplasty

COMMENTS

The surgical menu serves as a general site reference for the surgeon. Only the most common techniques are identified on a regional basis. Other techniques can be used for specific defects in a variety of body areas. The size and location of the defect, the condition of regional donor areas, and the preference of the surgeon generally dictate the selection of the technique(s).

Plate 10A

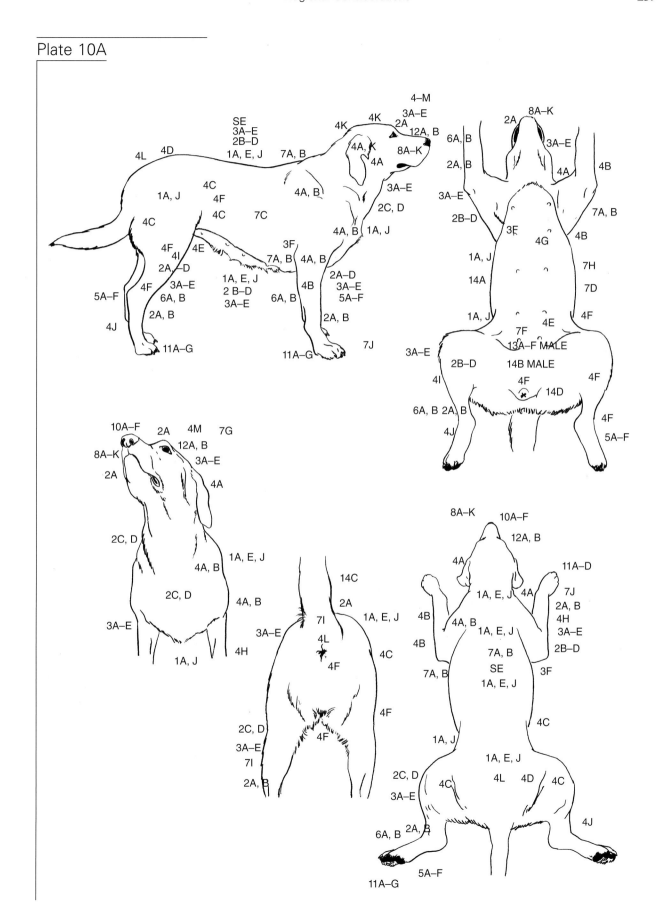

Plate 10B

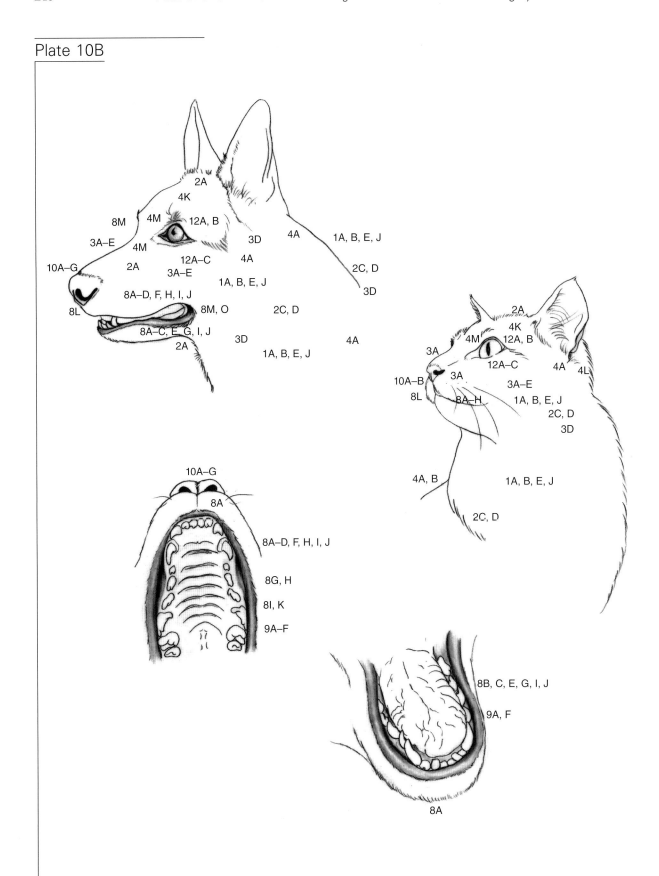

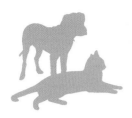

Tension Relieving Techniques

INTRODUCTION

Excessive tension during wound closure can result in circulatory compromise, retarded wound healing, dehiscence, and skin necrosis. Tissue swelling, underlying hematomas, and increased collagenase activity within the 5-mm border of the wound edges also can contribute to sutures "cutting out" (see Chapter 6). Tension-relieving techniques are methods of reducing wound tension or distributing the tension more uniformly in order to prevent the complications associated with wound separation (see Chapter 6). In veterinary medicine, the most common method used to mobilize cutaneous margins for wound closure is undermining. However, studies have demonstrated that skin can stretch beyond its natural or "inherent elasticity" by the processes of mechanical creep and stress relaxation when continuous tension is applied over time to the cutaneous tissues. Skin stretchers (Skin Stretchers, Pavletic, Angell Animal Medical Center, Boston, MA) and tissue expanders are examples of techniques that mobilize skin for wound closure, using these processes. Skin stretchers can be used to stretch prior to wound closure; they also may be used postoperatively to reduce incisional tension (see Chapter 10).

Various suture patterns can be used to help offset and distribute tension during wound closure. Relaxing (release) incisions, V-Y advancement, and Z-plasty can be used to reduce tension on the incision. This section discusses techniques for assessing and minimizing skin tension for successful skin closure.

SKIN TENSION IN THE DOG AND CAT

Patient Variations

Skin differs in thickness, pliability, and tension in various body regions, and there are also variations between breeds and species. Bloodhounds and Basset hounds, for example, have ample loose skin over many body regions, whereas whippets and greyhounds have comparatively less skin. Whippets and greyhounds also have considerably thinner, less durable skin compared to other dogs. As a result, skin repairs can be more problematic in these canine patients.

Dogs and cats have a similar cutaneous distribution, although feline skin appears to be more pliable and the limbs more flexible than the average dog. Extremely obese animals can lose considerable skin laxity from heavy deposits of fat beneath the dermis (Fig. 9-1). As discussed in Chapter 10, the skin is stretched in obese animals, potentially making wound closure more problematic.

Surgical Considerations

Skin over the dorsal and lateral surfaces of the trunk is pliable in a craniocaudal and dorsoventral direction. The excision and closure of small wounds in this area is not critical. As one removes larger areas of skin in an elliptical fashion, the length of the incision is best

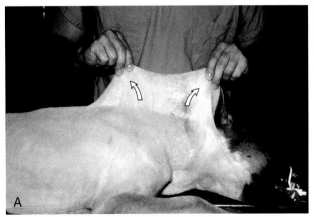
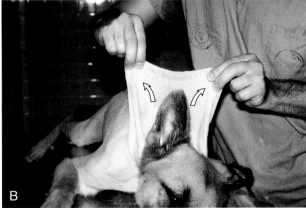

FIG. 9-1 (A, B) Example of skin laxity in a German shepherd cross. Lines of tension have limited use in areas where ample elastic skin prevails.

created (when feasible) parallel to the lines of greatest tension: this facilitates mobilizing the more elastic skin for apposition of the cutaneous borders of the wound created. If the elliptical excision is created at an angle to the lines of tension, angular tension lines may promote closure in a curvilinear fashion. The flank and axillary skin folds are elastic and mobile skin areas that adjust to limb motion. Although this skin would be considered a potential "donor" area for wound closure, the closed donor site is more prone to dehiscence in an active pet. The author avoids using this area for most closure techniques.

> Closure of wounds resulting in intersecting incisions is occasionally necessary, creating a T junction. Placed under tension from various traction forces, wound dehiscence most commonly begins at this weakest point of the closure, at the "T" intersection. For this reason, closure of wounds in a linear or curvilinear fashion is preferable.

The middle and distal portion of the extremities have a paucity of loose skin. However, skin can be mobilized to a limited degree in a craniocaudal plane whereas little skin can be elevated in a proximal-distal direction (Fig. 9-2). As a result, small advancement flaps can be created perpendicular to the limb axis to close small defects. Alternatively, the versatile transposition flap can be used to mobilize loose skin when created parallel to the axis of the limb (Fig. 9-3). Care must be exercised to avoid closing wounds under excessive tension that may result in compromise to the circulation and lymphatic drainage to the distal extremity below the closure site.

> Excessive circumferential skin tension on the lower extremity can result in a "biological tourniquet," effectively compromising venous and lymphatic return from the distal extremity. Swelling will then collapse arterial circulation. Partial wound closure with no circumferential tension always is preferable to complete closure under questionable tension.

Under these circumstances, wounds are better left (partially) open than closed under excessive tension. Release incisions also can be used to offset local incisional tension (Fig. 9-4).

> The author has developed a variation of the standard release incision: the hidden release incision. (See Plate 21.)

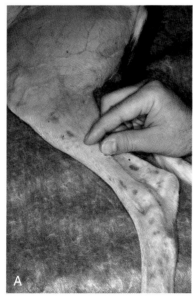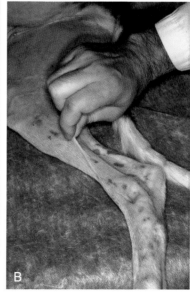

FIG. 9-2 (A) Note the inability to grasp any loose skin in a proximal-distal direction on the rear limb of a greyhound. (From Pavletic MM. 1990. Skin flaps in reconstructive surgery. *Vet Clin No Am* 20:81.) (B) A ridge of skin can be elevated in the cranial-caudal plane. This parallel fold of skin can be used for transposition flap elevation. This fact is contrary to the tension lines noted in Plate 1. (From Pavletic MM. 1990. Skin flaps in reconstructive surgery. *Vet Clin No Am* 20:81.)

FIG. 9-3 (A) Lower extremity defect in a cat. (B) A transposition flap was elevated parallel to the limb axis with the base or pedicle of the flap based distally. Carefully measured prior to elevation, the available loose circumferential skin allowed for closure of the donor and recipient beds.

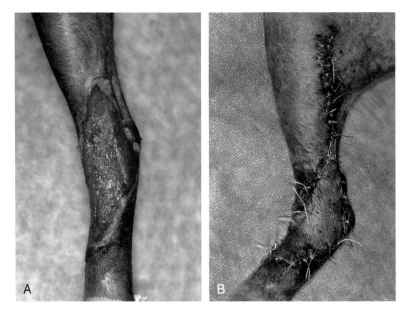

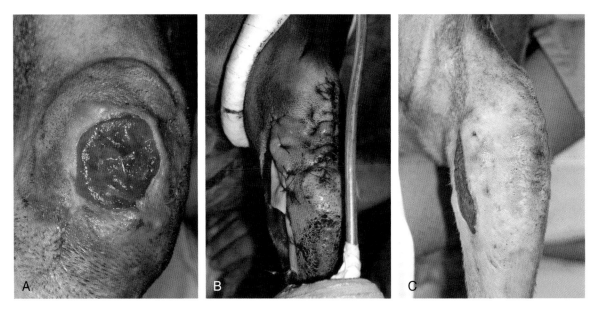

FIG. 9-4 (A) Pressure sore overlying the left elbow. Note the exposed orthopedic wire used to repair the fracture.

(B) Release incision made over the lateral surface of the elbow region, creating a bipedicled advancement flap. The flap was advanced over the elbow defect and sutured into position. The lateral donor defect is left open to heal by second intention. A Schroeder-Thomas splint was used to immobilize the elbow until suture removal.

(C) Healing of the lateral release incision occurred without complication. Use of the thicker lateral skin is preferable over the thinner medial skin of the extremity. Bilateral release incisions also can be used to facilitate closure of problematic elbow defects.

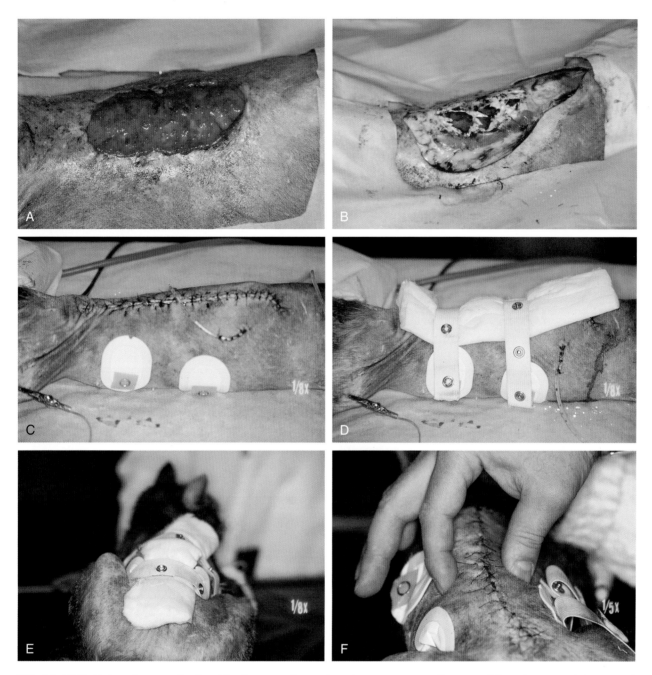

FIG. 9-5 (A) Radiation ulcer over the dorsal lumbar area of a cat. A carcinoma was surgically removed from the area and the surgical field irradiated. A slowly expanding radiation ulcer developed several months later.

(B) Wide resection of the ulcer and bordering epithelialized scar. Tissues resected did not reveal tumor recurrence, based on histopathologic analysis.

(C) Wound closure was accomplished, but the incision was under moderate tension.

(D) Two pair of skin stretcher pads were applied lateral to the incision, followed by application of elastic cables over a protective cotton dressing. A mild amount of tension was applied to each cable; cables were not adjusted prior to reexamination of the patient the following day.

(E) Dorsal view of the patient, 24 hours after surgery.

(F) Uncoupling of the stretcher cables at 24 hours. Note the relaxation of the skin along the border of the incision. Pads and cables were removed 72 hours after surgery; skin sutures were removed by day 14.

Harnessing the Viscoelastic Properties of Skin

As discussed in Chapter 1, the skin, and dermis in particular, is a viscoelastic medium, based on the physical properties of collagen and the surrounding mucopolysaccharide ground substance. Regional variations in skin thickness and pliability primarily are the result of collagen fiber size and weave. While skin normally stretches and deforms during normal physical activity and pregnancy, research has demonstrated that these inherent properties also can be harnessed to promote wound closure. Skin can be "prestretched" within hours to promote wound closure under less tension. A skin-stretching device (Skin Stretchers, Pavletic) also can be used to effectively offset incisional tension postoperatively (Fig. 9-5).

Those techniques discussed in this chapter offset skin tension by a few basic mechanisms. Incisional techniques (release incisions, Z-plasty, V-Y-plasty) divide collagen fibers and partially reduce tension in a fashion similar to cutting a rubber band. Z-plasty and some local flap techniques transpose additional skin into a skin tension plane perpendicular to an incision. Simply undermining skin will improve elastic advancement of skin by dividing underlying, restricting hypodermal/fascial attachments to the dermis. Skin can then be shifted or directed into adjacent defects by taking advantage of its regional and directional elastic properties (Fig. 9-6).

Tension suture patterns and walking sutures reduce tension, in large part, by distributing tension more uniformly to the surrounding cutaneous tissue surface by variable degrees. Skin stretchers recruit the viscoelastic properties of regional skin by distributing tension over the comparatively large footprint of contact between the skin pad and skin surface. Tension sutures also achieve some incisional tension reduction in a similar fashion.

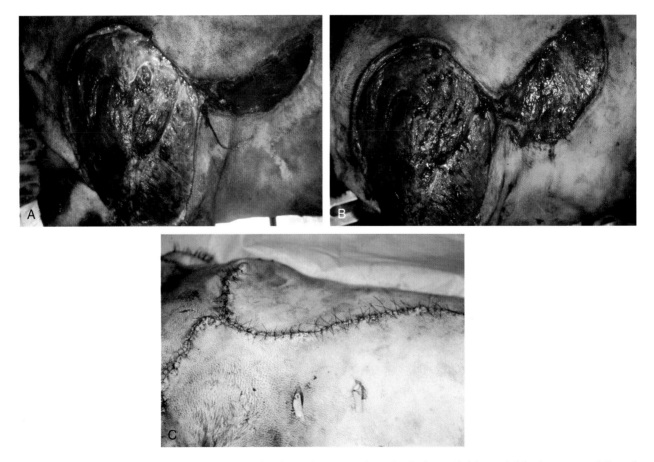

FIG. 9-6 (A) Multiple skin wounds: the dog was tied to the car bumper and accidently dragged. (B) Initial debridement was followed by wet-to-dry dressings. (C) The large left shoulder and thoracic wound was closed by directing the adjacent elastic skin toward the center of this large wound. (See Plate 28).

In face of excessive tension, tension sutures cannot accentuate skin deformation as effectively as skin stretcher pads due to their small point of contact with the skin and limitations in their physical placement in the areas surrounding the surgical site. Unlike skin stretchers, skin sutures placed under great tension can "cut-out" and cause circulatory compromise to the skin.

Selection and use of the following techniques will depend upon the individual circumstances of a given wound closure, the condition of the skin, and regional circulation. With experience, surgeons develop their own preference(s) for the techniques listed.

Positioning of the patient on the surgery table can have a significant effect on wound closure. For example, a common error in closing a large skin defect over the dorsal-lateral pelvic area is the placement of the patient in sternal recumbency, with the rear limbs in a "frog leg" position. This greatly reduces dorsal skin tension, facilitating closure. The postsurgical problem is discovered by the surgeon only after surgery is completed: skin closure tension results in the abduction of the rear limb(s), necessitating immediate revision of the closure.

This can be avoided by closing the defect with the patient in lateral recumbency (giving a true picture of regional skin tension). Thoughtful preoperative planning can prevent this problem regardless of patient positioning.

Suggested Readings

Bailey JV, Jacobs KA. 1983. The mesh expansion method of suturing wounds on the legs of horses. *Vet Surg* 12:78–82.

Hamilton HL, McLaughlin SA, Whitley RD, et al. 1998. Surgical reconstruction of severe cicatricial ectropion in a puppy. *J Am Anim Hosp Assoc* 34:212–217.

Johnston DE. 1990. Tension relieving techniques. *Vet Clin No Am* 20:67–80.

Pavletic MM. 1986. Undermining for repair of large skin defects in small animals. *Mod Vet Pract* 76:13–16.

Pavletic MM. 1990. Skin flaps in reconstructive surgery. *Vet Clin No Am* 20(1):81–103.

Pavletic MM. 1994. Surgery of the skin and management of wounds. In: Sherding RD, ed. *The Cat: Diseases and Clinical Management*, 2nd ed., 1969–1997. New York: Churchill Livingstone.

Pavletic MM. 2003. Pedicle grafts. In: Slatter DH, ed. *Textbook of Small Animal Surgery*, 3rd ed., 292–321. Philadelphia, PA: WB Saunders.

Pavletic MM. 2003. Skin and adnexa. In: Slatter DH, ed. *Textbook of Small Animal Surgery*, 3rd ed., 250–273. Philadelphia, PA: WB Saunders.

Swaim SF. 1979. A "walking" suture technique for closure of large skin defects in the dog and cat. *J Am Anim Hosp Assoc* 12:597–599.

Swaim SF, Henderson RA. 1997. *Small Animal Wound Management*, 2nd ed. Baltimore, MD: Williams and Wilkins.

Vig MM. 1985. Management of integumentary wounds of extremities in dogs: an experimental study. *J Am Anim Hosp Assoc* 21:187–192.

Plate 11   **Tension Lines**

DESCRIPTION

Dominant lines of skin tension in the dog. (Redrawn from Irwin DHG. 1966. Tension lines in the skin of the dog. *J Sm Anim Pract* 7:595–598.)

SURGICAL CONSIDERATION

(A) Ventral view, lines of greatest tension.
(B) Dorsal view, lines of greatest tension.
(C) Lateral view, lines of greatest tension.

COMMENTS

The lines of tension illustrated were determined by the use of stab incisions in canine cadaver skin. Separation of wound edges indicated the direction of tension "bands." Although similar studies in human cadavers have been considered somewhat inaccurate, these anatomic maps do serve as general guidelines for the small animal surgeon. It must be noted that many small- to moderate-sized skin defects can be closed perpendicular to these tension lines since ample loose skin is available for wound closure. For example, tension lines of the limbs would suggest wound apposition should be performed parallel to these bands to facilitate closure. However, there is greater loose skin around the circumference of the limbs compared to the proximal-distal direction. (See Chapter 1.)

Plate 11

TENSION LINES

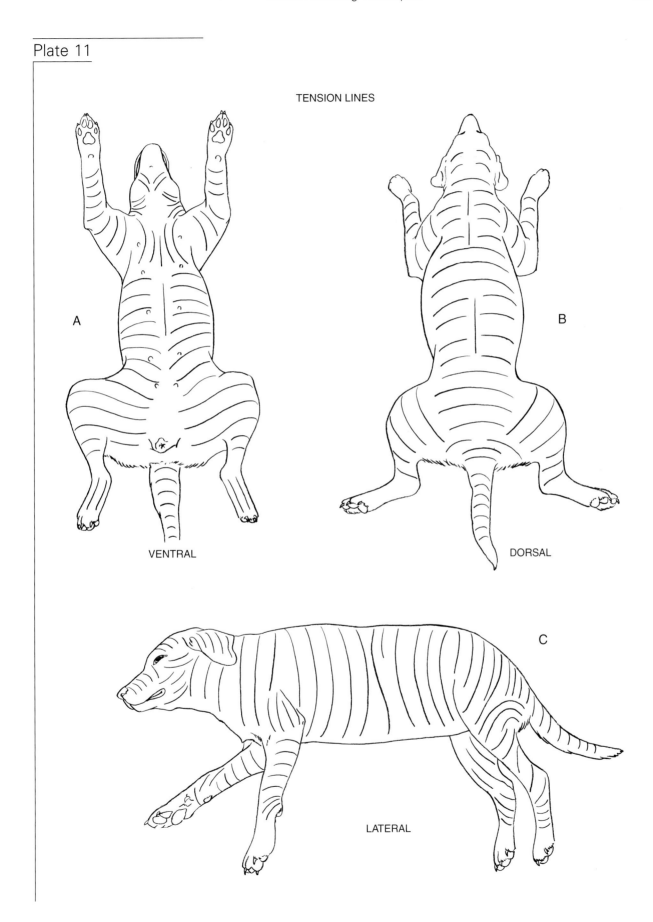

A

VENTRAL

B

DORSAL

C

LATERAL

Plate 12	**Effects of Skin Tension on Wound Closure**

DESCRIPTION

Elliptical excision and the effects of skin tension.

SURGICAL TECHNIQUE

(A) Elliptical excision *perpendicular* to lines of greatest tension results in widening of the defect as a result of elastic retraction of the skin borders.

(B) Elliptical excision is ideally performed parallel to lines of greatest tension and result in little distraction of wound margins. The closure takes advantage of the looser skin in the opposite direction. The surgeon will note less tendency for the wound to spread open from elastic retraction.

(C) Elliptical excision created at an angle to the lines of tension causes disparate traction of the incision. Closure of the wound will assume a wavy or curvilinear appearance.

COMMENTS

Closure of a skin defect is primarily determined by the size, shape, and location of the wound. In elective procedures, such as excision of skin tumors, the surgeon may be able to take advantage of regional skin laxity and elasticity to minimize tension on the closure. Cosmetic closure includes positioning the scar so that hair will grow over the region while minimizing excessive tension on the closure that could later result in expansion of the width of the scar. (From Burges AF. 1975. *Elective Incisions and Scar Revision*. Boston: Little Brown & Co. Modified with permission.)

Plate 12

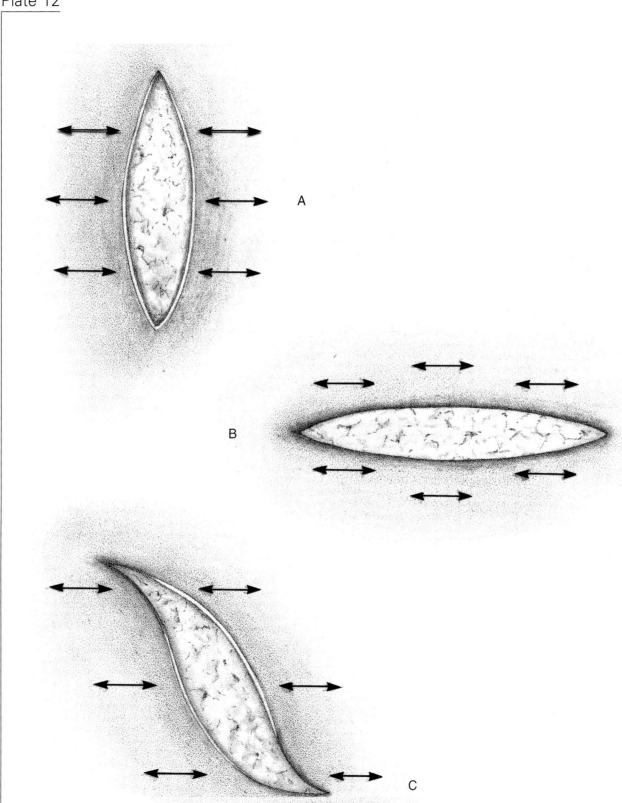

A

B

C

Plate 13 **Patient Positioning Techniques**

DESCRIPTION

When closing defects over the back, ventral abdomen, or lateral surface of the trunk of a large animal, undermining and advancement of skin may be impaired by the animal's weight, which can pin mobile skin against the surgery table. This can significantly impair wound closure. Sandbags, beaded "vacuum" bags, or rolled-up towels can be placed ahead and behind the surgical region, to elevate the skin trapped against the table.

POSITIONING TECHNIQUES

(A) Padded support placement beneath the cranial sternum and pelvis for closure of a large wound overlying the back.

(B) Padded supports beneath shoulders and pelvis for ventral thoracic and abdominal wound closure. This is ideal for unilateral or bilateral chain mastectomies when closure tension occasionally is a problem.

(C) Padded supports are placed beneath the lateral pelvis and shoulder for closure of large lateral thoracic or abdominal wall defects.

COMMENTS

Veterinary surgeons can note a dramatic improvement in the ability to mobilize skin using the appropriate positioning of the patient, as illustrated. This is most commonly noted in larger dogs during unilateral or bilateral chain mastectomy. The surgeon can further reduce skin tension in the inguinal or axillary/sternal regions by loosening rope ties used to secure the respective hind limbs/forelimbs.

Plate 13

A

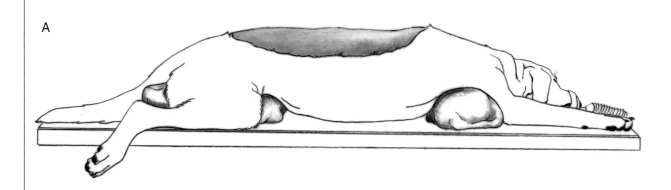

B

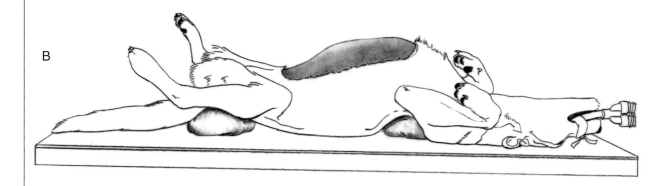

C

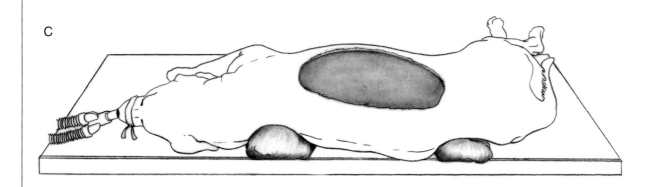

Plate 14   # Undermining Skin

DESCRIPTION

The loose skin over the neck and trunk in the dog and cat permits the veterinary surgeon to close many skin defects by undermining alone. The key to the successful surgical elevation of skin is preserving its blood supply. This requires the preservation of the direct cutaneous vessels and associated subdermal (deep) plexus. The following points can be employed by the clinician as general guidelines for undermining skin in small animals.

SURGICAL TECHNIQUE

(A) Skin should be undermined below the panniculus muscle layer, when present, to preserve the subdermal plexus and associated direct cutaneous vessels.

(B) Skin without an underlying panniculus muscle layer (middle and distal portion of the extremities) should be undermined in the loose areolar fascia beneath the dermis to preserve the subdermal plexus.

(C) Preserve direct cutaneous arteries and veins whenever possible during undermining.

(D) Skin closely associated with an underlying muscle should be elevated by including a portion of the outer muscle fascia with the dermis rather than undermining between these structures. This may help minimize injury to the subdermal plexus.

COMMENTS

Avoid direct injury to the subdermal plexus by using atraumatic surgical technique. Avoid or minimize the surgical manipulation of skin recently traumatized until circulation improves as noted by the resolution of contusions, edema, and infection.

Blunt-tipped Metzenbaum scissors are almost universally employed for undermining skin by alternately opening and closing the scissor blades to separate the loose areolar connective tissue. Dense fascial attachments are cut or snipped. A scalpel blade is best reserved for undermining skin adhered to the underlying fascia by dense scar tissue. This situation is most commonly seen in a 1- or 2-cm border of skin around chronic granulation beds.

Plate 14

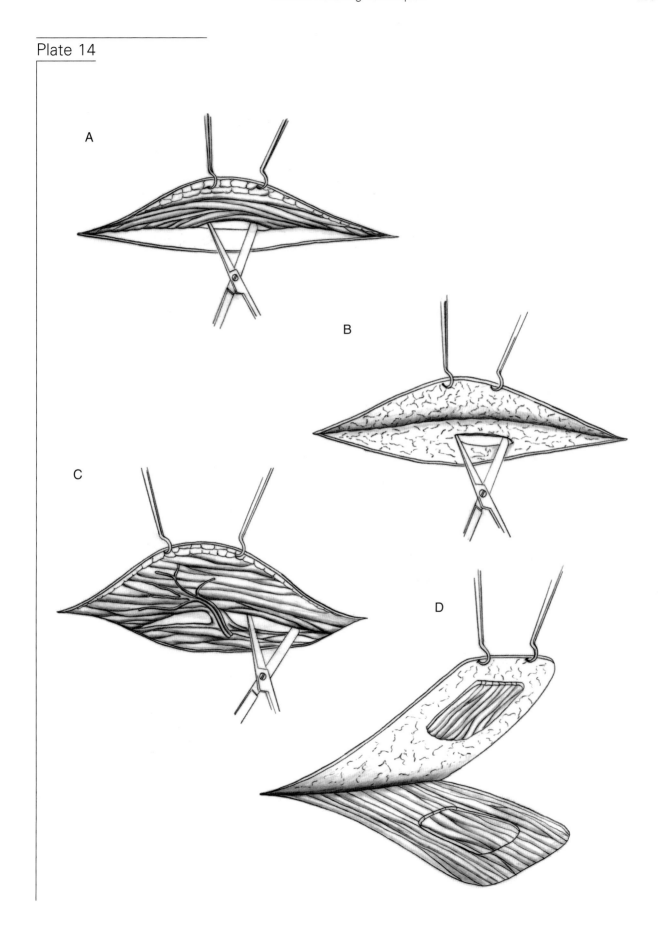

| Plate 15 | **Geometric Patterns to Facilitate Wound Closure** |

DESCRIPTION

Cutaneous wounds of an irregular shape can be converted to a simpler geometric pattern to facilitate wound closure. Similarly, a cutaneous lesion can be excised by selecting a geometric pattern that best conforms to its shape.

SURGICAL TECHNIQUE

(A) Triangular closure resulting in a Y-shaped scar.

(B) Rectangular closure resulting in an X-shaped scar.

(C) Elliptical closure resulting in a linear scar.

(D) Crescent closure resulting in a U-shapeded scar.

(E) Circular excision resulting in a linear scar; dog-ears may be noted. Large dog-ears can be excised (see Chapter 21).

COMMENTS

The surgeon should not rely solely on the use of simple geometric designs as the preferred method of wound closure. There are many circumstances where skin flaps may be more reliable for closure of the skin defect. Regional skin laxity or elasticity dictates, to a considerable degree, the method(s) of closure. (See Plate 28, Skin "Directing" for Maximum Coverage.)

It generally is preferable to close wounds in a linear or curvilinear fashion, since wound dehiscence is most likely to occur when two incisions intersect (X or Y closures). The point of intersection is a common location for incisional separation due to the difficulty in accurately suturing this area and the increased susceptibility to additional distracting forces.

Plate 15

A

B

C

D

E

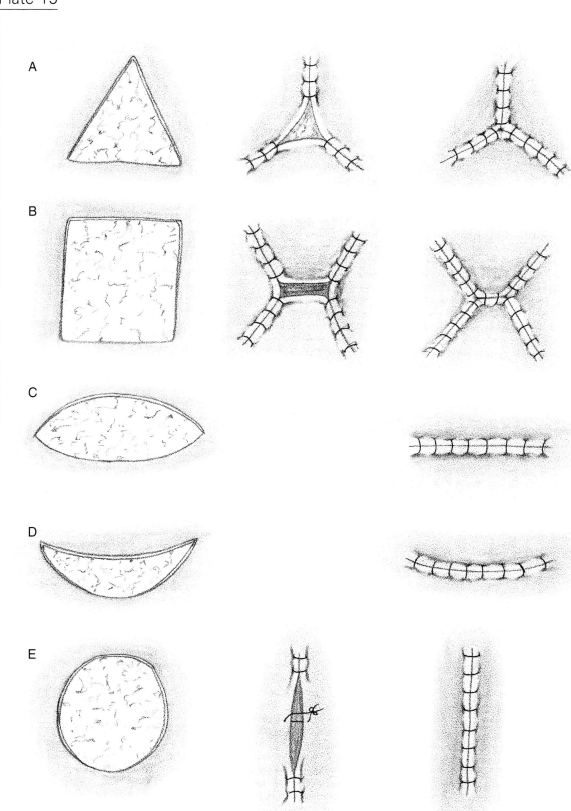

Plate 16   **V-Y Plasty**

DESCRIPTION

V-Y advancement is a lengthening procedure occasionally used to relieve minor tension to a limited area. Conversely, Y-V closure can be used to increase local skin tension. Both techniques are used to alter tension to a narrow band of skin where minor tension modification is desirable.

SURGICAL TECHNIQUE

(A) A V incision is made no closer than 3 cm from the skin incision (as a general guideline). The edges are carefully undermined, if necessary.

(B) Closure of the outer incision edges beginning at the tip of the V incision pushes the inner triangular skin flap forward to reduce tension within the plane of the incision.

(C) A Y configuration is created with advancement of the triangular flap.

COMMENTS

V-Y plasty is marginally effective in relieving skin tension; it cannot dramatically reduce tension over a wide area. It may be most effective for minor tension adjustments, especially in eyelid surgery. It is a very simple technique to execute.

Plate 16

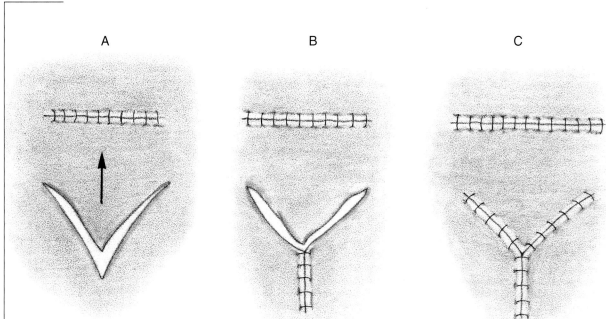

A   B   C

Plate 17   Z-Plasty (Option I)

DESCRIPTION

Z-plasty is used to (1) alter skin tension adjacent to an incision, (2) lengthen restrictive scars, and (3) change the direction of a linear scar into a less discernable pattern. In the latter case, the human eye has greater difficulty following a zigzag design compared to a linear scar, especially one that crosses a natural skin line or fold in a relatively hairless area. As a result, Z-plasty can change the position of the scar into a less conspicuous skin fold or line. The conventional Z-plasty technique involves forming two equilateral triangles. Each limb and the central member of the Z incision are equal in length; each limb extends at a 60-degree angle form the central member. Theoretically, the net length gained along the restrictive skin zone is approximately 75%.

SURGICAL TECHNIQUE

(A) Diagram illustrating the theoretical gain associated with Z-plasty. The theoretical gain in length is the difference in length between the long diagonal and the short diagonal. AB − CD = net gain. (In practice, the actual gain is less than the theoretical gain).

(B) A "Z" is drawn onto the skin. Each limb of the Z and the central member are equal in length. Each limb is drawn at a 60-degree angle to the central member. The Z design is positioned so that the central member overlies the restrictive scar (shaded area). The thin scar band is normally excised.

(C–E) Each triangular flap (I and II) is undermined and rotated into the opposing donor beds. The tip of each flap can be trimmed (rounded) to preclude the occasional necrosis noted in this area. Lastly, the individual flaps are sutured into place.

COMMENTS

Most Z-plasty procedures are used to increase the length of a skin area, thereby improving mobility. Lengthening restrictive scar bands or zones of tension perpendicular to a sutured incision under excessive tension is the most common use in veterinary medicine. Z-plasty actually is the simultaneous transposition of two equilateral triangular local flaps. As each flap is transposed, additional skin is placed in the previously restricted zone from the immediate area. The resultant scar also is more pliable than the previous linear scar. One or two standard transposition flaps actually may be more capable of lengthening more diffuse restrictive scars.

Z-plasty is somewhat confusing to clinicians unfamiliar with its design and execution. Practicing Z-plasty designs on thin sheets of elastic cloth or foam rubber is the best way to understand this procedure before attempting its use in a clinical situation.

Human reconstructive surgery textbooks demonstrate multiple variations in this standard Z-plasty technique. However, in veterinary surgery the basic equilateral triangle design employing 60-degree angles is sufficient for most situations where Z-plasty is indicated. Although the creation of wider angle flaps 70–90 degrees, can increase the theoretical length of gain to 100% and 120%, respectively; transposing these wider flaps is more difficult, except for areas of thin, elastic skin.

Experimental studies in dogs have indicated that *theoretical gains* in length, based on geometric measurements, were different from the actual gain achieved. For example, Z-plasty on the trunk of dogs has demonstrated that the actual gain of a 60-degree angle Z-plasty with 8-cm limbs was 28% less than theoretical measurements (a 45% gain as opposed to 73%). As the limb length decreased, the percentage of gain decreased. A Z-plasty with 1-cm limbs had 45% less gain than calculated (73% gain, less 45%, equals a total gain of 28%).

For Z-plasty to work properly, the skin in the base of the flaps created must be loose and elastic enough to rotate and stretch into its new position. If skin is under tension perpendicular to the central member of the Z, it may be impossible to transpose these flaps.

Plate 17

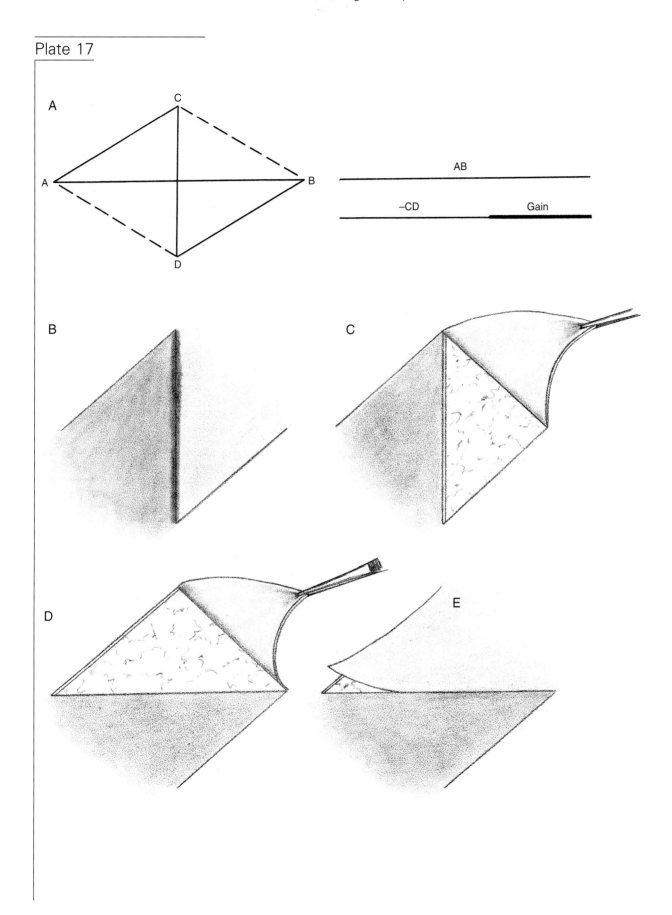

Plate 18   **Z-Plasty (Option II)**

DESCRIPTION

Z-plasty can be used to reduce tension on wound closures otherwise difficult or impossible to close in a given area.

SURGICAL TECHNIQUE

(A) The 60-degree angle Z-plasty is drawn onto the skin, with the central member of the Z parallel and overlying the line of greatest tension. It is desirable to create the Z incision no closer than approximately 3 cm from the primary incision. Each triangular flap is gently undermined.

(B) As the primary incision is sutured closed, each flap will begin to transpose into its appropriate position.

(C) Upon completion of the closure of the incision, the Z-plasty incisions are sutured to complete the procedure. The tips of each flap can be trimmed (rounded) to preclude the occasional necrosis noted in this area.

COMMENTS

See Plate 17. Placement of the Z-plasty incision must take into consideration regional blood supply, especially major direct cutaneous arteries.

Plate 18

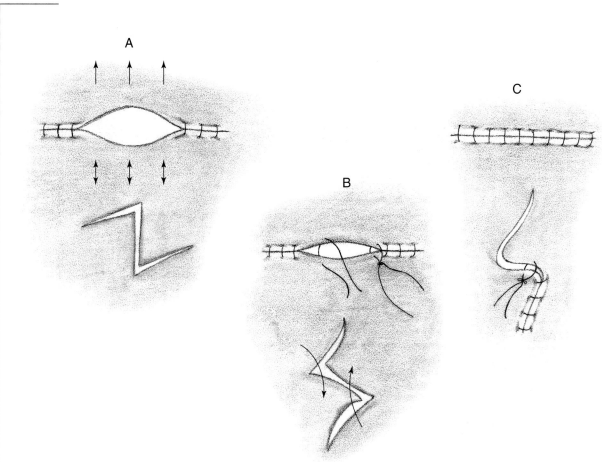

Plate 19   **Multiple Z-Plasties**

DESCRIPTION

Multiple small Z-plasties have been advocated for use in those areas where insufficient skin is present for using a single large Z-plasty procedure. Multiple small Z-plasties have a cumulative effect in lengthening restrictive areas.

SURGICAL TECHNIQUE

(A) Small 60-degree angle Z-plasties are created using the design illustrated.

(B) Paired flaps are individually elevated beginning at one end of the incision, transposed, and sutured into place.

COMMENTS

Experiments in dogs have shown that a single large 8-cm Z-plasty provides a greater gain in length compared to a series of eight 60-degree-angled Z-plasties with 1-cm limbs (see Plate 17). However, in areas with sparse hair growth, the resultant scar may be superior to one large Z-plasty.

Plate 19

A

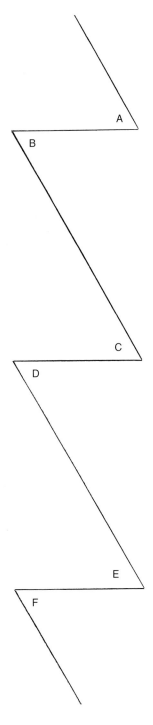

Plate 20   **Relaxing/Release Incisions**

DESCRIPTION

A relaxing or release incision is, by design, a skin incision created parallel to the length of a wound to facilitate closure of the primary defect. This bipedicle flap is carefully undermined and advanced over the wound. A secondary defect is created by this maneuver, which may be either closed primarily by undermining adjacent skin or left open to heal by second intention.

SURGICAL TECHNIQUE

(A) Illustration of a wound in which the line of greatest tension (perpendicular to the length of an elongated defect) is located at the widest portion of the defect.

(B) If the skin edge bordering the wound is thickened or fibrotic, it should be excised with a scalpel blade to improve marginal pliability. A skin incision is then created parallel to the primary defect in a staged fashion, beginning in the center of the zone of greatest tension. In this example, the width of the flap approximates the width of the wound. The cutaneous borders of the wound and bipedicle skin flap created can be gently undermined to facilitate their advancement.

(C) Towel clamps may be used to initially oppose wound borders. The relaxing incision is extended lengthwise in increments (dotted line in diagram B) as required to relieve tension on the remaining portion of the wound.

(D) Upon closure of the wound, the secondary defect can be left open to heal by second intention. If sufficient skin is available, the adjacent skin can be undermined and the secondary defect closed directly.

COMMENTS

The release incision is a simple and useful procedure to immediately decrease incisional skin tension. A second relaxing incision can be created on the opposite side of a wound if necessary. No guidelines are available to describe how close the relaxing incision should be to the wound. In practice, most relaxing incisions are created 3–10 cm from the wound border, depending on the size of the wound, the regional skin laxity, and the intended position of the secondary defect.

Relaxing or release incisions may seem to be a paradox: closing one defect at the expense of creating a second wound appears illogical. However, there are occasions where closure of a wound that exposes essential tendons, ligaments, nerves, and vessels justifies primary closure in exchange for a defect in a relatively unobtrusive location. Wound closure may be essential to prevent contamination and infection of surgical implants while creating a wound over a muscle surface where second intention healing can occur more easily. Skin coverage over a bony prominence may be necessary for proper healing compared to a defect created in a "protected" region.

Other wounds susceptible to external trauma and infection can be closed primarily at the expense of creating a secondary defect in an area where an epithelialized scar is less susceptible to future injury or where such a wound would be easier to manage postoperatively. Lastly, chronic nonhealing wounds (as a result of recurrent trauma, radiation, etc.) may heal primarily by using single or paired relaxing incisions (two bipedicle advancement flaps) that have adequate circulation for healing, while creating a secondary defect in a region with sufficient circulation to heal by second intention. Most of these secondary defects, left unsutured, will heal within 3 to 6 weeks.

Plate 20

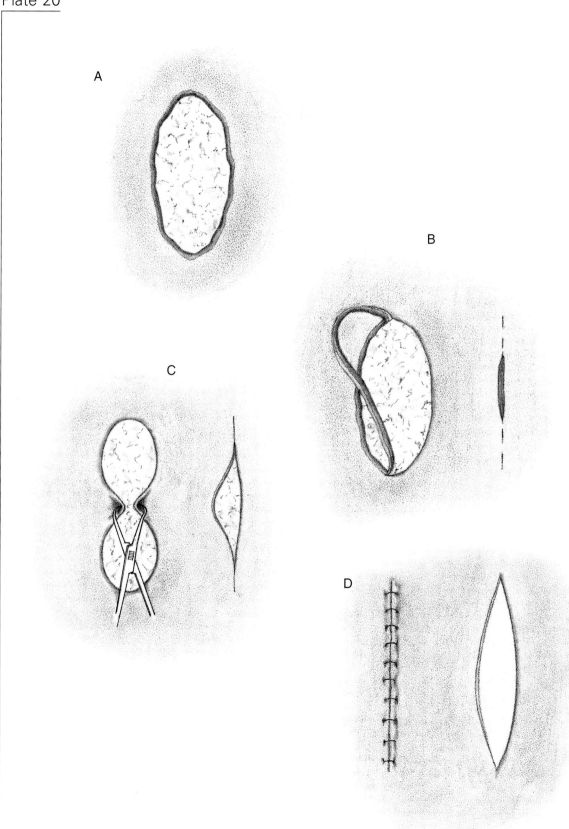

| Plate 21 | The "Hidden" Intradermal Release/Relaxing Incision |

DESCRIPTION

The standard skin release incision is created by incising through the epidermis and dermis. If regional skin tension is not excessive, this incision can be resutured, usually by undermining the adjacent skin to offset the deficit associated with advancing the bipedicled advancement flap. The author's dermal release incision is useful for similar cases, thereby eliminating the need for resuturing a full-thickness incision.

In place of incising the skin through its surface, a no. 15 scalpel blade is used to gently incise the dermis via the hypodermis. Care is taken not to cut through the thin, overlying epidermal layer. As a result, modest skin relaxation can be obtained without the need to suture the skin, creating an additional scar.

SURGICAL TECHNIQUE

(A) The skin bordering the wound is undermined and elevated with one or more skin hooks. The area for creating the dermal release is identified (see guidelines in Plate 20). A no. 15 scalpel blade is used to incise the dermis with a few delicate strokes to avoid incising completely through the epidermis. Scalpel strokes are repeated until a dermal gap can be seen (visualization is easier in thicker skin). The dermal release incision is made no closer than 3 cm to the cut skin margin.

(B) The epidermal surface is viewed as the dermis is progressively incised. The blade can be seen tenting the epidermal surface during this process. In this illustration, the epidermal surface remains intact: traction on the skin demonstrates the dermal gap or *release* created (dashed lines).

(C) Completion of the incisional closure, revealing the modest tension relief achieved. Because the epidermis is preserved, no suturing is required when using this technique.

COMMENTS

Properly executed, the "hidden" dermal release incision provides a modest gain in skin laxity. This dermal release technique does not provide the degree of skin relaxation noted when the release incision is left open to heal by second intention (see Plate 20). Yet, it is a useful way to reduce tension in those cases requiring a comparatively modest reduction in wound closure tension. If the surgeon inadvertently perforates the epidermis, the area can be sutured. There are three modest advantages of this technique: no suturing is required; open wound care is not required, unlike open release incisions; no visible scar is noted with preservation of the epidermal surface.

Plate 21

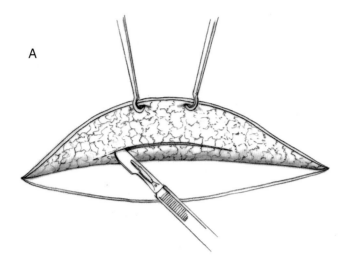

A

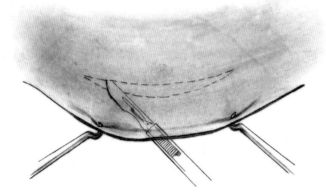

B

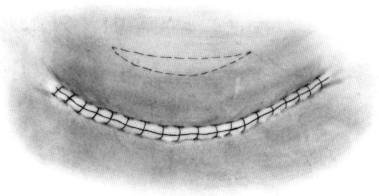

C

Plate 22	**Multiple Release Incisions for Extremity Wounds**

DESCRIPTION

Multiple relaxing incisions have been described for closing wounds involving the lower extremities. Multiple small stab incisions can be placed parallel to the long axis of the wound in a staggered fashion to promote skin advancement without the creation of a single, large secondary defect. The single relaxing incision, however, maximizes skin advancement, creating two bipedicle flaps and a single donor defect.

SURGICAL TECHNIQUES

Multiple Relaxing Incisions

(A) Skin sutures, stay sutures, or towel clamps are used to intermittently attempt apposition of the wound borders during the meshing procedure. Skin borders are carefully undermined.

(B) Mesh incisions are placed no closer than 1 cm from the skin edge. In general, they are approximately 1 cm long, and no closer than 1 cm apart. If additional rows are required, holes are made approximately 1–2 cm from the initial row in a staggered fashion. A greater number of holes are usually required at the widest area of the defect under greater tension. When sufficient tension has been relieved, the skin borders are sutured. A medicated nonadherent dressing is applied to the wound before the limb is immobilized in a bandage or splint.

Single Relaxing Incision

(C) In this example, illustrating a nonhealing wound involving the forelimb, a relaxing incision is made along the caudal aspect of the limb.

(D) The interposing skin is undermined and the two bipedicle flaps are advanced over the prepared wound bed and sutured together. The solitary defect created on the caudal aspect of the limb (dotted line) generally is managed as an open wound to promote wound contraction and epithelialization.

COMMENTS

Although multiple incisions have been used clinically, there is a significant risk of circulatory compromise to the incised skin by accidental division of direct cutaneous vessels and impairment of the cutaneous microcirculation traveling parallel in the skin. A wider dispersion of the multiple incisions would be preferable to minimize this risk, although the gain in tension relief would be less. A single, long, relaxing incision generally provides maximum tension relief compared to multiple, small release incisions, and it may be less likely to cause major circulatory compromise to the skin adjacent to the defect.

Plate 22

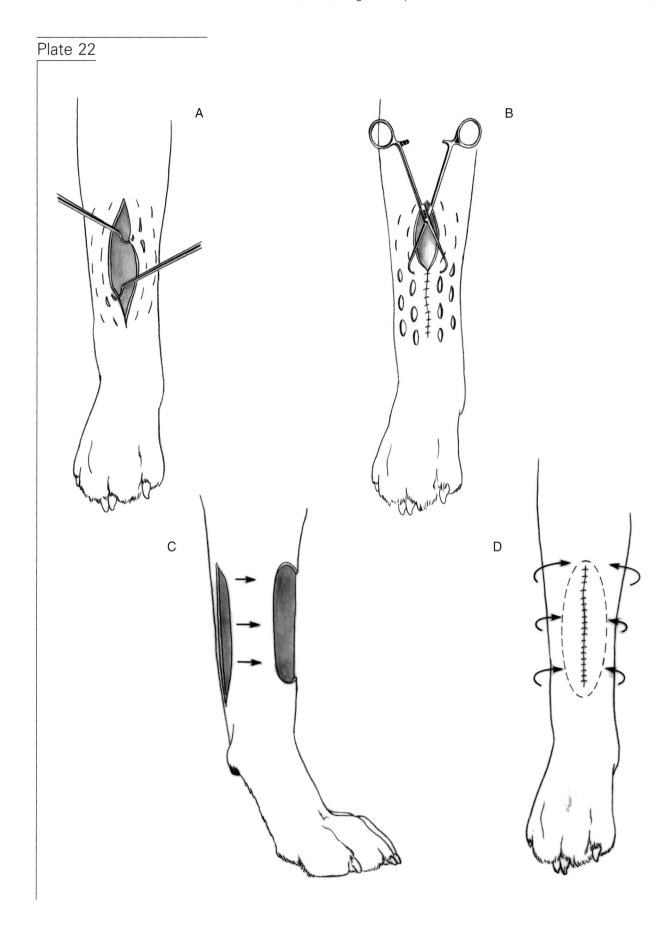

Plate 23   **Walking Suture Technique**

DESCRIPTION

The walking suture technique, popularized by S.F. Swaim, is a method of distributing tension sutures over a wide surface area when skin undermining and suture closure techniques alone are insufficient for wound apposition. Individual "walking" sutures pull the skin toward the defect in small increments. Multiple sutures have a cumulative effect in maintaining the undermined skin in position as it is advanced to the center of the defect.

SURGICAL TECHNIQUE

(A) 2-0 or 3-0 absorbable suture material is usually selected. Suturing begins at the distant limits of the undermined skin. The skin is elevated as the needle is inserted into the dermis. Sutures may pass through portions of the panniculus muscle to gain access to the dermis.

(B) The needle is then inserted into the underlying muscle fascia, generally or 2 or 3 cm closer to the midpoint of the wound. Deep placement of the needle into connective tissue is necessary when suture material is placed into a granulation bed in order to prevent suture pull-out.

(C) Walking sutures are no closer than 2 or 3 cm apart. After the "deep" row of sutures is tied, a second series of walking sutures are staggered with the first row.

(D) The skin on the opposite side of the wound can be advanced or "walked" in similar fashion.

(E) Completion of the wound closure. Note the skin depressions or dimples created from this buried suture pattern. A bandage can be used to control dead space with or without evacuation drains.

COMMENTS

Walking sutures are a simple and effective method to stretch skin over a wide defect and anchor the skin into position as gains in skin advancement are made. However, not all wide defects require the use of walking sutures.

Skin "dimples" or indentations are noted over the location of walking sutures. These disappear in time with absorbable suture materials. The two greatest concerns voiced with the use of walking sutures are the potential for circulatory compromise to direct cutaneous vessels and the subdermal plexus and the potential for formation of separate seromas or abscesses that would be difficult to drain separately. Careful placement of sutures and avoiding excessive numbers of walking sutures can minimize circulatory compromise. Clinical results to date have shown that multiple fluid pockets are not a major postoperative complication.

Skin stretchers (Skin Stretchers, Pavletic Angell Animal Medical Center, Boston, MA) may be used to prestretch the skin alone or in conjunction with walking sutures, in order to facilitate skin advancement. Skin stretching also may be used to promote wound closure without the use of walking sutures (see Plate 31 and 32).

Plate 23

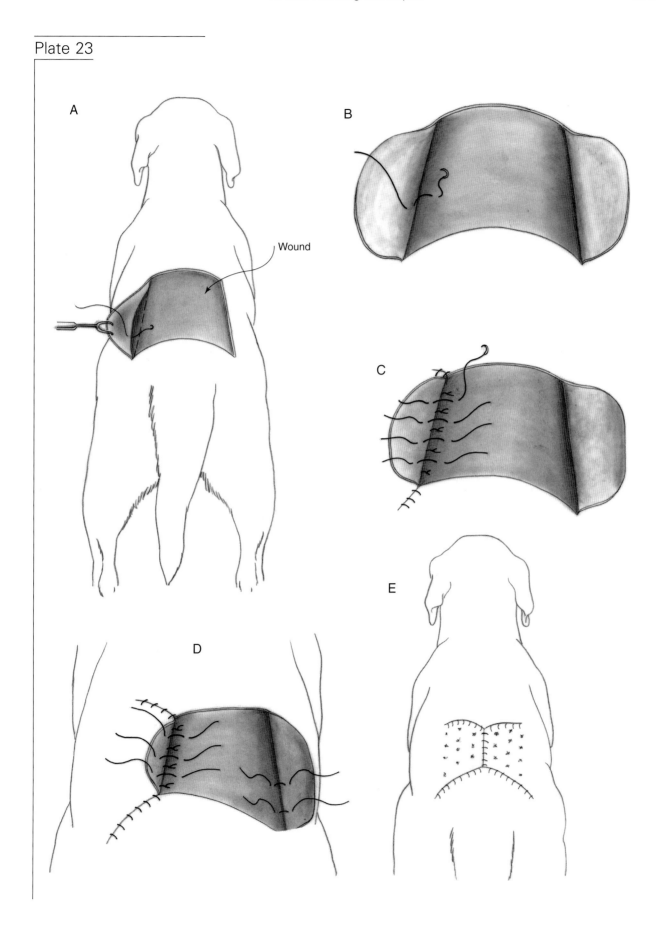

A

Wound

B

C

D

E

Plate 24   **Skin Stretchers to Offset Incisional Tension**

DESCRIPTION

Skin stretchers (Pavletic) can be used to offset incisional tension after wound closure. Skin pads, positioned on opposing sides of the incisional segment under tension, are connected with a segment of elastic cable. Pads may be left in position for 3–5 days, unless conditions dictate their prolonged placement.

SURGICAL TECHNIQUE

(A)   A large flank laceration has been prepared for debridement and surgical closure. The skin has been clipped liberally in preparation for skin stretcher pad application.

(B, C)   Closure was accomplished with using an absorbable intradermal suture pattern followed by alternating simple interrupted and vertical mattress skin sutures. Drains may be advisable to help prevent seroma formation.

(D)   Skin pads are secured approximately 5 cm from the incision (see Plate 31) using cyanoacrylate adhesive.

COMMENTS

Skin pads have a large "footprint" of surface area contact with the skin, compared to retention sutures (Plate 26). Pad size can be adjusted according to the location of the wound, size of the patient, and degree of adherence required. Larger pads naturally have a larger surface area, thereby facilitating adherence to the skin when elastic (tension) cables are applied.

Because of the large surface area of contact with the stratum corneum and the ability to place them at variable locations around the wound, skin pads are capable of recruiting a larger area of elastic skin to offset incisional tension. The use of this device can accelerate mechanical creep and stress relaxation, often within hours of application, in a fashion similar to the presuturing technique (Plate 30).

Plate 24

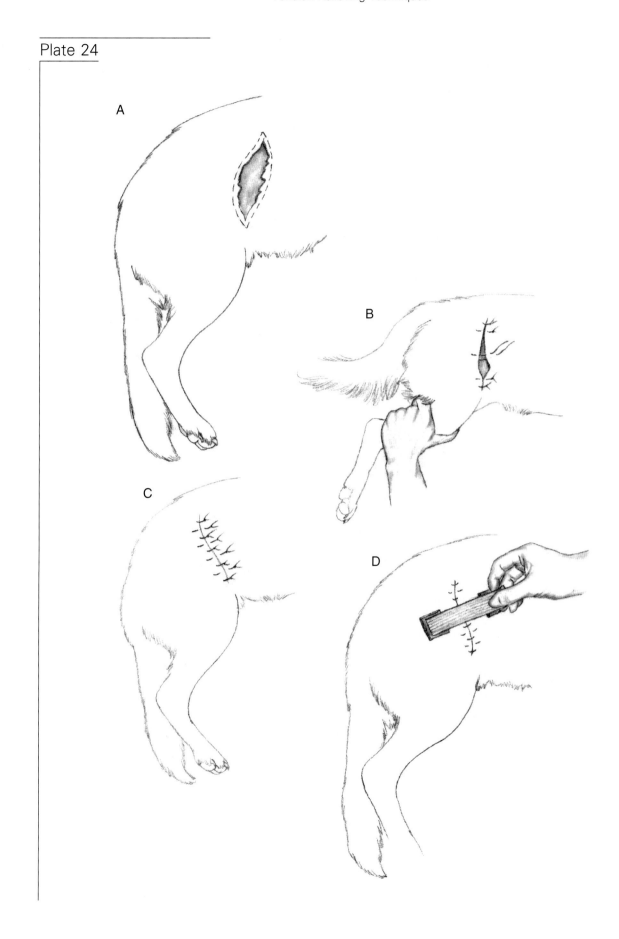

Plate 25   "Tension" Suture Patterns

DESCRIPTION

The simple interrupted suture pattern is the simplest and most common pattern used for accurate apposition of skin. Skin staples also can achieve closure rapidly and effectively. However, wounds under moderate tension may require a suture pattern that is better able to maintain tissue apposition and distribute skin tension and that is less likely to cut through the skin edges.

Vertical mattress sutures and the "far-near-near-far" or "far-far-near-near" suture techniques are useful tension suture patterns. Because they are placed perpendicular to the incision, they cause minimal circulatory compromise, unlike the horizontal mattress suture, which has greater potential for impairing local cutaneous blood flow. Vertical mattress sutures may be used alone or alternated with simple interrupted skin sutures. This combines the tension-reducing capacity of the mattress suture with the cosmetic advantages of the simple interrupted pattern, which more accurately aligns the skin borders directly.

Intradermal sutures may also reduce tension along a suture line and accurately appose the skin. Intradermal sutures can be followed by simple interrupted sutures for added security.

Towel clamps are quite useful for opposing skin edges under tension, while allowing the surgeon to tie sutures. The two-point contact of towel clamps causes minimal trauma.

SURGICAL TECHNIQUE

(A) The continuous intradermal suture pattern is placed in the deep dermal surface.
(B) The interrupted intradermal suture pattern is placed in the deep dermal surface.
(C) The vertical mattress suture pattern.
(D) Horizontal mattress suture pattern. In this example, the suture is placed through short segments of soft rubber tubing stents (see also Plate 26).
(E) The "far-far-near-near" suture pattern.
(F) The "far-near-near-far" suture pattern.

COMMENTS

Reverse cutting needles should be used to reduce the likelihood of sutures "cutting out." Taper point needles generally are more difficult to pass through skin but produce a circular hole that is more resistant to this problem. Because of increased collagenase activity within 5 mm of the wound border, sutures are better placed outside this zone to reduce the risk of dehiscence. Keeping the skin clean and dry will help prevent tissue maceration that may promote dehiscence from suture cut-out.

Selection of suture material for skin closure is largely a matter of personal preference. Absorbable suture material is commonly used for intradermal patterns (3-0 or 4-0), whereas monofilament or braided nonabsorbable materials are employed for skin closure (2-0 or 3-0). The author's preference for skin sutures is swaged-on monofilament nylon or polypropylene because of its strength, elasticity, and low coefficient of friction. Size 2-0 is occasionally used in the thicker skin over the back of the dog, whereas size 3-0 is used for most other wounds. Small-diameter materials enable the surgeon to place greater numbers of sutures. However, finer suture materials (4-0, 5-0) are used only for cosmetic closure where there is an absence of skin tension. Cotton bandages can help to protect the wounds and limit motion. Areas subject to motion (joint surfaces) also may benefit from additional external support to reduce the possibility of separation of apposed wound borders.

Plate 25

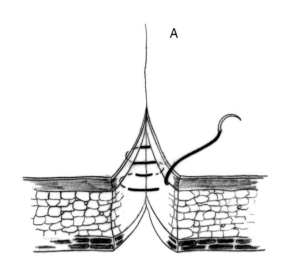

A

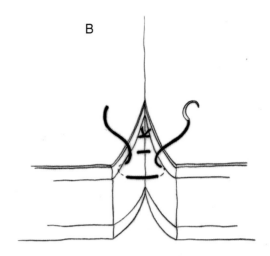

B

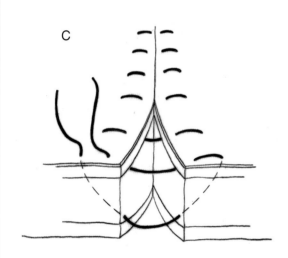

C

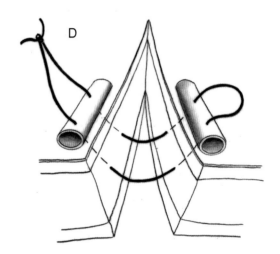

D

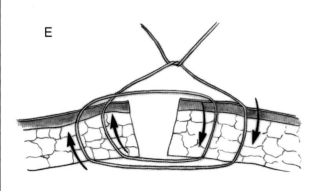

E

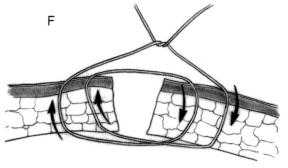

F

Plate 26   **Retention Sutures**

DESCRIPTION

Retention, stay, or echelon sutures provide a secondary suture line at a distance from the primary closure to relieve excessive tension on the healing wound and prevent cutaneous dehiscence. In small animal surgery, soft rubber tubing, Penrose drains, and buttons have been incorporated into the retention suture pattern as bolsters to prevent sutures from cutting into the skin under stress. Suture materials are usually 00 to 0 diameter.

SURGICAL TECHNIQUE

(A) Vertical mattress retention sutures (echelon pattern) placed around a length of Penrose drain (Penrose drain stents).

(B) Large, interrupted, retention sutures with skin bolsters or bumpers to prevent cutting into the skin. (*Note:* In cases in which the patient is obese and prone to abdominal dehiscence after laparotomy, retention sutures may be incorporated through all layers of the abdominal wall or deep fascial layers prior to standard closure of the laparotomy incision (see also Plate 27).

COMMENTS

Retention sutures are not routinely required except for wounds under moderate tension. They can be employed in the primary closure or set back from the incision line as secondary support. When used alone they are usually removed 3 or 5 days later as swelling and skin tension decrease. Retention sutures can be left in for a longer period of time, if warranted. A continuous line of firm tubing connected with a series of mattress sutures should be used with caution, especially when a firm bandage is applied over the entire closure. In this situation, bandage materials may compress the tubing into the skin, compromising cutaneous circulation from the drain to the incision. It may be better to use soft tubing or multiple short segments of soft tubing to avoid this situation. A noninvasive, alternative consideration would be skin stretchers (see Plate 24).

Plate 26

A

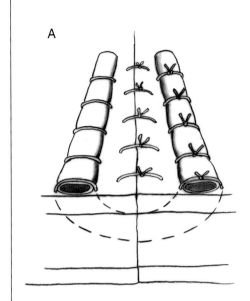

B

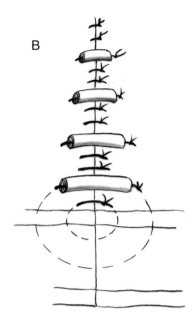

Plate 27   **Stent**

DESCRIPTION

A stent, by definition, is any material used to hold tissue in place, control dead space, or to provide support to a wound after closure. The most common wound stent in veterinary medicine employs rolls of soft cotton gauze that are secured over a closure site.

SURGICAL TECHNIQUE

(A) After wound closure, soft sterilized rolls of self-adherent gauze are laid over the wound. There are three common options to secure the gauze roll over the wound, as described below.

(B) Through-and-through retention sutures, incorporating all tissue closure layers, can be tied over the gauze rolls.

(C) Suture loops or eyelets can be placed 3–4 cm from the incision: suture material or umbilical tape is placed through opposing loops in a "shoelace" fashion.

(D) A continuous zigzag pattern is commonly used to secure the stent into position.

COMMENTS

Wound stents are more commonly employed in large animal surgery to protect wounds from environmental contamination and external trauma. They are not routinely used in small animal surgery. Soft gauze rolls have the potential to promote incisional infection unless they are kept dry and unsoiled. Of the two most common suture techniques used to secure stents, technique C gives the surgeon easier access to the gauze rolls for replacement, should contamination occur.

Plate 27

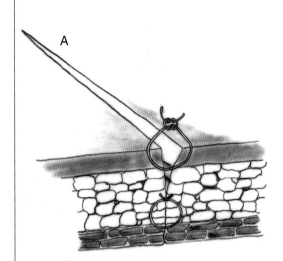

A

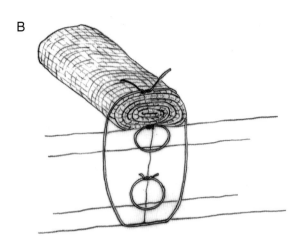

B

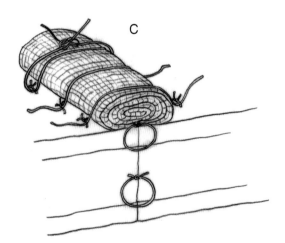

C

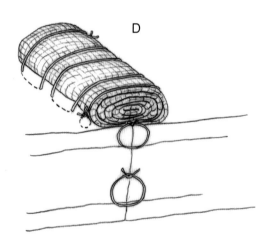

D

Plate 28 Skin "Directing" for Maximum Coverage

DESCRIPTION

When attempting closure of large irregular wounds, skin tension is manually assessed to determine areas where loose, elastic skin can be undermined and advanced over the defect. Smaller areas of the wound may be easily undermined and closed directly by taking advantage of the loose skin available. However, simple closure maneuvers may limit the ability to maximize use of the elastic skin to cover major (or more important) portions of the defect.

The loose skin available for wound coverage is determined by lifting the skin surrounding the wound and pushing the loose elastic skin border toward the central area of the major defect. This will better determine how to "direct" surrounding skin for maximum coverage.

When the surgeon has an estimation of whether undermining alone can achieve optimal wound coverage, it must be determined whether a skin flap employing the elastic donor area(s) would afford better wound coverage over undermining alone, such as that achievable with axial pattern flaps.

SURGICAL TECHNIQUE

(A) This is a clinical example of a skin wound as a result of an automobile accident.

(B) No flap design was determined to give better wound coverage than undermining. The temptation to initially suture the smaller area closed was rejected, since this maneuver would have restricted advancement of the most elastic skin to cover the largest skin defect overlying the shoulder.

(C) Directing the most mobile skin over the largest area of the defect provides maximum wound coverage. The smaller area was easily closed by undermining the dorsal skin bordering this defect.

COMMENTS

The surgeon should not rule out using a combination of closure techniques including undermining, tension-relieving techniques, skin flaps, second intention healing, and skin grafts. Closure should be accomplished in the simplest fashion that will restore regional integrity with the least stress to the patient. Lastly, determine which technique(s) can achieve the best cosmetic results without creating additional difficulties in achieving these goals.

If a flap is considered as an option for closure, the surgeon should attempt to reduce the total surface area of the wound with simple closure techniques in order to shorten the length of the flap required for final coverage. Shorter flaps naturally have a greater likelihood to survive completely.

Plate 28

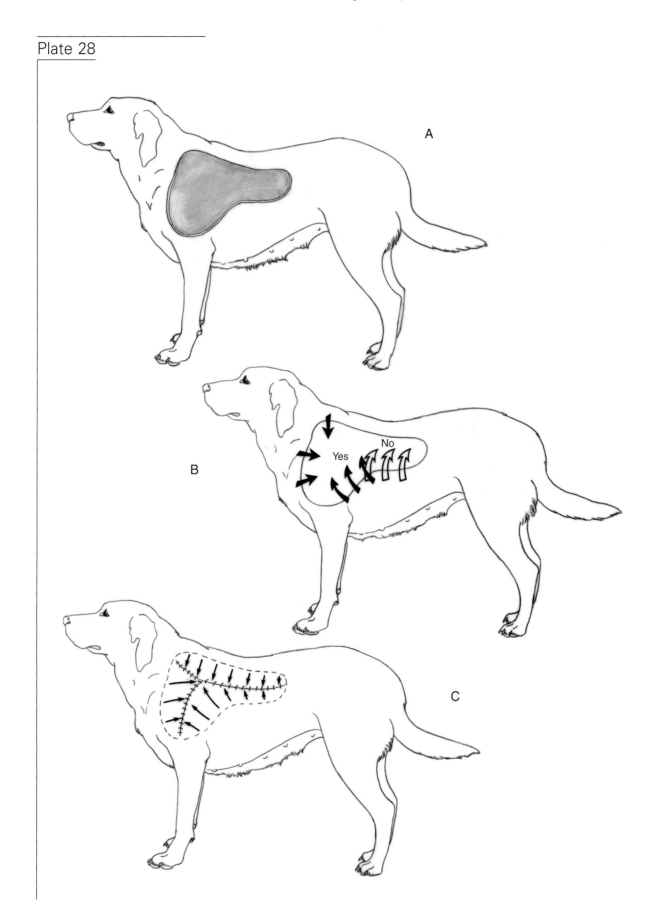

Plate 29   **Relaxing Incision to Reduce Flap Tension**

DESCRIPTION

Improperly designed flaps occasionally result in a flap too short to completely cover a wound. A line of tension can be noted along the length of the extended flap (line of greatest tension). A small, carefully placed, stab incision can reduce tension thereby preserving cutaneous circulation.

SURGICAL TECHNIQUE

(A) A no. 11 or no. 15 scalpel blade is used to make a small stab incision perpendicular to the line of greatest tension (located from the pivot point of the flap to its most distant edge). The resultant wound heals by second intention.

(B) A similar alternative is to incise the neighboring cutaneous surface in line with this tension band.

COMMENTS

Care must be taken to avoid dividing direct cutaneous vessels or creating unnecessarily long flap incisions that may compromise cutaneous vascular channels in the flap. The dermal surface of the flap can be inspected to assure the stab incision will not divide any direct cutaneous vessels. The latter technique (B) can avoid this potential complication. V-Y or Z-plasty could be substituted for the technique in (B).

Plate 29

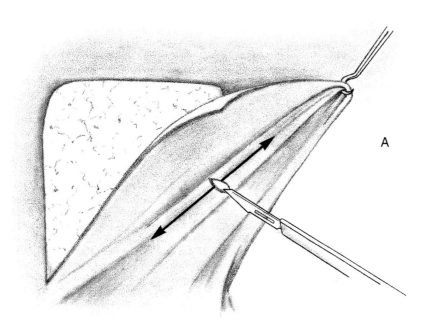

A

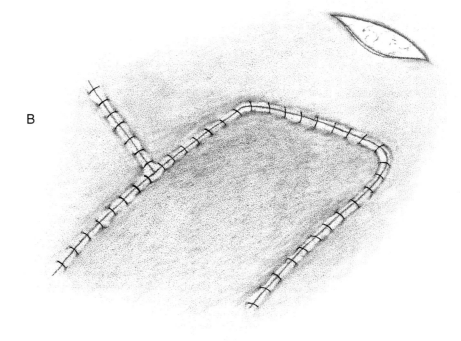

B

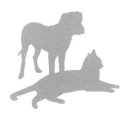

Skin-Stretching Techniques

PHYSIOLOGY OF SKIN STRETCHING

Surgeons rely on the inherent elastic properties of the skin to close wounds secondary to trauma or the removal of diseased tissues. The skin's inherent elasticity can vary between species, individuals, body regions, patient age, body conformation, and pathologic conditions involving the cutaneous tissues. To minimize tension during basic wound closure, surgeons may attempt to place incisions parallel to lines of maximum tension. The undercutting of skin margins can further mobilize skin, although the combined effects of excessive undermining and wound closure under tension can result in circulatory compromise.

Skin is capable of further extension beyond its inherent elasticity from the application of a stretching or tension force over time. This phenomenon, termed *mechanical creep*, is complimented by *stress relaxation* or the progressive reduction in force required to keep the stretched dermal collagen fibers at a given length. During this process, tissue fluid is slowly displaced from around the randomly arranged convoluted dermal collagen filaments as they progressively align and compact longitudinally in the direction of the stretching force. This increase in cutaneous length can be measured within minutes after load application: the greater the force applied to the skin, the sooner maximal extension can be achieved over time.

There are a number of natural examples of skin expansion beyond its normal estimated limits in humans and animals including advanced pregnancy, obesity, and the expansion of large subcutaneous neoplasms. This form of cutaneous surface area enlargement is the result of *biologic creep*, a slower physiologic mechanism of tissue accommodation (Fig. 10-1).

The basic concept of surgically expanding skin, described by Neumann in 1957, led to the development of the modern tissue expander by Radovan and Austad in the 1970s. Recruitment of skin from tissue expansion is the result of a combination of acute stretch, the recruitment of adjacent elastic skin, and true expansion as a result of the biomechanical properties of stress/relaxation previously described (Fig. 10-2).

In the literature, various devices have been used experimentally and clinically to stretch human skin. These systems involve the insertion of needles, metallic loops, or other invasive cutaneous anchoring techniques. Sutures or elastic bands are used to connect anchors and are periodically tightened. Unfortunately, the force becomes concentrated on a small area of skin, risking tissue tearing, pain, and infection. Due to this limited skin-anchor interface, care must be taken to limit the "cable tensions" generated. The simplest and most effective device for animal use is the skin-stretcher cable system discussed in this chapter. This externally applied device disperses cable tension over a large footprint on the skin surface area. Skin will not tear with this painless device.

PRESUTURING

The technique of presuturing is another surgical method that in part uses the biomechanical properties of mechanical creep and stress relaxation to facilitate the closure of skin wounds. Presuturing relies on the use of tension mattress sutures to imbricate the skin on opposing sides of cutaneous lesions. The sutures primarily exert their effect on the healthy skin immediately adjacent to the proposed surgical site. The force required to close surgical wounds can be markedly reduced within 24 hours after suture application, based on studies performed in swine, with positive benefits noted as early as 2.5 hours after application in humans and pigs (Plate 30). Skin stretchers can be used as an alternative to the presuturing technique (Plate 32).

SKIN STRETCHERS

The externally applied, noninvasive skin-stretching device described in this chapter is capable of rapidly stretching skin, both adjacent to and distant from a surgical site in animals (Fig. 10-3). Unlike those techniques used to manipulate skin bordering wound margins, this method and device has the capability of achieving significantly greater cumulative gains in skin mobilization by recruitment from large surface areas of skin. This device can be employed to close moderate to large wounds prior to elective surgical procedures or during the course of open wound management (see Plate 31 and 32). Postoperatively, the device also can be used to reduce incisional tension (see Plate 24).

The basic device, as it is presently designed, applies continuous, adjustable tension to skin by means of the following two components:

1. Adherent skin pads or anchors applied to opposing sides of a surgical site.
2. Adjustable, elastic tension straps or cables that engage the skin pads.

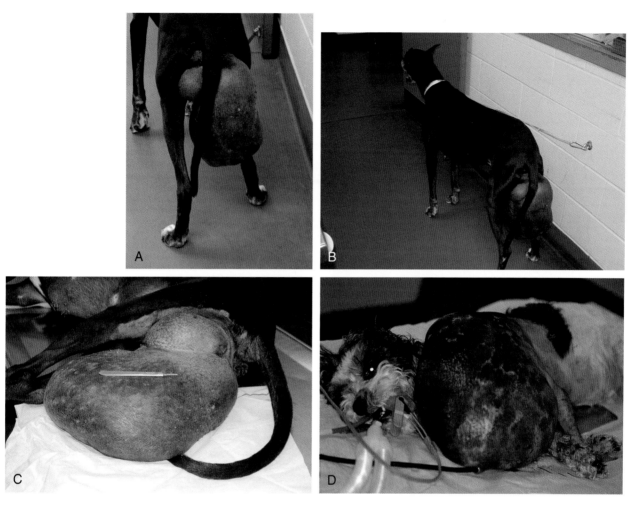

FIG. 10-1 (A–C) Massive lipoma attached to the skin below the vulva, 1 year-plus in duration. Note how the skin overlying the tumor has increased its surface area by "biologic creep. " Lipoma enlargement, coupled with gravitational pull, played a role in this process. The mass was successfully removed.

(D) Small terrier with recurrent infiltrative lipoma involving the left upper forelimb. The skin overlying the area has increased its surface area by slow biologic creep. Infiltrative lipomas usually are problematic to remove; recurrence is likely unless surgical margins can be obtained.

Skin pads and the cable devices are made in a variety of embodiments, depending upon the size of the wound, amount of skin recruitment desired, and their intended use.

The predetermined cutaneous sites for pad application are prepared by removing hair and cleaning the skin with a surgical soap and isopropyl alcohol swabs. The skin is allowed to dry completely before pad application. Multiple adherent pads can be applied to the skin local to and distant from the surgical site, depending on the amount of skin available or required for recruitment. Skin pads can be contoured to the natural curvature of the body region: alternatively, small scissor cuts can be used to improve skin surface contact. Cyanoacrylate adhesive is used to enhance pad adherence to the skin as needed.

The pile pad surface attached to the elastic cables engage the paired cutaneous "hook" pads positioned on opposite sides of the surgical site. The elastic cable is attached to one pad and stretched prior to engaging the opposing pad in order to generate moderate cable tension. As the skin areas progressively stretch from the force applied, cable tension is adjusted every 6 to 8 hours to generate optimal tension forces during the

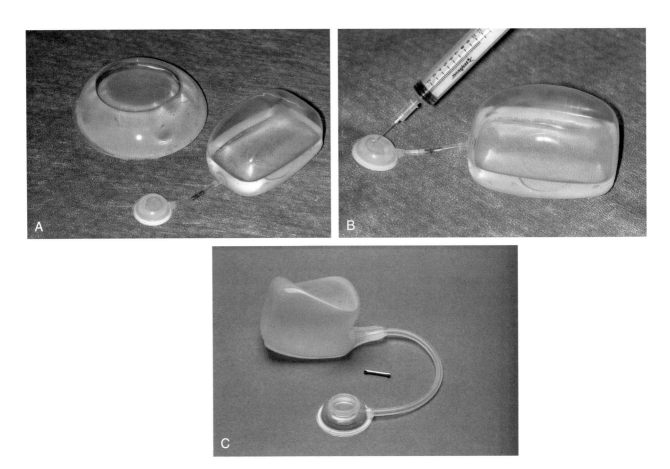

FIG. 10-2 (A, B) Tissue expanders can be purchased or specially designed in a variety of shapes and sizes. Sterile saline or lactated Ringer's solution is used to progressively inflate the reservoir through an injection port connected by a silicone tube. (C) Basic components of a tissue-expander kit include a metallic splice, enabling the surgeon to shorten the extension tube to the appropriate length.

brief period of application. Elastic cable also helps maintain the position of any dressings or bandages placed over the surgical site: wounds can be easily inspected at the time of cable adjustment. Sufficient skin may be recruited within 48 hours after application, although the devices were maintained up to 96 hours in some subjects (Fig. 10-4).

Upon completion of the stretching procedure, elastic cables are removed; skin pads are peeled from the skin surface or removed with a glue solvent on the anesthetized patient. Pads left on the skin will begin to separate within days after application, as the outer corneal layer desquamates. After surgical preparation of the patient, the recruited skin is advanced to close the skin wound. Generally, little or no cutaneous undermining is required in small animal patients. As noted, skin pads and cables also can be used postoperatively over a 2- to 5-day period to offset excessive incisional tension (see Plate 31).

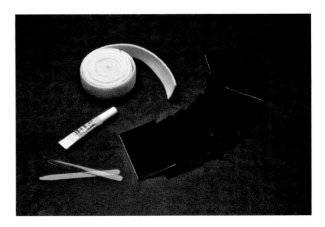

FIG. 10-3 Components of the skin-stretching kit, including self-adherent skin pads, elastic connecting cable, supplemental glue, and glue applicators.

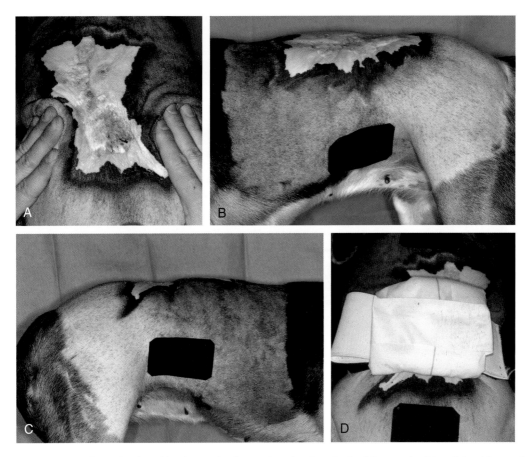

FIG. 10-4 (A) Burn scar overlying the dorsal lumbar and pelvic regions in a beagle. the inherent elasticity of the skin was insufficient for wound closure without resorting to extensive undermining of the skin.

(B, C) Application of large skin pads onto the left and right sides of the dog.

(D) Attachment of a wide elastic cable to the left and right pads, under moderate tension. A second set of pads was applied caudal and cranial to the epithelialized burn scar. A cotton pad was placed beneath both sets of cables to prevent irritation to the scar surface.

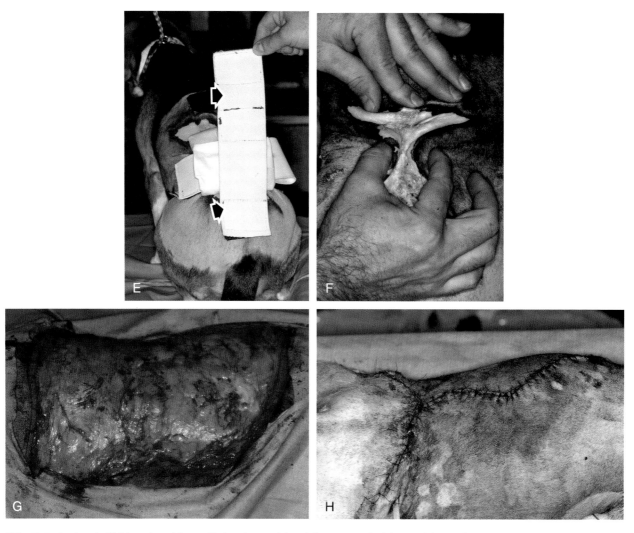

FIG. 10-4 *Continued* (E) Note the cable, applied to the caudal pad, being stretched forward for application to the remaining cranial pad (arrows). Cables were adjusted every 6 hours for a total of 72 hours.

(F) After 72 hours, note the skin bordering the lesion is approximated with minimal effort.

(G) Complete surgical removal of the scar. Incisions were made in the adjacent skin.

(H) Wound closure was accomplished with minimal cutaneous undermining.

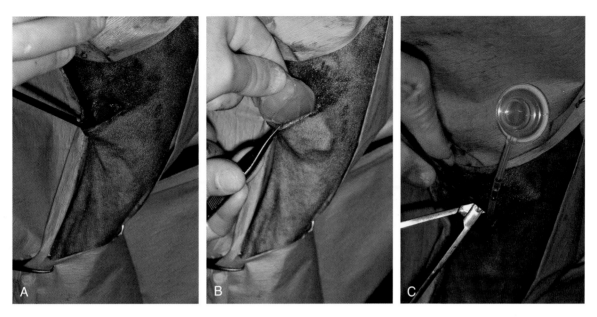

FIG. 10-5 (A) Undermining the skin in preparation for tissue expander insertion. The pocket size should be limited to the minimum area needed to accommodate this implant.

(B) Placement of a collapsed 100-cc tissue expander into a pocket created over the lateral tibial region.

(C) Proximal pocket created to accommodate injection port.

Today, the author uses skin stretchers for nearly all large skin defects involving the trunk and cervical area. It is a fast, efficient, and economical method of closing problematic wounds. It reduces surgical trauma to the patient by reducing the need for more invasive closure techniques.

SKIN EXPANDERS

Tissue expansion is based upon the inherent ability of skin to respond to mechanical stresses. Small animal veterinarians have long noted the ability of skin to stretch and accommodate to underlying expanding tumors. Inflatable skin expanders can mimic this physiologic process.

During tissue expansion, a variable change is noted in epidermal thickness. Epidermal mitosis temporarily increases following each inflation: the intercellular distance increases and the basal lamina displays increased undulation. The dermis displays a variable decrease in thickness during expansion. Large, compact bundles of collagen fibers are oriented in an orderly fashion over the implant surface, forming a dense, fibrous capsule (Plate 33).

The subcutaneous fat decreases. Skeletal muscle above or below the expander can undergo pressure atrophy without loss of function. Initially, this muscle has the capability of regaining mass after implant removal. A transient neuropraxia may be noted in nerves immediately adjacent to the expander.

Interestingly, the vascular supply to the overlying skin and compressed musculature remains intact. Cir-

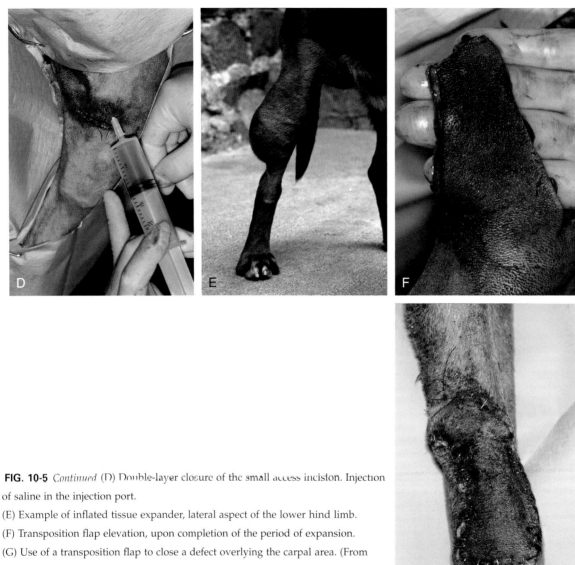

FIG. 10-5 *Continued* (D) Double-layer closure of the small access incision. Injection of saline in the injection port.

(E) Example of inflated tissue expander, lateral aspect of the lower hind limb.

(F) Transposition flap elevation, upon completion of the period of expansion.

(G) Use of a transposition flap to close a defect overlying the carpal area. (From Spodnick G, Pavletic MM. 1993. Controlled skin expansion to mobilized skin in the distal extremities. *Vet Surg* 22:436.)

culation to the skin demonstrates enhancement similar to what is seen with delayed flap procedures. Experimental studies indicate a greater viability of "expansion" flaps compared to acutely raised and delayed flaps. Skin expanders are best employed for secondary reconstructive surgery rather than for acute post-trauma construction. Skin showing irritation prior to surgery is best avoided in tissue expansion. Skin expanders have potential use in small animals, particularly for lower extremity defects in dogs (Fig. 10-5).

Despite the relative simplicity of their use, tissue expanders have failed to gain popularity in veterinary medicine. This is likely due to the cost of the implants and the general lack of familiarity with their use by veterinarians. Moreover, there are a variety of reconstructive techniques that can be used in place of this device. Nonetheless, it can be a valuable option in closing some of the more challenging extremity wounds occasionally encountered.

Suggested Readings

Johnston D. 1990. Tissue expanders. *Vet Clin No Am* 20:227–234.

Keller WG, Aron DN, Rakich PM, et al. 1994. Rapid tissue expansion for the development of rotational skin flaps in the distal portion of the hindlimb of dogs: an experimental study. *Vet Surg* 23:31–39.

Liang MD, Briggs P, Heckler FR, et al. 1988. Presuturing: a new technique for closing large skin defects: clinical and experimental studies. *Plast Reconstr Surg* 81:694–702.

Pavletic MM. 2000. Use of an external skin-stretching device for wound closure in dogs and cats. *J Am Vet Med Assoc* 217(3):350–354.

Spodnick G, Pavletic MM. 1993. Controlled skin expansion to mobilize skin in the distal extremities of dogs. *Vet Surg* 22:436–443.

Plate 30   **Presuturing Technique**

DESCRIPTION

The presuturing technique employs large mattress sutures to stretch skin on opposing sides of an elective surgical site prior to the actual procedure. Skin can stretch by the processes of mechanical creep and stress relaxation when continuous tension is applied to the skin over time. Research in a swine model, and subsequent clinical studies in humans, indicate that this technique can reduce skin tension and thereby facilitate wound closure within 24 hours after application.

SURGICAL TECHNIQUE

(A) In this illustration, the presuturing technique will be used to reduce skin tension prior to surgical removal of this cutaneous lesion. Using reverse cutting needles, 0 or 00 suture materials may be used for presuturing. Lidocaine anesthetic blocks, sedation, or light anesthesia are used to reduce patient discomfort during suture placement. Vertical mattress suture "bites" are applied approximately 3–5 cm from the proposed borders of resection. The number of sutures employed will vary with the length of the proposed surgical site. Application is performed 24 hours prior to surgery.

(B) As the sutures are tied, the skin around the immediate surgical area is placed under tension.

(C) A cross-sectional view of the presutured area. Imbrication of the skin places tension on the adjacent skin.

COMMENTS

The presuturing technique underscores the potential for skin to deform or stretch beyond the boundaries of its inherent elasticity. Presuturing is effective only in those body regions where elastic skin is somewhat limited, such as the extremities. As such, its practical use is limited to smaller skin defects. Presuturing will not be effective or even necessary in most body regions where elastic or redundant skin is present.

Skin stretchers (Plate 32) can be a more effective substitute for the presuturing technique described above. The adjustable cables permit the veterinarian to maintain moderate to high levels of skin tension continuously to enhance gains in skin mobilization for successful wound closure. The presuturing technique is not adjustable and its stretching effects are limited to the skin immediately adjacent to the site of suture placement. Nonetheless, this simple, economical preoperative stretching technique can be useful in some wound closure situations.

Plate 30

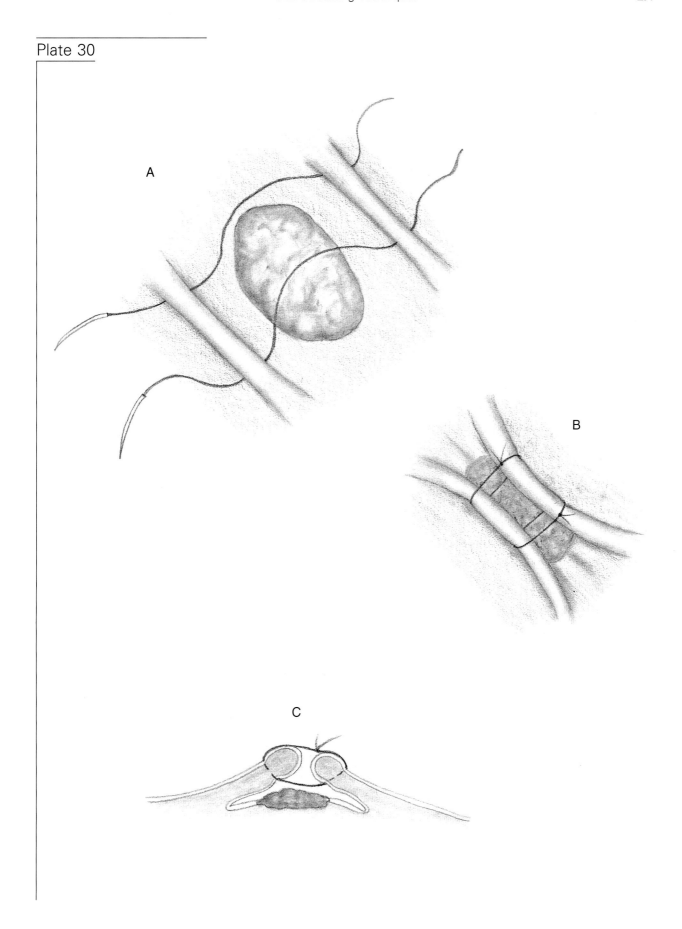

A

B

C

| Plate 31 | **Application of Skin Stretchers** |

DESCRIPTION

Skin under the continuous application of tension (load) over time can deform beyond its natural or inherent extensibility by the processes of mechanical creep and stress relaxation. Unlike the presuturing technique (Plate 30), the skin stretchers developed by the author employ externally applied adhesive pads. Elastic cables are attached to cutaneous pads that have been placed on opposing sides of a surgical site. The surgeon can adjust the elastic force applied to the skin to maintain a continuous high-tension load in order to accelerate skin stretching or deformation. In 24–96 hours the mobilized or recruited skin is used to close the cutaneous defect.

SURGICAL TECHNIQUE

(A) Illustration of a skin wound. The fur has been liberally clipped around the area. Surgical soap and water are used to remove cutaneous oils and debris. Isopropyl alcohol can be used to swab the skin to further clean the skin and facilitate drying. The skin must be completely dry before skin pad application. A marking pen can be used to mark the proposed sites of pad application.

(B) The hooked pads can be applied to the skin after peeling off the protective tab. However, a commercially available cyanoacrylate glue is best applied to enhance its adherence to the skin in the dog and cat. A thin layer of cyanoacrylate glue is spread onto the base of the pad and applied immediately to the designated skin site.

(C) Note the long axis of the rectangular pads have been placed parallel to the direction of tension in order to minimize the potential for pad separation or displacement. Pads are placed approximately 10–20 cm from the wound margins. An additional row or tier of pads can also be applied outside this suggested zone, if additional skin recruitment is required or feasible (e.g., the trunk). In this illustration, one elastic cable has been attached to paired pads. A small protective bandage has been placed over the wound surface.

(D) Completion of cable application. A mild amount of tension is applied to each cable. The tension then is increased every 6 to 8 hours as the skin stretches. One end of the elastic cable is disengaged from a skin pad, stretched, and recoupled to the skin pad, as illustrated.

(E) At the completion of the procedure (24–96 hours), skin pads can be peeled off the skin. Nail polish remover can be used to facilitate their separation (although the author has found this to be unnecessary). Manual removal of the pads normally is performed, although this maneuver may strip the outer corneal layer of the skin. (This outer epithelial layer reforms rapidly.) In this example, all four sides of this rectangular wound were advanced to accomplish closure. Note that two pads and a short segment of stretcher cable were reapplied postsurgically in order to reduce incisional tension.

COMMENTS

As a general observation, the greatest gains in skin mobilization occur by 72–96 hours. Occasionally, skin pads will separate from the skin, necessitating their reapplication with additional adhesive. The greatest gains in skin stretching are in body regions where it is possible to mobilize large surface areas, both local and distant to the surgical site. The neck and trunk are most amenable to effective use of skin stretchers. Skin stretchers are least effective in the lower extremities. The amount of undermining required, at the time of wound closure, usually is minimal after the use of skin stretchers. As noted, skin stretchers also can be used to reduce incisional tension postoperatively for a few (3–5) additional days. In Plate 32, skin stretchers are used to stretch skin prior to elective surgical procedures to facilitate closure.

Plate 31

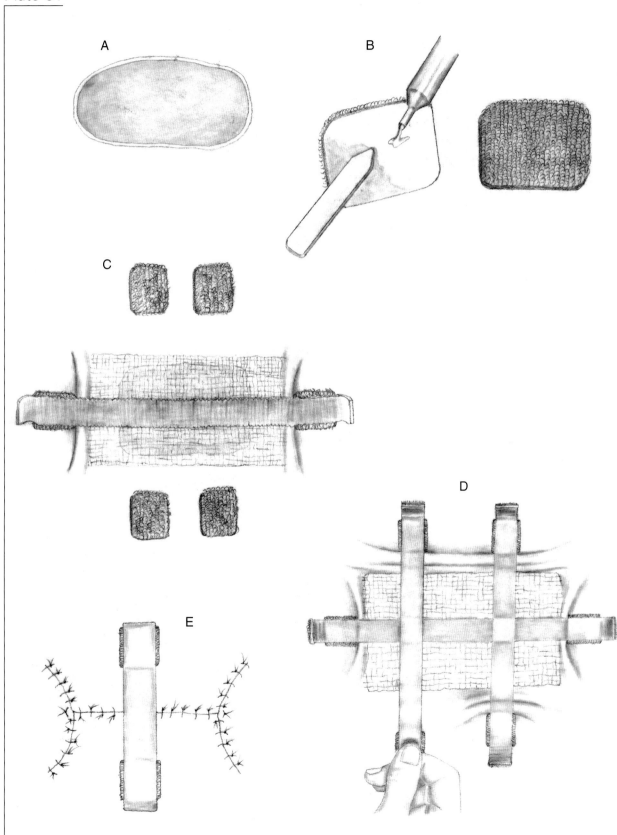

Plate 32	**Skin Stretcher Substitution for Presuturing**

DESCRIPTION

Skin stretchers can be quite effective in recruiting skin prior to elective surgical procedures. This is particularly true when removing diseased skin, including neoplasms.

SURGICAL TECHNIQUES

(A) In this example, a large neoplasm overlying the ilium requires removal. Skin stretcher pads have been applied around the lesion.

(B) Dorsal view of the stretcher pads.

(C) Elastic cables cross over to the opposing (paired) pads.

(D) Dorsal and lateral views of the elastic cables applied under moderate tension. Cable tension is increased every 6–8 hours for 24–96 hours before surgery. Skin pads are stripped off the patient after anesthetic induction.

(E) After resection of the mass, the wound is closed using an intradermal suture pattern followed by simple interrupted sutures. Vertical mattress sutures can be alternated with a simple interrupted pattern if tension is present at a given point of wound closure. Skin stretchers can be used to further offset skin tension as previously noted (Plate 24). A closed vacuum drainage system may be employed to control dead space.

COMMENTS

Skin mobilization is optimal over the neck and trunk of the dog and cat. Stretchers are least effective in the lower extremities, where minimal loose skin is available. Skin stretchers can be very useful to prestretch the thoracic and abdominal skin prior to unilateral or bilateral chain mastectomies.

Plate 32

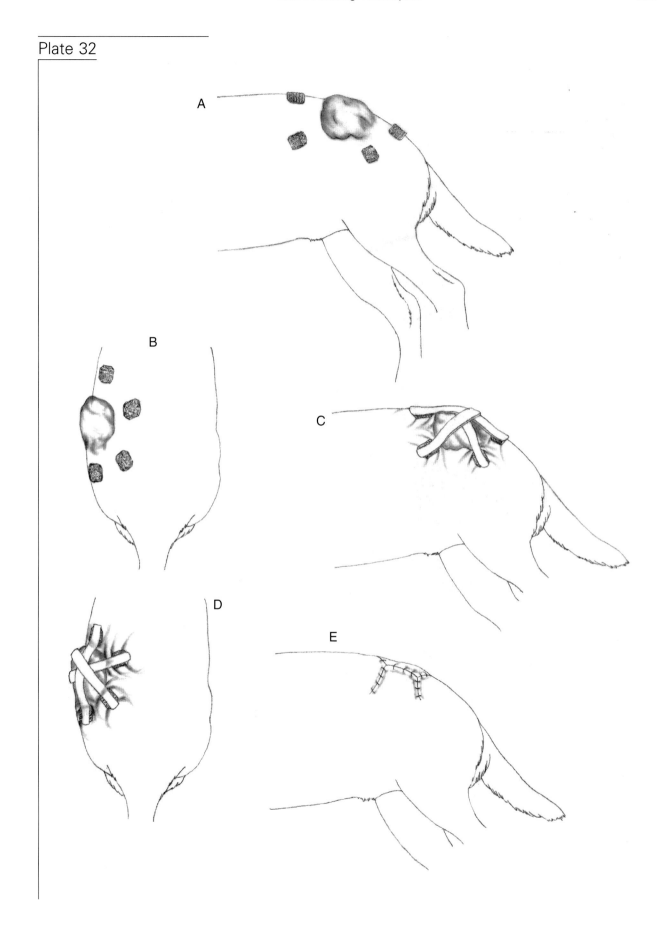

Plate 33   **Skin Expanders**

DESCRIPTION

Skin expanders are inflatable devices comprised of an expandable silicone elastomer bag, silicone connecting tube, and a self-sealing inflation reservoir that serves as an injection port. There are, however, other tissue expanders designed with an injection port incorporated in the reservoir. Self-inflating tissue expanders also have been used in humans. The basic unit described in this plate is the most practical design for veterinary patients. Controlled inflation of this device is capable of creating sufficient donor tissue to elevate an advancement of transposition flap to close an adjacent skin defect (traumatic or surgically induced).

SURGICAL TECHNIQUE

(A) In this example, a skin incision is made for the insertion of a 100-cc tissue expander (length: 6.0 cm; width: 4.7 cm; height: 5.3 cm; Mentor Corporation, Goleta, CA) in a medium-sized dog. Metzenbaum scissors are used to develop a pocket of sufficient size to accommodate the collapsed expander. Note the access incision is positioned for eventual incorporation into the flap incision. The incision is not affected by the inflated expander.

(B) The index finger is inserted into the pocket to assess its size and feel for fascial bands that require division.

(C) The collapsed expander bag is partially folded and moistened with sterile saline to facilitate its insertion. The thick silastic base is positioned against the limb. The connecting tube is cut centrally and trimmed to the appropriate length for placement of the inflation reservoir in a subcutaneous pocket dorsal to the incision. The ends of the connecting tube are joined by a metallic connecting insert. Two small 3-0 monofilament nonabsorbable ligatures are used to secure the tube ends from leakage or separation. Care is taken to avoid creation of a large pocket that may cause the components of the expander to migrate. The incision is closed with a subcuticular suture pattern and skin sutures.

(D) View of the tissue expander during expansion. A 23- to 25-gauge hypodermic needle is inserted into the inflation reservoir at an angle. A butterfly needle may be used for injection to compensate for patient movement. Sterile saline is injected. From the author's research using 100-ml expanders, initial expansion can be instituted beginning 48 hours after insertion. Injection rates of 10–15 ml every 2 days are equally successful. Flap elevation is initiated 48 hours after the last injection.

(E) Upon completion of expansion, the planned skin flap is incised beginning at the level of the original skin incision. Care is taken to avoid damaging the expander during its removal. The tube connector is separated to drain the saline from the reservoir, and the unit is withdrawn. In this case, a single pedicle advancement flap is being created to cover the craniomedial skin defect created by the simultaneous removal of diseased skin. In some cases, a distally based transposition flap can be created for lower limb defects (inset). (See Plate 36.) In this example, a dorsally based transposition flap is inadvisable since the access incision would be at the base of the flap, interfering with normal cutaneous circulation.

COMMENTS

There are a variety of standard expanders of variable sizes and shapes for surgical implantation. Specialized designs can be ordered from manufacturers. At present, the cost of these implants is high and can amount to several hundred dollars, depending on the size and design of the expander. High cost and a lack of familiarity with these devices have discouraged some veterinarians from using them. It must be kept in mind that they can be autoclaved and reused multiple times with appropriate care.

Skin expanders require a degree of skin laxity to accommodate the mass of the collapsed unit. For skin expanders to be effective, implants must be of sufficient size to exert their stretching effect on the overlying skin. The loose elastic skin of the neck and trunk would preclude the need and effective use of skin

Plate 33

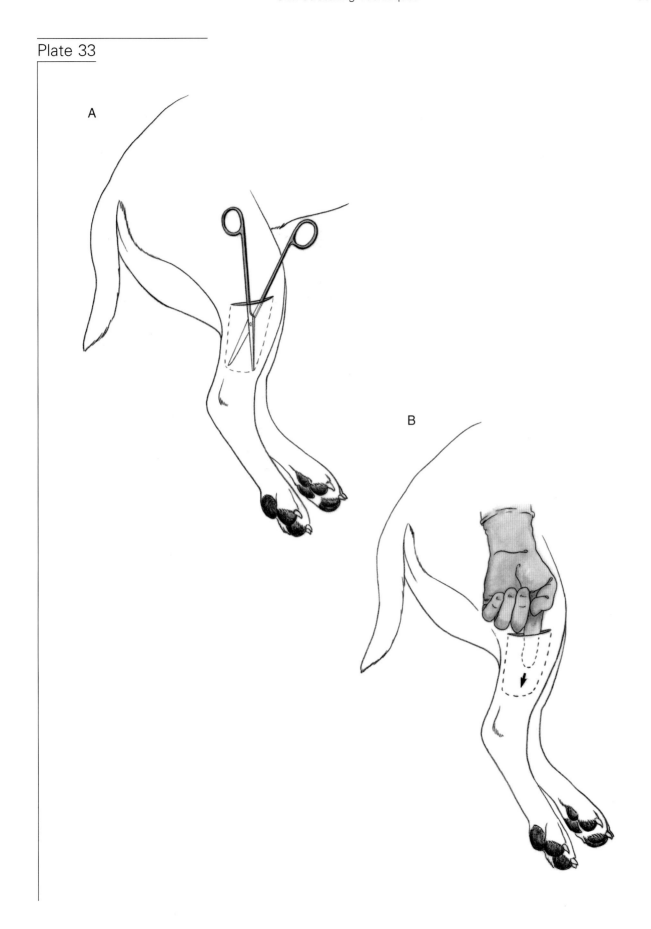

A

B

Plate 33

(Continued)

expanders in most cases. The greatest clinical potential for skin expanders is in moderate-sized defects of the middle to lower extremities, where primary closure is not feasible and alternate closure options are less satisfactory.

It is unrealistic to expect a skin expander to be effectively employed for large defects of the extremity. They do not permit one-stage surgical reconstruction and are best used for secondary restorative procedures rather than in acute traumatic injuries.

The size of the implant generally is determined by the size of the defect. The flat base of the implant generally corresponds to the net gain expected. Not all body regions, however, can accommodate a skin expander of the size required to achieve coverage. It is possible to select two or more small expanders to accomplish this goal. Skin expanders can be hyperinflated beyond their designated volume capacity by 20%–25% for additional tissue gains. The 100-cc expander used in medium-sized dogs, placed in the mid- to lower tibial and radial region, were very effective experimentally. It would be possible to employ two such expanders in some situations where additional skin is desirable.

Variable rates of inflation have been used in human surgery. Although a slow rate of expansion may be preferable in elective reconstruction surgical procedures where time is not critical, other situations demand more rapid rates of expansion. The author's research demonstrated that 100-cc expanders can be inflated with equal efficacy within 2 weeks, using an alternate-day injection schedule. We elected not to partially inflate the expander upon initial implantation although it can be performed to slightly stretch loose skin overlying the implant, potentially saving 2 days. However, a more cautious rate would be indicated in delicate cutaneous tissues, especially those previously compromised by trauma. Their use in previously irradiated tissues is best avoided.

Owners can be trained to inject the expander or the patient can be handled on an outpatient basis. Clinical guidelines for expansion rates in humans include change in skin coloration (ischemia or cyanosis) and patient discomfort. In the author's study, no patient displayed discomfort during injection. Skin blanching or cyanosis was not noted. Unimpeded hair growth of the expanded skin, compared to the regional skin, suggested skin circulation and viability were not compromised throughout the procedure.

The advancement flap design is simple to execute if the expander can be satisfactorily positioned adjacent to the recipient area. When used for advancement as illustrated, at least one-third of the circumference must be preserved to provide an adequate base to support circulation to the flap. The transposition flap can be rotated into lower extremity defects, thus enabling the surgeon to develop a donor source proximal to the recipient area. As noted, the initial skin incision used for insertion of the implant should not be incorporated into the base of the skin flap. The author has seen circulatory compromise in flaps that incorporated a linear scar perpendicular to the length of the flap body.

Complications noted with skin expanders include dehiscence, implant extrusion, seroma, infection, implant failure (leakage), and skin necrosis. A thick, fibrous capsule forms around the implant, which reduces the pliability of the flap created. Skin expanders take time to develop and require two surgeries to complete flap transfer. In most situations, skin flaps and free grafts can close wounds very effectively and more economically than skin expanders (at least with respect to their initial cost). Moreover, large skin defects necessarily require flap or grafting procedures. Skin expanders do enable the surgeon to create full-thickness donor skin of similar color, hair growth, and texture adjacent to a defect where no flap can be otherwise employed. They have the greatest potential for some defects involving the extremities (especially distal) and perhaps the rostral facial area. Skin expanders clearly have a place in veterinary surgery, although its niche is smaller than for human patients.

Plate 33

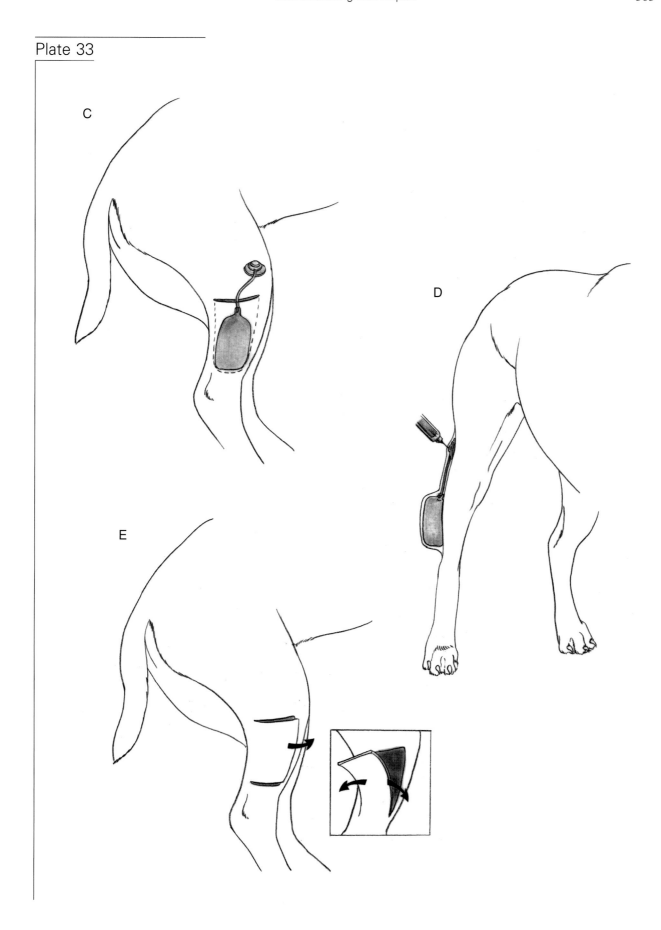

C

D

E

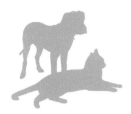

Local Flaps

INTRODUCTION

A pedicle graft or skin flap is a partially detached segment of skin and subcutaneous tissue: the base or pedicle of the flap maintains circulation to the skin during its elevation and transfer to a recipient location. Pedicle grafts developed adjacent to the recipient bed are termed local flaps. They represent one of the most practical methods of closing defects that cannot be approximated by simple undermining and suturing. The effective use of these flaps usually depends on forming a flap in a neighboring area in which loose, elastic skin prevails. Any secondary defect created by the transfer of the flap to the defect can be closed directly. Local flaps are both simple and economical to perform. They are more likely to maintain a similar pattern of hair growth and color than distant flaps. Local flaps have been effectively used to close defects in dogs, cats, birds, and other species. The 90-degree transposition flap is particularly useful in this context.

Local flaps are classified according to their method of transfer: flaps that advance in a forward direction are *advancement flaps* and those that rotate or pivot into position are *rotating flaps*. Most local flaps are based over the subdermal plexus circulation unless a direct cutaneous artery and vein are fortuitously included in the base of the flap.

Ideal donor areas have ample skin available to elevate a flap without creating a secondary defect (donor bed) unamenable to simple closure. Donor sites subject to excessive motion and stress should be avoided whenever possible, as they are prone to wound dehiscence or can compromise local mobility. Exceptions include cases in which closure of a wound for the protection of exposed structures has priority over the creation of a secondary defect. The secondary defect, in turn, can be closed by undermining and primary closure, a second flap, a free graft, or healing by second intention.

Local flap procedures begin with assessment of lines of greatest versus least tension. Local flaps are designed to advance or rotate into place. An advancement (sliding) flap is developed parallel to lines of *least* tension, to facilitate its forward stretch over the wound. A 90-degree transposition flap is aligned parallel to the lines of greatest tension, to obtain the bulk of the flap required to cover the defect. When the transposition flap is rotated into place, the donor site can be closed directly because minimal tension lines are perpendicular to the suture line.

Factors that maximize the circulation to the pedicle graft should be considered during flap planning. Large flaps should include a direct cutaneous artery and vein whenever possible. Unfortunately, the consistent development of axial pattern flaps requires predictable anatomical landmarks and proper patient positioning. When possible, it may be beneficial to position the base of local flaps in the direction of known, direct cutaneous vessels arborizing in their general vicinity, thus improving the perfusion pressure to the pedicle graft.

Increasing the width of a pedicle graft does *not* increase its total surviving length. Flaps created under the same conditions of blood supply survive to the same length regardless of flap width. Increasing the width of the pedicle graft only permits the chance of including direct cutaneous vessels in the flap. Moreover, the cutaneous circulation differs regionally, and a set length/width ratio is not applicable. Narrowing of a pedicle can reduce blood perfusion to the body of the flap and increase the likelihood of necrosis. Procedures that narrow the pedicle, such as the back-cut technique (counterincisions) are best avoided. Axial pattern flaps are an exception to this rule, as long as the direct cutaneous artery and vein are preserved. Creating unduly long subdermal plexus flaps also can result in necrosis. As a rule, the author recommends the following:

1. Create flaps with a base slightly wider than its body to avoid inadvertent narrowing of the pedicle.

2. Limit flaps to the size required to cover the recipient bed without undue tension.

Two or more small flaps may be preferable to a single, large pedicle graft whose effective circulation at the end of the flap may be questionable.

> A key point in skin flap survival is to keep the length of a skin flap to a minimum. In other words, *keep the flap as short as possible* to close a given wound without excessive tension.

The surgeon should consider the use of bipedicled flaps when longer flaps are required. A "delay procedure" should be considered when there is a concern regarding the flap's circulation and survival if transferred in a single stage to the recipient site. Careful planning and meticulous, atraumatic surgical technique are necessary to prevent excessive tension, kinking, and circulatory compromise to the flap.

All measurements of the defect and proposed flap are recorded in centimeters. As a precaution, a cloth or foam rubber template of the flap can be made to represent the proposed dimensions of the defect and the additional skin required for the flap to reach the recipient bed from the proposed donor site. The flap template is positioned over the defect, and the base of the flap model is held in a fixed position as the model is transferred to the proposed donor site. This procedure is repeated until the template is an accurate model for successful flap transfer. The flap is drawn on the skin with a marking pen to provide reference lines for the skin incision. Once one becomes familiar with certain flap techniques, the measurements can be drawn directly on the skin without resorting to the templates.

Atraumatic surgical technique is essential to the successful execution of local flaps. Their comparatively limited blood supply from the subdermal plexus requires greater care in their development and transfer. Skin hooks and Adson-Brown forceps are best used to manipulate the skin flaps. In general, flaps should be kept as short as possible in order to assure optimal perfusion to the distant edge.

ADVANCEMENT FLAPS

The single pedicle advancement flap, bipedicle advancement flap, and the V-Y advancement flap are examples of pedicle grafts moved forward into a wound without lateral movement. The single pedicle advancement flap (sliding flap) is probably the most common local flap employed in veterinary medicine because of its simple design and lack of a secondary defect requiring closure (Fig 11-1). Paired single-pedicle advancement flaps can be employed to close square or rectangular defects, resulting in an H closure design (H-plasty). (See Plate 34.) V-Y advancement is a triangular, single pedicle advancement technique primarily employed to relieve tissue tension; it has limited efficacy in wound closure.

The bipedicle advancement flap is constructed by making a skin incision parallel to the long axis of a defect, with a flap width generally equal to the width of the defect. (See Plate 35.) The undermined skin segment is advanced into the recipient bed. The bipedicle advancement flap has the advantage of two sources of circulation to maintain a longer flap body. The relaxing (relief or release) incision used to aid in wound closure is a bipedicle advancement flap by design (Fig 11-2). (See Plate 20.)

It must be noted that advancement flaps, despite their simple design and application, have limitations that preclude their routine use. The advancement flap primarily relies upon wound coverage by *stretching* over the defect. As a result, an opposing elastic retraction occurs along the length of the flap. Excessive retraction can promote dehiscence or distortion of the

distant wound margin. This must be anticipated before a single pedicle advancement flap is employed in cases in which postoperative tension could distort neighboring structures (e.g., eyelid margins). In these areas, a transposition flap would be a better option.

> The single pedicle advancement flap (SPAF) primarily closes wounds by stretching over the defect. Postoperatively, the collagen fibers will exert a traction force that has the potential to distort the recipient bed. The bottom line is use this flap with caution around areas where mild retraction of the flap could distort function. *This problem is most commonly noted when a SPAF is elevated perpendicular to the eyelid margin to close a problematic cutaneous eyelid defect. Consider the use of a 90 degree transposition flap in its place.*

ROTATING (PIVOTING) FLAPS

Rotation flaps, transposition flaps, and interpolation flaps are the three basic flaps that rotate on a pivot point. The rotation flap is a semicircular flap that rotates into the adjacent recipient bed (see Plate 39). Single or paired flaps can be employed to close triangular defects. As a general rule, no secondary defect is created with the rotation flap in the dog or cat .

The transposition flap is a rectangular pedicle graft commonly rotated within 90 degrees of the wound's axis. (See Plates 36 and 37.) The transposition flap is the most useful of the rotating flaps (Figs. 11-3 through 11-9). Z-plasty, a modification of the transposition flap, is discussed in Chapter 9. A modification of the transposition flap technique is exemplified by the forelimb fold flap (see Plate 40).

> The 90-degree transposition skin flap is by far the most useful flap technique available to close a variety of the small- to moderate-sized problematic wounds.

The interpolation flap is a rectangular flap rotated into a nearby, but not immediately adjacent, defect. (See Plate 38.) A portion of the flap must pass over the skin between the donor and recipient beds. The exposed subcutaneous surface of this flap segment is usually left

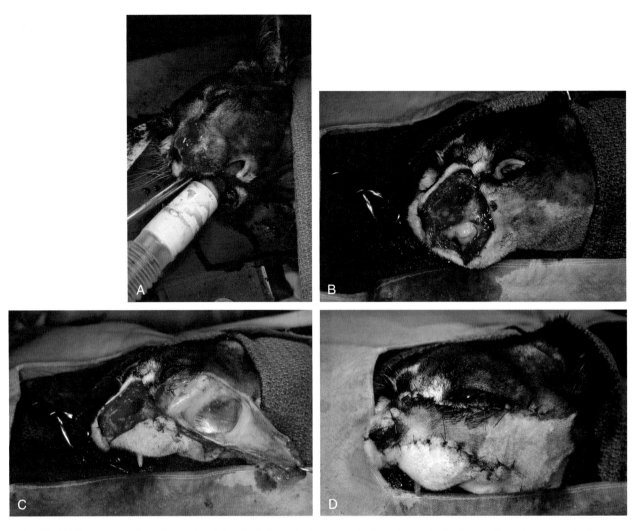

FIG. 11-1 (A) Squamous cell carcinoma involving the left nasal planum and adjacent skin. (B) Wide resection of the mass, including underlying bone. (C) Closure of lower gingival-labial mucosal defect. Staged elevation of a single pedicle advancement flap below the platysma muscle layer. (D) Closure of this wound, with the advancement flap, underscores the considerable cutaneous elastic advancement present in most feline patients.

FIG. 11-2 (A) Bipedicle advancement flap used to cover a large skin defect overlying the calcaneus. A Schroeder-Thomas splint was used to immobilize the tarsal area until incisional healing was complete. (B) A release incision is a bipedicle advancement flap by design. Note that the flap provides durable full-thickness skin coverage over this potentially problematic bony prominence. The exposed lateral (donor area) and medial granulation beds quickly healed by second intention.

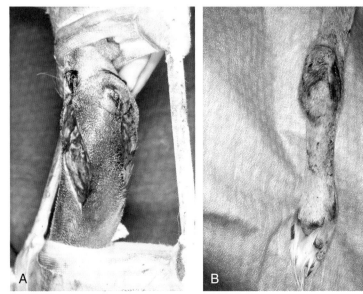

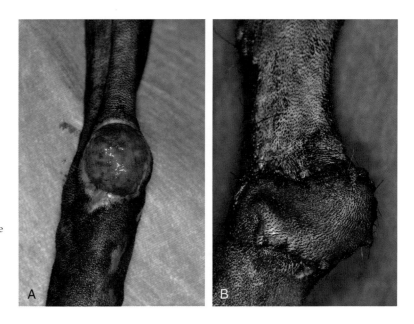

FIG. 11-3 (A) Skin loss over the calcaneus in a Doberman. Skin loss of this magnitude over a bony prominence is unlikely to heal by second intention without surgical intervention. (B) Sufficient circumferential skin was available to facilitate closure of this defect, using a 90-degree transposition skin flap. The donor area closed primarily. See Figure 11-2 as an alternative option, depending on the availability of loose, elastic skin.

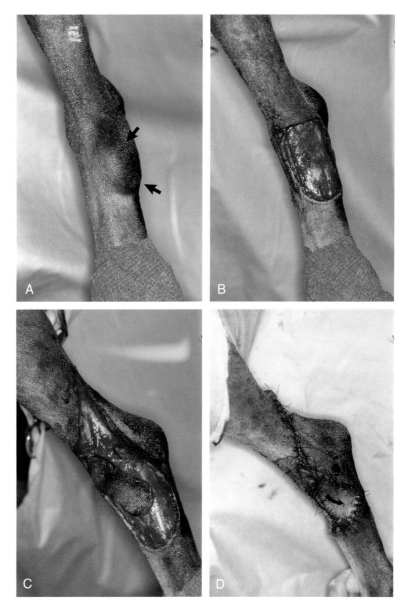

FIG. 11-4 (A) Cutaneous neoplasm involving the distal left tibiotarsal area. (B) Excision of the mass. (C) Rotation of a 90-degree transposition flap. (D) Closure of the donor and recipient beds. Developed after careful measurement, the transposition flap can be effectively employed for many of the smaller- to moderate-sized defects of the limbs.

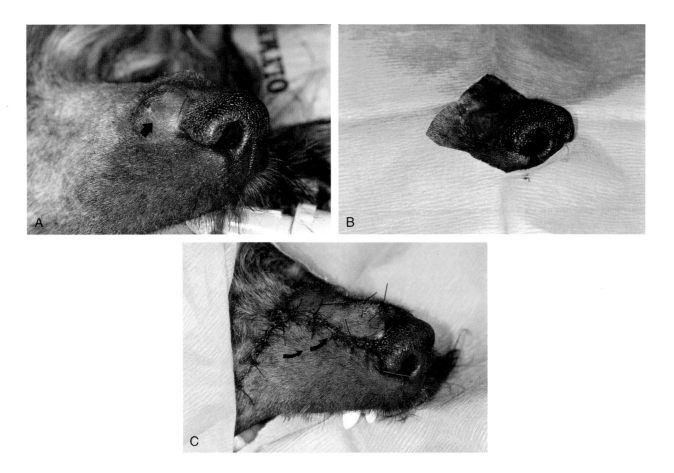

FIG. 11-5 (A) Benign neoplasm involving the right nasal region. (B) Resection of the tumor. (C) Closure with a 90-degree transposition flap. Note that skin laxity of the muzzle is at a right angle to the axis of the skull. The 90-degree transposition flap is ideally suited to closing smaller problematic defects in this general region.

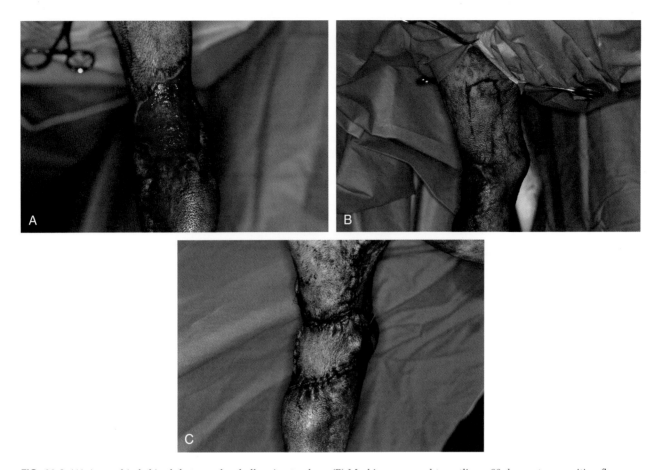

FIG. 11-6 (A) Antecubital skin defects can be challenging to close. (B) Marking pen used to outline a 90-degree transposition flap, parallel to the long axis of the limb. (C) Successful closure. An Elizabethan collar was used to prevent licking. Severe exercise restriction was imposed until suture removal 2 weeks later.

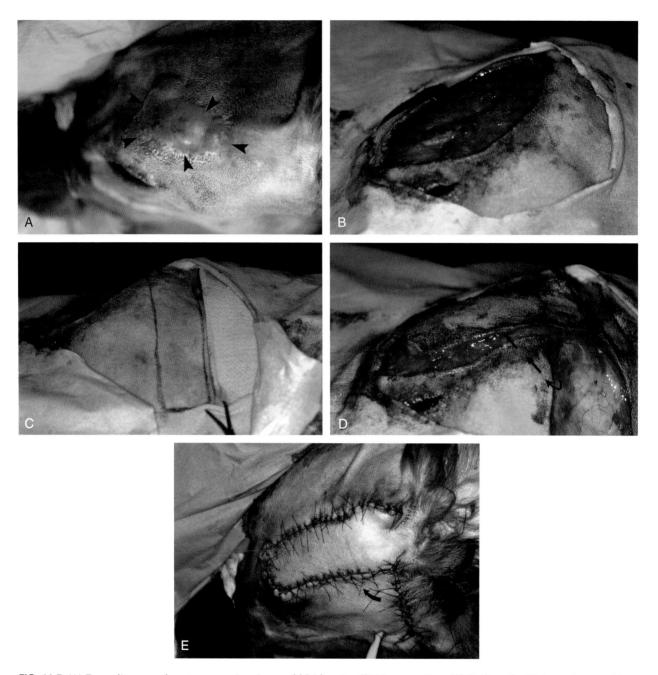

FIG. 11-7 (A) Expanding granulomatous mass in a 1-year-old Irish setter. (B) Mass resection. (C) Outline of a 90-degree transposition flap along the left lateral facial area. (D) Rotating the flap into position. Based on local tissue elasticity, the skin flap could be shortened 2 cm to help assure complete flap survival. (E) Closure was achieved without distorting the function of the upper eyelid. Due to the surgical dead space, a drain is important to prevent seroma formation.

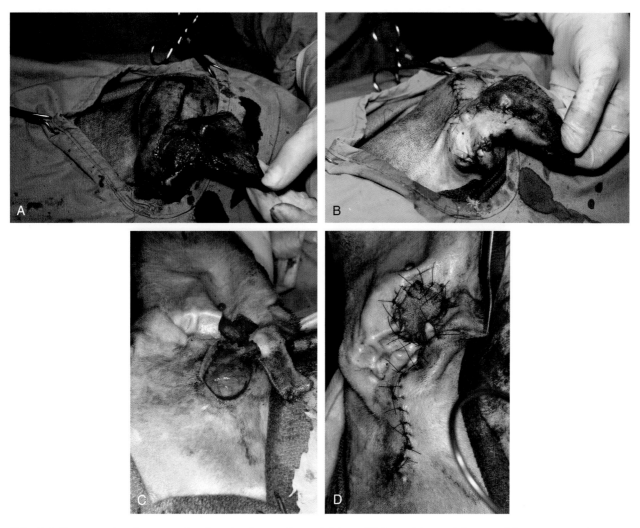

FIG. 11-8 Two examples of transposition flaps for closure of pinnal defects. (A) Loss of the caudal aspect of the pinna secondary to a bite wound in a German shepherd. Note the incisional outline of the flap. (B) Completion of closure. Note the effectiveness of this simple flap technique to reconstruct the pinna. (C) Resection of a small mast cell tumor, including the underlying cartilage proximal to the external ear canal. Elevation of a transposition flap. (D) Successful closure (see Plate 132).

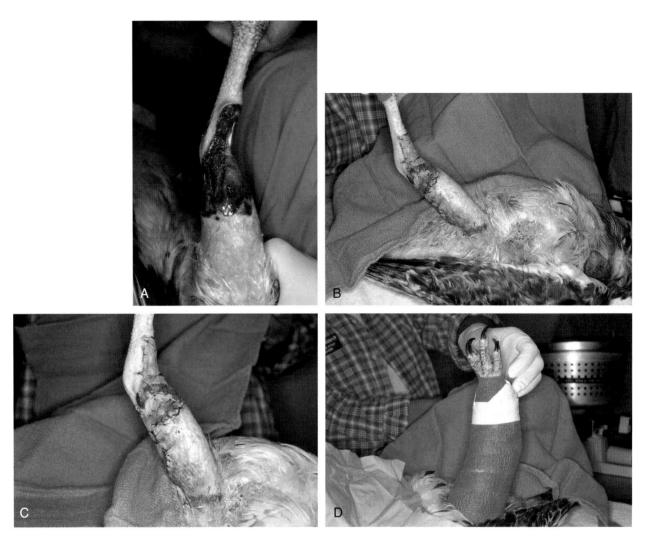

FIG. 11-9 (A) Limb wound in a red-tailed hawk. Open wound management was performed until a healthy granulation bed formed.

(B) Closure of the wound was accomplished with a 90-degree transposition flap (upper area) and a full-thickness free graft (lower area). The free graft was harvested from the left lateral thorax.

(C) Complete survival of the graft and flap. The small remaining defect healed by second intention healing.

(D) The grafted leg was protected with a partial fiberglass cast. The rehabilitated hawk was later released. Note how flap and graft techniques are applicable to a variety of species.

open, although it may be covered temporarily with a free graft. This redundant portion of the flap is later excised once healing onto the recipient defect is complete. A second option is the use of a bridge incision discussed in Chapter 13, Plate 55. Interpolation flaps are uncommonly employed in veterinary medicine, although this general design is employed in tubed flaps and some axial pattern flap techniques.

Think local flap first before considering more elaborate flap techniques. For example, a dorsal cranial defect can be closed by a caudal auricular axial pattern flap (CAAPF). Half the length of the CAAPF is needed simply to traverse the area between the base of the flap and the caudal border of the defect. In contrast, a smaller transposition flap developed adjacent to the pinna can cover the defect completely. The transposition flap is smaller, easier to elevate, and the time associated with skin closure is less.

Suggested Readings

Hunt GB. 1995. Skin-fold advancement flaps for closing large sternal and inguinal wounds in cats and dogs. *Vet Surg* 24:172–175.

Hunt GB, Tisdall PLC, Liptak JM, et al. 2001. Skin-fold advancement flaps for closing large proximal limb and trunk defects in dogs and cats. *Vet Surg* 30:440–448.

Pavletic MM. 1990. Skin flaps in reconstructive surgery. *Vet Clin No Am* 20:81–103.

Pavletic MM. 1994. Surgery of the skin and management of wounds. In: Sherding RD, ed. *The Cat: Diseases and Clinical Management*, 2nd ed., 1969–1997. New York: Churchill Livingstone.

Pavletic MM. 1998. Skin. In: Bojrab MJ, ed. *Current Techniques in Small Animal Surgery*, 4th ed. Philadelphia, PA: Lea and Febiger.

Pavletic MM. 2003. Pedicle grafts. In: Slatter DH, ed. *Textbook of Small Animal Surgery*, 3rd ed., 292–321. Philadelphia, PA: WB Saunders.

Stanley BJ, Read RA, Egar CE, et al. 1991. Bilateral rotation flaps for the treatment of chronic nasal dermatitis in four dogs. *J Am Anim Hosp Assoc* 27:295–299.

Plate 34 **Single Pedicle Advancement Flap**

DESCRIPTION

The single pedicle advancement flap is the simplest of the local flaps by design. Flap width equals the width of the defect; flap length is dictated by the amount required to stretch and advance the flap into the defect without excessive tension.

SURGICAL TECHNIQUE

(A) The skin is gently grasped to assess regional skin tension. The index finger is used to push the skin toward the center of the defect to determine final flap orientation.

(B) Two slightly *diverging* skin incisions are made equal to the width of the defect in a staged fashion. The flap is carefully undermined and the skin progressively incised until the flap is sufficiently mobile to stretch over the defect.

(C) The flap is sutured into position to complete the transfer. Half-buried horizontal mattress sutures are placed in the corners of the flap to minimize circulatory compromise to the flap corners.

(D) An alternate technique is to use two single pedicle advancement flaps on each side of the wound. This technique is called H-plasty based on the resulting H-shaped closure achieved.

COMMENTS

Although the single pedicle advancement flap is a simple flap technique to master, it has significant limitations dictated by the availability of loose elastic skin immediately adjacent to the defect. The single pedicle advancement flap does not bring additional "loose" skin to the wound site; successful closure requires the flap to stretch over the defect. There is a tendency for the advancement flap to retract due to the inherent elastic nature of the skin. This must be anticipated before it is used in areas where postoperative tension can distort neighboring structures (e.g., eyelid). Because the flap is supplied by the subdermal plexus, flap length should be kept to a minimum. H-plasty, using two shorter advancement flaps may be advisable to avoid closure with a single, long advancement flap. A disadvantage of H-plasty is the greater amount of suturing required and the formation of two "incisional intersects," which are more prone to dehiscence.

Although the use of Burow's triangles has been advocated to prevent dog-ear formation and to improve flap mobility, they are rarely required to prevent dog-ears or puckers and are minimally effective in relieving tension. Only flaps created with the thicker, less-elastic skin of the neck and back in the dog are likely to benefit most from their use in minimizing dog-ears. Even then, most dog-ears flatten in time without surgical removal.

Plate 34

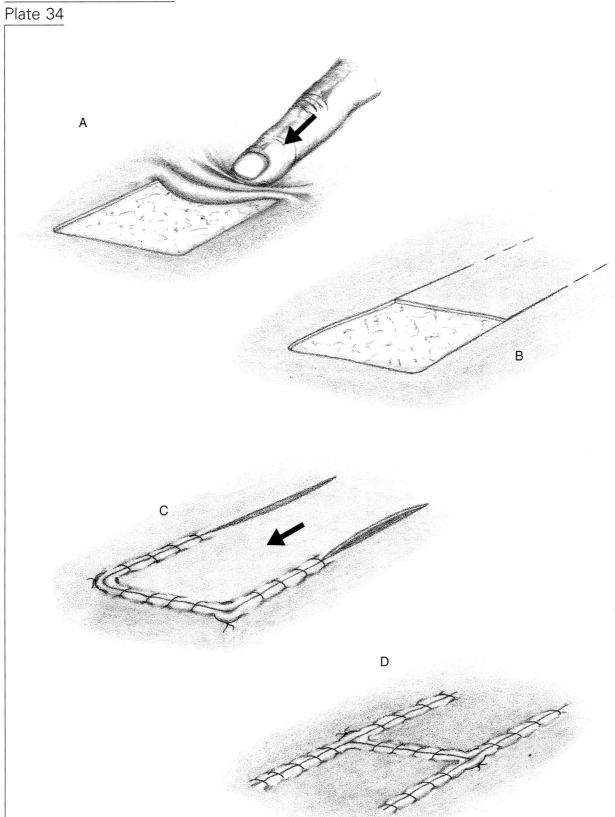

A

B

C

D

Plate 35   **Bipedicle Advancement Flap**

DESCRIPTION

The bipedicle advancement flap is a local flap constructed with two bases or pedicles. Each pedicle is a source of circulation to the body of the flap. The circulation is derived from the subdermal plexus, unless a direct cutaneous artery is incorporated into one pedicle. The bipedicle advancement flap is constructed by making a skin incision parallel to the long axis of the wound, with the flap width generally equal to the width of the defect. The undermined flap is advanced into the recipient bed and sutured. The donor defect created is usually closed primarily.

SURGICAL TECHNIQUE

(A) Flap orientation is determined by the shape and location of the defect in relation to the availability of potential donor sites. It is generally preferable to develop bipedicle advancement flaps parallel to the long axis of the defect, taking advantage of areas where loose elastic skin prevails. Digital manipulation of the skin (arrows) is used to assess skin tension and the feasibility of using this technique.

(B) The proposed flap is drawn onto the skin with a marking pen. Flap width generally equals the width of the wound; flap length equals the length of the defect. However, avoid unusually narrow flaps that may have questionable circulation. Flap advancement (arrow) can be facilitated by curving the outer "relaxing incision" slightly outward so that the convex side of the incision is away from the defect. If the wound is a long-standing granulation bed, it may be necessary to excise the scar-laden inner border of the flap to improve its mobility.

(C) The flap is carefully undermined, advanced over the wound, and sutured into place.

(D) The secondary defect (donor bed) generally is closed by undermining the remaining skin border and closing the wound primarily.

COMMENTS

Bipedicle advancement flaps can be created on each side of a defect. Bilateral application of this flap may be advisable when the wound is too wide for unilateral application of this technique. Although bipedicle advancement flaps have two sources of circulation, the "central body" of the flap can undergo ischemic necrosis if flaps are excessively long. This may be avoided by creating flaps that are as short as possible, minimizing surgical trauma during flap elevation and transfer, and incorporating a direct cutaneous artery and vein into one pedicle when feasible. It may not be possible to close the donor site after flap transfer by undermining when there is a lack of loose, elastic skin available. The area may be left open to heal by second intention, closed with a free graft, or closed with an additional local flap.

The relaxing or release incision employed to relieve tension on a closure site is a bipedicle advancement flap by design. Relaxing incisions are frequently left open to heal by second intention in those cases in which the excessive tension at the closure site is considered more important than the secondary defect created at another location. These secondary defects may be more suitable to contraction and epithelialization when they are in a body area less subject to trauma and have a better blood supply than the closure site in question. (See Plate 20: Relaxing/Release Incisions, in Chapter 9).

Plate 35

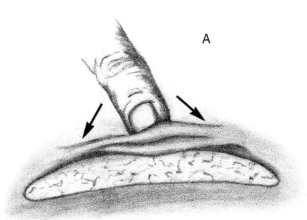

A

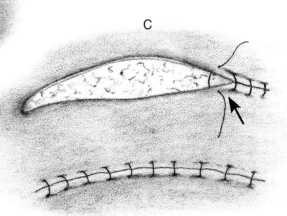

B

C

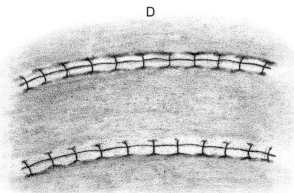

D

Plate 36   **Transposition Flap (90 degrees)**

DESCRIPTION

The transposition flap is a local flap technique with a wide variety of uses. It is a rotating flap that is applicable in most body regions in the dog, cat, and other species, including birds. When it is based on the subdermal plexus as its primary source of circulation, its size is more limited than axial pattern flaps.

SURGICAL TECHNIQUE

(A) Local skin tension is assessed by grasping between the thumb and index finger the skin adjacent to the defect to determine the laxity and elasticity present. The elevated skin fold indicates a transposition flap can be created parallel to this cutaneous ridge without sacrificing the ability to close the donor bed.

(B) The width of the flap, which equals the width of the defect, is measured and marked off along the baseline. This corresponds to the pivot point of the flap. The base or pedicle of the transposition flap is aligned along the lower border of this defect (upper dashed line). The transposition flap is developed within 90 degrees to the long axis of the defect (lower dashed line), depending on the loose, elastic skin available for wound closure.

(C) Flap length is determined by measuring from the pivot point to the most distant portion of the defect. This measurement, in turn, begins at the established baseline. Two parallel lines are drawn using the measured length dimension.

Plate 36

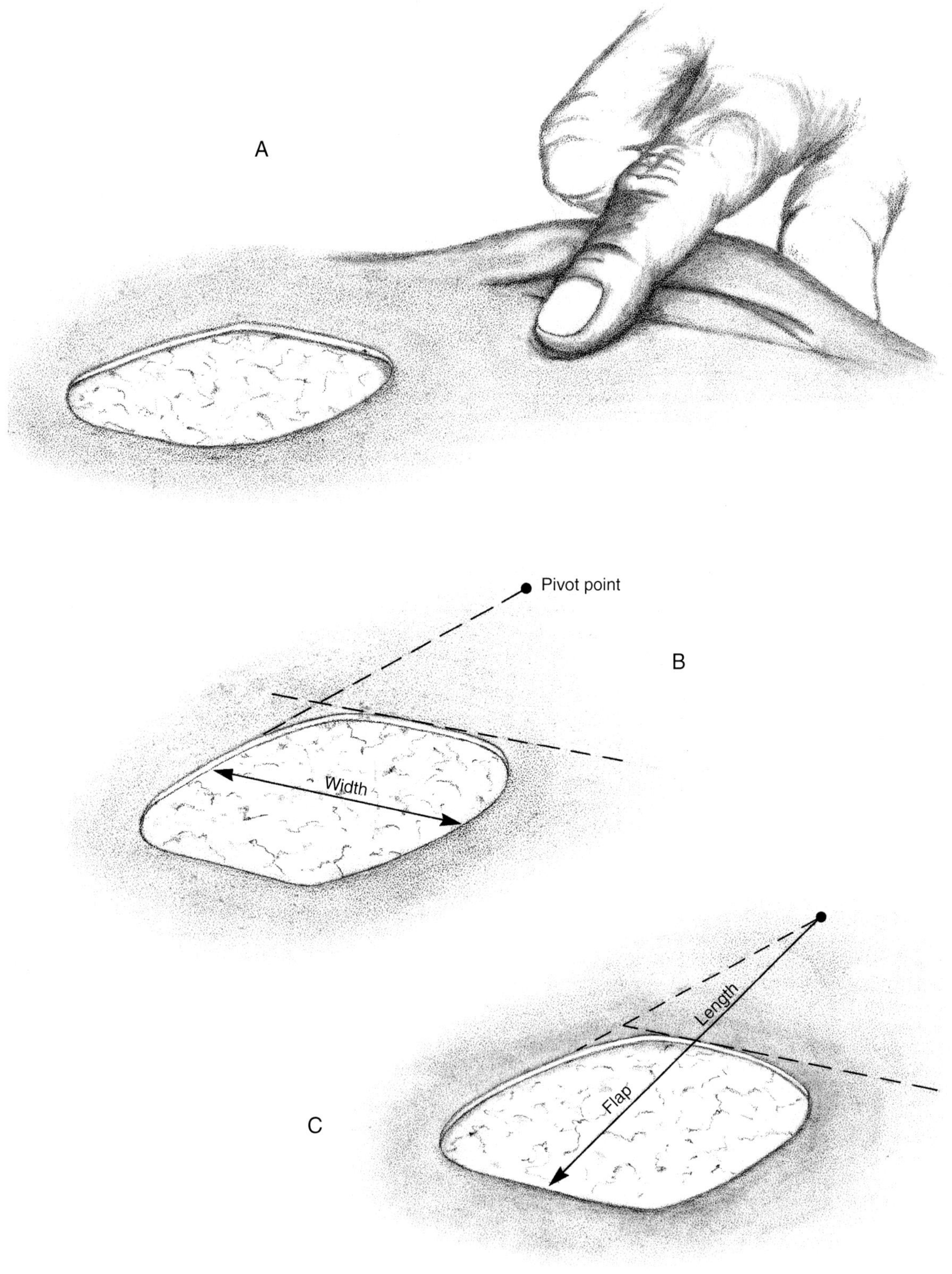

A

Pivot point

B

Width

Length

Flap

C

Plate 36

(Continued)

(D) The flap is drawn with a marking pen prior to incising the skin. (Note that the transposition flap shares a common border with the defect.) The skin is carefully undermined using Metzenbaum scissors. Thin triangular "tips" of skin created during the elevation of the flap are trimmed or rounded off since they are prone to ischemic necrosis.

(E) The flap is sutured into place using a simple interrupted suture pattern.

(F) The donor bed is closed in a similar fashion. A half-buried horizontal mattress suture is used to appose the junction of the flap and donor bed closure.

COMMENTS

The transposition flap is a rotating flap by design and is considered by the author to be the most versatile of the local flaps for wound closure. Although transposition flaps can be pivoted up to 180 degrees to cover a defect, a considerable loss of flap length occurs as it bends and kinks to extreme rotation. As a result, most transposition flaps are developed within 90 degrees to the axis (length) of the wound. Transposition flaps bring additional skin to the defect, unlike the single pedicle advancement flap, which relies upon the stretching of the elastic skin. For this reason, transposition flaps are best employed for wounds in which postoperative skin tension could cause distortion or compromise function. The transposition flap is adaptable to smaller defects of the limbs by developing the flap *parallel* to the length of the limb in order to take advantage of the limited circumferential skin laxity present in the dog and cat. While there is a certain degree of skin elasticity around wounds involving the trunk, which can compensate for small errors in flap dimension, measurements for flap development and transfer on the extremities must be precise. A 1-cm error in measurement can result in the inability to completely close the donor or recipient site.

On occasion, the surgeon may note a variable amount of skin elasticity along the distant border of the cutaneous defect. *Note:* Whenever possible, it is advisable to shorten the premeasured flap accordingly to improve the probability of maintaining adequate circulation to the terminal flap border.

Plate 36

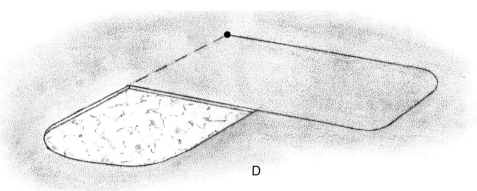

D

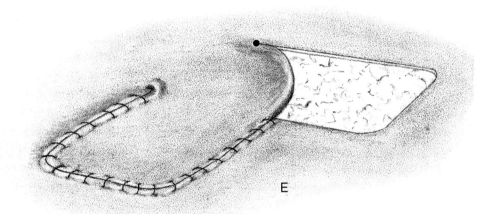

E

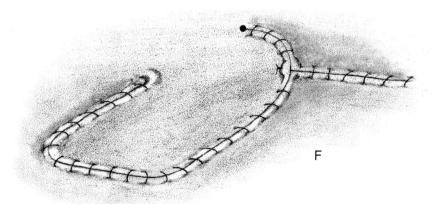

F

Plate 37   **Transposition Flap (45 degrees)**

DESCRIPTION

The 45-degree angle transposition flap is developed at a more acute angle to the axis of the defect compared to the preceding right-angle variation. Its use is more commonly associated with closure of triangular defects.

SURGICAL TECHNIQUE

(A) Flap development is similar to the 90-degree angle transposition flap. The flap is created at a 45-degree angle to the axis of the defect.

(B) The flap is pivoted and sutured into the prepared recipient bed.

(C) The donor site is closed primarily after undermining the bordering cutaneous tissue.

COMMENTS

The 45-degree angle transposition flap variation generally is used to close triangular wounds where local skin immediately adjacent to this wound is ample to support its development. The 90-degree angle transposition flap, however, has greater ability to bring additional loose skin into defects from its (slightly) more distant donor site. As a result, the 90-degree transposition flap is better able to close wounds that require more skin for closure or wounds in which wound tension must be avoided to prevent regional distortion and functional impairment.

Plate 37

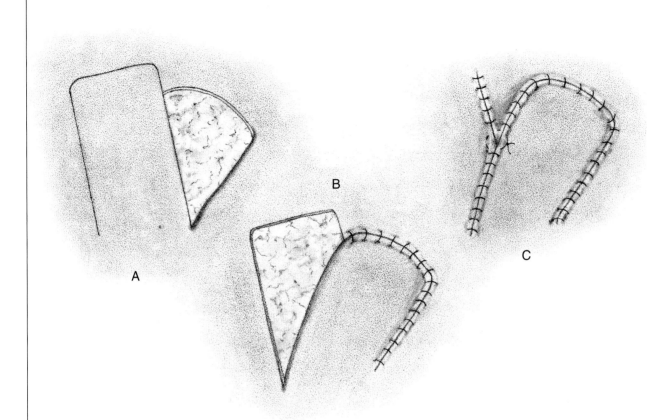

A

B

C

Plate 38   **Interpolation Flap**

DESCRIPTION

The interpolation flap is a variation of the transposition flap, but it lacks a common border with the defect. As a result, a portion of the flap must traverse an area of skin interposed between the donor and recipient beds. The design and execution of the interpolation flap is nearly identical to a transposition flap. However, the length of the interpolation flap must include the additional length required to extend over the intervening skin segment.

SURGICAL TECHNIQUE

(A) Local skin tension is assessed by grasping between the thumb and index finger the skin adjacent to the defect and determining the laxity and elasticity present. The donor location is positioned to use the (loose) skin ridge grasped (dashed line).

(B) The width of the flap, which equals the width of the defect, is measured and marked off at the predetermined baseline (dashed line). Note the base of the flap is aligned with the lower border of this defect. Flap length is determined by measuring from the pivot point (distant edge of the proposed pedicle or base) to the most distant portion of the defect. (*Note:* Flap length includes the additional amount required to traverse the interposing skin.) This measurement in turn is marked from the baseline.

(C) The flap is drawn with a marking pen prior to incising the skin. The two parallel lines forming the flap are equal to the length measurement in (B).

Plate 38

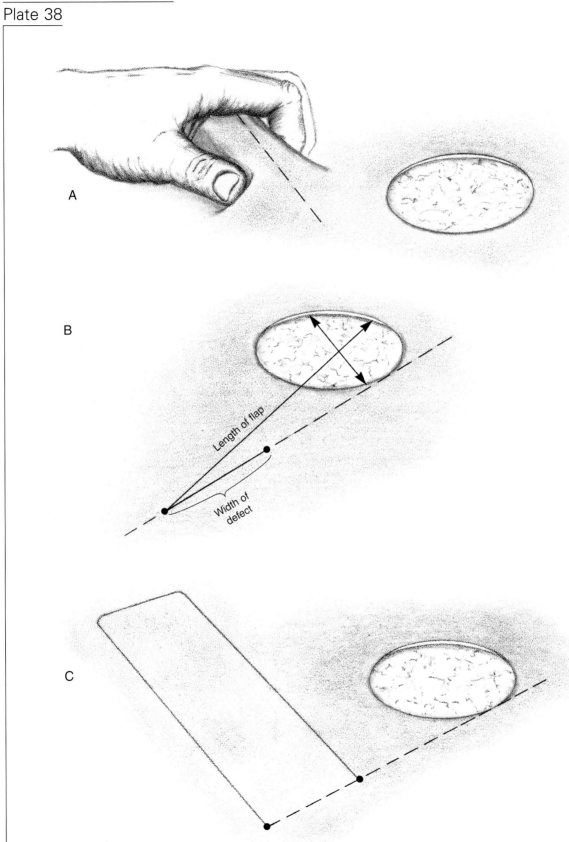

A

B

Length of flap

Width of defect

C

Plate 38

(Continued)

(D) The skin is then carefully undermined with Metzenbaum scissors and rotated into position. The flap is sutured into place with a simple interrupted suture pattern. The donor bed is closed in a similar fashion. A small triangular segment of skin is excised to facilitate donor bed closure.

(E) The redundant portion of the flap, overlapping the interposing skin between the donor and recipient sites, is excised in approximately 14 days once the flap has completely healed to the wound bed. Skin incisions are sutured to complete the transfer.

COMMENTS

Like the transposition flap, the interpolation flap is a rotating flap by design. It is uncommonly used in veterinary surgery because, unlike their human counterparts, dogs and cats have a greater availability of loose skin. However, the execution of the interpolation flap technique is similar to that used for axial pattern flap coverage of distant recipient areas.

The exposed portion of the interpolation flap is subject to local infection, but a granulation surface will form on the exposed skin surface within a matter of days. The eventual excision of the redundant flap segment will control this condition. Unless the distant portion of the interpolation flap has healed over the wound with formation of collateral vascular channels to support this flap segment, severance of the pedicle could result in necrosis. Two weeks is a general clinical guideline for this maneuver.

An alternative to leaving a portion of the flap exposed would be formation of a bridge incision between the donor and recipient beds to which the flap borders are sutured (see Plate 56 in Chapter 13). Therefore, it may not be necessary to excise the redundant flap segment except for cosmetic purposes. Tubing the exposed portion of the interpolation flap or application of a split thickness skin graft to the exposed dermal surfaces are less practical options to consider for this local flap technique.

Plate 38

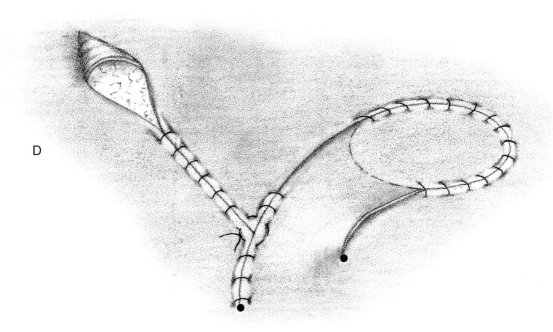

D

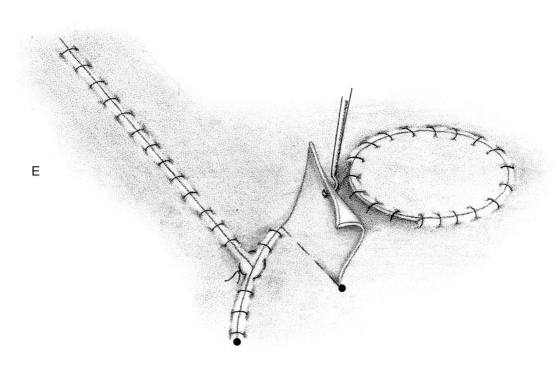

E

Plate 39   **Rotation Flap**

DESCRIPTION

The rotation flap is a semicircular flap most commonly used for closing triangular defects. In humans, the incision arc is four times the length required to rotate the flap into the defect. In veterinary practice, a curved incision is created in a stepwise fashion, and the flap is undermined until it covers the wound without excessive tension.

SURGICAL TECHNIQUE

(A) Skin tension is assessed by grasping the adjacent skin between the thumb and index finger. The rotational flap will be positioned to take full advantage of this loose skin. A marking pen can be used to draw a circle that incorporates the triangular wound.

(B) The skin is incised over the outlined semicircle and undermined in increments until the flap rotates and stretches over the defect without undue tension.

(C) The flap is secured with a simple interrupted sutured pattern.

COMMENTS

The rotation flap in design and execution combines the properties of the transposition flap and advancement flap: skin rotates and stretches to close the triangular wound without creating a secondary defect requiring a separate closure. A variation of the rotation flap usage includes paired rotation flaps created on each side of a wide triangular defect (a variation of H-plasty employing two single pedicle advancement flaps).

Similarly, two rotation flaps can be employed to close rectangular areas by closing the two triangular surface areas formed by a diagonal line across opposing corners of the defect. Because of the loose elastic skin in the dog and cat, most rotation flaps do not require complete elevation of the arc outlined with the marking pen. The author finds no particular advantage in the use of this technique over the transposition flap.

Plate 39

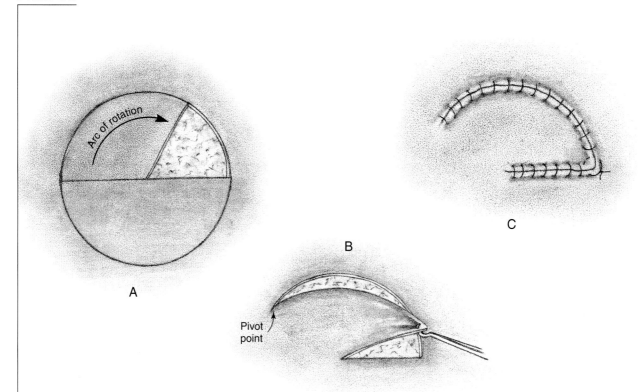

A

B

Pivot point

C

Plate 40   **Forelimb Fold Flap**

DESCRIPTION

The forelimb skin fold, loosely overlying the triceps musculature, can be elevated as a transposition flap and used to close skin wounds in the adjacent axillary area of the dog and cat.

SURGICAL TECHNIQUE

(A) The forelimb skin fold is grasped to determine the amount of skin that can be harvested as a skin flap. Manipulation of the limb will help determine the width of flap that can be elevated without creating excessive tension upon closure of the donor site. Symmetrical lateral-medial skin incisions are outlined with a marking pen and reassessed before incising the prepared skin. Incisions are connected in a U fashion, proximal to the elbow.

(B) The flap is carefully undermined and elevated. An axillary wound has been prepared for flap placement.

(C) The flap is transposed and sutured into position.

(D) The donor area is sutured, completing the transfer procedure.

COMMENTS

Described by Hunt, this transposition flap technique uses the thin, elastic skin fold of the forelimbs. Paired forelimb fold flaps can be transposed to cover larger defects that encroach on the axillary and sternal areas of the dog and cat. Flap size and length will vary with the body conformation of the individual patient.

Plate 40

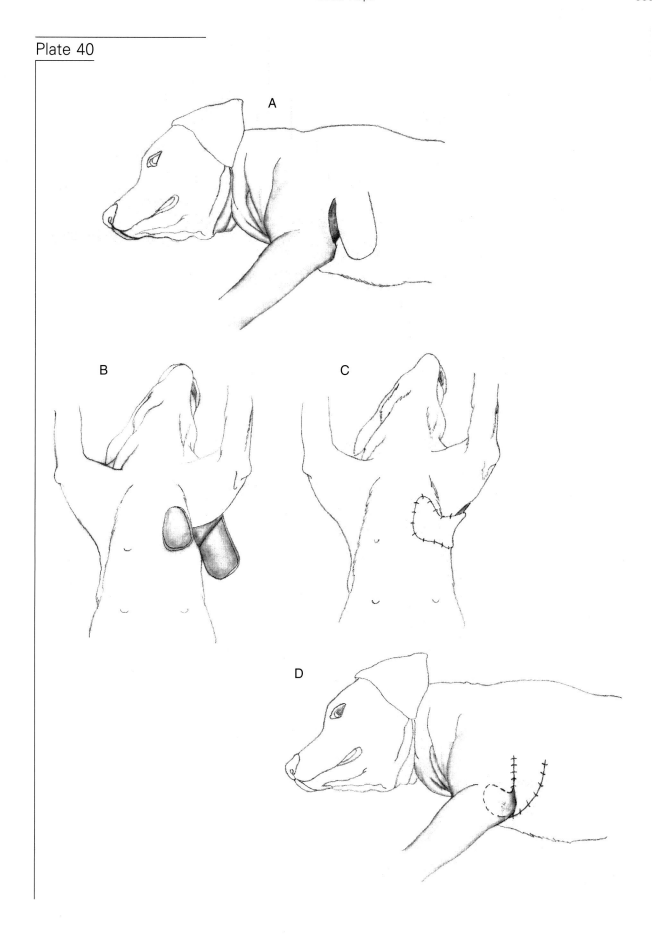

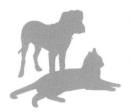

Distant Flap Techniques

DISTANT FLAPS

Distant flaps are constructed at a distant location from a skin defect. They are used almost exclusively for wounds that involve the middle to lower extremities. The skin of the lateral thorax and abdomen are the most frequently used donor sites. Distant flaps are subdivided into *direct flaps* and *indirect flaps*, based on the method used to transfer the distant flap to the recipient bed.

Distant flap techniques were originally developed for use in human patients and were modified for use in the dog and cat. They provide full-thickness skin coverage for wounds and a means of successfully transplanting skin without resorting to the more exacting surgical skills and postoperative care required for successful coverage with a free graft. Like other multistaged surgical procedures, they are time-consuming and expensive to perform. In the case of direct flaps, there are some canine and feline (especially) patients who will not tolerate having a limb immobilized against their chest or abdomen for an extended period of time.

Over the past several years, new reconstructive surgical techniques have evolved that are simpler and more economical to perform. Axial pattern flaps and refinements in free graft transplantation have largely replaced the need for distant flaps. Nonetheless, there are occasional cases in which these procedures can be used effectively (see Figure 18-5.) Elevation of massive skin losses overlying the knee, for example, may be amenable to elevation to a lateral abdominal wall (direct) flap. In one reference (White 1999), an external fixator was used to maintain the hind limb in a fixed position while using this direct flap technique to close a skin defect over the stifle area.

DIRECT FLAPS

Direct flaps include the single pedicle (hinge flap) and the bipedicle (pouch flap) designs developed for using the middle to lower lateral surface of the thorax or abdomen. The affected limb is lifted and the recipient bed is sutured to the elevated flap (Fig. 12-1). The pedicles are eventually divided in stages to complete the transfer in a 2- to 3-week time frame, provided that vascularization and healing occur between the flap and the wound bed. Direct flaps are used successfully in small animals, although cats are better anatomically suited to this technique than dogs because of their size, flexible limbs, and the ample loose, elastic skin available over the trunk. However, some cats in particular, poorly tolerate the immobilization of their limbs in an elevated position (see Plates 41 and 42).

Direct flaps have the disadvantage of requiring prolonged immobilization of the affected limb to assure flap survival and healing over the wound. The author has noticed mild muscle atrophy of the limb until normal use of the leg is regained. Dermatitis secondary to skin-to-skin contact and moisture accumulation requires the doctor's close attention. Because multiple stages and prolonged hospitalization are required to complete their transfer, the cost to the owner is moderate. The transplanted skin assumes the same hair growth characteristics despite its new location on the limb (Fig. 12-2).

> Today, direct flaps are considered for problematic extremity wounds in which other flap and grafting techniques are not feasible or in which their use is hampered by the wound's location and size.

INDIRECT FLAPS

Indirect flaps are almost entirely of the tubed-flap design, in which a bipedicle flap is sutured into a tube prior to its eventual transfer to the recipient bed after a delay procedure. (see Plate 43). Tubing the flap prevents it from healing to the donor bed, minimizes infection, and facilitates eventual transfer to the recipient bed. Most long tubed flaps require a 2- or 3-week "delay" to enhance their circulation before one pedicle can be severed and advanced toward the defect. Although tubed flaps can be "walked" great distances by periodically severing each pedicle alternately and advancing the freed end toward the recipient bed at 2-week intervals, it is both time consuming and impractical. Each successive step increases the likelihood of partial flap necrosis from an ineffective delay period, accidental kinking or twisting of the intact pedicle, trauma, or infection. As a result, tubed flaps are best developed close enough to the recipient bed to allow their immediate application to the wound after the initial delay period. Tubed flaps shrink or contract prior to their transfer and should be made larger than the recipient bed and longer than the length required to reach the defect: increasing the size by 25% of the exact measurements taken helps compensate for the shrinkage factor. Like direct flaps, the color and quality of hair growth after transplantation of the flap are maintained despite its new location (Fig 12-3).

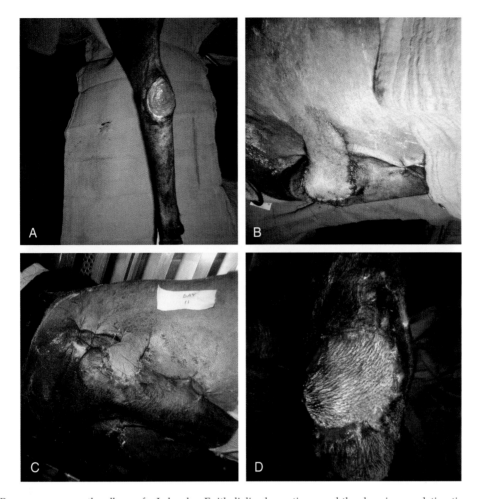

FIG. 12-1 (A) Pressure sore over the elbow of a Labrador. Epithelialized scar tissue and the chronic granulation tissue were resected; within days, a healthy granulation bed formed, suitable for closure.

(B) Application of a single pedicle direct flap, elevated from the lateral thorax. Although successful results were obtained, the prolonged bandaging, hospitalization, and staged transfer were costly. Today, a thoracodorsal axial pattern flap likely would be the best method to close this difficult wound.

(C) By day 11, the flap has healed onto the underlying granulation surface.

(D) By day 14, the pedicle was divided in stages: one-half the pedicle, 2 days apart. Following division and closure of the donor area, the incised edge was sutured to the wound border, completing the transfer. The elbow was protected with a padded bandage for an additional 2-week period. Close follow-up assured the distant flap was not traumatized. Soft padded bedding was advised.

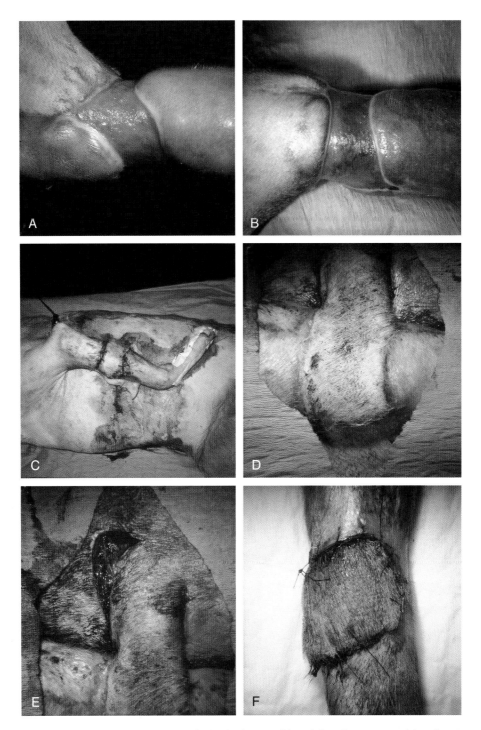

FIG. 12-2 (A, B) Circumferential degloving injury to the forelimb of a mixed-breed dog. Contracture of this chronic wound resulted in distal limb edema. Lateral (A) and medial views (B). The epithelialized border was resected prior to direct flap application.

(C) Elevation of a single pedicle direct (hinge) flap. Securing the limb to the side required an elaborate bandage, as noted in Plates 41 and 42.

(D) At 2 weeks, the hinge flap has healed to the lateral half of the wound.

(E) The pedicle is extended and partially divided.

(F) Approximately 3 days later, the remaining half of the pedicle was divided and the remaining half of the flap was sutured to the medial side of the defect. Partial necrosis of the terminal flap occurred; second intention healing of this site completed the closure. Today a mesh graft would be one of the best choices for closing this wound. (From Pavletic MM. 1985. Pedicle grafts. In: Slatter DH, ed. *Textbook of Small Animal Surgery*. Philadelphia, PA: WB Saunders.)

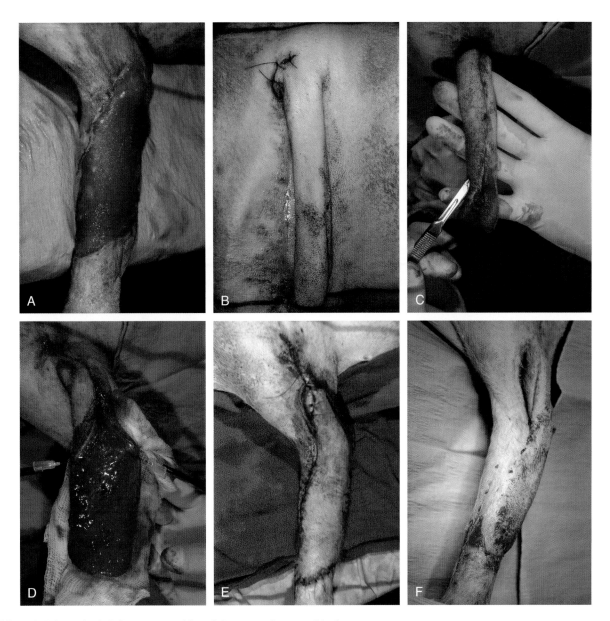

FIG. 12-3 (A) Forelimb defect in a mixed-breed dog, secondary to vehicular trauma.

(B) Staged elevation of an (indirect) delayed tube flap developed over the left shoulder region. At week 3 the final segment of the proximal pedicle was divided.

(C) The tubed flap was carefully incised over the "seam" of the tube.

(D) The partially contracted tube was opened.

(E) The flap was sutured into position.

(F) The end of the flap necrosed: second intention healing of this area occurred without incident. The distal tube segment of the healed flap site was resected 1 month after transfer to the recipient bed. This wound today could have been closed more easily and effectively with a mesh graft, thoracodorsal axial pattern flap, or, possibly, the brachial axial pattern flap.

THE DELAY PHENOMENON

Large flaps (without inclusion of direct cutaneous vessels) gradually developed in two or more stages prior to transfer are more likely to survive than pedicle grafts transplanted at the first operation. The physiologic mechanism(s) of augmenting flap survival is called the *delay phenomenon*. The improved circulation after a delay procedure can help offset the hazards of torsion and tension upon flap transfer. This delay effect also may contribute to skin flap survival with the use of tissue expanders: expanders in the latter phases of inflation create episodes of ischemia that may enhance neovascularization of the overlying skin.

Studies have focused on the microcirculatory mechanisms that account for delay and the optimal time for flap transfer. Selective division of the nerve, artery, and vein in neurovascular island flaps of rats has demonstrated that both denervation (sympathectomy) and ischemia play major roles in the delay phenomenon. Although the exact delay mechanism still is unclear, sustained vasodilation is currently believed to be the cause of improved flap survival. Delay is a two-phase response, the second phase being vasodilation of microcirculation from causes other than changes in the flap's sympathetic innervation.

Angiography and functional studies employed to examine the developing circulation within canine tubed flaps (8–10 cm long, 3–3.5 cm wide) as well as tubed flaps in rabbits have demonstrated that vessels in the subcutaneous tissue (corresponding to the subdermal plexus) increased in size and number with parallel reorientation or main vascular channels to the long axis of the flap. The longitudinal vascular arrangement in delayed flaps is most evident in loose-skinned research subjects (dog, rat, rabbit).

If ischemia and denervation are the stimuli for effective delay, tubed flaps of variable length, located in different regions of the body and on different animals, have variable circulatory efficiency. Flaps with adequate circulation do not benefit appreciably from a surgical delay compared with ischemic flaps. As a result, the variable tubed flaps employed clinically and experimentally suggest that the shorter delay period employed for short-tubed flaps (2 weeks or less) may be insufficient for long-tubed flaps with greater ischemia.

The optimal time for transfer varies among species; for example, the maximum delay effect in rabbits and swine occurs in 8–10 days, whereas rats required up to 6 weeks. One-week, 2-week, and 3-week time intervals have been suggested as satisfactory before flap transfer in the dog. A 3-week delay is the safest interval for the dog, based on Hofmeister's research. At 18 days, the author divides one half of the pedicle; the second half is severed 3 days later to complete the delay. Long-tubed flaps may also require staged elevation to avoid an ischemic crisis from immediately tubing the bipedicle flap.

Sphygmomanometer cuffs, rubber-padded intestinal clamps, and Penrose drain tubing have been employed to "train" a tube to rely on vascular support from one pedicle by applying these compressive devices around the opposite pedicle. Compression can be applied for progressively longer periods of time until the tubed flap circulation can survive on the unclamped pedicle. As noted, delayed tube flaps have been largely abandoned for clinical usage in veterinary and human reconstructive surgery with the advent of axial pattern flaps, myocutaneous flaps, and improvements in free-grafting techniques. However, deciphering this phenomenon may hold the key to selecting drugs that may mimic this physiologic response in order to salvage skin flaps with serious circulatory compromise. Although a variety of drugs have shown promise in improving survival of failing flaps, results have been inconsistent, and at times refuted by subsequent studies.

Suggested Readings

Pavletic MM. 1990. Skin flaps in reconstructive surgery. *Vet Clin No Am* 20:81–103.

Pavletic MM. 1994. Foot salvage and delayed reimplantation of severed metatarsal and digitial pads, using a bipedicled direct flap technique. *J Am Anim Hosp Assoc* 30:539–549.

Pavletic MM. 1994. Surgery of the skin and management of wounds. In: Sherding RD, ed. *The Cat: Diseases and Clinical Management*, 2nd ed., 1969–1997. New York: Churchill Livingstone.

Pavletic MM. 1998. Skin. In: Bojrab MJ, ed. *Current Techniques in Small Animal Surgery*, 4th ed. Philadelphia, PA: Lea & Febiger.

Pavletic MM. 2003. Pedicle grafts. In: Slatter DH, ed. *Textbook of Small Animal Surgery*, 3rd ed., 292–321. Philadelphia, PA: WB Saunders.

Spodnick G, Pavletic MM. 1993. Controlled tissue expansion to mobilize skin in the distal extremities in dogs. *Vet Surg* 22:436–443.

Swaim SF, Henderson RA. 1997. *Small Animal Wound Management*, 2nd ed. Baltimore, MD: Williams and Wilkins.

Swaim SF, Henderson RA, Sutton HH. 1980. Correction of triangular and wedge shaped skin defects in dogs and cats. *J Am Anim Hosp Assoc* 16:225–232.

White RN. 1999. Management of proximal pelvic limb skin laceration in a dog using a skin flap and an external fixator. *J Sm Anim Pract* 40:84–87.

Plate 41	**Direct Flap: Single Pedicle (Hinge) Flap**

DESCRIPTION

The hinge flap is a single pedicle, direct flap generally used to close limb defects at or below the elbow or knee. (It is rarely used to resurface large defects involving the pinna.) The base of this pedicle graft can be positioned dorsally or ventrally on the middle to lower lateral region of the thorax or abdomen. The affected limb is elevated to the trunk and the defect positioned beneath the flap.

SURGICAL TECHNIQUE

(A) The affected limb is lifted up to the lateral surface of the trunk to determine the proper location for flap development. The width of the flap equals the dorsoventral borders of the defect, including any epithelialized wound borders that require excision. An additional 1 or 2 cm is added to this measurement to offset elastic contraction and stretching of the flap associated with limb placement. The flap is carefully drawn onto the skin of the donor site. Flap length is determined from the desired location of the flap base to the most distant edge of the defect. A cloth template is useful to determine this measurement.

(B) The flap is incised and elevated beneath the cutaneous trunci muscle. The donor bed is partially closed. Epithelialized wound borders are excised to assure complete flap coverage of the entire defect.

(C) The flap is sutured to the wound borders.

Plate 41

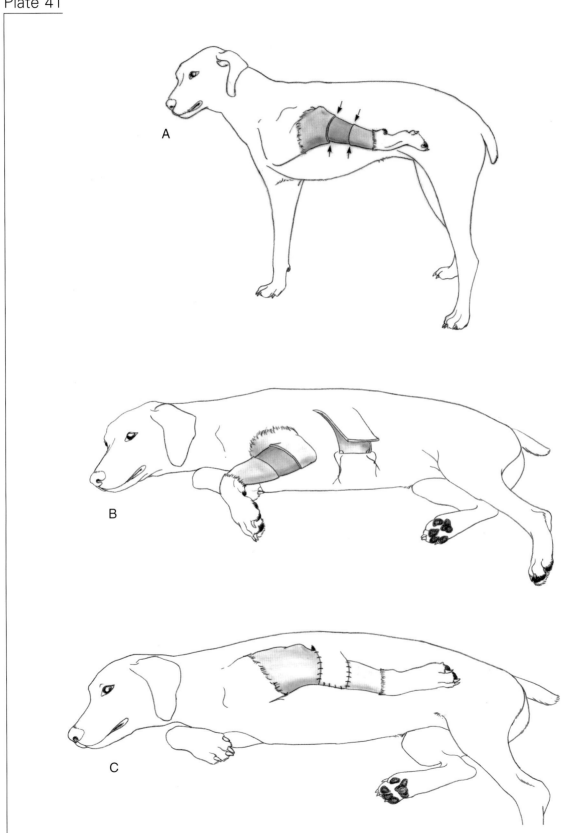

Plate 41

(Continued)

(D) To prevent shifting and slippage of the extremity from beneath the flap, elastic adhesive tape is folded over the lower extremity and continued around the circumference of the trunk. Two or three large stay or retaining sutures (size 1-0 or 2-0) are additionally placed through the skin adjacent to the defect and into the skin of the trunk to prevent the limb from shifting ventrally and placing tension on the flap pedicle. Cotton padding is placed between the limb and trunk to prevent moist dermatitis.

(E) Soft cotton padding, self-adherent gauze, and elastic adhesive tape encompass the limb and trunk. An access window may be cut into this protective wrap later for local wound care and for replacement without removing the entire bandage. Local bandage changes generally are performed every 2 or 3 days. Excitable or uncooperative patients should be sedated and restrained to avoid struggling during local wound care.

(F) The pedicle is divided in stages 10–14 days after surgery unless healing between skin edges and the underlying wound bed is incomplete. One-half of the pedicle is divided (dotted line) followed by the remaining half 2 or 3 days later (asterisks). The freed border is sutured to the opposing wound border. Removal of a portion of the granulation bed may be necessary to facilitate closure of the donor site.

COMMENTS

Division of the flap pedicle can be performed more rapidly than the suggested guidelines indicate, although there is a greater likelihood of necrosis. Considering the time and cost invested in this procedure, the few extra days required for delayed pedicle division is a practical investment. Elevated limbs tend to rotate outward, making proper flap application more difficult. Carefully applied bandages can help offset this effect. Hinge flaps, like other distant flap techniques, require a wound bed with sufficient vascularity to support flap survival when the pedicle is completely divided. For example, this flap would be a poor choice to close an ischemic wound bed secondary to radiation therapy.

Hinge flaps are better suited for defects on the lateral surface of the limbs, although carefully designed (ventrally based) trunk flaps can be folded to cover medial defects. The single pedicle can be lengthened slightly before final division of the pedicle to cover any remaining medial defect. Long pedicle extensions are likely to suffer a degree of necrosis due to insufficient circulation. (See Plate 42, Direct Flaps: Bipedicle [Pouch] Flap to determine which of these two direct flap techniques is preferable.)

Plate 41

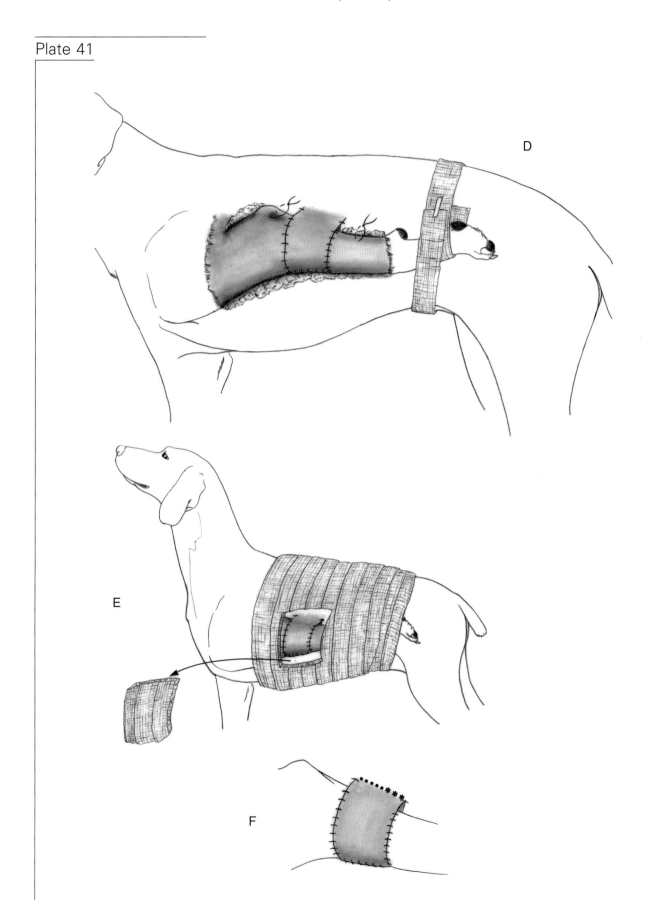

Plate 42   # Direct Flap: Bipedicle (Pouch) Flap

DESCRIPTION

The pouch flap is a bipedicle direct flap beneath which the limb wound is positioned. Its development, location, and execution is similar to that of the hinge flap.

SURGICAL TECHNIQUE

(A) The injured limb is lifted to the lateral surface of the trunk to determine the location of flap placement. The limb is flexed to simulate the maneuver required to comfortably position the extremity defect beneath the proposed pouch flap. The affected limb and donor area are thoroughly clipped of fur.

(B) The width of the flap corresponds to the dorsoventral dimension of the limb defect. It is advisable to create a flap 1 or 2 cm wider than measured to offset elastic contraction and stretching of the flap associated with limb placement. The proposed flap is carefully drawn onto the skin of the donor area. Two parallel incisions are extended in increments.

(C) The pedicle graft is undermined beneath the cutaneous trunci muscle. Sufficient room is created for limb placement beneath the flap without excessive tension, yet allowing optimum contact between the opposing surfaces. Epithelialized wound borders are excised to provide complete flap coverage. The flap is sutured to the proximal and distal borders of the limb defect. The ventral openings formed by "tenting" of the flap serve as drainage sites for the surgical area.

Plate 42

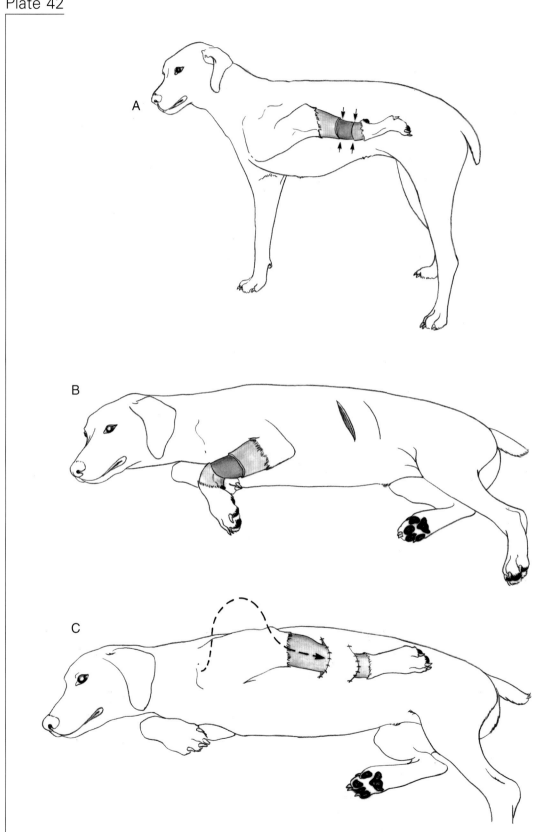

Plate 42

(Continued)

(D) To prevent shifting and slippage of the extremity from beneath the flap, elastic adhesive tape is folded over the lower extremity and continued around the circumference of the trunk. Two or three large stay or retaining sutures are additionally placed through the skin adjacent to the defect and into the skin of the trunk to prevent the limb from shifting ventrally and placing tension on the flap pedicles. Cotton padding is placed between the limb and trunk to prevent moist dermatitis.

(E) Soft cotton padding, self-adherent gauze, and elastic adhesive tape encompasses the limb and trunk. An access window may be cut into this protective wrap later for local wound care and replacement without necessarily removing the entire bandage (see Plate 41). Local bandage changes generally are performed every 2 or 3 days. Excitable or uncooperative patients should be sedated and restrained to avoid struggling during local wound care.

Plate 42

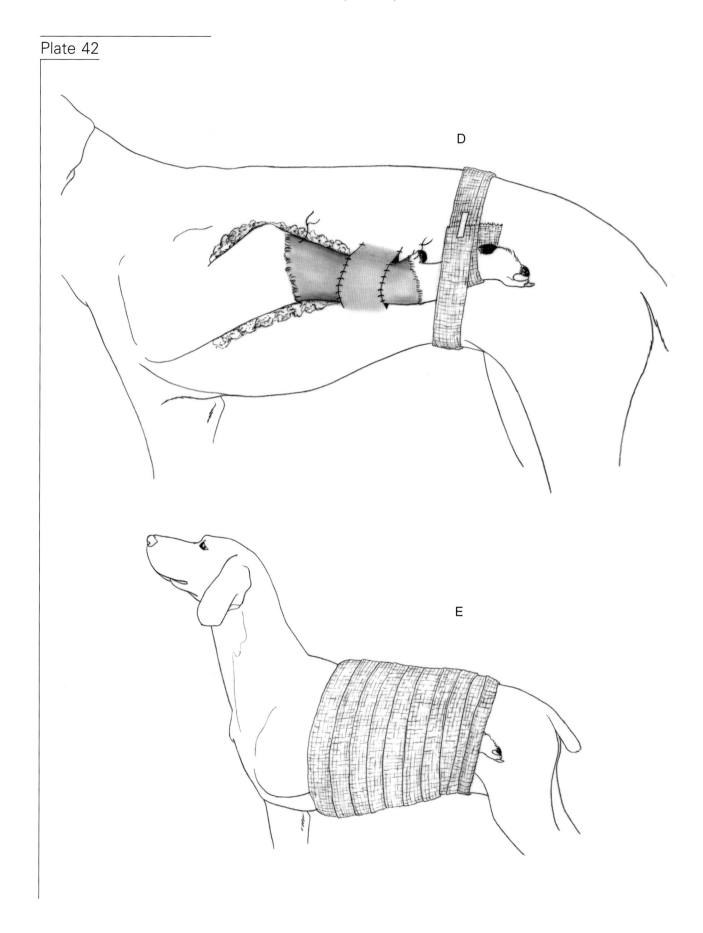

Plate 42

(Continued)

(F) Pedicles are divided into stages beginning 10–14 days after surgery unless healing between the skin edges and underlying wound bed in contact with the flap is incomplete. One-half of the lower pedicle is divided (asterisks), followed by division of the second half 2 days later (dotted line). Delayed division of the upper pedicle is then repeated in similar fashion beginning 2 days after the preceding procedure (circular and oval dots). The freed edges of the flap are sutured to the opposing wound border with each division.

(G) The donor site usually is laden with granulation tissue. Excision of portions of the wound bed may be required to facilitate closure. In the event of a circumferential wound to the limb, the length of each pedicle can be extended beyond the suggested margins in (G). Each extended pedicle flap is wrapped medially to close the remaining defect. Unless circulation from the wound bed to the flap is adequate, partial necrosis of the ends of the medially placed pedicles may be noted.

COMMENTS

The advantages and disadvantages of pouch flaps and hinge flaps are nearly identical. They are tedious, time consuming, multistaged procedures. Maintaining the limb in a fixed position is a challenge in the uncooperative patient, and mild muscle atrophy can be expected upon release of the limb. However, muscle mass is eventually regained with exercise.

When dealing with more proximal limb defects, it may be impossible to flex the limb of the dog sufficiently to tuck the extremity into the pouch created. This maneuver is less of a problem in the cat. The hinge flap is best used when an unduly long flap is not required to cover a given defect and is more commonly used for defects that cannot be positioned beneath a bipedicle flap. Both pouch and hinge flaps are ideally suited for lateral defects of the extremities.

Elevated limbs have a natural tendency to rotate outward, which occasionally makes application to wounds more difficult. Carefully applied bandages can reduce this effect. Pouch flaps, like other distant flap techniques, require a wound bed with sufficient vascularity to support its survival after complete division of both pedicles. (See Plate 41, Direct Flap: Single Pedicle [Hinge] Flap, to determine which of these two direct flap techniques is preferable.)

Plate 42

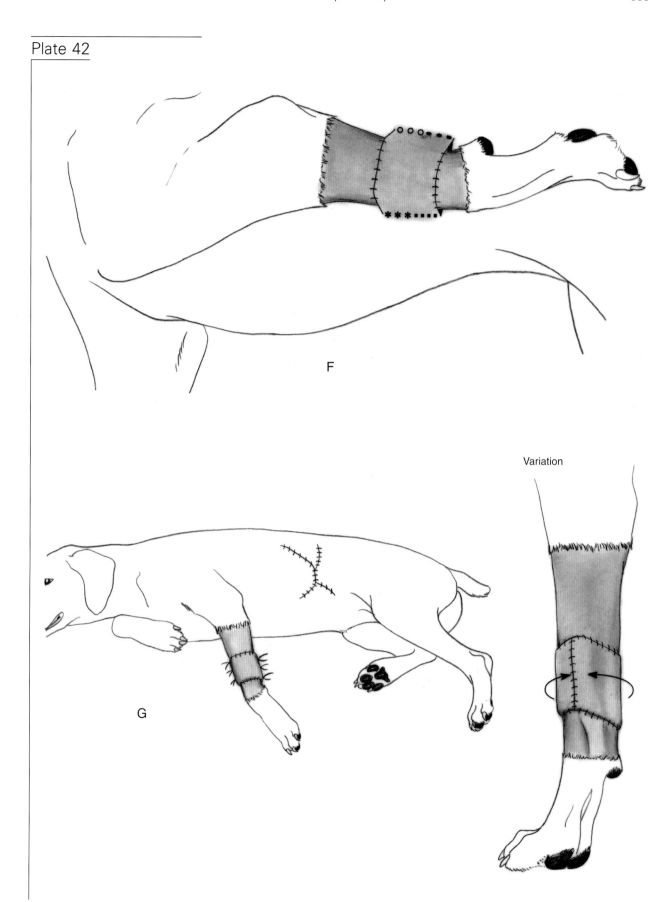

F

G

Variation

| Plate 43 | **Indirect Flap: Delayed Tube Flap** |

DESCRIPTION

Indirect flaps are almost entirely of the delayed tube flap design in which a bipedicle flap is sutured into a tube prior to its eventual transfer to the recipient bed. A delay period prior to transfer is used to enhance circulation to those flaps in which adequate blood flow to portions of the flap is questionable. This is particularly important for long flaps whose circulation is based on the subdermal plexus.

SURGICAL TECHNIQUE

(A) Delayed tube flaps are best developed close enough to the defect to allow its immediate application (tumbling) to the wound after the initial delay period. Loose, elastic skin is required for flap development and donor bed closure. Tube flaps can be rotated up to 180 degrees as long as care is taken to avoid excessive kinking or twisting of the transfer pedicle.

Flap width equals the width of the wound: an additional 2 or 3 cm are added to this measurement to offset flap "shrinkage" secondary to fibrosis and loss of skin elasticity. Additional width should be considered to assure no circumferential tension is present when the flap is sutured into the tube configuration. Flap length is determined by measuring from the base of the flap closest to the wound (transfer pedicle) and the length required to arc or rotate the flap into its new position. This is best determined with the use of a foam rubber model. An additional 2 or 3 cm are also added to this measurement to offset flap shrinkage.

(B) Two parallel incisions are made based on these measurements. Alternatively, central pedicle(s) can be created temporarily to protect the central area of a long flap from necrosis. This central pedicle is divided in 1 week and the tubed flap maintained for an additional 2-week delay period.

(C) The bipedicle flap borders are sutured together, creating a tube. The donor bed is undermined and closed directly. Alternatively one (or both) sides of the donor bed can be converted to an advancement flap to facilitate closure if necessary. Three weeks is the delay period for long tube flaps.

(D) The pedicle farthest from the defect is divided in two stages. On day 19, one-half of the pedicle is divided and sutured back into place temporarily with the patient under sedation with a 2% (subcutaneous) lidocaine block to the pedicle area to be divided. On day 21, the remaining half of the pedicle is divided and flap transfer can be initiated under general anesthesia. However, final severance of the remaining half of the pedicle can be postponed for a longer period of time if tube swelling or ischemia are recognized.

A variation of this technique is the creation of a "pancake" extension on the end of the tube (outer dashed line) beyond the normal level where the pedicle is divided (inner dashed line). This round skin extension may be used to cover a wider defect without necessarily using the entire body of the tube flap.

(E) The recipient site is prepared for surgery prior to final division of the pedicle. Epithelialized borders are excised. The tube is incised along the original incision line, carefully dissected open, and sutured into place. Care is taken to avoid unnecessary tension, twisting, or kinking of the transfer pedicle.

(F) The redundant portion of the tube flap is usually excised when the flap has healed completely to the wound bed. The author usually divides the pedicle, in stages, no sooner than 4 weeks after transfer.

Plate 43

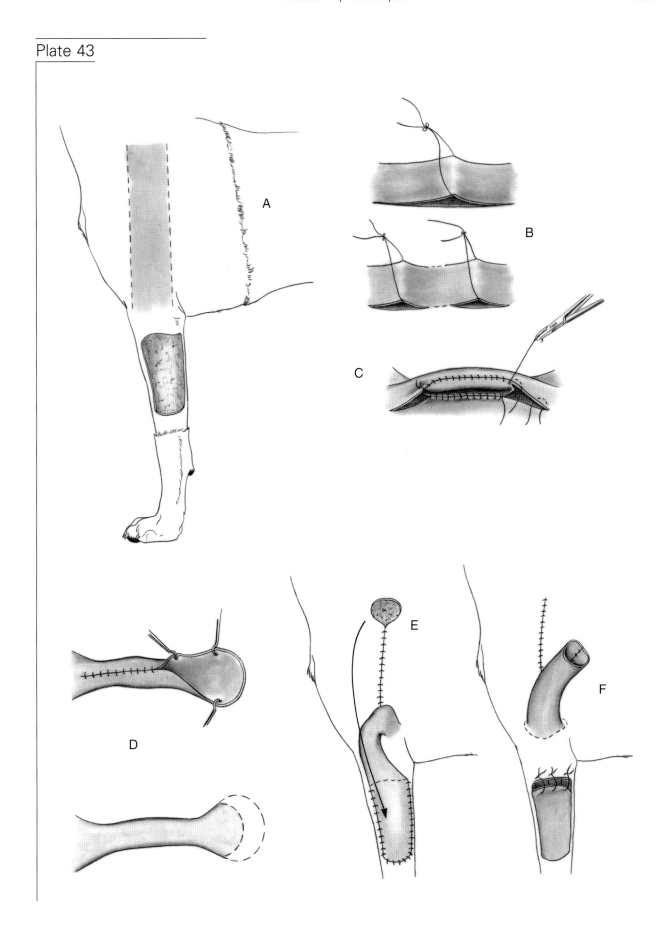

Plate 43

(Continued)

COMMENTS

Delayed tubed flaps are used to transfer skin to a distant recipient site if there is no immediate need to cover an area. They are used almost exclusively for lower limb defects and employed only if simpler methods of skin transfer are unable to close the defect satisfactorily. In this clinical example, a brachial axial pattern flap, thoracodorsal axial pattern flap, or free graft technique would be preferable options for closure.

Tubed flaps are moved by migration in dogs and cats by one of three techniques: *caterpillaring*, *waltzing*, or *tumbling*. *Caterpillaring* entails moving one end of the flap close to the other; in essence, doubling the flap on itself. After a second delay procedure, the other pedicle is severed, and the freed end is extended toward the defect. *Waltzing* requires the alternate movement of each pedicle in a lateral motion, whereas *tumbling* entails severing one pedicle and extending it forward, thereby advancing the flap directly toward the defect. Of the three, tumbling is the most direct method of transfer, especially when it is developed close to the defect, thus enabling immediate application of the flap to the recipient bed after a single delay period.

Although modifications in the basic design have been reported, the standard technique illustrated is satisfactory for most cases requiring this procedure. Removal of subcutaneous fat has been advocated to facilitate the tubing of flaps in obese human patients but this is rarely considered necessary in the dog. Moreover, the removal of subcutaneous fat and the associated panniculus muscle can inadvertently damage the subdermal plexus and the associated vasculature, significantly compromising flap circulation. If adipose tissue might impair tubing, the flap should be designed so that it is wide enough to avoid this problem.

Each pedicle does not necessarily have the same circulatory contribution to the flap body. The "dominant" pedicle, which has greater blood perfusion, is best preserved, whereas the nondominant pedicle can be divided with less danger of distal flap necrosis after the delay procedure. Unfortunately, flap design is usually dictated primarily by the defect and available donor tissue. The final flap design is a compromise between these factors.

Tube necrosis can occur at the vascular interface between the two pedicles; this does not occur at the center of a tubed flap unless the circulatory contribution of each pedicle is equal. In general, there is no immediate need to divide the transfer pedicle after successful flap transfer. Although staged division of the tube can be instituted 10 to 14 days after transfer, the author generally waits a minimum of 1 month. Excluding cosmetic considerations and possible dermatitis, the tubed transfer pedicle can be retained on the patient indefinitely. It may be preserved (as a spare tire) if future regional reconstructive surgery is anticipated (e.g., local tumor recurrence). It, too, can be employed for additional coverage of any portion of the wound that remains uncovered, or it can be left intact to maintain flap circulation in those wounds lacking the circulation required to support pedicle graft survival (e.g., chronic radiation wounds, etc.). In these situations, a bridge incision (see Plate 56) could be used to eliminate a free-standing tube segment. Postoperatively, the tube must be protected from trauma and supported with a soft cotton bandage, depending on its position on the body. Soft cotton rolls are usually taped on each side of the tubed flap, followed by a soft cotton bandage over the area, until the flap is transferred. A bandage applied after flap transfer should place no pressure on the flap. Elizabethan collars are advisable to prevent self-mutilation.

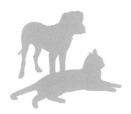

Axial Pattern Skin Flaps

INTRODUCTION: AXIAL PATTERN FLAPS

An axial pattern flap is a pedicle graft that incorporates a direct cutaneous artery and vein into its base. The vessels extend up the length of the flap to a variable degree, the terminal branches of which supply blood to the subdermal plexus. As a result, axial pattern flaps have better perfusion as compared to pedicle grafts, whose circulation is derived from the subdermal plexus alone (subdermal plexus flaps). Experimental studies and clinical trials have demonstrated that large axial pattern flaps can be safely elevated and transferred in a single stage for closure of major cutaneous defects within their general radius.

There are several axial pattern flaps that have been formally researched and designed for clinical use in the dog. They are based on the following direct cutaneous arteries: the omocervical artery, thoracodorsal artery, lateral thoracic artery, superficial brachial artery, caudal superficial epigastric artery, cranial superficial epigastric artery, deep circumflex iliac artery, genicular artery, caudal auricular artery, lateral caudal (tail) artery, and superficial temporal artery. The caudal superficial epigastric artery (Figs. 13-1–13-3) and thoracodorsal artery (Figs. 13-4–13-6) have the greatest clinical promise for axial pattern development, both in the cat and dog (see Table 13-1). Other axial pattern flap techniques, such as the genicular (Fig. 13-7), cranial superficial epigastric (Fig. 13-8), and deep circumflex iliac (Fig. 13-9) (dorsal and ventral branches) are effective for a more selective group of defects based on their size and location. A variation of the ventral deep circumflex iliac, the flank fold flap (Fig. 13-10), can be useful for defects involving the caudal abdomen and inguinal area.

Axial pattern flaps are generally rectangular in shape (standard peninsula configuration), although they can be modified with a right-angle extension (L, or hockey-stick configuration). The right-angle design enables the surgeon to cover irregular or wider defects that may not be completely covered by the standard peninsular design. Furthermore, this latter design can avoid encroachment upon the other side of the patient whereby the opposite direct cutaneous vessels may be necessarily sacrificed during flap elevation.

Axial pattern flap development and transfer requires careful planning. Measuring and drawing the flap on the patient's skin prior to surgery minimizes errors. Alcohol-resistant marking pens (VWR markers, VWR Scientific, San Francisco, CA) are preferable when isopropyl alcohol is used for surgical preparation of the skin. Alternatively, skin staples may also be used to silhouette the outlined flap to avoid losing the markings of the predrawn flap. Because axial pattern flaps rotate into adjacent defects, guidelines for local transposition flap measurement and transfer are equally applicable to their planning.

ISLAND ARTERIAL FLAPS

Island arterial flaps can be developed from axial pattern flaps by dividing the cutaneous pedicle but preserving the direct cutaneous artery and vein entering the newly created "skin island." Although island arterial flaps have considerable mobility tethered to the direct cutaneous vessels, their routine clinical use is unnecessary. One exception involves large defects that encroach upon the origin of a direct cutaneous artery and vein. Under these circumstances, it is possible to rotate an island arterial flap (the base of which shares a common border with the wound) 180 degrees over the defect (Fig. 13-8 and 13-9).

Island arterial flaps have potential for use in free flap development and transfer, using present-day microvascular surgical techniques; however, the surgical training, skill, equipment, and cost involved in microvascular surgery restrict such techniques to the largest academic institutions. Fortunately, most wounds can be handled more easily with the reconstructive techniques covered in this textbook.

REVERSE SAPHENOUS CONDUIT FLAPS

A variation of the axial pattern flap, the reverse saphenous conduit flap, has clinical application for wounds involving the tarsal and metatarsal areas of the dog. This flap is based over the saphenous artery and medial saphenous vein, which supply small direct cutaneous vessels to the overlying skin. Upon division from the femoral artery and vein, circulation flows in reverse fashion through the saphenous vessels via anastomoses with collateral vascular tributaries (Fig.13-11).

SECONDARY AXIAL PATTERN FLAPS

A secondary axial pattern flap is a modification of the axial pattern flap design. Skin segments positioned over vessels or tissue containing a major artery and

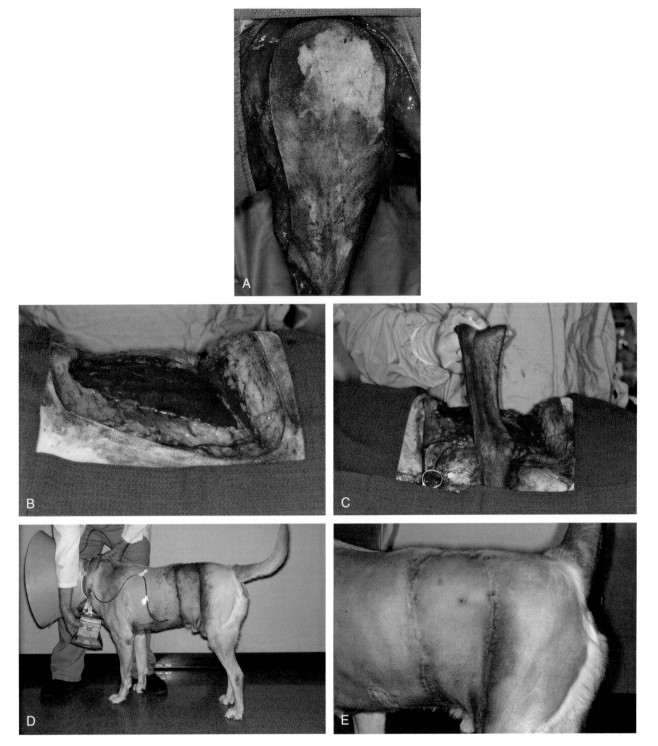

FIG. 13-1 (A) Wide resection of fibrosarcoma involving the left flank and lateral abdomen. (B) The external abdominal oblique muscle also was resected. (C) Elevation of the left caudal superficial epigastric axial pattern flap. (D) Closure of the wound. 35W skin staples were used to secure the flap. The drain was secured to the dog's collar. Tape strips applied to the vacuum tubing were secured to the thoracic skin with staples. (E) Complete survival of the flap.

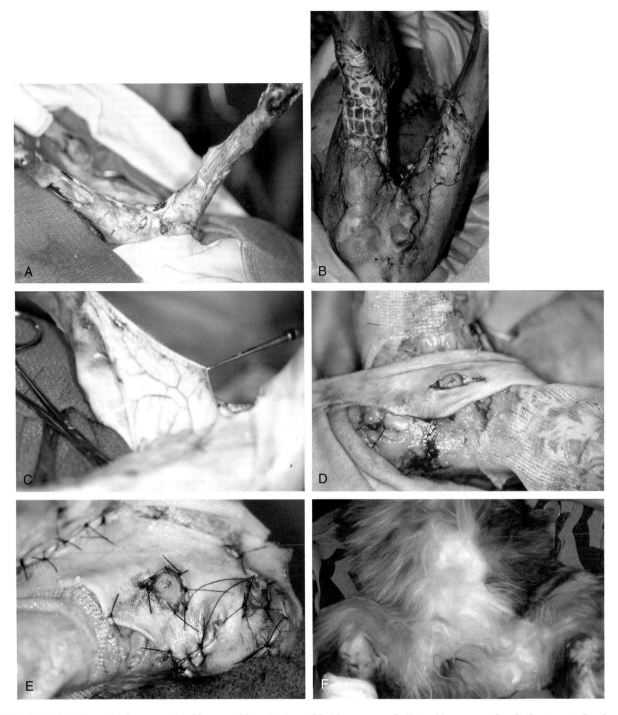

FIG. 13-2 (A, B) Extensive burn sustained by a cat. Necrotic tissue debridement was facilitated by warm saline baths in a sterilized stainless steel bucket (Fig. 7-15). Wound closure was attempted when a healthy granulation bed formed. Contractures in the popliteal areas were released; mesh grafts were applied to the rear extremities.

(C) Elevation of a caudal superficial epigastric axial pattern flap. Note branching of the epigastric vasculature.

(D) A slit was created in the flap, between branches of this direct cutaneous artery and vein, to accommodate the prepuce and penis.

(E) The flap was carefully fashioned around the anus and prepuce.

(F) The patient a few months later, completely rehabilitated. The medical and surgical management of the wounds (flaps/grafts) and an additional operation to release a scar stricture/contracture involving the anus and right forelimb, respectively, were costly. Several years after the surgery, the patient is in excellent health.

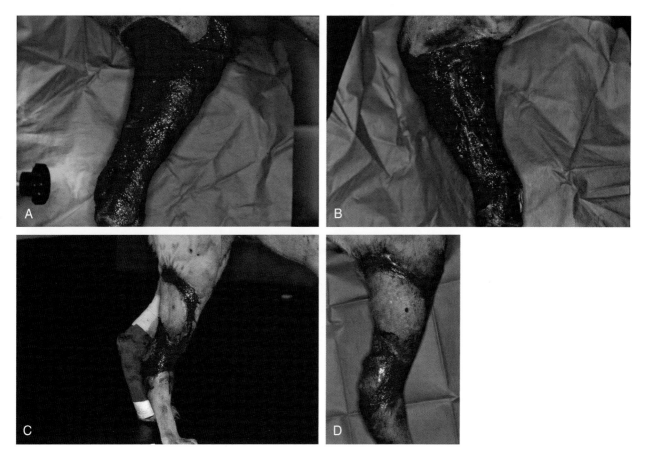

FIG. 13-3 (A, B) Massive circumferential loss of skin from the rear leg of a German shepherd, secondary to vehicular trauma. (C, D) Successful coverage with two caudal superficial epigastric axial pattern flaps, in a double-helix fashion. The second flap was delayed for approximately 5 days to allow mobilization of additional abdominal skin with skin stretchers. This maneuver was needed to assure the ventral abdominal donor site could be closed after recruitment of both flaps, which accounted for the skin of the entire ventral abdomen. Areas of exposed granulation tissue rapidly epithelialized from the borders of the flaps.

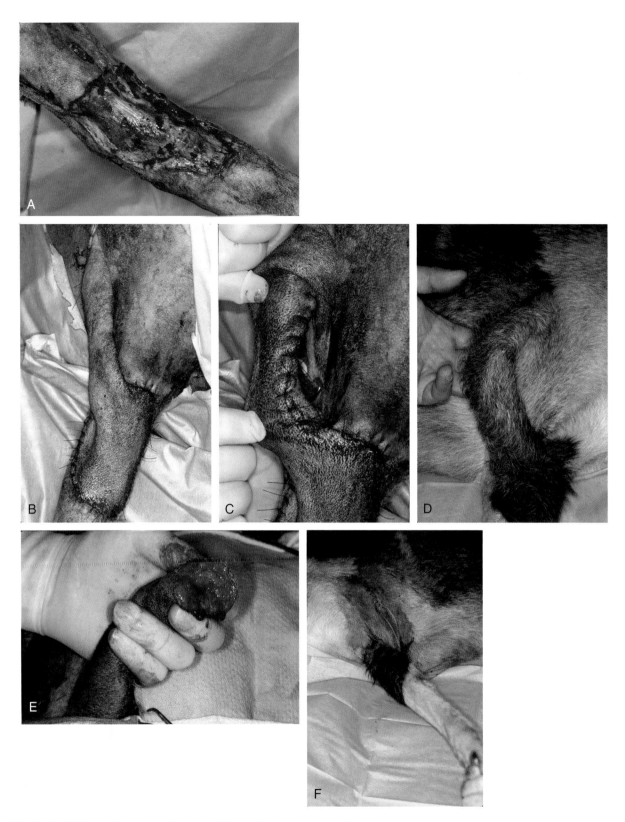

FIG. 13-4 (A) Nonhealing, traumatic antecubital defect in a German shepherd.

(B) Tubed thoracodorsal axial pattern flap coverage of the defect.

(C) Close-up view of the tubed pedicle. At the time of surgery, a tubed transfer was considered easier to position the flap, compared to a bridge incision.

(D, E) Two months after transfer, the tubed pedicle was divided at both ends to complete the transfer. The dorsal end of the flap was divided first, and the thoracodorsal vessels were ligated. Note the "reverse" bleeding from the cut end of the tube.

(F) Completion of the tube resection.

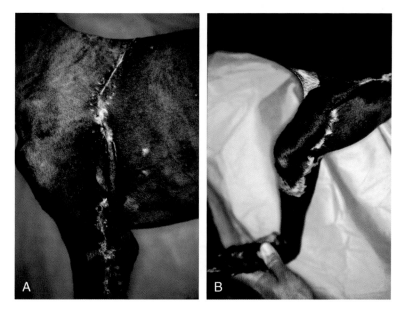

FIG. 13-5 (A) Thoracodorsal axial pattern flap used to close a massive skin loss over the elbow region, secondary to infection. A small portion of the terminal flap underwent necrosis, necessitating debridement and resuturing. Note early epithelialization of the exposed granulation bed. (B) Healing of the area was complete within 4 weeks after surgery. The flap provided a durable coverage to the elbow region of this greyhound.

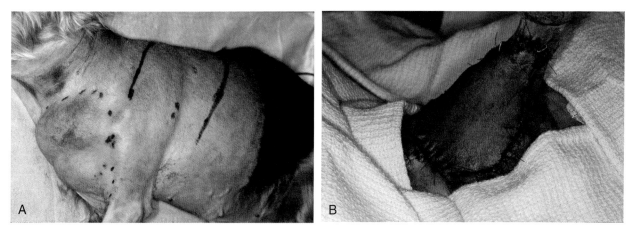

FIG. 13-6 (A) Mast cell tumor involving the left shoulder region. (B) Wide excision was followed by rotation of the adjacent thoracodorsal axial pattern flap. The patient later underwent radiation therapy and chemotherapy.

TABLE 13-1
Summary of guidelines for axial pattern flap development.

Artery	Anatomic Landmarks	Reference Incisions	Potential Uses*
Cervical cutaneous branch of the omocervical artery	Spine of the scapula Cranial edge of the scapula (cranial shoulder depression) Dogs in lateral recumbency, skin in natural position, thoracic limb placed in relaxed extension Vessel originates at location of the pre-scapular lymph node	*Caudal incision*: spine of the scapula in a dorsal direction *Cranial incision*: parallel to the caudal incision equal to the distance between the scapular spine and cranial scapular edge (cranial shoulder depression) *Flap length*: variable; contralateral scapulohumeral joint	Facial defects Ear reconstruction Cervical defect Shoulder defect Axillary defects
Thoracodorsal artery	Spine of the scapula Caudal edge of the scapula (caudal shoulder depression) Dog in lateral recumbency, skin in natural position, thoracic limb in relaxed extension Vessel originates at caudal shoulder depression at a level parallel to the dorsal point of the acromion	*Cranial incision*: spine of the scapula in a dorsal direction *Caudal incision*: parallel to the cranial incision equal to the distance between the scapular spine and caudal scapular edge(caudal shoulder depression) *Flap length*: variable; can survive ventral to contralateral scapulohumeral joint	Thoracic defects Shoulder defects Forelimb defects Axillary defects
Superficial brachial artery	Flexor surface of elbow Humeral shaft Greater tubercle	*Incision Lines*: Flap base includes flexor surface of elbow, anterior one-third Lateral and medial incisions parallel humeral shaft Flap is progressively tapered approaching greater tubercle *Flap Length*: Variable, flap ends at level of greater tubercle	Antebrachial defects Elbow defects
Caudal superficial epigastric artery	Midline of abdomen Mammary teats Base of prepuce	*Medial incision*: abdominal midline In the male dog, the base of the prepuce is included in the midline incision to preserve the adjacent epigastric vasculature *Lateral incision*: parallel to medial incision at an equal distance from the mammary teats *Flap length*: variable: may include the last four glands and adjacent skin	Flank defects Inner thigh defects Stifle area Perineal area Preputial area
Cranial epigastric artery	Hypogastric region Abdominal midline Mammary teats Base of prepuce	*Base of flap*: location in hypogastric region *Medial incision*: abdominal midline *Lateral incision*: parallel to midline incision at an equal distance from mammary teats *Flap length*: glands 2, 3, 4; anterior to prepuce	Closure of wounds overlying sternal region
Deep circumflex iliac artery (dorsal branch)	Cranial edge of wing of ilium Great trochanter Dog in lateral recumbency, skin in natural position, pelvic limb in relaxed extension Vessel originates at a point cranioventral to wing of the ilium	*Caudal incision*: midway between edge of wing of ilium and greater trochanter *Cranial incision*: parallel to caudal incision equal to the distance between the caudal incision and cranial edge of the iliac wing *Flap length*: dorsal to contralateral flank fold	Thoracic defects Lateral abdominal wall defects Flank defects Lateral/medial thigh defects Defects over the greater trochanter
Deep circumflex iliac artery (ventral branch)	Anatomic landmarks of flap base are the same as dorsal branch of deep circumflex iliac artery Shaft of femur	*Caudal incision*: Extends distally, anterior to cranial border of femoral shaft *Cranial incision*: Parallel to caudal incision *Flap length*: proximal to patella	Lateral abdominal wall defects Pelvic defects Sacral defects—as an island arterial flap

TABLE 13-1
Summary of guidelines for axial pattern flap development. *Continued*

Artery	Anatomic Landmarks	Reference Incisions	Potential Uses*
Genicular	Patella Tibial tuberosity Greater trochanter	*Base of the flap:* 1 cm proximal to the patella and 1.5 cm distal to tibial tuberosity (laterally) *Flap borders:* extend caudodorsally parallel to the femoral shaft. Flap terminates at the base of the greater trochanter	Lateral or medial aspect of the lower limb, from the stifle to the tibiotarsal joint
Lateral caudal arteries (left and right)	Proximal third of tail length Transverse processes of vertebrae	*Incision:* dorsal or ventral midline skin incision, depending on intended flap usage; careful dissection along deep caudal fascia of the tail; vessels located lateral and slightly ventral to transverse processes, in proximal tail region; amputation of tail at third to fourth intervertebral space, preserving skin *Flap length:* proximal third of tail length	Perineum, caudodorsal trunk
Caudal auricular	Wing of atlas Spine of the scapula	*Base of flap:* palpable depression between lateral aspect of wing of atlas and vertical ear canal: flap centered over wing of atlas *Width of flap:* central "third" of lateral cervical area over lateral aspect of wing of atlas: in cats, dorsal border close to dorsal midline *Flap length:* up to spine of scapula (survival length variability)	Facial area Dorsum of head Ear
Reverse saphenous conduit flap**	Inner thigh Tibial shaft	*Proximal incision:* central third of inner thigh at level of patella; ligate saphenous artery and vein at level of femoral artery and vein *Cranial and caudal incisions:* skin incisions extended distally in converging fashion, 0.5–1.0 cm cranial and caudal to cranial and caudal saphenous artery and medial saphenous vein; flap undermined beneath saphenous vasculature; ligate and divide peroneal artery and vein *Flap length:* variable, base of flap at level of anastomosis of cranial branches of medial and lateral saphenous veins	Defects of tarsometatarsal regions *Note:* use of flap requires intact collateral blood to lower extremity
Superficial temporal	Caudal edge of zygomatic arch Lateral border of caudal orbital rim	*Base of Flap:* level of zygomatic arch; flap *Width of Flap:* approximates width of zygomatic arch *Incisions:* parallel incisions from landmarks, extending over dorsum of head towards opposing landmark, to the mid-dorsal orbital rim of the opposite eye. Undermine below frontalis muscle layer	Defects over dorsal nasal area, lateral facial area
Lateral thoracic	Axillary skin fold Deep pectoral muscle	*Base of Flap:* axillary skin fold; Ventral border: parallel to dorsal border of deep pectoral muscle Dorsal border: below origin TDA *Flap length:* terminates at/before costal arch; second teat not included	Elbow; axilla, upper extremity

*Major defects only
**Axial pattern flap variation

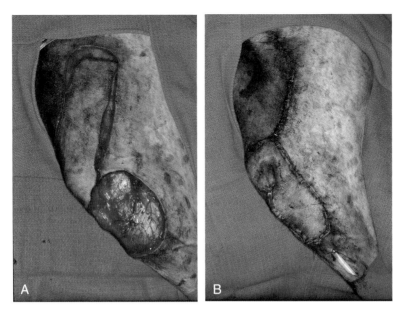

FIG. 13-7 (A) Elevation of a genicular axial pattern flap to close a skin defect secondary to sarcoma removal. (B) The flap was successfully transposed into the defect.

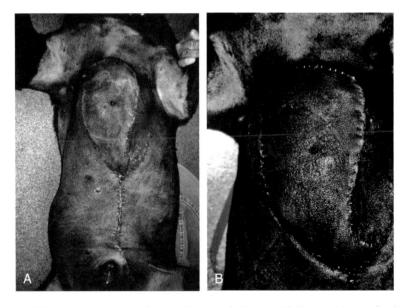

FIG. 13-8 (A, B) Wide mast cell tumor resection over the sternal area and closure with the cranial superficial epigastric axial pattern flap, island arterial flap variation. Today, the author would have used skin stretchers to prestretch the skin of the thorax 72 hours prior to excision to facilitate wound closure. Nonetheless, the cranial epigastric axial pattern flap can be useful for closing the more challenging skin defects in this area.

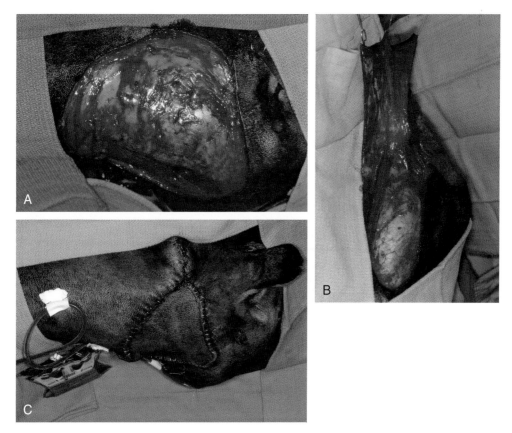

FIG. 13-9 (A) Excision of a chronic granulomatous lesion overlying the left dorsolateral pelvic region.

(B) Elevation of a deep circumflex iliac axial pattern flap, island arterial flap variation, based on the ventral branch of this vessel. Note the base of the flap shares a common border with the defect, thereby creating an island arterial flap.

(C) A small dorsal portion of this skin defect was closed by direct apposition of the adjacent skin margins. The bulk of the defect was successfully closed with this flap.

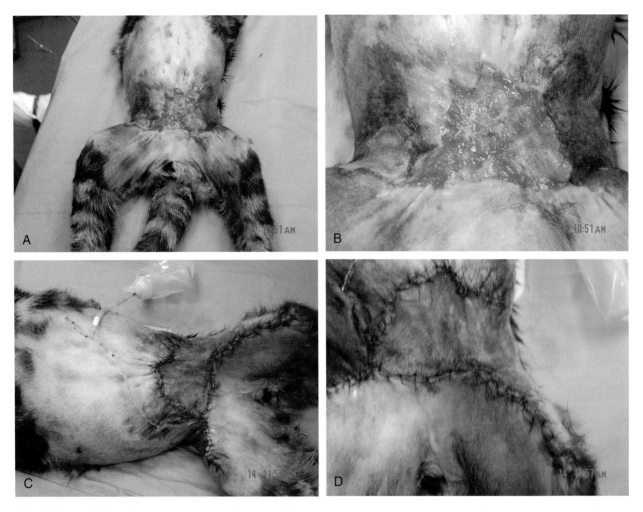

FIG. 13-10 (A, B) Cat with lower abdominal wall defect: dehiscence secondary to sarcoma resection. The wound contracted and epithelialized minimally after a period of open wound management. (C, D) Closure of the defect with the left flank fold flap. The primary source of circulation to this flap is derived from the ventral branch of the deep circumflex iliac artery and vein. This technique is a variation of the axial pattern flap.

FIG. 13-11 (A, B) Example of the reverse saphenous conduit flap for closure of a metatarsal defect. The other common method of closing large defects in this area is a full-thickness mesh graft using a no. 15 scalpel blade to create the holes.

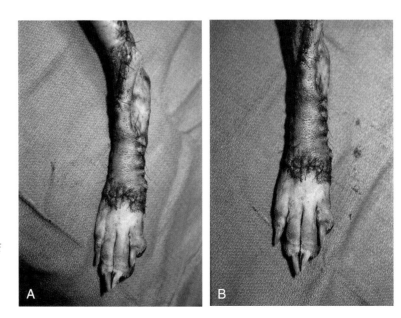

368

vein can be transferred as a unit at a later time. Once circulation is established between the dermal circulation and underlying vasculature, the elevated skin island tethered by the long vessels can be rotated into a regional defect or transferred using microvascular surgical techniques. One example of a secondary axial pattern flap includes skin segments developed over an omental pedicle that includes the epiploic vessels. Unfortunately, two-staged development and transfer is slow and comparatively expensive. It cannot be used for immediate closure of wounds, unlike the other flap and free graft techniques discussed in this book.

> Flap guidelines are simply that: guidelines. Use of the longest variations of *any flap* includes the risk of partial necrosis of its terminal end, secondary to ischemia. Traumatic surgical technique, improper flap elevation and transfer, infection, and insufficient postoperative care can contribute to circulatory compromise to the terminal end of the flap. In most axial pattern flaps, this usually amounts to the last few centimeters. Debridement and resuturing may be required for full-thickness skin loss. In some cases, skin loss is partial thickness, with resultant survival of a portion of the dermis: resection is not necessary in these cases. If the terminal end of a longer flap is considered vital to the closure of a problematic area, a delay procedure (see Chapter 12) may should be considered.

Suggested Readings

Anderson DM, Charlesworth TC, White RAS. 2004. A novel axial pattern skin flap based on the lateral thoracic artery in the dog. *Vet Comp Orthop Traumatol* 17:73–77.

Aper R, Smeak D. 2003. Complications and outcome after thoracodorsal axial pattern flap reconstruction of forelimb skin defects in 10 dogs, 1989–2001. *Vet Surg* 32:378–384.

Cornell K, Salisbury K, Jakovljevic S, et al. 1995. Reverse saphenous conduit flap in cats: an anatomic study. *Vet Surg* 24:202–206.

Degner DA, Bauer MS, Cozen SM. 1993. Reverse saphenous conduit flap: a case report in a cat. *Vet Comp Ortho Traumatol* 6:175–177.

Fahie MA, Smith MM. 1997. Axial pattern flap based on the superficial temporal artery in cats: an experimental study. *Vet Surg* 26:86–89.

Fahie MA, Smith MM. 1999. Axial pattern flap based on the cutaneous branch of the superficial temporal artery in dogs: an experimental study and case report. *Vet Surg* 28:141–147.

Henney LHS, Pavletic MM. 1988. Axial pattern flap based on the superficial brachial artery in the dog. *Vet Surg* 17:311–317.

Hunt GB. 1995. Skin fold advancement for closing large sternal and inguinal wounds in cats and dogs. *Vet Surg* 24:172.

Jackson AH, Degner DA, Jackson IT, et al. 2003. Deep circumflex iliac cutaneous free flap in cats. *Vet Surg* 32:341–349.

Kostolich M, Pavletic MM. 1987. Axial pattern flap based on the genicular branch of the saphenous artery in the dog. *Vet Surg* 16:217–222.

Lidbetter DA, Williams FA, Krahwinkel DJ, et al. 2002. Radical lateral body-wall resection for fibrosarcoma with reconstruction using polypropylene mesh and a caudal superficial epigastric axial pattern flap: a prospective clinical study of the technique and results in 6 cats. *Vet Surg* 31:57–64.

Mayhew PD, Holt DE. 2003. Simultaneous use of bilateral caudal superficial epigastric axial pattern flaps for wound closure in a dog. *J Sm Anim Pract* 44:534–538.

Pavletic MM. 1980. Caudal superficial epigastric arterial pedicle grafts in the dog. *Vet Surg* 9:103–107.

Pavletic MM. 1980. Vascular supply to the skin of the dog. A review. *Vet Surg* 9:77–82.

Pavletic MM. 1981. Canine axial pattern flaps, using the omocervical thoracodorsal, and deep circumflex iliac direct cutaneous arteries. *Am J Vet Res* 42:391–406.

Pavletic MM. 1982. Combined closure techniques for a large skin defect in a cat. *Feline Pract* 12:16–22.

Pavletic MM. 1994. Surgery of the skin and management of wounds. In: Sherding R, ed. *The Cat: Diseases and Clinical Management*, 2nd ed., 1969–1997. New York: Churchill Livingstone.

Pavletic MM. 1998. Skin. In: Bojrab MJ, ed. *Current Techniques in Small Animal Surgery*, 4th ed., 585–603. Baltimore, MD: Williams & Wilkins.

Pavletic MM. 2003. Pedicle grafts. In: Slatter DH, ed. *Textbook of Small Animal Surgery*, 3rd ed., 292–321. Philadelphia, PA: WB Saunders.

Pavletic MM, MacIntire D. 1982. Phycomycosis of the axilla and inner brachium in a dog. Surgical excision and reconstruction with a thoracodorsal axial pattern flap. *J Am Vet Med Assoc* 180:1197–1200.

Pavletic MM, Watters J, Henry RW, et al. 1982. Reverse saphenous conduit flap in the dog. *J Am Vet Med Assoc* 182:380–389.

Reetz JA, Seiler G, Mayhew PD, Holt DE. 2006. Ultrasonographic and color-flow Doppler ultrasonographic assessment of direct cutaneous arteries used for axial pattern skin flaps in dogs. *J Am Vet Med Assoc* 228:1361–1366.

Remedios AM, Bauer MS, Bowen CV. 1989. Thoracodorsal and caudal superficial epigastric axial pattern skin flaps in cats. *Vet Surg* 18:380–385.

Saifzadeh S, Hobbenaghi R, Noorabadi M. 2005. Axial pattern flap based on the lateral caudal arteries of the tail in the dog: an experimental study. *Vet Surg* 34(5):509–513.

Smith MM, Carrig CB, Waldron DR, et al. 1992. Direct cutaneous arterial supply to the tail of dogs. *Am J Vet Res* 53:145–148.

Smith MM, Payne JT, Moon ML, et al. 1991. Axial pattern flap based on the caudal auricular artery in dogs. *Am J Vet Res* 52:922.

Spodnick GS, Hudson LC, Clark GN, et al. 1996. Use of a caudal auricular axial pattern flap in cats. *J Am Vet Med Assoc* 208:1679–1682.

Stiles J, Townsend W, Willis M, et al. 2003. Use of a caudal auricular axial pattern flap in three cats and one dog following orbital exteneration. *Vet Ophthalm* 6:121–126.

Plate 44	**Four Major Axial Pattern Flaps of the Canine Trunk**

DESCRIPTION

The comparative positions of the omocervical (O), thoracodorsal (T), deep circumflex iliac (dorsal branch) (DD), and caudal superficial epigastric (C) axial pattern flaps are illustrated.

SURGICAL CONSIDERATIONS

(A) The left side of the dog demonstrating the relative location of the respective axial pattern flaps.

(B) The right side of the dog shows the flap extending from the opposite side. Note the standard peninsula and right angle (L hockey-stick) variations.

(C) The position of the underlying superficial cervical branch of the omocervical artery (O), thoracodorsal artery (T), dorsal branch (DD) of the deep circumflex iliac artery and its ventral branch (DV) of the deep circumflex iliac artery, and the caudal superficial epigastric artery (C) are illustrated.

COMMENTS

Careful measurement of the defect and flap are required. measurement tapes are ideal for this purpose. The peninsula flap design has a greater length than the right-angle design. However, the latter shape can cover a wider regional defect if the inner flap angle is sutured to itself. Advantages of each technique is discussed individually in this chapter.

Plate 44

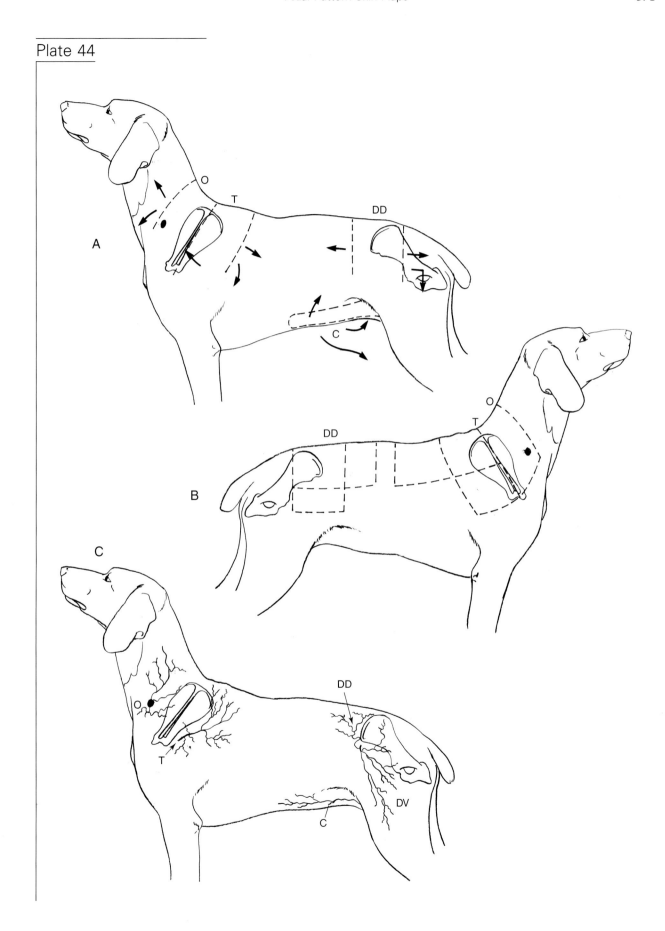

| Plate 45 | **Skin Position and Axial Pattern Flap Development** |

DESCRIPTION

The proper position of the skin in relation to the underlying anatomic structures is essential to locating the direct cutaneous arteries for appropriate axial pattern flap development on the canine trunk.

SURGICAL CONSIDERATIONS

(A) Outline of the omocervical and thoracodorsal axial pattern flaps requires the skin overlying the scapula to remain in a natural position in relation to the underlying scapula. The forelimb is placed in relaxed extension. The skin over the scapula is grasped, lifted, and allowed to spontaneously retract to its natural undistended position before outlining the flap with a felt-tipped marking pen.

(B) The elevation of the deep circumflex iliac axial pattern flap similarly requires placement of the hind limb in relaxed extension. The skin overlying the lateral pelvis is grasped, lifted, and allowed to retract into its natural position. The flap is outlined on the skin using the anatomic landmarks discussed in this chapter.

COMMENTS

The donor area must be thoroughly clipped. Cleansing the skin with isopropyl alcohol–impregnated gauze sponges will help to remove natural oils that impair use of felt-tipped marking pens. Alcohol-resistant marking pens are preferable since the flap outline is less likely to rub off during the surgical preparation of the skin (VWR Marker, VWR Scientific, San Francisco, CA).

Plate 45

A

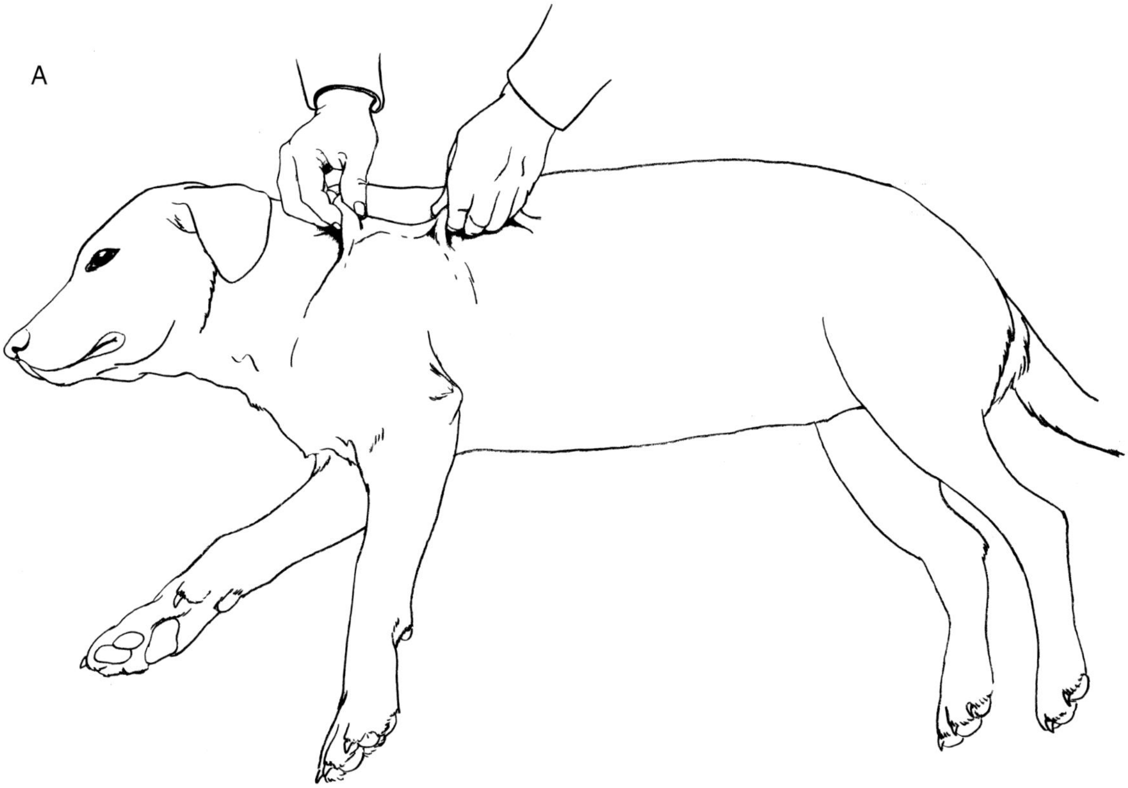

B

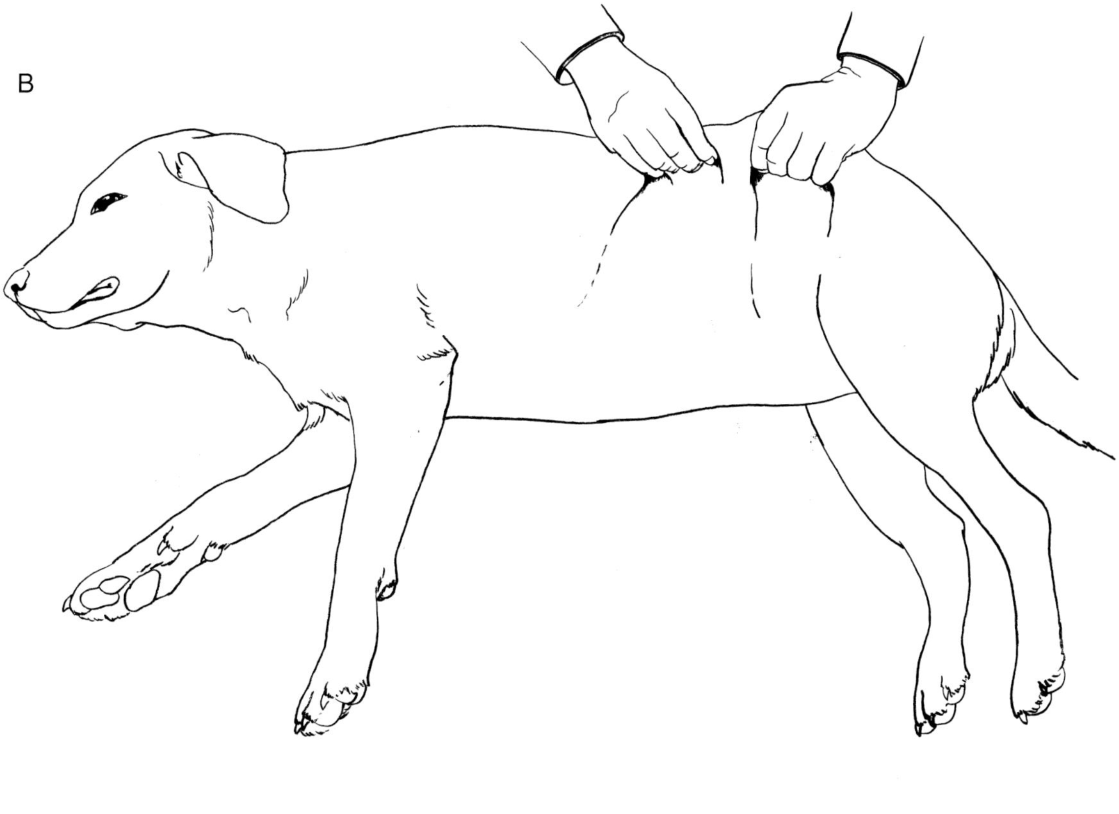

| Plate 46 | **Omocervical Axial Pattern Flap** |

DESCRIPTION

The omocervical axial pattern flap incorporates the superficial cervical branch of the omocervical artery and its associated vein. The vessels originate adjacent to the prescapular lymph node and arborize dorsally just cranial to the scapula.

SURGICAL TECHNIQUE

(A) The anesthetized patient is placed in lateral recumbency. The forelimb is placed in relaxed extension perpendicular to the trunk. The cervical and thoracic skin is grasped, lifted, and allowed to spontaneously retract to normal position to assure the loose skin is not shifted or distorted in relation to the anatomic landmarks (see Plate 45). A line is drawn over the spine of the scapula with a marking pen, forming the caudal border of the flap (arrow). The cranial shoulder depression is palpated. The cranial incision is drawn on the skin, parallel to the caudal incision site, equal to the distance from the cranial shoulder depression (prescapular lymph node) to the caudal incision line.

(B) The reference lines are extended to the dorsal midline and down the opposite side to the contralateral scapulohumeral joint (B_1). Alternatively, the right angle (hockey-stick) design can be created as required. Note that this variation does not extend down to the contralateral scapulohumeral joint: this surface area is "converted" to the angular extension (B_2).

(C) The flap is undermined below the level of the sphincter coli superficialis muscle, beginning at the distant end of the flap. Care must be taken to avoid any trauma to the direct cutaneous vessels. Elevation of long omocervical axial pattern flaps necessitates division of the opposite omocervical direct cutaneous artery and vein.

(D) The omocervical axial pattern flap can be rotated into a variety of positions.

(E) As the flap is being sutured into the recipient bed, the donor site is closed with a subcuticular pattern followed by skin sutures or staples. Drains are employed to control dead space and reduce the likelihood of seroma formation.

COMMENTS

The omocervical axial pattern flap has potential use for large skin defects within its arc of rotation, including wounds involving the face, head, ear, shoulder, neck, and axilla. The more robust thoracodorsal axial pattern flap is preferred over the omocervical flap for the closure of defects within their mutual areas of coverage.

Plate 46

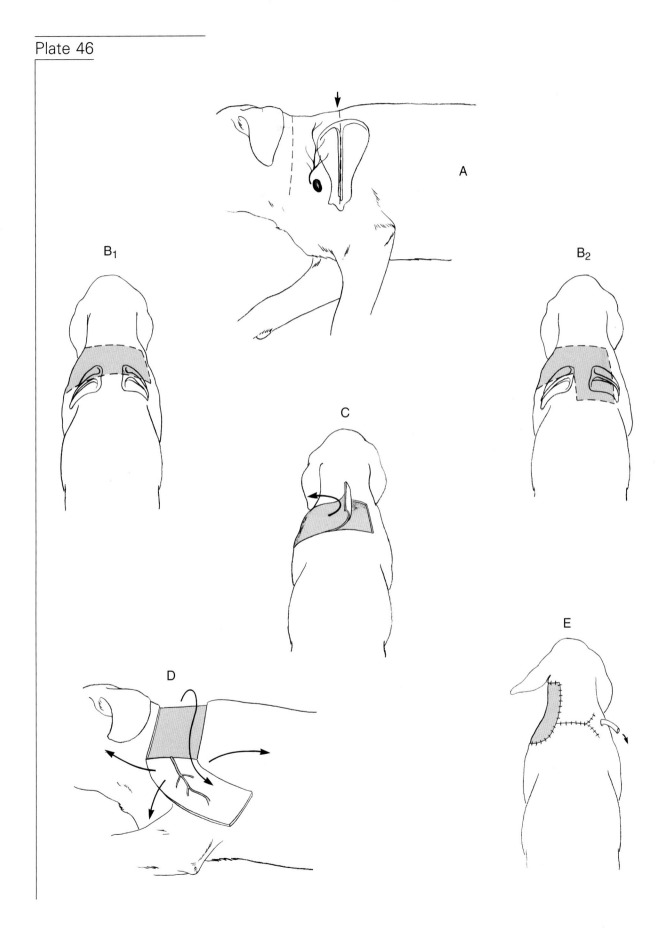

A

B₁   B₂

C

D

E

Plate 47 **Thoracodorsal Axial Pattern Flap**

DESCRIPTION

The thoracodorsal axial pattern flap is based upon the cutaneous branch of the thoracodorsal artery and associated vein. The moderately sized thoracodorsal direct cutaneous artery arborizes in a dorsal direction behind the scapula.

SURGICAL TECHNIQUE

(A) With the dog in lateral recumbency, the lateral cervical and thoracic skin is grasped, lifted, and allowed to spontaneously retract to a normal position. The forelimb is placed in relaxed extension perpendicular to the trunk (see Plate 45). A felt-tipped marking pen is used to draw a line over the spine of the scapula, forming the cranial border of the flap. (The thoracodorsal vessel that originates at the caudal shoulder depression is palpated.) The caudal incision is drawn onto the skin parallel to the cranial incision, equal to the distance from the cranial incision to the caudal shoulder depression. The reference incision lines extend to the dorsal midline.

(B) The standard peninsular (B_1) or hockey-stick (L) configuration (B_2) can be created, depending on the location and size of the defect.

(C) The flap is elevated below the level of the cutaneous trunci muscle, beginning at the end of the flap. Great care must be taken to avoid injury to the thoracodorsal artery and vein: subcutaneous fat frequently obscures the ability to visualize them. The thoracodorsal flap can be pivoted into a variety of defects. The flap may be partially tubed to reach a distant defect or sutured to a bridge incision to traverse the skin interposed between the donor and recipient sites.

COMMENTS

Note that the peninsular design can extend down to the contralateral scapulohumeral joint, whereas the hockey-stick variation is shortened to accommodate the angular extension. Both flap configurations, however, have similar surface areas. Thoracodorsal axial pattern flaps of considerable length can be developed to cover defects involving the shoulder, forelimb, elbow, axilla, and thorax in the dog and cat. Development of long thoracodorsal axial pattern flaps may necessitate division of the opposite cutaneous branch of the thoracodorsal artery and vein. When feasible, it is preferable to position forelimb defects for immediate flap transfer rather than repositioning the patient intraoperatively. The thoracodorsal axial pattern flap is a robust flap capable of covering a variety of defects in the dog and cat. Distal limb coverage is dependent upon body conformation and limb length for the dog. In the cat, this flap can extend to the level of the carpus.

Plate 47

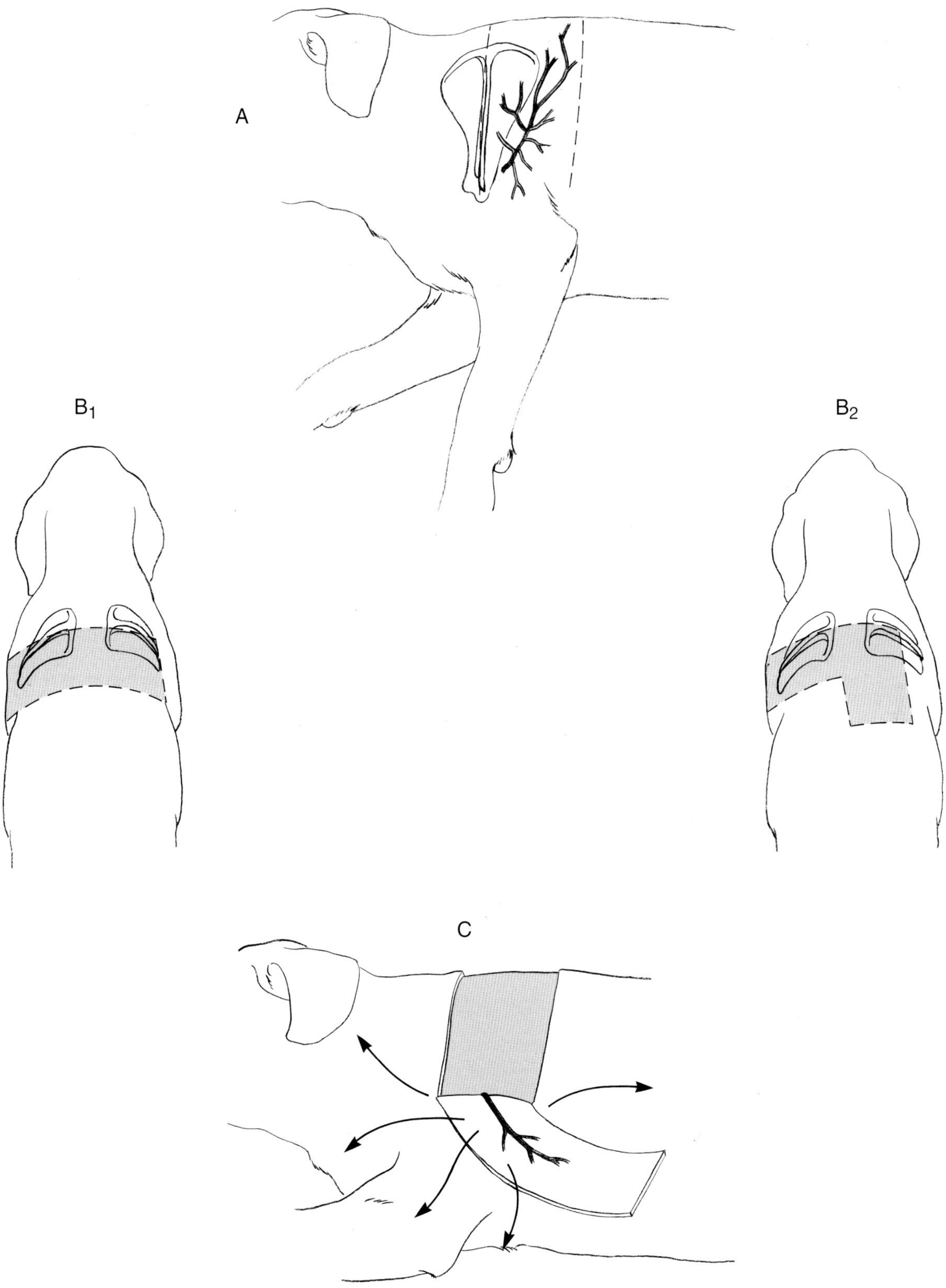

A

B₁

B₂

C

| Plate 48 | **Lateral Thoracic Axial Pattern Flap** |

DESCRIPTION

The lateral thoracic artery [LTA; see (A) below] arises from the caudal aspect of the axillary artery, adjacent to the cranial border of the first rib. The cutaneous branch extends in a caudal direction, supplying the cutaneous trunci muscle and overlying skin caudal to the axillary skin fold. The LTA is noted to enter the skin cranial and ventral to the origin of the thoracodorsal artery. The resultant flap has potential for closing defects involving the elbow region and other problematic wounds within its arc of rotation.

SURGICAL TECHNIQUE

(A) Outline of the LTA axial pattern flap. The *ventral margin of the flap*, caudal to the axillary skin fold (ASF), follows the palpable (dorsal) border of the *deep pectoral muscle*. This border is outlined with a marking pen. The dorsal border of the flap is drawn parallel to the outlined ventral flap border, beginning slightly ventral to the origin of the TDA (see Plate 47, Thoracodorsal Axial Pattern Flap). The outlined flap inclines toward the nipple of the second mammary gland, which is not included into the body of the flap. The distal end of the flap terminates at the level of the costal arch.

(B) Elevation of the lateral thoracic axial pattern flap for closure of a defect overlying the lateral elbow region. A small segment of interposing skin (crosshatched area) or a bridge incision can be used to facilitate flap placement onto the recipient bed.

(C) The flap, sutured into place.

COMMENTS

The size and distribution of the lateral thoracic artery was somewhat inconsistent in the study performed by Anderson. This has been the author's experience in previous anatomic studies, and this should be considered when using this technique. Doppler may be useful in confirming the presence of this vessel prior to surgery. This small axial pattern flap would be useful for closure of problematic wounds in the elbow region, based on its proximity to the area. The skin is not as thick as the skin associated with the more dorsally located thoracodorsal axial pattern flap, a consideration in heavy, large-breed dogs. Failure of this flap would not preclude using the thoracodorsal axial pattern flap. In this report, it was suggested that dogs with underdeveloped or ill-defined skin folds may be a poor candidates for use of the lateral thoracic axial pattern flap. (From Anderson DM, Charlesworth TC, White RAS. 2004. A novel axial pattern skin flap based on the lateral thoracic artery in the dog. *Vet Comp Orthop Traumatol* 2:73–77.)

Plate 48

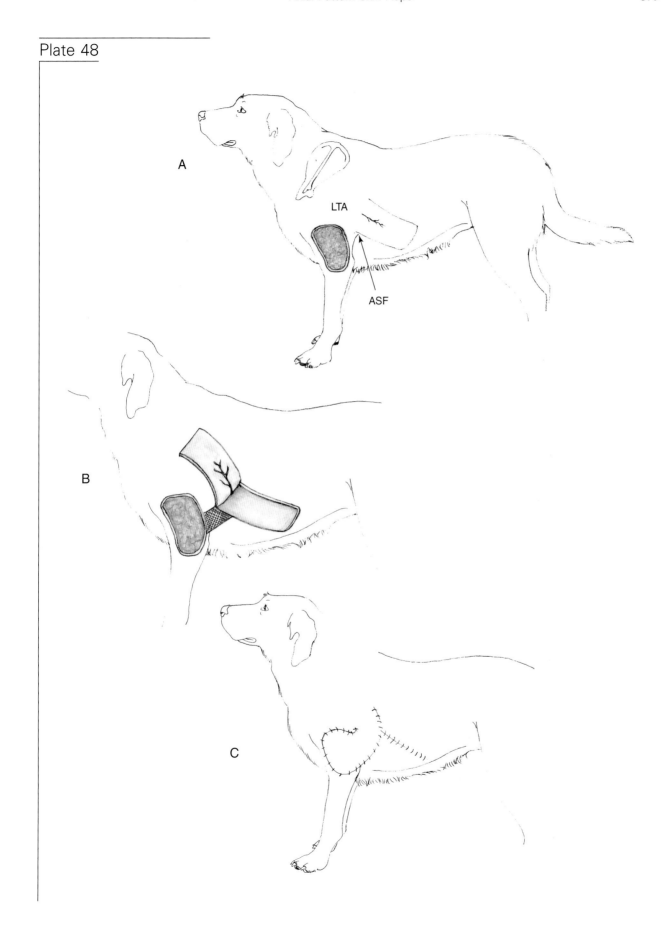

A

LTA

ASF

B

C

| Plate 49 | **Superficial Brachial Axial Pattern Flap** |

DESCRIPTION

The superficial brachial artery branches from the brachial artery, approximately 3 cm proximal to the elbow joint in the average-sized dog. A cutaneous branch of this vessel supplies the craniomedial antebrachium. This small, direct cutaneous artery lies medial to the cephalic vein. The axial pattern flap based over this vessel has special use for closure of antebrachial wounds.

SURGICAL TECHNIQUE

(A) The anatomic landmarks for flap outline include the elbow, humerus, and scapulohumeral joint. The anesthetized patient is placed in dorsal recumbency, with the affected forelimb supported in an elevated position. The entire limb is clipped and vacuumed.

(B) The base of the flap is centered over the anterior third of the flexor surface of the elbow. Lateral and medial incision lines are drawn proximally, parallel to the humeral shaft. However, the lines are drawn to gradually converge, tapering the flap proximally in order to facilitate closure of the donor bed. Both lines are connected at or below the proximal point of the greater tubercle.

    The flap is elevated from the end of the flap toward its base. Care is taken to avoid injury to the subdermal plexus, superficial brachial vasculature, and adjacent cephalic vein.

(C) The flap is rotated laterally into the adjacent defect and sutured into position.

COMMENTS

Note that proximal antebrachial defects that approach the base of the superficial brachial axial pattern flap can be closed by its island flap variation. The vessel is capable of supporting an axial pattern flap of sufficient size to cover major defects involving the midantebrachium and elbow. In general, flap length and subsequent survival preclude its use for coverage of the carpal area. Because of the small size of this vessel, meticulous surgical technique is critical in the preservation of the microcirculation to the flap.

Plate 49

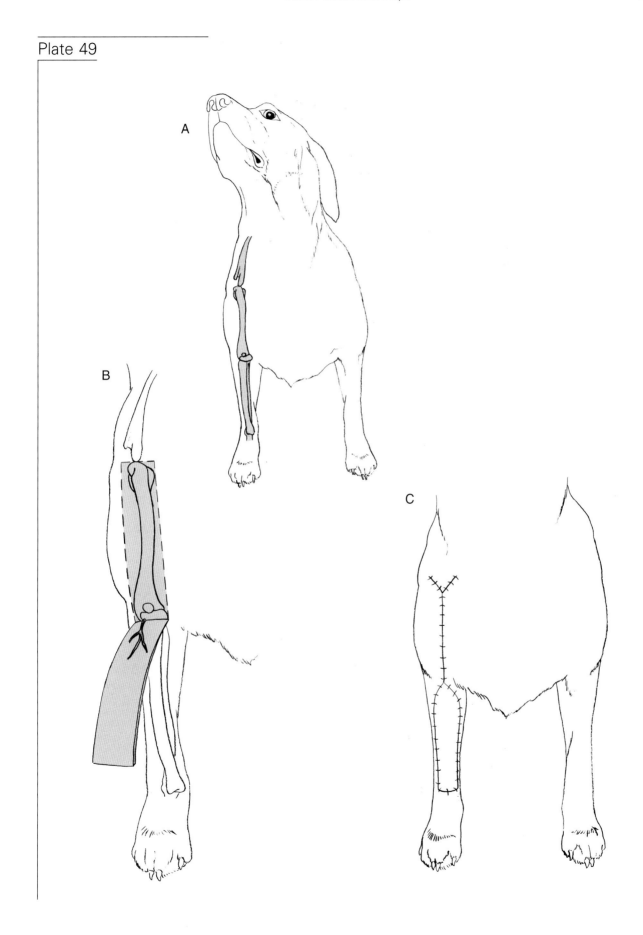

Plate 50	**Caudal Superficial Epigastric Axial Pattern Flap**

DESCRIPTION

This flap includes the last three or four mammary glands (glands two through four in the cat) and is nourished by the caudal superficial epigastric vessels arising at the inguinal canal. The wider arc of rotation of this flap facilitates its placement for closure of a number of caudal trunk and pelvic extremity wounds.

SURGICAL TECHNIQUE

(A) A midline abdominal incision is drawn with a felt-tipped pen, beginning just behind the last mammary teat and continued in a cranial direction. In male dogs, the midline incision must incorporate the base of the prepuce to preserve the epigastric vasculature (inset). If a rear limb defect requires coverage, the leg can be suspended in extension and prepared in routine fashion for the surgical transfer of the skin flap. Depending on the length required, the reference incision line is drawn between glands one and two or glands two and three and continued as the lateral incision, parallel to the medial incision line, at an equal distance from the mammary teats.

(B) The flap is undermined below the supramammarius muscle and above the aponeurosis of the external abdominal oblique muscle progressively in a caudal direction. The epimysium of the superficial pectoral muscle (closely attached to portions of the overlying skin) may be included with the flap in order to assure the subdermal plexus is not traumatized. The caudal superficial epigastric flap can be rotated into a variety of positions when care is taken to preserve the direct cutaneous vessels from excessive kinking or twisting.

(C) This example demonstrates its use for coverage of a medial thigh defect.

COMMENTS

Wider flaps are possible if adequate skin remains to close the donor bed. Because mammary tissue is functional in its new location, ovariohysterectomy is recommended. Ovariohysterectomy can be performed through the medial incision at the time of flap elevation.

The caudal superficial epigastric axial pattern flap is a highly versatile pedicle graft for closure of major skin defects of the caudal abdomen, flank, inguinal area, prepuce, perineum, thigh, and rear limbs. Flap length and width will vary according to the patient's body conformation, the availability of loose skin, and the size required to reach/cover a given defect. Long bodies and short limbs in some dogs, for example, enable the surgeon to develop a flap of sufficient size to extend along the length of the limb. In cats, and dogs with shorter limbs in relation to body length, the caudal superficial epigastric axial pattern flap can extend at or below the level of the tibiotarsal joint. An ample amount of loose, elastic skin in patients enables the surgeon to create wider flaps than the guidelines suggest for flap development.

Plate 50

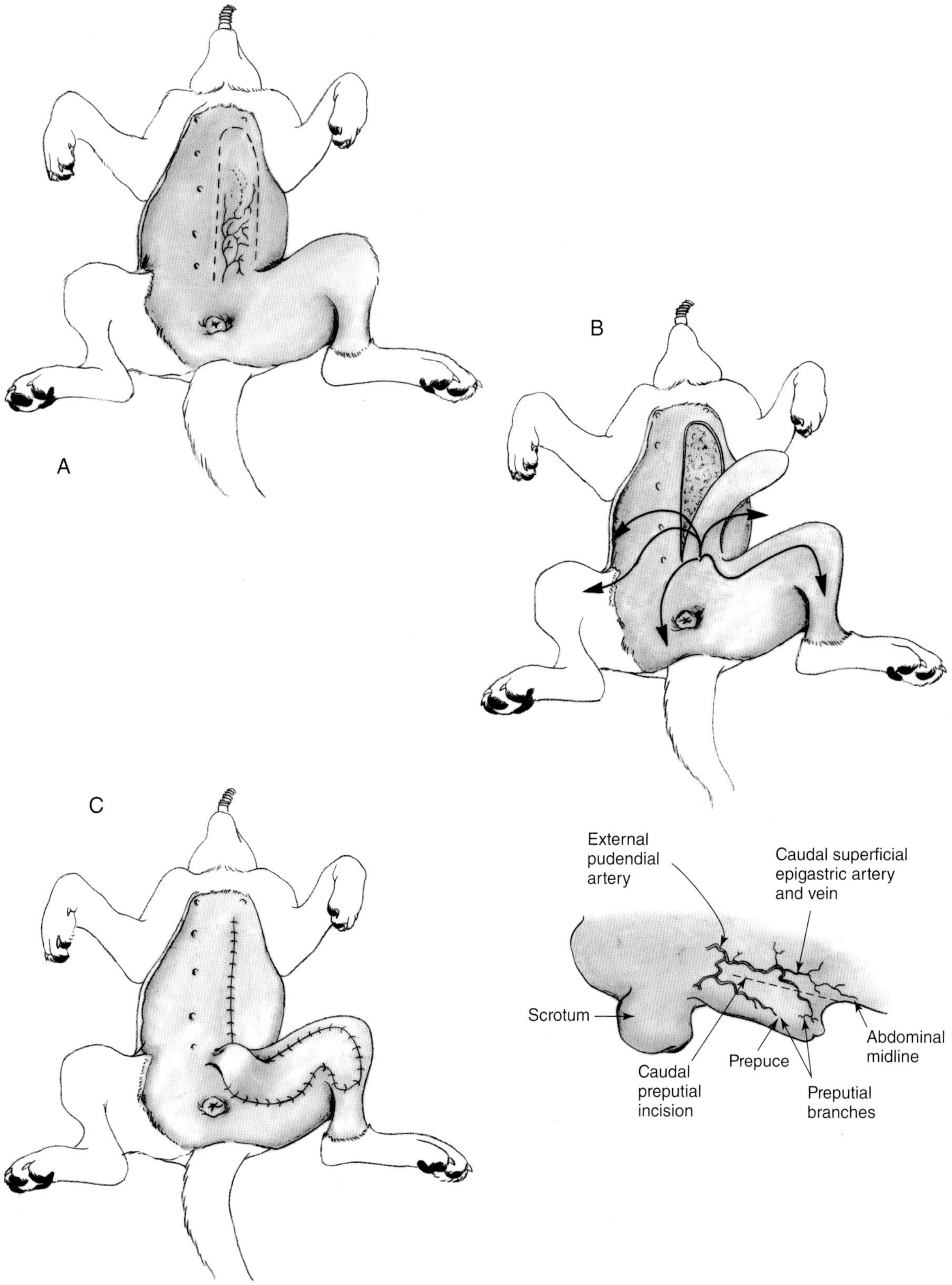

A

B

C

External
pudendal
artery

Caudal superficial
epigastric artery
and vein

Scrotum

Abdominal
midline

Caudal
preputial
incision

Prepuce

Preputial
branches

| Plate 51 | **Cranial Superficial Epigastric Axial Pattern Flap** |

DESCRIPTION

The cranial superficial epigastric axial pattern flap is based over the short cutaneous branches of the cranial superficial epigastric artery located in the hypogastric area caudal to the ventral border of the thoracic cage.

SURGICAL TECHNIQUE

(A₁) The flap is outlined with the patient in dorsal recumbency: a large skin defect is overlying the sternal region of this patient. Depending on the size of the patient, the base of the flap is located in the region of the cranial epigastric vessel, entering the skin lateral to the abdominal midline and a few centimeters caudal to the cartilaginous border of the ventral thorax. The midline of the abdomen serves as the central border of the flap. Like the caudal superficial axial pattern flap, the distance from the midline to the mammary teats serves as the reference of measurement for the lateral incision. The flap length includes the mammary glands three, four, and possibly five. In the male, the end of the flap should be situated cranial to the prepuce due to the risk of necrosis and difficulty associated with closure of flaps extended parallel to the length of the prepuce (see inset).

(B₁) The flap is elevated in a cranial direction beneath the panniculus muscle layer, beginning at the terminal end of the outlined flap. Great care should be taken as undermining approaches the hypogastric origin of the cranial epigastric artery and vein. In this example, a peninsular flap design is employed.

(A₂) In this second variation, an island arterial flap is outlined for elevation. Note that the caudal border of the defect encroaches on the base of the flap, in essence dictating that a cranial epigastric island arterial flap is required to close this sternal wound.

(B₂) Closure of the defect after pivoting the island arterial flap into position. Additional care must be taken to avoid stretching or kinking of the cranial epigastric vessels to which this island flap is tethered.

COMMENTS

The cranial epigastric artery and vein are not nearly as long as the caudal superficial epigastric vessels. As a result, the perfusion pressure of these smaller direct cutaneous arteries cannot sustain the flap dimensions of the caudal superficial epigastric axial pattern flap. Keeping the flap length as short as possible to accomplish wound closure is advisable since a variable degree of flap necrosis occasionally is noted. The location of the cranial superficial epigastric vessels is less predictable than the caudal superficial epigastric artery and vein. In one research subject, a second or supplemental direct cutaneous artery and vein were noted caudal to the small cranial epigastric artery. Although this flap lacks the size and versatility of the caudal superficial epigastric variation, it can be very useful for closure of large skin defects overlying the sternum. Readers should review the use of skin stretchers (see Plate 31): the author has successfully closed similar wounds in this area without the need of the cranial superficial epigastric axial pattern flap.

Plate 51

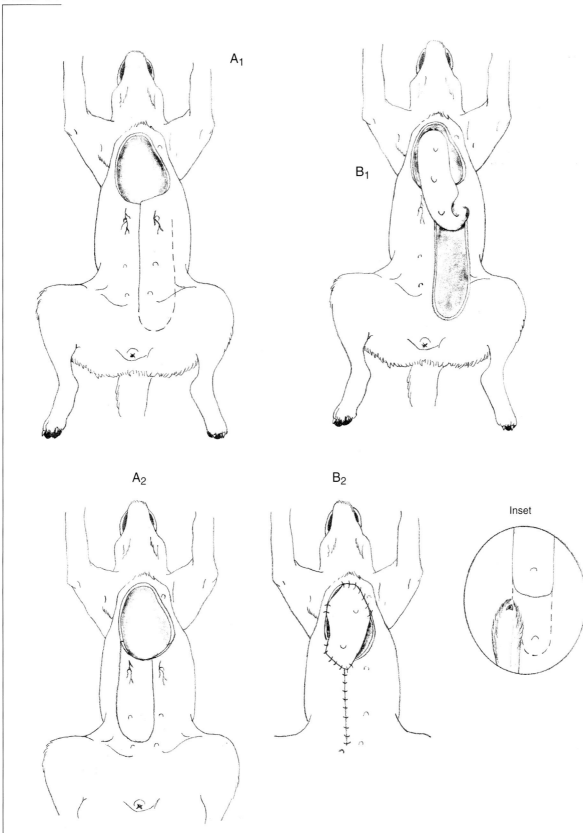

A₁

B₁

A₂

B₂

Inset

| Plate 52 | **Deep Circumflex Iliac Axial Pattern Flap: Dorsal Branch** |

DESCRIPTION

The deep circumflex iliac artery (and paired vein) exits the lateral abdominal wall, cranioventral to the wing of the ilium. It divides to form a dorsal and ventral branch. Each vessel can be used independently for axial pattern flap development.

SURGICAL TECHNIQUE

(A) With the dog in lateral recumbency, the lateral thoracic and abdominal skin is grasped, lifted, and allowed to spontaneously retract to a normal position. The hind limb is placed in relaxed extension perpendicular to the trunk (see Plate 45). A felt-tipped marking pen is used to draw the caudal reference incision line between the cranial border of the wing of the ilium and the greater trochanter. The cranial incision is drawn parallel to the caudal reference incision line and equal to the distance between the iliac border and caudal incision line.

(B) The reference lines are extended to the dorsal midline. At this point, the standard peninsula design can be created, depending on the location and size of the defect.

(C) Alternatively, the flap can be created at a right angle. Note the similar surface area in comparison to the peninsula flap design.

(D) Flaps are elevated below the level of the cutaneous trunci muscles and fascia, beginning at the distant border of the flap. The resultant flap can be rotated into a variety of defects encountered within its arc of rotation.

COMMENTS

The shorter dorsal branch has general application for defects involving the ipsilateral flank, lateral lumbar area, caudal thorax, lateral thigh, and pelvic area. The author finds this flap especially useful for major skin defects overlying the greater trochanter and associated lateral pelvic area.

Plate 52

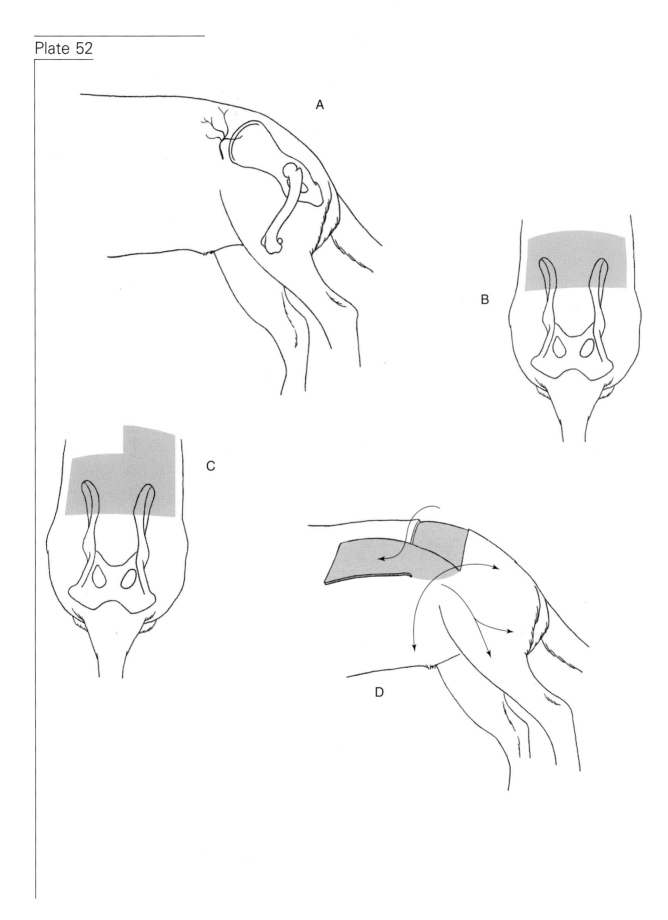

| Plate 53 | **Deep Circumflex Iliac Axial Pattern Flap: Ventral Branch** |

DESCRIPTION

The ventral branch of the deep circumflex iliac artery extends down the lateral flank and craniolateral thigh for axial pattern flap development.

SURGICAL TECHNIQUE

(A) The dog is positioned as previously discussed in Plate 52. Landmarks for establishing the width of the flap are identical. The caudal incision line is drawn from the midpoint between the wing of the ilium and greater trochanter and directed distally, cranial to the border of the femoral shaft. The cranial incision line extends from the established base point (in relation to the wing of ilium), extending down the flank/thigh region, parallel to the caudal flap border. The flap terminates above the patella by a connecting line drawn between the cranial and caudal flap borders.

(B) The deep circumflex iliac flap (ventral branch) in its peninsular or island arterial flap configurations can be used to close defects within its 180-degree arc of rotation.

(C) The island arterial flap is elevated, beginning at the distal border, and carefully pivoted over the preserved direct cutaneous artery and vein. It is important to fully assess skin tension and elasticity prior to surgery. Flap dimensions may require modification to assure closure of the donor bed can be achieved without difficulty. Excessive wound tension upon closure of the donor site will compromise limb function and increase the risk of dehiscence.

(D) The island arterial flap is sutured over the dorsal pelvic surface. Drainage is established to prevent seroma formation.

COMMENTS

Perhaps the greatest use of the ventral flap is in the creation of an island flap for closure of major sacral and lateral pelvic skin wounds that preclude the use of the dorsal branch of the deep circumflex iliac artery for axial pattern flap development.

The hind limb flank fold flap (Plate 54) is a variation of the ventral deep circumflex iliac axial pattern flap. The flank fold region includes the territory of this direct cutaneous artery, but the flap size is limited to the confines of the flank fold for transposition into inguinal defects.

Plate 53

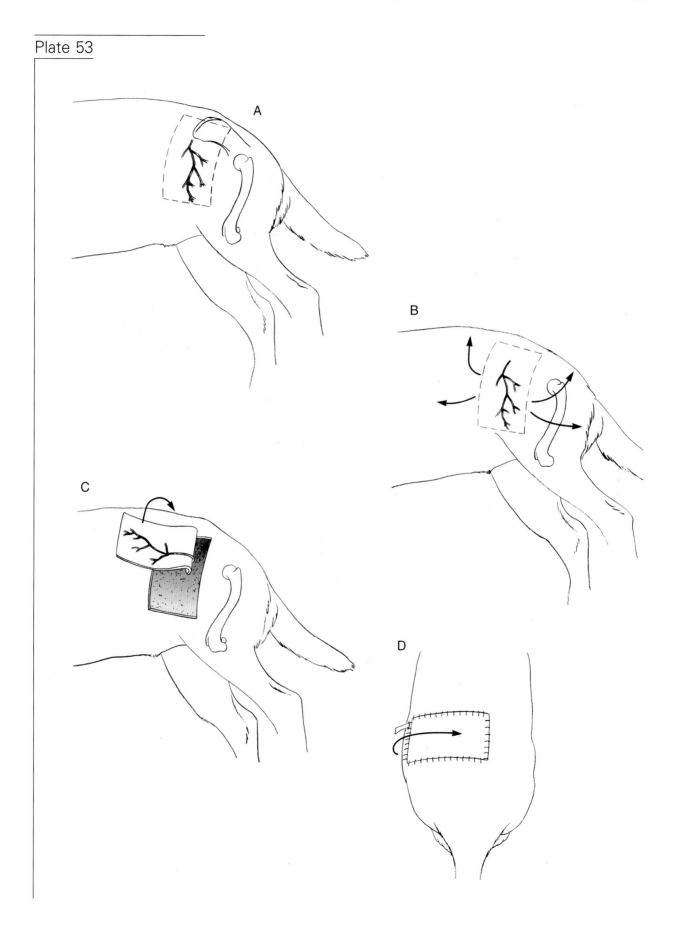

Plate 54   **Flank Fold Flap: Hind Limb**

DESCRIPTION

The dog and cat have a natural fold of skin located in the flank area, dorsal and anterior to the knee. The lower branches of the ventral branch of the deep circumflex iliac artery supply this cutaneous area. It is possible to elevate and transpose this fold of skin (as reported by Hunt) to cover defects in the inguinal area, especially when the caudal superficial epigastric axial pattern flap is not feasible.

SURGICAL TECHNIQUE

(A) The flank fold can be gently grasped to determine the amount of skin that can be harvested. The leg is manipulated during this maneuver, to assure that sufficient skin is present to permit closure of the donor site without undue tension. The lateral to medial (dashed line) U-shaped fold flap is drawn onto the clipped skin.

(B) A caudal inguinal defect is noted in this example. Note the relationship of this wound to the proposed flank fold flap.

(C) The flap is elevated; the small patch of skin (lined area) is resected to allow the transposition of the flap.

(D) The elastic flank fold flap is sutured into position.

(E) Lateral view of the limb, after transposition of the flap and closure of the donor site.

COMMENTS

This flank fold flap is a more restricted variation of the ventral deep circumflex iliac axial pattern flap. It can be effectively used to close the more difficult wounds encountered in the inguinal area. This thin, elastic skin can conform readily to wounds in this area. Careful measurement of the flap is required in this area. Excessive tension during closure of the donor site can result in restricted movement of the involved limb, risking dehiscence: open flank wounds can be quite difficult to close.

Plate 54

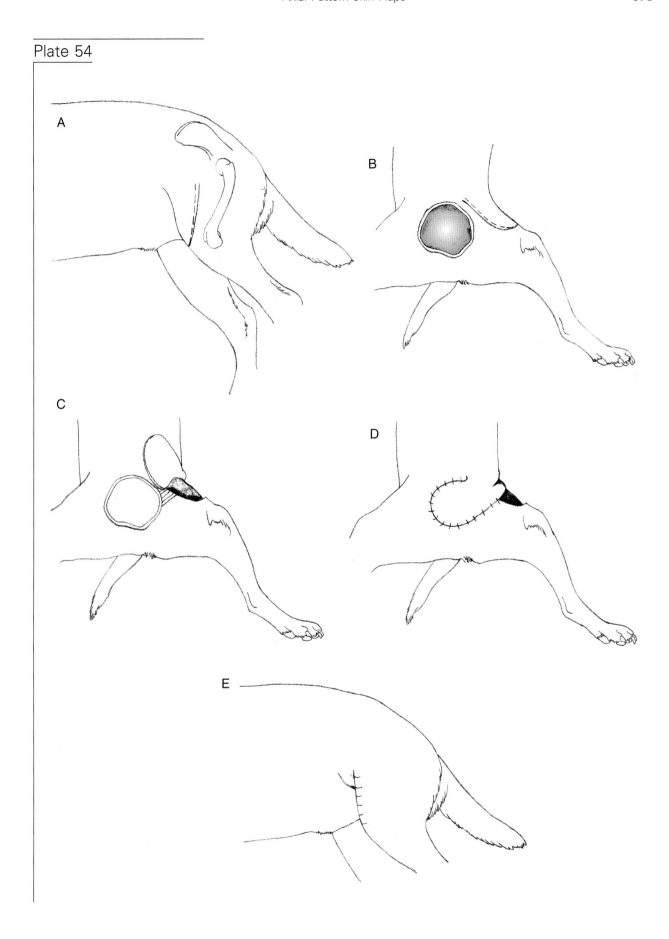

Plate 55   # Genicular Axial Pattern Flap

DESCRIPTION

The genicular axial pattern flap originates over the short genicular branch of the saphenous artery and medial saphenous vein. The genicular artery extends cranially over the medial aspect of the stifle and terminates over its craniolateral surface.

SURGICAL TECHNIQUE

(A) The dog is placed in lateral recumbency and the rear limb is clipped and prepared for surgery in routine fashion. The base of the flap is marked with a felt-tipped pen at a point 1 cm proximal to the patella and 1.5 cm below the tibial tuberosity. Two lines are extended on the lateral thigh parallel to the femoral shaft to the base of the greater trochanter.

(B) The flap is carefully elevated by undermining the skin in the loose areolar fascial plane beneath the dermis.

(C) In this example, the flap is rotated into the lower limb defect and sutured into place. The donor site is closed with a subcuticular pattern and skin sutures to minimize the risk of dehiscence.

COMMENTS

The genicular artery, like the superficial brachial artery, is not a large vessel capable of supporting circulation to a large segment of skin. However, it usually is sufficient to support flaps for closure of wounds of the lateral or medial tibial regions, as well as flaps capable of extending distally to the level of the tibiotarsal joint, depending upon the individual conformation of the canine patient. Keeping skin flaps as short as possible to accomplish wound closure helps assure complete flap survival.

Plate 55

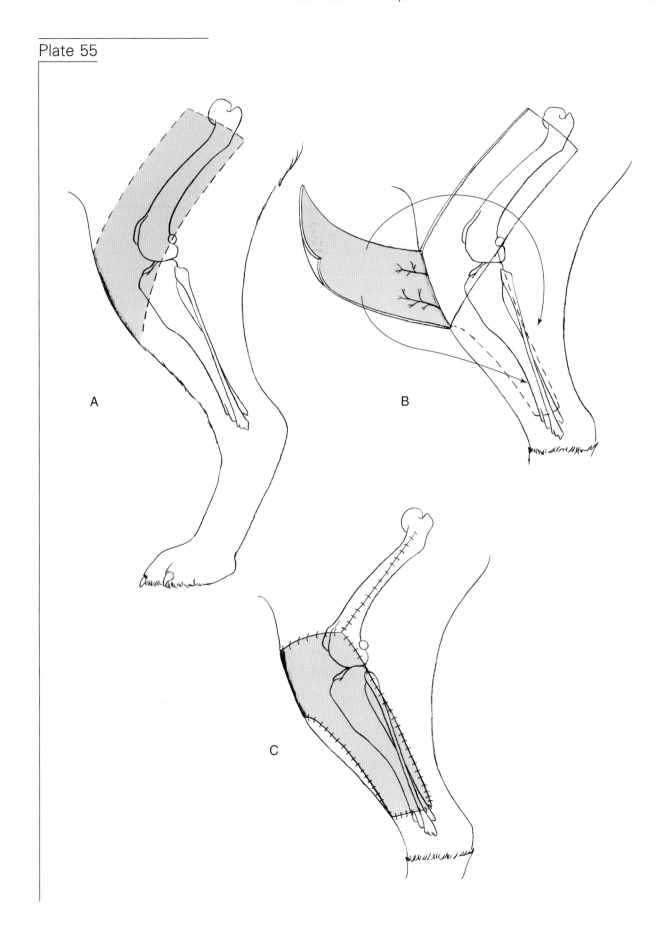

Plate 56   **Reverse Saphenous Conduit Flap**

DESCRIPTION

The reverse saphenous conduit flap incorporates branches of the saphenous artery and medial saphenous vein, which in turn supply and drain the overlying skin by means of direct cutaneous vessels. By division of vascular connections with the femoral artery and vein, blood flow is maintained in reverse by distal anastomotic connections (1) between the cranial branch of the saphenous artery and the perforating metatarsal artery by way of the medial and lateral plantar arteries and (2) between the cranial branch of the medial saphenous vein and the cranial branch of the lateral saphenous vein, and other venous connections with the cranial and caudal branches of the medial saphenous veins distal to the tibiotarsal joint.

SURGICAL TECHNIQUE

(A)   Measurements are taken to determine the flap required to reach and cover the lower limb defect. The flap width is tapered distally, owing to the limited skin available for flap development. A skin incision is generally made across the central third of the inner thigh, at or slightly above the level of the patella.

(B)   Metzenbaum scissors are used to expose the underlying saphenous artery, medial saphenous vein, and nerve (at the level of the femoral artery and vein) prior to their ligation and division. Two incisions are extended distally in convergent fashion, 0.5–1.0 cm cranial and caudal to the borders of the cranial and caudal branches of the saphenous artery and medial saphenous vein, respectively. The flaps are undermined beneath the saphenous vasculature. To avoid injury to the caudal branch of the saphenous artery and medial saphenous vein during progressive raising of the pedicle graft, a portion of the medial gastrocnemius muscle fascia is included with the flap. Below this point, the tibial nerve merges with the descending caudal branches of the saphenous artery and medial saphenous vein and can be preserved by meticulous dissection between these structures. Ligation and division of the peroneal (fibular) artery and vein are necessary to facilitate flap mobility. Flap elevation is completed proximal to the anastomosis between the cranial branch of the medial saphenous vein and the cranial branch of the lateral saphenous vein.

(C, D)   The donor bed is initially closed with interrupted subcuticular sutures, then with simple interrupted skin sutures, using 3-0 suture material at the end of the transplantation. The "transfer pedicle" can be tubed to traverse the skin between the donor and recipient beds. Care is taken to ensure that the tubed pedicle is not under undue tension on extension of the tibiotarsal joint.

(E$_{1,2}$)   A bridge incision connecting the donor and recipient beds is an optional method to traverse the skin between donor and recipient beds.

COMMENTS

Slightly longer flaps are possible, if required. The resultant flap with a distally based pedicle has potential for use in major cutaneous defects at or below the tarsus, especially wounds overlying the metatarsal surface. When the reverse saphenous conduit flap is considered for use on skin defects secondary to extensive trauma, angiography should be considered to ensure that anastomotic connections are intact and that the saphenous artery and medial saphenous vein are not the major routes of circulation to the lower limb. Based on anatomic studies, the vascular supply and general guidelines for flap development in the cat are remarkably similar to the dog.

Plate 56

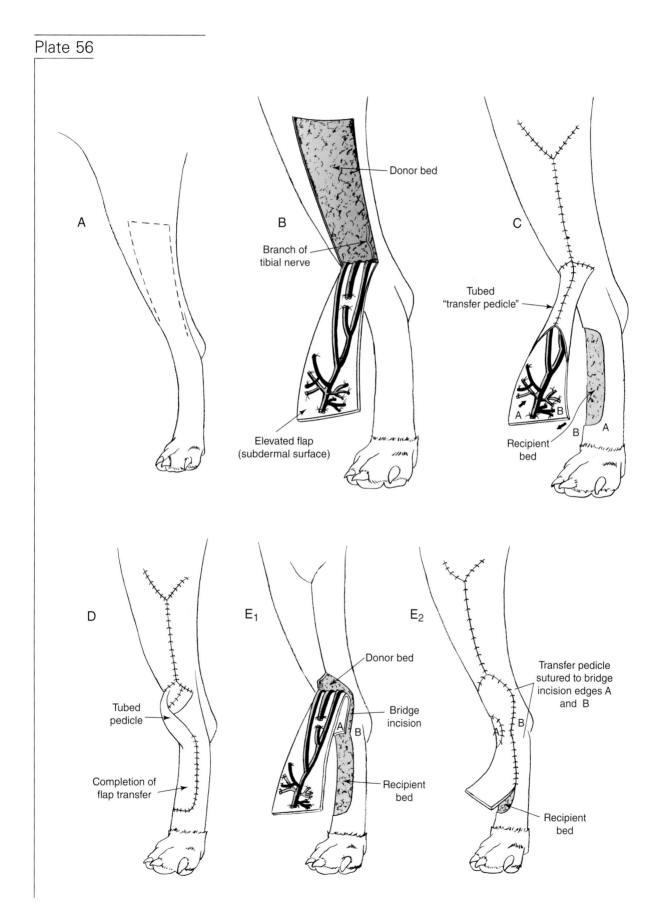

A

B

Donor bed

Branch of
tibial nerve

Elevated flap
(subdermal surface)

C

Tubed
"transfer pedicle"

A B

B A

Recipient
bed

D

Tubed
pedicle

Completion of
flap transfer

E₁

Donor bed

Bridge
incision

A B

Recipient
bed

E₂

Transfer pedicle
sutured to bridge
incision edges A
and B

A B

Recipient
bed

Plate 57   **Caudal Auricular Axial Pattern Flap**

DESCRIPTION

The caudal auricular axial pattern flap incorporates the sternocleidomastoid branches of the caudal auricular artery and vein located in the palpable depression between the lateral aspect of the wing of the atlas and the vertical ear canal.

SURGICAL TECHNIQUE

(A₁) The anesthetized patient is placed in lateral recumbency. The forelimb is placed in relaxed extension, thereby positioning the scapula perpendicular to the trunk. The skin is grasped and lifted to assure there is no distortion of the cervical skin to the underlying anatomic landmarks. The flap base is centered over the palpable lateral wing of the atlas. Two parallel lines are positioned in the central one-third of the lateral cervical profile of the dog. Wider flaps are possible. The two lines are connected to complete the outline of the flap, at the level of the scapula.

(A₂) The general outline of the flap in the cat is similar to the dog. The flap is centered over the lateral border (wing) of the atlas. Based on the feline anatomy, the dorsal line (border) of the flap is closer to the dorsal midline. The ventrolateral incision is positioned at the same distance measured from the dorsal line to the point of entry of the caudal auricular artery (a palpable depression at the midpoint between the base of the pinna and lateral wing of the atlas).

(B₁) The flap is elevated in a caudal to cranial direction beneath the sphincter colli superficialis muscle layer to preserve the vascular integrity of the skin. Care is taken to preserve the auricular cutaneous vessels entering the flap between the vertical ear canal and wing of the atlas.

(B₂) The elevated flap can be rotated into a variety of positions within its arc of rotation. In this example, the flap has been rotated rostrally to close a large facial defect secondary to wide tumor resection in a cat. The flap spans any interposing skin between the donor and recipient site with a bridge incision or the flap can be partially tubed to "caterpillar" over this region. Vacuum drains are ideally suited for controlling dead space and fluid accumulation, although Penrose drains may be satisfactory.

COMMENTS

Described by MM Smith et al., the caudal auricular axial pattern flap can be used to reconstruct the ear, dorsum of the head, or extend further rostrally to close defects overlying the orbital area as illustrated in (B₂). Like other flaps, keeping the flap as short as possible reduces the likelihood of partial flap necrosis that occasionally is noted when the caudal auricular axial pattern flap is extended to the cranial and midscapular regions. In the more rostral areas of the head, the surgeon must keep in mind that simpler (local) transposition flaps, created in the lateral facial area or dorsal aspect of the head, can be used to close small to moderate defects. Like other axial pattern flaps, a variable portion of these flaps are utilized simply to span over interposing skin in order to achieve closure of a defect. Despite this caveat, the caudal auricular axial pattern flap is a useful technique to close many of the more challenging wounds resulting from trauma or tumor resection.

Plate 57

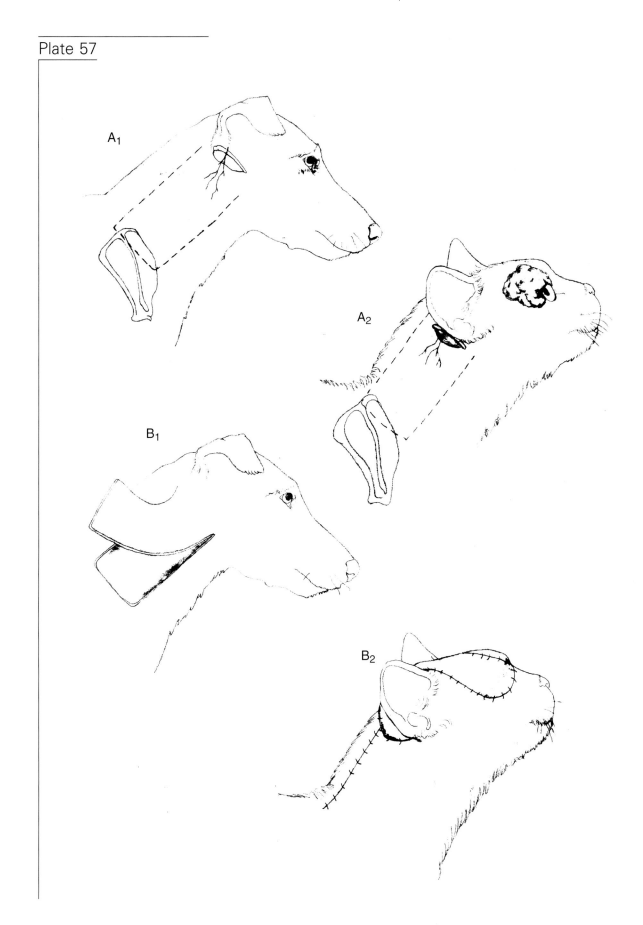

A₁

A₂

B₁

B₂

Plate 58	**Superficial Temporal Axial Pattern Flap**

DESCRIPTION

The cutaneous branch of the superficial temporal artery can be developed into an axial pattern flap using the skin over the temporal muscle area. The flap has potential use for facial defects within its arc of rotation. General guidelines for the dog and cat are identical.

SURGICAL TECHNIQUE

(A) General outline of the flap, dorsal view. The flap is outlined on the skin prior to incising it.

(B) Lateral view. The base of the flap is located at the level of the zygomatic arch. The width of the flap approximates the length of the zygomatic arch: the caudal orbital rim is the rostral border of the flap, and the caudal aspect of the zygomatic arch represents the caudal flap margin. Flap length, based on research by Fahie et al., is the mid-dorsal orbital rim of the opposite eye (see A). The flap is elevated deep to the frontalis muscle to help preserve its blood supply. The flap is elevated from the distant end of the flap toward its base.

(C) The flap rotated over the dorsal muzzle to close a large skin defect after tumor resection.

COMMENTS

As noted, anatomic landmarks and guidelines for this flap are identical in the dog and cat. Inclusion of the frontalis muscle makes this flap somewhat a hybrid between a myocutaneous flap and axial pattern flap. However, the muscle is included to help preserve the vasculature rather than contributing to the circulation to the overlying skin.

Use of the superficial temporal axial pattern flap may be most useful for midfacial defects. Lateral facial defects may be closed with a simpler local flap (advancement or transposition), depending on the size and location of the wound. Care must be taken to avoid wide flaps that could compromise function of the upper eyelid(s). Skin tension in this region should be closely assessed prior to elevating this flap.

Plate 58

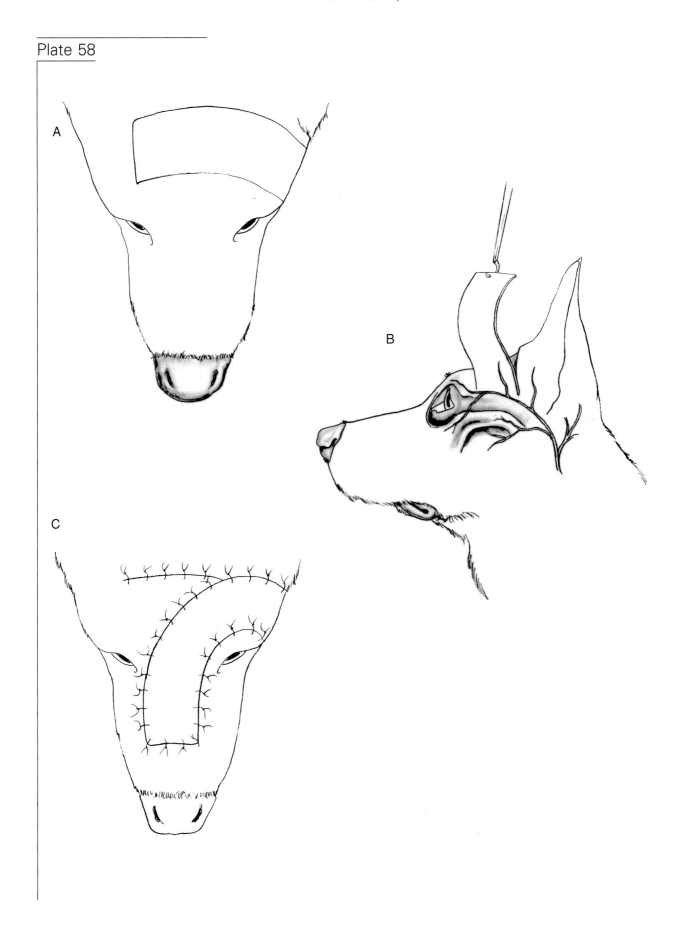

Plate 59	**Lateral Caudal (Tail) Axial Pattern Flap**

DESCRIPTION

The caudal gluteal arteries give rise to the lateral caudal arteries, which contribute circulation to the length of the tail skin. Each vessel resides in a lateral location, ventral to the transverse processes of the caudal vertebrae in the proximal tail region; in the distal tail, the vessels course dorsal to the transverse processes. Based on these two direct cutaneous arteries and associated veins, the tail skin can serve as a source of skin for difficult wounds associated with the perineum and caudodorsal pelvic region.

SURGICAL TECHNIQUE

(A₁) Profile of the tail, demonstrating the caudal tail vessels and related anatomy. The dashed line illustrates the limits of the proximal one-third of the tail. In this example, the length of the flap is limited to this designated length.

(B₁) A dorsal midline incision is made in preparation for coverage of a dorsal pelvic defect.

(C) Dissection is directed down to the level of the deeper tail fascia. The subcutaneous tissue interface is carefully freed from this fascial plane, thereby helping to preserve the integrity of caudal tail vessels in the subcutis. Upon completion of the procedure, the tail proper is amputated at the caudal third or fourth intervertebral space.

(D) The flap is advanced over the caudodorsal aspect of the pelvis in this example.

(A₂) In this example, the flap was developed as noted in A₁–D. A ventral midline incision effectively "bi-valves" the flap. Each half is supplied by its own lateral caudal artery and vein.

(B₂) In this example, the bi-valved flap is employed to close a perianal defect.

COMMENTS

By highlighting the direct arterial blood supply to the tail, MM Smith et al. established an effective method of harvesting this source of skin with a greater probability of flap survival. The entire tail length potentially can be used for flap development, although the circumference of the proximal one-third of the tail is the largest source of skin. In some dogs, the proximal tail can provide a surprising amount of skin for closure of challenging wounds in the caudal pelvic area. Other flap techniques may potentially overlap the "cranial territorial limits" of this flap without the need to amputate the tail (a point of contention for some owners) Nonetheless, the lateral caudal axial pattern flap can be very useful for closing cutaneous defects within its arc of rotation especially in those cases when disease/trauma preclude the effective use of other closure options.

    This axial pattern flap can be elevated using a ventral incision alone, if the surgeon does not wish to "bi-valve" the flap. However, the dorsal approach is technically easier to perform, and partially dividing the flap down the middle allows the surgeon to wrap the flap around the anus at the time of wound closure.

Plate 59

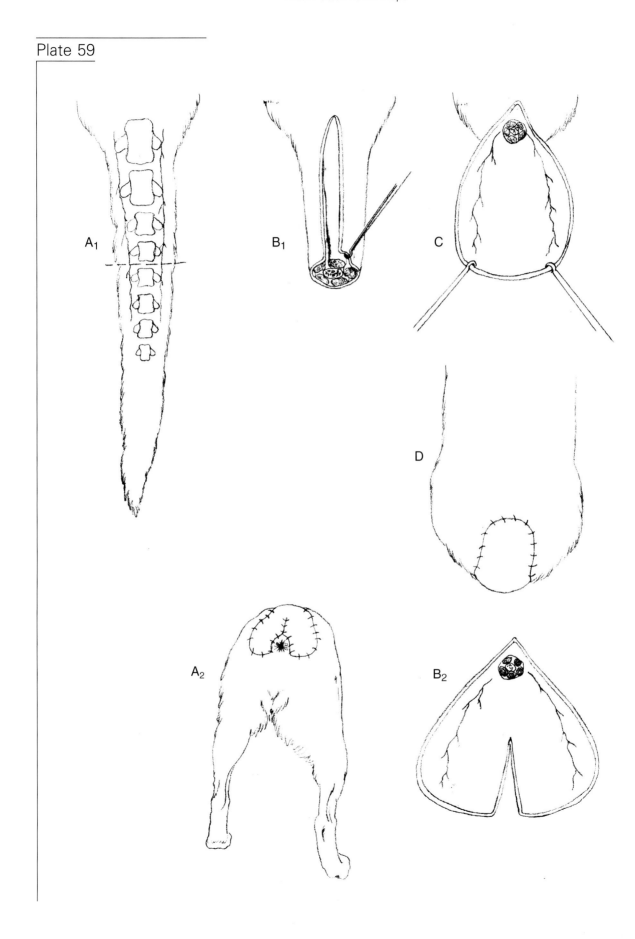

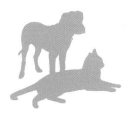

Free Grafts

FREE SKIN GRAFTS

Free grafts are segments of skin completely detached from one area of the body and used to resurface another body area lacking an epithelial surface. Free grafts lack a vascular attachment upon transfer to the recipient graft bed. They must survive by absorbing tissue fluid from the recipient bed by capillary action during the initial 48 hours after transplantation. During this period, capillaries from the recipient bed unite with the exposed graft plexuses to reestablish vital circulation. New capillaries later grow into the graft and the vascular channels remodel. In addition, fibrous connective tissue forms to hold the graft securely in place. Grafts assume a pink color in 48 hours if circulation is adequate. Grafts with venous obstruction have a cyanotic hue until circulation improves.

Any accumulation of material such as pus, serum, blood, hematoma, or foreign matter between the graft and recipient bed will delay or prevent graft revascularization. This delay often results in graft necrosis. Motion between the graft and the recipient bed has a similar effect. Fibrinolysis secondary to bacterial infection destroys the early fibrin "glue" between the graft and the bed, resulting in motion and graft necrosis. Improper contact between the graft and the recipient bed prevents proper surface-to-surface interdigitation and poor graft revascularization. This occurs if the graft is stretched over the bed like a drum skin or if an excessively large graft is applied to form graft folds that lack proper recipient bed contact. Nonviable grafts are white or black in appearance when assessed after sufficient time has progressed for their revascularization.

Although free skin grafts require a vascularized recipient bed for survival, granulation tissue is not necessary before a graft is applied. Healthy muscle, periosteum, and peritenon can support a skin graft. Healthy pink granulation tissue, however, is an excellent recipient bed for skin grafts. Pale, collagen-laden chronic granulation tissue has a poor vascular supply and should be excised to promote formation of healthy granulation tissue. Contamination and infection should be controlled, and any "epithelial cover" can be excised with a scalpel blade before graft application. Skin grafting in dogs, cats, and birds can be highly successful once the surgical details on graft harvesting, application, and bandaging are mastered. Fortunately, the learning curve is not particularly steep.

Antibiotics and Skin Grafting

All granulation beds are contaminated with bacteria. Surgeons have their preference for whether to use topical and systemic antibiotics in skin-grafting procedures. Surgeons occasionally culture the granulation bed prior to skin grafting to assure appropriate treatment can be instituted prior to graft application. (The author does not culture wound beds before grafting in most routine clinical cases.) In humans, group A beta-hemolytic streptococci (*Streptococcus pyogenes*) is the biggest culprit for graft dissolution. Topical and systemic penicillin can be used to control this organism prior to grafting. Other organisms, including *Pseudomonas* sp. and *Klebsiella* occasionally are problematic for graft survival.

The following is the author's method: Once a healthy granulation bed is obtained, apply a heavy layer of silver sulfadiazine or triple antibiotic ointment over the recipient bed, followed by a nonadherent dressing and protective bandage. This should take place 24–48 hours prior to grafting. Place most patients on a broad-spectrum antibiotic, usually Cephazolin (Novaplus, Sandoz Inc., Broomfield, CO), 20 mg/kg TID, prior to surgery and postoperatively for 1 week.

At the time of surgery, cover the recipient bed with sterile gauze when fur is clipped. Thoroughly cleanse the skin and graft bed with a chlorhexidine-saline (or lactated Ringer's solution) in a 1:40 dilution.

Use gauze sponges to gently scrub the granulation bed. After transfer to the recipient bed, cover the graft with a layer of triple antibiotic ointment, followed by a nonadherent dressing and protective bandage wrap.

CLASSIFICATION OF FREE GRAFTS

Free grafts can be classified according to the source of the graft, the graft thickness, and the graft shape or design. Although autogenous grafts are used for permanent free graft coverage in small animals, allografts (homografts) and xenografts (heterografts) can be used as temporary biologic dressings until an autogenous graft can be successfully applied. Free grafts can be harvested as full- or split-thickness skin grafts. Split-thickness grafts are harvested with razor blades, graft knives, or a dermatome. Graft knives and razors are difficult to master and rarely harvest the quantities of split-thickness skin grafts required for larger skin wounds that occasionally justify their use. Uniform thickness and adequate harvesting of split-thickness grafts require the use of the more expensive gas- or electric-powered dermatomes.

Grafts usually are applied immediately after harvesting. Under unusual clinical circumstances, the harvested skin can be temporarily refrigerated until application can be completed.

GRAFT THICKNESS

Graft thickness varies according to the amount of dermis included with the overlying epidermis. The donor bed of a split-thickness graft bed can be excised and closed, or it may be left to heal by adnexal regeneration and epithelialization. Thin split-thickness grafts "take" more readily than full-thickness grafts, but they lack durability and proper hair growth, and they are more susceptible to secondary graft contraction. Full-thickness grafts are preferred by many veterinarians for these reasons. From the author's experience, properly prepared full-thickness grafts can achieve survival rates comparable to thinner grafts in the dog and cat. Free grafts can be applied as a sheet over the entire recipient bed, or they can be cut into various shapes or patterns.

> The full-thickness hand or scalpel mesh graft is a highly effective technique for closing defects involving the lower extremities (see Plate 67).

PARTIAL-COVERAGE GRAFTS

Punch grafts, pinch grafts, strip grafts, stamp grafts, and mesh grafts are commonly used as partial-coverage grafts to increase the total recipient surface area that a small graft harvest can cover.

Although these grafts can vary in thickness, they are frequently full-thickness grafts. With these grafts, open spaces between the graft perimeters allow for drainage until the granulation tissue bed is covered by the advancing sheet of epithelial cells originating from the graft. For this reason, partial-coverage grafts are useful for recipient beds with low-grade infections. Small grafts also conform to irregular recipient beds and are simple to apply. Widely placed graft segments unfortunately can produce an epithelialized surface that lacks the functional and cosmetic results achieved

with the more complete coverage of full-thickness grafts. The author prefers to use full-thickness mesh grafts to close wounds of the lower extremities and to use punch or strip grafts for smaller wounds that are not located over areas where durability is essential (Fig. 14-1 and 14-2). Thin split-thickness mesh grafts are used for extensive body defects, particularly those resulting from burns (Fig. 14-3).

> Punch, pinch, and strip grafts are primarily used to facilitate epithelialization of problematic wounds. They lack the durability achieved with sheet grafts and [Q]mesh grafts which cover the majority of the wound with full-thickness skin.
>
> *Punch graft "Induction":* There have been several cases, over the years, in which punch graft placement dramatically induced the processes of wound contraction and epithelialization in chronic open extremity wounds (see Fig. 14-1). Epithelialization from the perimeter of the wound quickly expands toward the center of the wound, oftentimes more so than the epithelial contributions of the punch grafts themselves. The cause of this dramatic healing process remains unclear. Grafts may enhance the release of cytokines to promote epithelialization or possibly they serve as anchors for more effective myofibroblastic contraction.

Of the various grafting techniques discussed, full-thickness skin grafts harvested manually are most useful in closing moderate skin defects involving the extremities. Full-thickness and split-thickness grafts, meshed with a scalpel blade, are practical and effective in providing a more durable skin coverage in small animals than are punch and strip grafts. Hair growth is fair, but does not achieve the density provided by a skin flap (Figs. 14-1–14-6).

DERMATOMES

There are several dermatomes available commercially for human use. The Brown Electric dermatome has been the most commonly used unit in veterinary practice. The author has used the Zimmer Electric Dermatome (Zimmer USA, Warsaw, IN) and has found this instrument to be superior in its ability to harvest split-thickness skin grafts in the dog and horse (Fig. 14-7). Although uncommonly used on a routine basis, large practices may find this instrument worthwhile to have on hand.

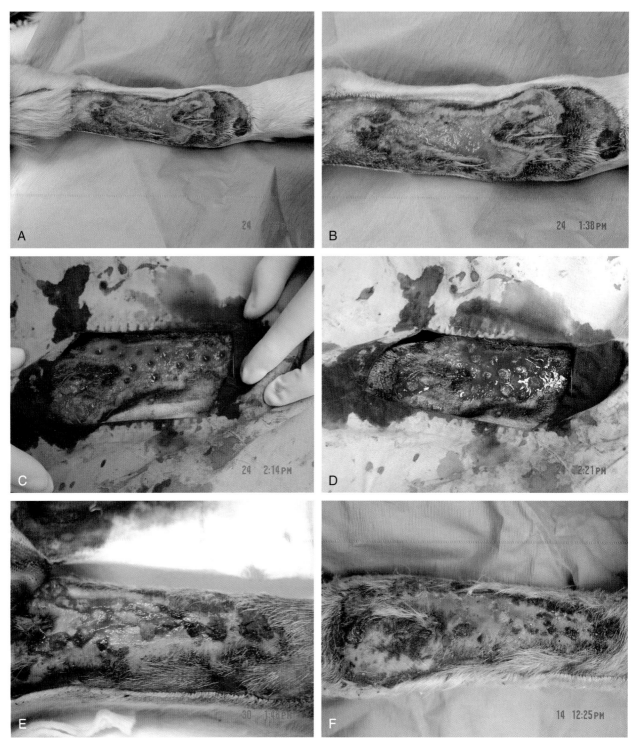

FIG. 14-1 *See legend on opposite page.*

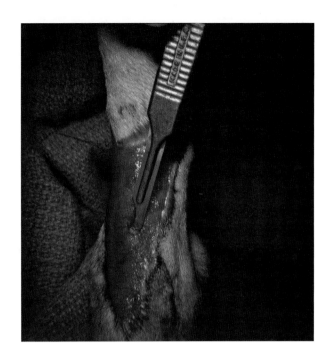

FIG. 14-2 Pinch graft application. This technique is used for thinner granulation beds. A no. 15 blade is used to make a small pocket for insertion of a small pinch graft.

FIG. 14-1 (A) Chronic, fibrotic forelimb wound of several months duration. Multiple topical wound-healing stimulants and dressings were used in an attempt to promote second intention healing to no avail.

(B) Close-up view of the wound, note the perimeter of old epithelial coverage.

(C) A 4-mm disposable skin biopsy punch (Sklar Tru-Punch, Sklar Instruments, West Chester, PA) was used to create holes in the thick granulation bed, approximately 1 cm apart. Small iris scissors can be used to trim off the core of granulation tissue. Cotton swabs or topical compression with moistened sponges are used to control bleeding. A syringe and a 20-gauge needle can be used to flush clotted blood from the holes with sterile saline prior to graft insertion.

(D) A 6-mm biopsy punch was used to harvest skin plugs in the healthy skin more proximal to the wound. A single 3-0 nylon suture is used to close each donor hole. The punch grafts are kept between two moistened sponges prior to their insertion. The plugs are inserted, followed by the application of a nonadherent Adaptic pad (Adaptic, Johnson & Johnson) with a layer of triple antibiotic ointment applied over its surface. The Adaptic pad is stapled to the skin peripheral to the wound to prevent slippage beneath the outer protective bandage. The patient was discharged the same day.

(E) Recheck 5 days later. The wound has dramatically decreased in size as a result of wound contraction and epithelialization. The author has occasionally seen this phenomenon of rapid epithelialization and wound contraction after the use of punch grafts to promote epithelial coverage to lower extremity wounds and calls this phenomenon *punch graft induction.*

(F) Complete closure at a 2-week recheck. Prolonged use of an Elizabethan collar is advisable to prevent the patient from licking at the healed wound.

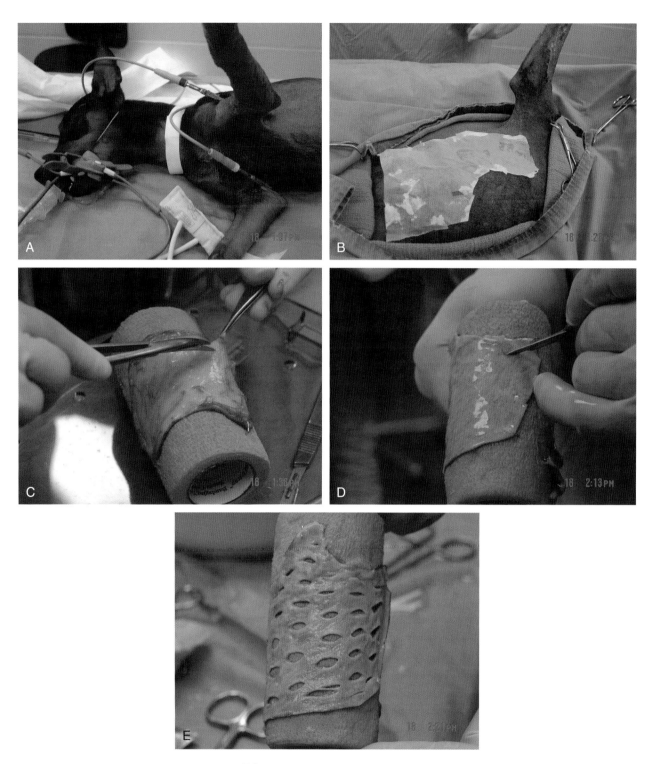

FIG. 14-3 *See legend on opposite page.*

PRESERVATION BY REFRIGERATION

In veterinary medicine, there is little need to refrigerate harvested skin: in most cases grafts are harvested and applied directly to the wound in one surgical procedure. If there is extra skin and the possible need for additional grafting, short-term refrigeration can be used to preserve the tissue (Fig. 14-8). In the event of a need to abort the grafting procedure, the skin can be refrigerated and reapplied at a later time in a more stable patient. In humans, excisional defects may be complicated by excessive bleeding or the graft may be necessarily delayed if the recipient bed is considered unsuitable for successful grafting. Careful planning can minimize these intraoperative errors.

Storage of grafts may reduce the phase of plasmatic imbibition by the production of anaerobic metabolites that stimulate early vascularization of the graft. This may be a benefit in those areas in which immobilization is problematic. In one limited study in horses, meshed skin grafts were refrigerated in a tissue culture medium composed of a balanced electrolyte solution with amino acids, vitamins, and dextrose (McCoy's 5A Medium, Flow Laboratories Inc, McLean, VA). Grafts were rolled in moistened gauze and placed in a sterile plastic container with 1.0–1.5 ml of McCoy's Medium per square centimeter of skin graft tissue; air was included in the container to support cellular metabolism. Grafts were refrigerated at 4°C. Graft acceptance was good to excellent up to the 3-week limit of the study. For humans, successful graft storage has been reported up to 6–8 weeks. McCoy's 5A Medium contains phenol red as an indication of catabolite production. A color change of cherry red to orange-yellow is an indication of catabolite buildup, necessitating replacement of half the media volume; complete change of the medium may have an adverse effect on graft survival.

In small animal surgery, careful preparation of the patient and recipient bed can eliminate the need for graft storage and the costs incurred with graft preparation/refrigeration.

INTRAOPERATIVE CONSIDERATIONS

Strict aseptic technique is mandatory. The harvested graft must be kept moistened at all times with sterile saline or lactated Ringer's solution. Unless immediately applied, harvested skin is placed in moistened gauze pads and secured to the surgery table cover with forceps to assure the sponge is not accidentally used and discarded. To save time, an assistant can close large donor sites while the surgeon prepares and applies the harvested graft to the recipient site.

FIG. 14-3 (A) Miniature pinscher with a large circumferential skin defect of the left forelimb, secondary to vehicular trauma.
(B) A template of the wound is created, using the absorbent paper liner from a package of sterile surgical gloves. The paper is applied to the wound surface, leaving an outline of the moist wound surface. The paper is trimmed and placed over the lateral trunk area, with care taken to help assure that a reasonable hair growth pattern of the extremity is maintained.
(C) The harvested graft is placed on a 4-inch roll of autoclaved Vetrap (3M Animal Care Products), exposing the subcutaneous surface of the skin. 35W skin staples (sutures are also acceptable) are used to position the graft onto the Vetrap. This greatly simplifies the removal of the subcutaneous tissues down to the dermal surface.
(D, E) Saline is applied to the graft periodically to prevent desiccation. Upon completion of the "defatting" process, a no. 15 blade is used to create a series of 1-cm stab incisions in a staggered row configuration. Upon completion, the "hand mesh graft" is positioned over the viable granulation bed.

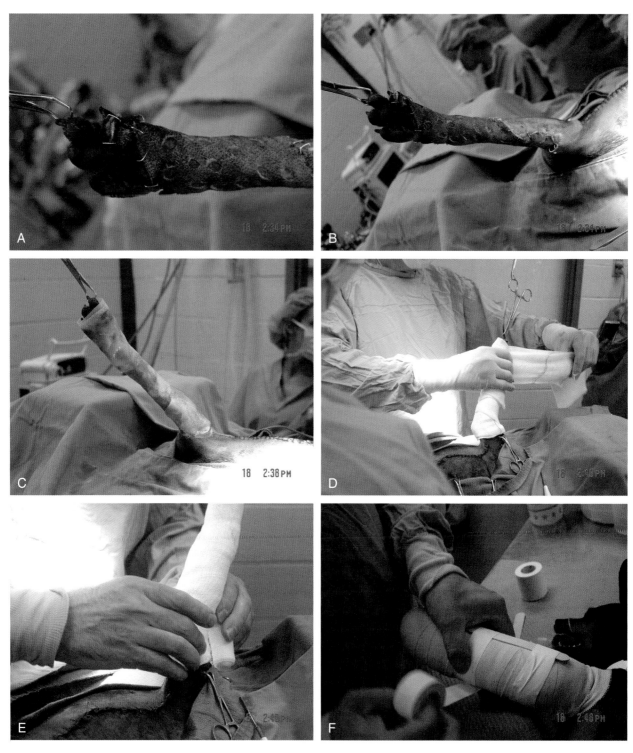

FIG. 14-4 *See legend on opposite page.*

410

BANDAGING TECHNIQUE FOR SKIN GRAFTS

Few bandages require more exact application than a bandage used to secure and immobilize a body region after application of a free graft. Most skin grafts are performed on the extremities. All three layers of a bandage are essential for a successful "take." Components of the bandage include the following (see Fig. 14-4):

1. *Ointment.* An antibiotic ointment (oil base) is applied to a nonadherent dressing uniformly. The ointment protects the graft from desiccation and helps to reduce bacterial proliferation. (The author normally prefers triple antibiotic ointment.)

2. *Nonadherent dressing.* The dressing overlaps the entire graft. It is applied evenly over the grafted surface, without wrinkles or folds. The nonadherent (or more properly called *low-adherent*) dressing helps prevent the bandage from sticking to the graft area during subsequent bandage changes. Skin staples or "tacking" sutures can be used to prevent shifting of the dressing. (The author prefers Adaptic, Johnson & Johnson.)

3. *Absorptive/padding layer.* Sterile 4 × 4 gauze sponges are unfolded to 4 × 8 lengths. Usually two sponges are spiraled around the circumference of the extremity to cover the dressing. Sterile self-adherent gauze is used to secure the pads around the extremity (or body part grafted). Layers of nonsterilized cast padding normally is used in conjunction with layers of roll gauze for the bulk of the bandage. This layering process is repeated until a thick, firm secondary layer of gauze and cotton is created to immobilize the graft against the recipient bed and discourage motion. The bandage is extended above the adjacent joint in the process of application.

4. *Elastic wrap.* An outer elastic wrap is applied to the bandage. Adhesive elastic is used to secure the bandage to the fur and skin to prevent slippage. (The author

---

FIG. 14-4 (A, B) Continuation of patient in Fig. 14-3. Graft application to the wound bed. Skin staples greatly facilitate graft application. Uniform tension is applied to the graft to assure it conforms to the wound bed without excessive tension; the stab incisions are allowed to gap slightly open to facilitate drainage from beneath the graft. The graft should directly contact the irregularities of the recipient wound bed. The graft slightly overlaps the adjacent skin bordering the wound bed; staples are used to secure the graft. Staples are also used to secure the graft to itself where the graft completes the circumference of the lower extremity defect.

(C) Triple antibiotic ointment is applied liberally to 3 × 8-inch Adaptic dressings (Johnson & Johnson). Each dressing is spiraled around the graft in a flat, uniform fashion. Staples are used to secure dressings to each other as well as to the skin bordering the grafted area.

(D) Sterile 4 × 8-inch surgical sponges are opened and spiraled over the Adaptic dressing (two layers).

(E) This can be followed by two or more layers of 4-inch wide cast padding (Specialist Cast Padding, BSN Medical, Brierfield, England) secured with roll gauze to form a firm bandage.

(F) Elasticon (Johnson & Johnson) forms the tertiary wrap. Note the tape overlaps the skin above the bandage for added security. Tongue depressors are added to the Elasticon with 1-inch surgical tape for added bandage rigidity.

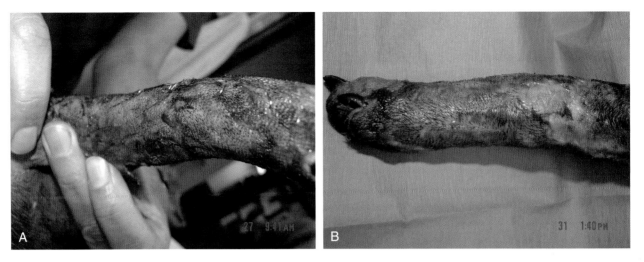

FIG. 14-5 (A, B) Continuation of the patient in Figs. 14-3 and 14-4. The graft at 1 week (lateral and medial views), with complete survival or "take."

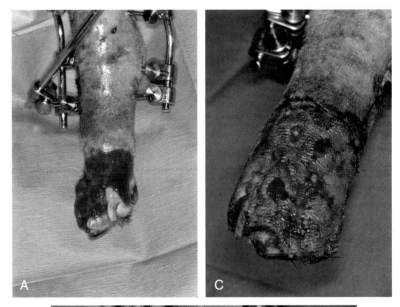

FIG. 14-6 (A, B) Hand mesh graft application to the lower extremity of a dog. External fixators used in fracture repair provide an additional "security anchor" for the graft bandage. (C) Approximately 5 days after graft application. Grafts that survive have a pink to lavender hue at the time of initial revascularization. Full-thickness mesh grafts are among the most useful techniques for closure of distal extremity defects.

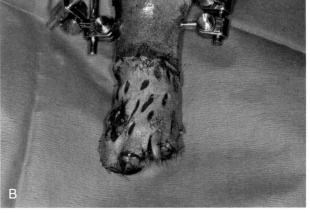

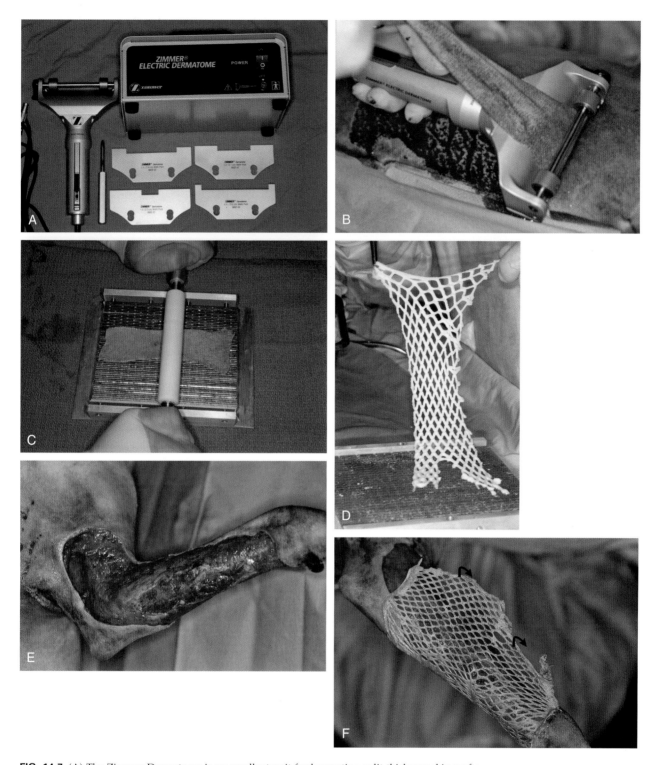

FIG. 14-7 (A) The Zimmer Dermatome is an excellent unit for harvesting split-thickness skin grafts.

(B) The width of the graft harvested is determined by which base plate is selected (A). Each plate has a slot that determines the amount of skin exposed to the dermatome blade.

(C) The Padgett Mesh Graft Expansion Unit (3:1 ratio). The Teflon roller compresses the graft into the staggered blades.

(D) The meshed skin graft elevated from the Padgett Expansion Unit.

(E, F) The graft can be expanded (stretched) up to three times the original surface area of the graft, depending upon the desired coverage.

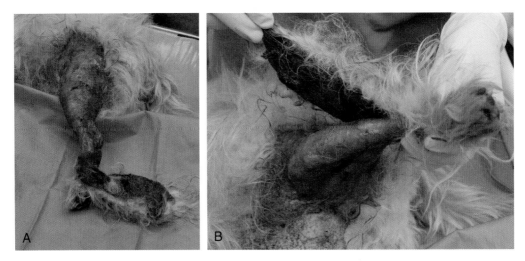

FIG. 14-8 (A, B) Fresh avulsion wound involving the rear leg of a small dog, as a result of a dog fight. This specific type of injury is occasionally referred to as a *degloving injury*, in which the skin is circumferentially avulsed or pulled distally in the fashion of removing a glove. Although this skin theoretically could be prepared (even preserved) and grafted back to the leg, it is best to discard this contaminated and traumatized tissue. The wound should be prepared for surgical closure using a freshly harvested skin graft. In this case, one or two caudal superficial epigastric axial pattern flap(s) also is an option (with or without the addition of a skin graft.)

prefers Elasticon, although a combination of Vetrap and Elasticon also can be used effectively.)

5. *Additional immobilization.* Slings, Mason metasplints, spicas, Schroeder-Thomas splints, tongue depressors, plywood coaptation splints, or reinforcement rods are used if additional rigidity or immobilization is necessary. Skin grafts applied over, or adjacent to, a joint surface usually require additional support or immobilization. A spica bandage/splint may be advisable for grafts applied to the proximal portions of the limb to avoid slippage and help restrict regional motion. Cats are quite adept at "flicking" bandages off their extremities, but cannot remove spica-style bandages (see Plate 5). Tie-over dressings can be effective in immobilizing grafts, especially in difficult areas (inner thighs, upper limbs, etc.).

6. *Postoperative care.* Bandages may be changed as early as 48 hours after graft application. However, it is safer to wait for a minimum of 3 days to assure the critical

48-hour period of the graft revascularization is not disturbed. Patients should be sedated and restrained during bandage changes to avoid accidental trauma to the graft site. General anesthesia is recommended for excitable/aggressive patients. Care must be taken not to pull or lift the graft from the underlying wound bed during dressing removal. In most cases, adherence of the topical dressing is the result of dried blood binding exposed areas of the granulation bed to the interstices of the dressing. These areas can be softened with warm saline and "unbuttoned" with gentle traction applied to the dressing. If the dressing is particularly tenacious, the dressing may be left on the graft followed by the addition of topical ointment *on top of this dressing*, before reapplication of the secondary and tertiary bandage layers. As noted in Chapter 4, VAC style devices (see Plate 1) also have been used to secure skin grafts.

The frequency of bandage changes varies with the patient and graft techniques used. Unless infection is a concern, bandage changes can be timed every 3–4 days after the initial change. Once healing is complete, bandaging can be discontinued (*usually by 2 weeks after mesh graft application*). However, the author has protected grafts up to 1 month, usually in conjunction with prolonged use of Elizabethan collars, in active patients with a propensity to lick or chew at themselves.

7. *Cage/run confinement.* Dogs and cats are confined to their cages. They are kept on a leash when taken outdoors to urinate and defecate. Minimal activity is essential to graft survival, especially in the first 48-hour period of graft revascularization. Minor soiling of the outer bandage does not necessitate a complete bandage change, as the heavy padding and the outer wrap usually limit the depth of contamination. However, bandages should not be allowed to get soaked with water or urine. A plastic bag can be applied temporarily to the bandaged foot when the dog is exposed to wet surfaces. It must be remembered that motion can result in bandage materials rubbing on the graft site. This has been recognized as a cause of graft failure in active patients.

With cooperative patients and compliant pet owners, the patient can be discharged from the hospital after the first bandage change. Again, the key factor is minimizing activity and local motion to assure graft survival.

Viable grafts assume a pink to lavender hue depending upon the state of vascularization. Dead skin assumes a white or black color. Early signs of superficial graft necrosis are discouraging, but not always catastrophic, because hair follicles and cutaneous adnexa in the deep portion of the graft may survive and may serve as a source for wound epithelialization.

Suggested Readings

Aragon CL, Harvey SE, Allen SW, et al. 2004. Partial-thickness skin grafting for large thermal skin wounds in dogs. *Compend Contin Edu Pract Vet* 26:200–212.

Pavletic MM. 1993. Surgery of the skin and management of wounds. In: Sherding RD, ed. *The Cat: Diseases and Clinical Management*, 2nd ed., 1991–1996. New York: Churchill Livingstone.

Pavletic MM. 1998. Skin. In: Bojrab MJ, ed. *Current Techniques in Small Animal Surgery*, 4th ed., 599–602. Philadelphia, PA: Lea & Febiger.

Pope ER. 1990. Mesh skin grafting. *Vet Clin No Am* 20:177–187.

Schumacher J, Chambers M, Hanselka DV, et al. 1987. Preservation of skin by refrigeration for autogenous grafting in the horse. *Vet Surg* 16:358–361.

Schumacher J, Ford TS, Brumbaugh GW, et al. 1996. Viability of split-thickness skin grafts attached with fibrin glue. *Can J Vet Res* 60:158–160.

Swaim SF. 1990. Skin grafts. *Vet Clin No Am* 20:147–175.

Swaim SF. 1997. *Small Animal Wound Management*, 2nd ed., 330–333. Baltimore: Williams and Wilkins.

Swaim SF. 2003. Skin grafts. In Slatter DH, ed. *Textbook of Small Animal Surgery*, 3rd ed., 423–476. Philadelphia, PA: WB Saunders.

White RAS. 1991. Skin grafting in the dog. *Waltham Focus* 1:2–8.

Plate 60	**Punch Grafts**

DESCRIPTION

Punch grafts are small circular full-thickness grafts used to seed a granulation bed with "epithelial islands." Suitable numbers are used to reepithelialize the interposing granulation surface. A biopsy punch can be used to harvest tissue and create holes in a thick granulation bed.

SURGICAL TECHNIQUE

(A) Fur is clipped sufficiently close to leave a short stubble that serves as an "angle guide" for plug harvesting. Adson-Brown forceps and a biopsy punch (6–10 mm) are used to harvest skin graft plugs. The pinch is angled parallel to the hair shafts. Scissors are used to lift and cut the skin plug from its subcutaneous attachments. Subcutaneous fat is trimmed from the base of each plug (inset). Harvested grafts are then placed between sponges moistened with sterile saline or lactated Ringer's solution. Donor beds are closed with individual sutures.

(B) A smaller biopsy punch (approximately 2 mm smaller) is used to cut circular holes into the thickened granulation bed to compensate for graft contraction upon harvesting and to allow grafts to fit more snuggly into each hole. Grafts are spaced about 1–2 cm apart. Rows are staggered using the same guidelines. Forceps and fine-tipped sharp-sharp scissors are used to remove the plug of granulation tissue. Sterilized cotton swabs are inserted (for 5 minutes minimum) into the individual granulation holes created to control hemorrhage.

(C) Harvested grafts are inserted into the granulation bed level to its surface. A sterile nonadherent dressing, antibiotic ointment, and firm cotton bandage is applied to the area to secure the grafts into their new position and immobilize the area. The bandage is changed 3–5 days postoperatively and every 2 or 3 days thereafter until epithelialization is complete.

COMMENTS

The punch graft technique is a modification of one technique designed for "correction" of male pattern baldness. Unlike humans, however, the purpose of punch grafts for animals is to promote wound epithelialization and not hair growth. The technique is simple to execute and is easily performed on an outpatient basis. Punch grafts are forgiving: partial loss of punch grafts can be remedied with a second set with minimal surgical time or skin required. Grafts can be harvested with a local lidocaine block and patient sedation.

Punch grafts are more applicable to thicker granulation beds that allow firm seating of the graft plugs. Moreover, graft insertion facilitates revascularization by exposing the base and sides of the plugs to the capillary bed of the recipient site. In thin granulation beds, harvested plugs are inserted into pockets created with a no. 15 scalpel blade, as described in Plate 61. Holes are created beginning at the lower border of the wound so that bleeding does not obscure the area as additional grafts are applied.

The major disadvantages of punch grafts include poor cosmetic results and an epithelialized wound surface that lacks the durability of flap or full-thickness graft coverage of the entire wound. They are best used for smaller wounds located in areas *not* subject to excessive wear or external trauma. In large wounds, the harvesting and insertion of multiple punch grafts is tedious. Under these circumstances, mesh grafts are comparatively easy to perform and provide a more suitable outcome.

Plate 60

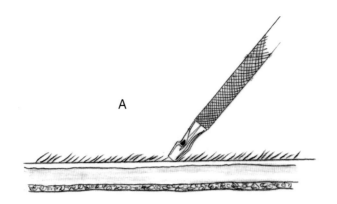

A

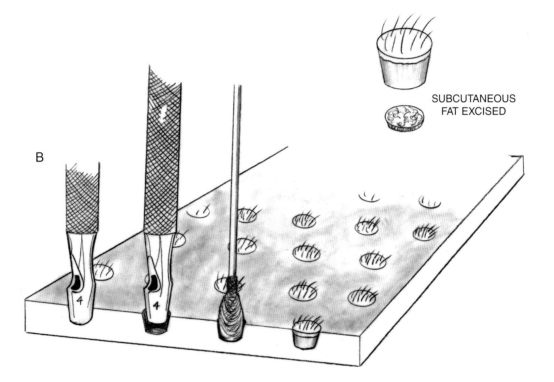

B

SUBCUTANEOUS
FAT EXCISED

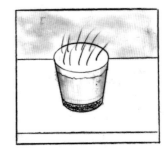

C

Plate 61　**Pinch Grafts**

DESCRIPTION

Pinch grafts (seed grafts) are a variation of the punch graft technique, although the method of harvesting the skin segments differs. Pinch grafts are inserted into angular pockets in the granulation bed formed with a no. 15 scalpel blade.

SURGICAL TECHNIQUE

(A) The skin is prepared for surgery in routine fashion. A hypodermic needle or curved suture needle is grasped with a needle holder. The needle is inserted into the skin and elevated. The "tented" skin segment is harvested with a scalpel blade (dotted line). Donor areas are closed with skin sutures. Subcutaneous fat is excised before wrapping the skin segments in gauze sponges, moistened with sterile saline or lactated Ringer's solution.

(B) A no. 15 scalpel blade is angled 30–45 degrees and stabbed into the granulation bed. Digital compression is used to control bleeding.

(C) The small grafts are inserted into the angular slits followed by application of a snug bandage (previously described under punch grafts).

COMMENTS

Stab incisions in the granulation bed are begun at the most dependent position to prevent hemorrhage from obscuring the entire surgical field. The incision is directed ventrally/distally to create a "gravity proof" pocket for the grafts. Hemorrhage must be controlled prior to insertion of the graft, otherwise the graft can float out with active bleeding. The depth of the stab incision is adjusted by the angle of blade insertion. Shallow granulation beds require a narrow angle, whereas a thicker bed may allow an angle up to 45 degrees.

Pinch grafts have the same general advantages and disadvantages as punch grafts, although harvesting is less uniform than the latter technique.

Plate 61

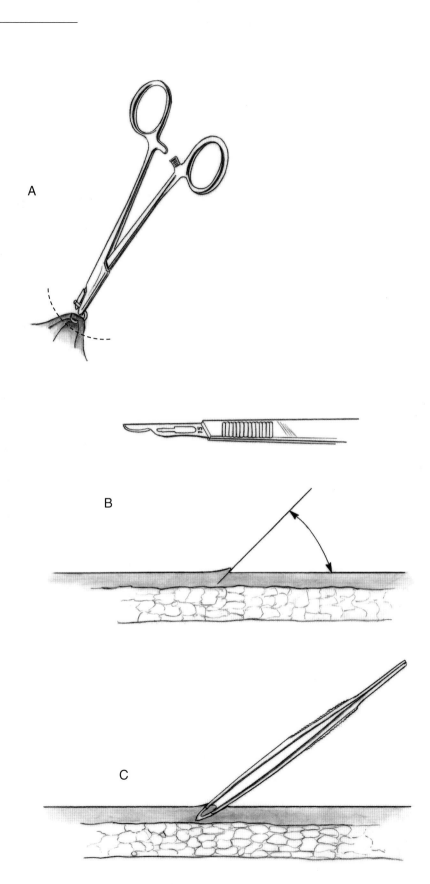

A

B

C

Plate 62   **Strip Grafts**

DESCRIPTION

Strip grafts are a variation of the punch graft technique. Narrow strips of harvested skin are placed in parallel grooves or furrows cut into the granulation surface. They are most commonly employed to cover longer wounds.

SURGICAL TECHNIQUE

(A) A rectangular segment of skin is harvested equal to the length (long axis) of the defect. The width of skin harvested is estimated by the number of strips required, the width of the skin strips, and the space between each strip upon their application to a recipient bed. All subcutaneous tissue is excised from the harvested skin graft. The harvested graft is divided into strips 3–5 mm wide. If necessary, wider strips can be developed.

(B) A no. 11 or 15 scalpel blade is used to cut furrows into the recipient granulation bed, approximately 2 mm deep and wide enough to accommodate the graft strips. Furrows or graft rows can be spaced 10–15 mm apart. Strips of gauze or umbilical tape are compressed into these grooves to control hemorrhage for 5 minutes. Grafts are laid into the depression formed upon removal of the gauze strips. A single suture can be placed on each end of the strip grafts. Alternatively, the surgeon can rely on the bandage alone to secure the grafts into the granulation furrows.

COMMENTS

Strip grafts, like punch and pinch grafts, are primarily employed to promote epithelialization of the wound. Their advantages and disadvantages are similar to those described for punch and pinch grafts. Strip grafts may be more applicable to long narrow wounds involving the extremities, although the selection among these three grafting techniques is largely the preference of the surgeon.

Plate 62

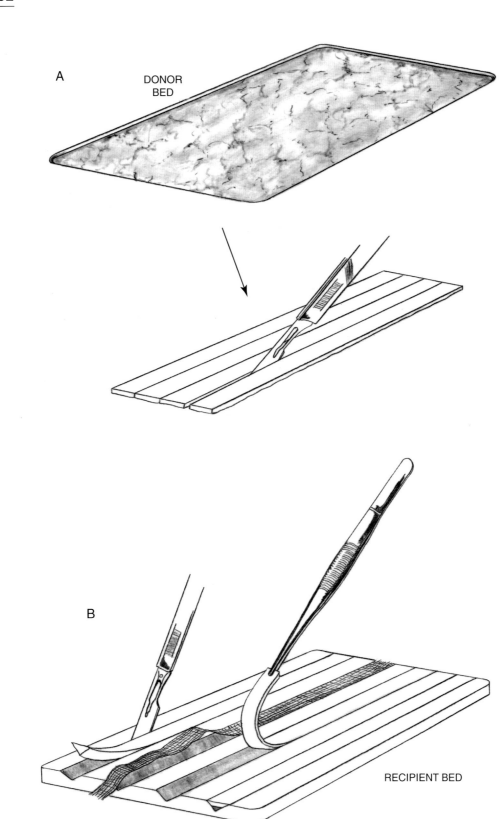

A   DONOR BED

B

RECIPIENT BED

Plate 63   **Stamp Grafts**

DESCRIPTION

Stamp grafts are yet another method of providing coverage to wounds by placing "postage stamp" segments of skin over a wound bed. Their borders serve as sources of epithelium for the exposed granulation surface between each stamp graft. When placed approximately 1 cm apart, stamp grafts serve the purpose of wound coverage; when placed at greater distances apart, they act more as skin islands to reepithelialize larger granulation beds.

SURGICAL TECHNIQUE

(A) Split-thickness or prepared full-thickness grafts (free of subcutaneous tissue) are cut into postage stamp–sized segments. Size can be somewhat varied.

(B) Grafts are laid onto the wound surface. Stamp grafts are commonly placed approximately 1 cm apart. Fine sutures can be placed in each corner to maintain the flaps' position until the fibrin "glue" forms between the wound bed and overlying graft. A nonadherent dressing and protective wrap are used to restrict motion.

(C) Alternatively, the surgeon can resect a thin portion of a wound bed to recess the graft, thereby reducing the likelihood of surface motion. This more tedious technique will necessitate control of hemorrhage before graft application. It is rarely required.

COMMENTS

Stamp grafts are yet another method of applying free grafts to wound beds. Drainage is provided by spacing them apart. They technically combine the advantages of the simpler punch, pinch, and strip grafting techniques with the greater coverage afforded by sheet and mesh grafting. It is the author's opinion that they have no significant advantages over mesh grafts and lack the simplicity of the punch, pinch, and strip techniques. Cosmetic results vary with their thickness and proximity of placement.

Plate 63

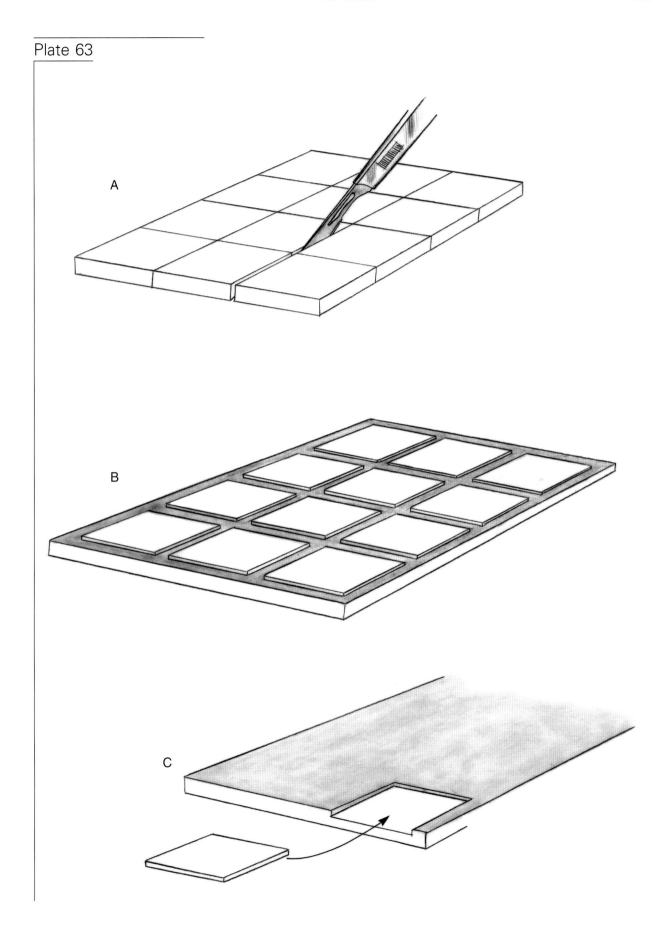

Plate 64   **Sheet Grafts**

DESCRIPTION

Sheet grafts are used to completely cover a recipient bed with a uniform layer of skin. Skin thickness can be varied according to the individual needs of the patient. When possible, full-thickness skin grafts are usually selected for their durability and hair growth. The vascular wound bed must be free of debris, epithelial coverage, and infection prior to graft application.

SURGICAL TECHNIQUE (FULL-THICKNESS GRAFTS)

(A) Using sterile paper (from a surgical glove package) or gauze, a template is made of the recipient bed by pressing the material onto the wound. When the material is lifted off the bed, it has the moistened impression of the defect. The template is positioned on the selected donor site and is oriented to match the hair growth at the recipient area. A marking pen can be used to outline the template onto the donor site, about 1 cm outside its border to assure adequate wound coverage. In general, a rectangular segment embracing these dimensions is removed to facilitate closure of the donor defect. Redundant (excessive overlapping) skin is excised during graft application.

(B) The graft is removed and the donor area closed. The graft is "defatted" by removing all subcutaneous tissue, including any panniculus muscle by using Metzenbaum scissors. Initial fat removal can be achieved by securing the harvested skin (dermal surface up) to a 4-inch roll of autoclaved Vetrap with skin staples (see Fig. 14-3). The graft also may be draped over the index finger, advancing Metzenbaum scissors across the graft for close fat excision from the dermis.

Some surgeons try to defat the graft with a scalpel blade during its harvest. The blade is used to cut the hypodermis from the dermis, rather than simply undermining the skin. A Zimmer Dermatome also could be set to remove a thick split-thickness skin graft to avoid the need to defat the graft.

The defatted dermal surface exposed assumes a cobblestone appearance after scissors resection of the hypodermal tissues. Hair follicles (appearing as dark flecks) can be seen within the dermis. When held to a light source, the resultant graft appears opaque. Grafts are periodically immersed in a bowl of sterile saline or lactated Ringer's solution to keep the graft moist, rinse off fragments of subcutaneous fat, and visualize strands of attached subcutaneous tissue requiring removal. It is useful to have a second bowl of saline for a final graft rinse before its placement onto the recipient bed.

(C) The graft is laid over the wound, enabling it to contact the irregular surface of the vascular recipient bed. One or more stab incisions can be made in the graft to promote drainage. The graft overlays the wound slightly to assure complete wound coverage. Simple interrupted sutures or skin staples are used to secure the graft border to the underlying skin overlapped. The graft is carefully bandaged.

COMMENTS

Although grafts prepared in this fashion are considered full-thickness grafts, in reality they vary in thickness depending upon the amount of dermis inadvertently removed during the removal of the subcutaneous tissues. Hair growth varies with the number of surviving hair follicles. The graft must be kept moist at all times during the procedure by periodically bathing the graft with cool, sterile saline or lactated Ringer's solution. Skin grafts must not be applied too loosely or too tightly. The graft must contact the wound bed uniformly. Properly applied, the graft has the mobility of the skin over the back of your hand when manipulated with your index finger. Surviving grafts initially assume a pink to lavender hue. As circulation improves, skin color becomes normal and hair growth resumes.

Overlapping the free graft border assures complete wound coverage and keeps the skin border from curling underneath which would prevent survival of the border line. However, it is not absolutely necessary to overlap the graft borders, especially in those cases where there is limited skin for wound coverage. With a successful "take," the overlapped skin border sloughs and will peel off during suture removal 7–10 days later.

The author favors mesh grafts over sheet grafts because of their better drainage. The multiple slits help prevent fluid accumulation; drain holes rapidly close upon a successful graft "take."

Plate 64

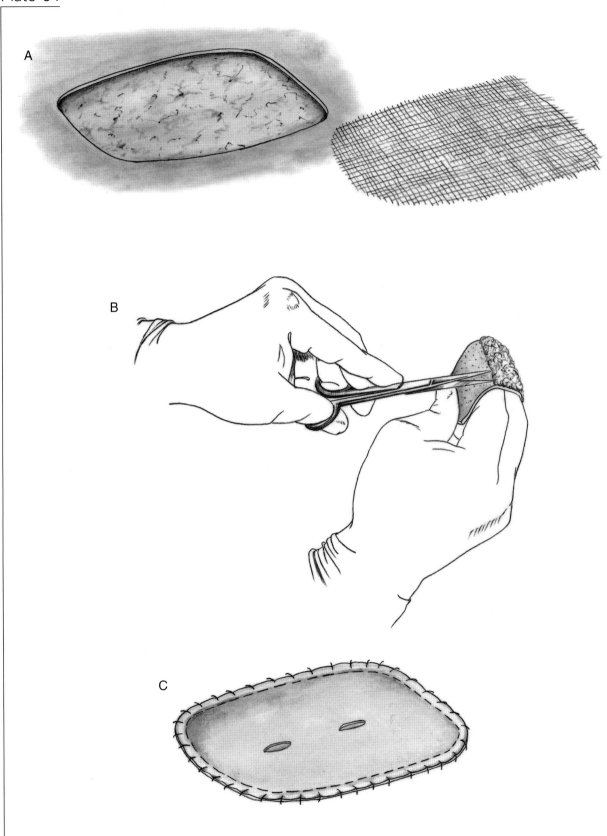

Plate 65   Dermatome: Split-Thickness Skin Graft Harvesting

DESCRIPTION

There are several dermatomes available commercially for harvesting split-thickness grafts. Use of the Brown Dermatome and newly redesigned Zimmer Dermatome are discussed.

SURGICAL TECHNIQUE

The surgeon must be familiar with the components and setting adjustments of any dermatome prior to surgery. Practice in its use can be obtained on fresh cadaver specimens. The width of the graft is adjusted on the dermatome. Graft thickness can be adjusted to between 0.015 and 0.030 inches thick depending on the thickness of the donor skin and the graft thickness desired. The author usually selects a graft 0.015 inches (0.38 mm) thick.

Basic preparation and use of the newer Zimmer Dermatome is similar to that of the Brown Dermatome. There is a single dial to easily set the depth (thickness) of the graft cut. Exchangeable base plates vary the exposure of the skin to the oscillating blade to control the width of the graft harvested.

The dermatome is ideally suited to harvesting skin from a long, flat surface. Selection of a donor site(s) is a matter of availability. In general, it is preferable to select a suitable donor site in a location or locations that are easily assessable and that do not require the intraoperative repositioning of the patient.

Sterile saline or lactated Ringer's solution can be injected beneath the skin to facilitate graft harvesting over irregular areas (e.g., ribcage). Sufficient fluid is injected to elevate the skin from the underlying structures that impede advancement of the dermatome or alter the angle of the oscillating blade.

Sterilized mineral oil (or a thin layer of a light topical ointment) is applied over the donor area to facilitate smooth advancement of the dermatome. A sterile water-soluble lubricant also can be substituted for mineral oil, although the author prefers an oil-based lubricant.

Two towel clamps are placed ahead, and two behind the path of the dermatome. Traction on the towel clamps by an assistant tightens the donor skin, facilitating the harvesting of the split-thickness graft. The blade is angled and pressed firmly onto the skin surface as the dermatome is engaged. The dermatome is advanced forward on its base. The graft is grasped with forceps as it emerges from the unit. The graft harvest can be terminated by angling the dermatome upward to cut the graft free of the donor site. The graft is kept moistened with sterile saline or lactated Ringer's solution during its application to the recipient bed.

COMMENTS

The Zimmer Dermatome is easy to use and cuts the skin of the dog remarkably well. It is superior to the Brown Dermatome. Graft knives are difficult to use in animals and have inconsistent results. Injection razors and safety razors can be modified to harvest small segments of skin, but the harvest is unrewarding for the larger wounds for which split-thickness grafts are most applicable. Long segments can be difficult to obtain from cats and small dogs. The relatively firm, flat surface of the epaxial muscles lateral to the dorsal spinous process and lateral thigh are among the best areas for harvesting long strips of skin. The skin is thicker over the back and more amenable to split-thickness skin graft harvesting. The lateral surface of the upper extremities also can be used. The flexible abdominal wall can be a difficult area from which to harvest skin with a dermatome. The ribs also limit the effective ability to harvest a graft from the lateral thorax despite injection of saline subcutaneously.

Thin split-thickness grafts have sparse hair growth and less durability than thicker grafts. Their primary clinical advantage in veterinary medicine resides in their ability to cover large wounds without sacrificing skin from the donor area. The partial-thickness defect created can reepithelialize within 3 weeks. It is possible to harvest additional thin split-thickness grafts from the same donor site upon healing.

Full-thickness grafts, properly prepared and applied, have a survival rate comparable to split-thickness grafts, with the added advantage of durability and better hair growth. When a graft is required, smaller- to moderate-sized defects usually are closed with full-thickness grafts; large defects can be closed with split-thickness grafts.

Plate 65

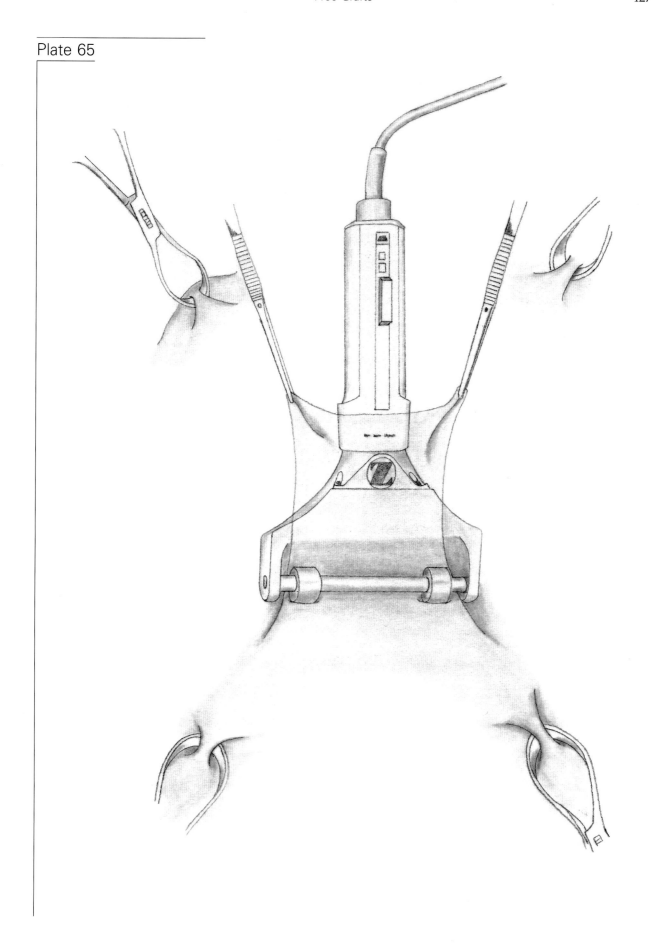

| Plate 66 | **Mesh Grafts (With Expansion Units)** |

DESCRIPTION

Harvested split-thickness grafts can be converted to a diamond on an "expandable steel" configuration using special mesh graft-expansion devices. The uniform coverage provided by machine mesh grafts is ideally suited for large surface wounds, wounds with irregular surface contours, or the presence of a low-grade infection for which postoperative drainage is critical to graft survival.

SURGICAL TECHNIQUES

(A) A split-thickness graft or appropriately prepared full-thickness graft is positioned on the mesh graft-expansion unit, dermal surface down.

    The Teflon rolling pin is rolled over the cutting bed with steady, firm, uniform pressure. The staggered cutting blades must completely cut through the entire thickness of the graft (Padgett Instruments, Kansas City, MO). Repeated application and roller compression are required to assure the graft is completely cut; the blades must be kept sharp for optional effectiveness.

(B) The graft is lifted off the expansion unit with forceps. Restrictive graft borders are cut off with scissors. The graft is applied over the wound bed, overlapping the wound borders when possible. Individual sutures or staples are used to secure the graft to the skin bordering the wound. Mesh grafts placed upon the central regions of a large wound can be carefully secured to the granulation bed with a few sutures. Care is taken to limit bleeding during this maneuver. The graft is kept moist with sterile saline or lactated Ringer's solution during the entire procedure. The wound is covered with a sterile bandage.

COMMENTS

Graft expansion using mesh graft–expansion units provides a uniform means of increasing the surface area of skin grafts. (There are mesh graft–expansion units other than the unit illustrated). Graft expansion is largely in the lateral direction in relation to the instrument. In small animal surgery, these grafts are primarily employed for large surface area defects with limited donor sites. For this reason, a dermatome is frequently employed to harvest split-thickness skin grafts, thus enabling the donor areas to reepithelialize without the complete loss of skin. However, full-thickness grafts can be meshed when the surgeon wishes to maximize graft coverage and provide optimum drainage. The malleable diamond or expandable steel design is ideally suited for wound beds with irregular surfaces and wounds with a low-grade infection for which optimal drainage can prevent pus or discharge accumulation beneath the graft. Although there are expansion units (Mesh Graft II Dermatome, Zimmer Manufacturing) that vary the mesh expansion ratio (3:1, 6:1, 9:1), the 3:1 ratio is selected as the most useful design for sufficient coverage to promote prompt epithelialization. Mesh grafts do not require maximum expansion unless optimum coverage is required. Because of the cost and infrequent need for a dermatome and mesh graft–expansion unit, most practitioners will not elect to purchase these surgical devices. Animals requiring expansion grafts are best referred to a local surgical referral practice or institution equipped with these specialized instruments.

Plate 66

A

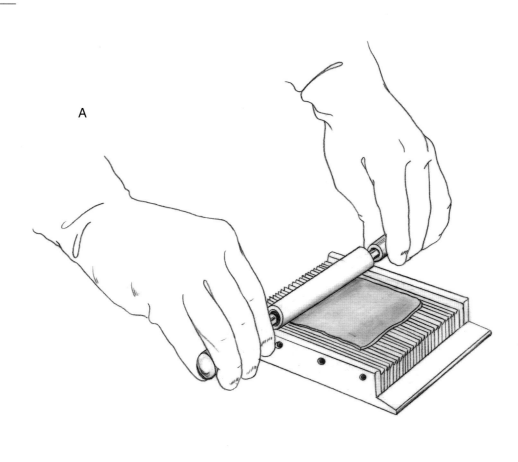

B

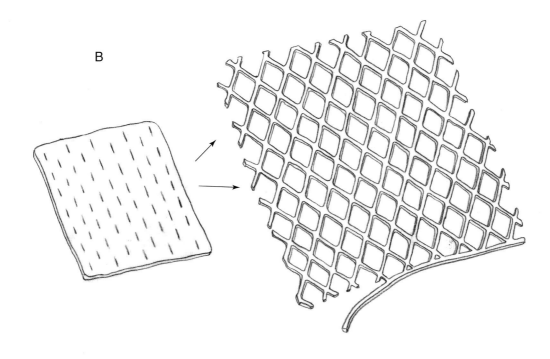

| Plate 67 | **Mesh Grafts (With Scalpel Blades)** |

DESCRIPTION

Multiple small (1 cm) incisions can be used to improve drainage beneath a graft and obtain limited expansion of its surface area for wider wound coverage. Hand meshing is generally used with full-thickness grafts.

SURGICAL TECHNIQUES

(A) See Plate 64, Sheet Grafts, for the technique of graft preparation. The prepared graft is laid on a firm sterilized flat surface. The author uses the bottom of stainless steel surgical trays. Sharp no. 15 scalpel blades are used to create small parallel incisions approximately 1 cm long and less than 2 cm apart, over the length of the graft. Subsequent parallel rows of drain holes are alternately staggered in similar fashion, less than 2 cm apart. The graft is stretched between the thumb and index finger to facilitate this procedure.

(B) The graft is sutured into place. Suturing or stapling one side of the graft enables the surgeon to slightly stretch the graft with the appropriate tension as the opposite side is secured (see Plate 64). This is repeated for the remaining sides and opposing corners. The author generally overlaps the graft borders slightly as described in Plate 52. A bandage is applied to secure the graft.

COMMENTS

"Hand" mesh grafts expand in one direction, but are not as expansible as grafts that have been meshed mechanically. Hand meshing is primarily employed to maximize drainage. The graft is stretched slightly to enable the slit to gape open a few millimeters. With a successful "take," these holes contract and epithelialize rapidly, frequently within a week after application. The author prefers full-thickness mesh grafts over other free grafting techniques for moderate-sized defects involving lower extremities. As noted in Fig. 14-3, harvested grafts can be secured to autoclaved Vetrap to remove the subcutaneous fat. Stab incisions are easily performed by pushing the no. 15 scalpel blade through the graft and into the underlying Vetrap.

Plate 67

A

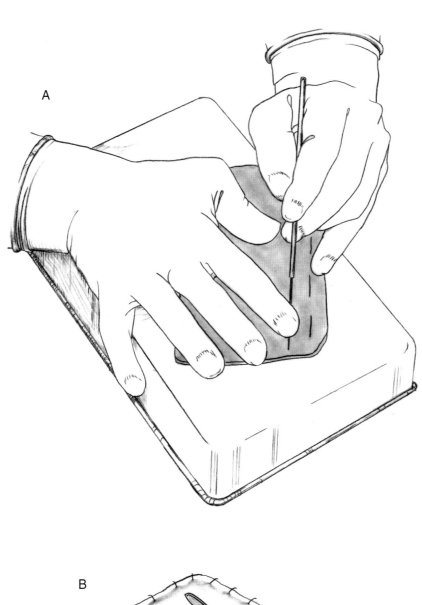

B

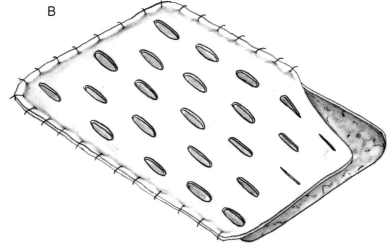

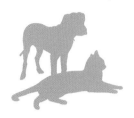

15

Facial Reconstruction

INTRODUCTION: FACIAL RECONSTRUCTIVE SURGERY

There are a variety of defects of the lips, cheek, and planum nasale encountered in the dog and cat. Defects resulting from trauma, chronic inflammation/infection, wide tumor resection, and congenital disorders are particularly challenging to the veterinarian faced with restoration of function of the oral cavity and achieving satisfactory cosmetic results for the concerned owner (Figs. 15-1–15-3).

Dogs are graced with large upper labial and buccal surfaces, which facilitate closure of moderate-sized defects. Cats, with their more refined facial conformation, lack the fullness and elasticity of the canine lips and cheeks. Although dogs generally present with the greater number of wounds and oral neoplasms of the lips and cheeks, the techniques discussed in this section are applicable to the dog and cat.

Selection of the most appropriate method of closure is based on the size and location of the defect, the donor tissues available for closure, and the inherent tissue elasticity unique to the species, breed, and individual patient. Skin defects of the face are generally closed with skin flaps (see Chapters 11 and 13). One novel closure noted in the literature used a pinnal flap to close an extensive facial burn in a dog (Swainson et al. 1998). Anatomic differences between breeds also can affect the method of closure. For example, the cocker spaniel's large lips and cheeks are more amenable to simpler closure techniques, whereas a collie's longer facial conformation may require a more elaborate restorative procedure.

Restoration of function is the primary goal of the veterinarian. Although our patients have no interest in the cosmetic outcome, most owners do have a variable degree of concern about their pets' appearance, especially as it pertains to the face. Most clients readily accept cosmetic imperfections when the potential outcome is discussed prior to surgery. Most cases involving wide tumor resection and single-stage reconstruction result in very acceptable cosmetic results, especially when the surgeon and client recognize the notable improvement in appearance compared to the injury or disease process being corrected (Fig. 15-4).

The large adjacent donor areas of skin and mucosa facilitate wound closure without resorting to multi-staged reconstructive procedures used in human plastic surgery (Figs. 15-5–15-7). Dense fur growth helps to cover scars and mask deficits. Unlike the flatter, completely exposed, hairless human face, the elongated muzzle of the dog and cat essentially divides the facial area into halves and makes any facial asymmetry less obvious to the human eye. This chapter will discuss wound closure techniques and corrective procedures for the variety of defects encountered in surgery (Fig. 15-8 and 15-9).

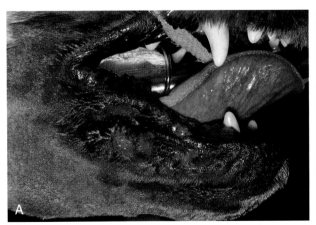 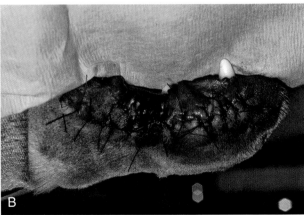

FIG. 15-1 (A) Lip fold pyoderma (labial fold intertrigo), secondary to chronic exposure of the lower labial skin to the overlapping upper labial tissues.

(B) Elliptical excision of the inflamed segment. The tissue may be removed with a scalpel blade with electrocautery to control the multiple bleeders normally associated with removal of this chronic inflammatory tissue. A surgical laser also may be used. It is recommended that both intradermal sutures and skin sutures are used together: healing may be delayed based on the location of the surgical incisions.

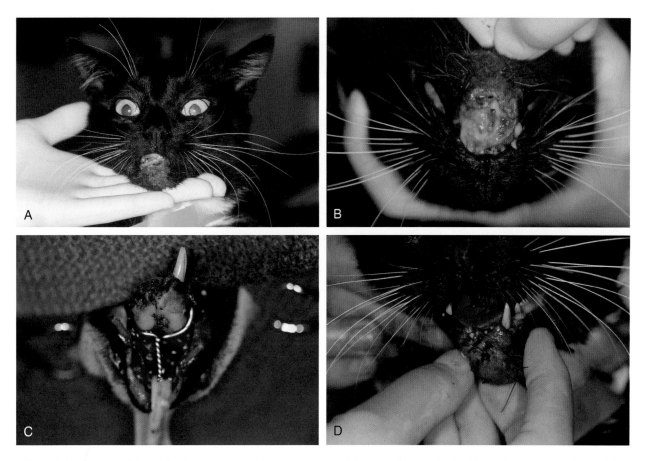

FIG. 15-2 (A) Lower labial avulsion in a stray cat. This wound is several days old. The cat also had lacerations and a partial avulsion of the tongue.

(B) Close-up view. Debridement and lavage were needed to prepare this wound for closure.

(C) A 22-gauge wire is suitable for realigning and stabilizing a separated mandibular symphysis. The author prefers to twist the wire ventrally, to avoid lingual laceration. Three to four wire twists are used to stabilize the wire: removal is easily performed under sedation.

(D) Completion of the closure. See Plate 68. (From Pavletic MM. 1990. Reconstructive surgery of the lips and cheek. *Vet Clin No Am* 20:201–226.)

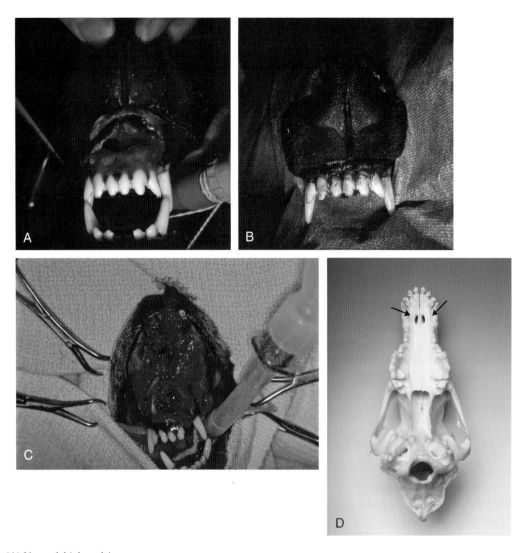

FIG. 15-3 (A) Upper labial avulsion.

(B) Closure is comparatively easy: gravity helps maintain tissue alignment whereas gravity has a tendency to pull lower labial avulsion closures apart. See Plate 69.

(C) Massive avulsion of the upper labial and nasal tissues.

(D) The incisive foramina (arrows) can be used to loop two absorbable sutures through the palate and into the septal tissues to stabilize the nasal area. These stabilizing sutures are tied in the oral cavity. The mucosal laceration is then closed, completing the procedure. (See Plate 69.)

436

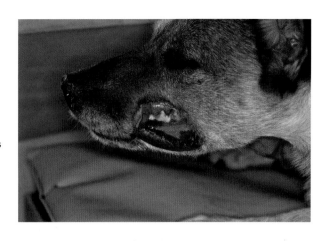

FIG. 15-4 Resection of a labial neoplasm. The surgeon elected to close the wound by apposing the adjacent muzzle skin to the remaining mucosa. Cosmetic results are poor; patient function was adequate, although leakage of oral contents occasionally was noted. A buccal rotational flap (Plate 74) could have resulted in improved cosmetic results and reduced the loss of oral contents from the labial defect.

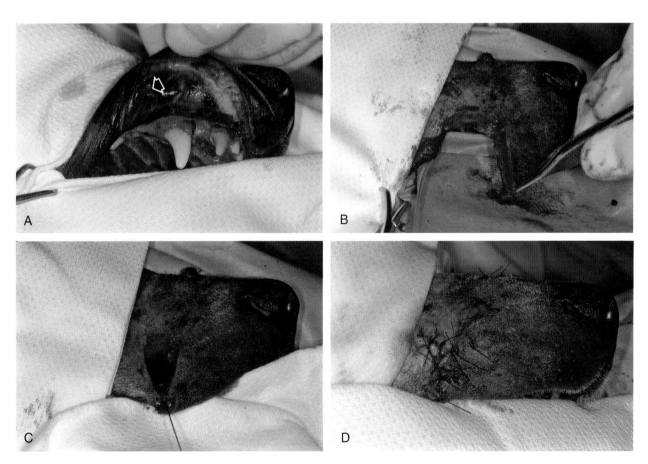

FIG. 15-5 (A) Upper labial melanoma. (B) Full-thickness rectangular resection (see Plate 71). (C) Initial apposition of the labial border. (D) Closure of the mucosa was followed by skin closure.

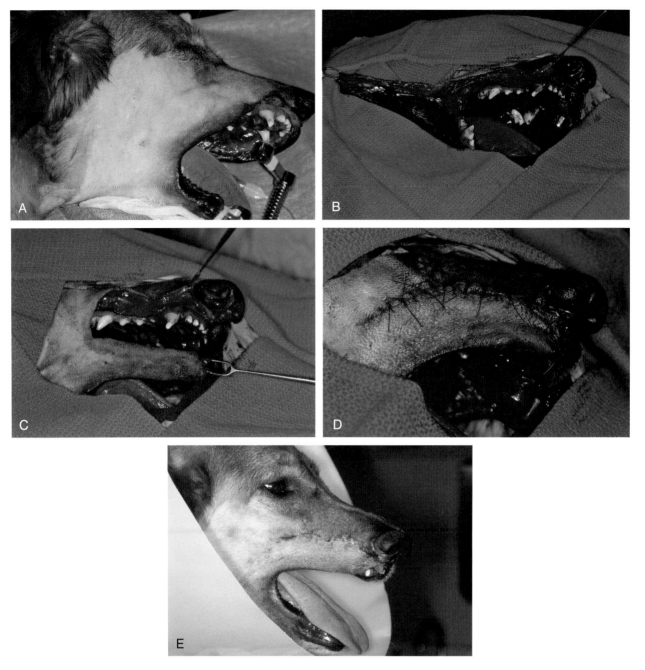

FIG. 15-6 (A) Stray golden retriever with a rostral labial defect. The owner reported food and water would run out of the labial defect.

(B) Elevation of the labial advancement flap.

(C) Forward advancement with a skin hook.

(D) Suture closure of the mucosal, musculofascial, and cutaneous layers.

(E) Note the small area of dehiscence at the time of suture removal, secondary to the dog rubbing his nose; a longer Elizabethan collar would have been advisable (From Pavletic MM. 1990. Reconstructive surgery of the lips and cheek. *Vet Clin No Am* 20:201–226.) (See Plate 72.)

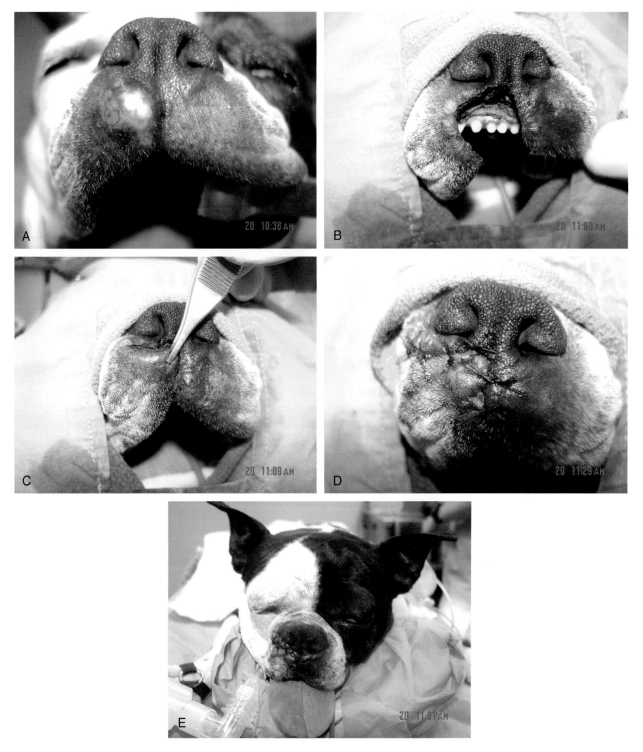

FIG. 15-7 (A) Labial mast cell tumor (grade II) resection.

(B) Excision with a CO$_2$ laser.

(C) Demonstration of one option, labial pivot flap (see Plate 80). This would have required partial resection of the labial border.

(D, E) A short labial advancement flap was better suited to closure of the surgical defect, still maintaining symmetry with the opposing half of the rostral labial area. This patient underwent subsequent radiation therapy.

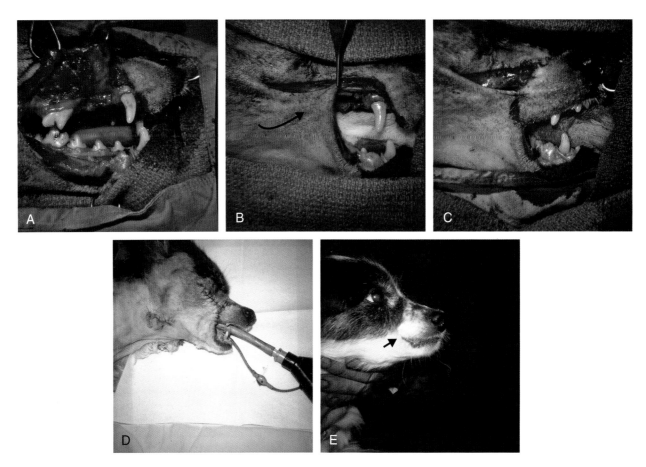

FIG. 15-8 (A) Wide labial excision of a diffuse squamous cell carcinoma, involving the upper lip and adjacent gingiva. To assure complete removal, the involved dental arcade and adjacent hard palate were excised with the involved labial tissue.

(B, C) With two-thirds of the upper lip resected, the cheek is rotated rostrally (arrow). A portion of the labial border is resected for apposition to the remaining rostral labial segment. The mucosal border of the rotated cheek is sutured to the palatal border and rostral mucosa of the rostral lip segment. This is followed by closure of the middle fascial layer and then by skin sutures. The jaw was manipulated intraoperatively to assure that a reasonable range of motion was preserved during closure.

(D) Completion of closure. Lymph node biopsy was negative for metastatic disease

(E) The patient had no recurrence 1 year after follow-up. Note the new oral commissure is advanced forward using this technique (arrow) (see Plate 74).

Anatomic Considerations

A basic understanding of the anatomy of the lips and oral cavity is essential to the understanding of the techniques discussed in this section. The lips (labia oris) form the anterior and most of the lateral boundaries of the vestibule. The upper and lower lips (labia maxillaria et mandibularia) join caudally at acute angles, forming the commissures of the lips (commissurae labiorum). A deep, straight cleft, the philtrum, marks the union of the halves of the upper lips rostrally. The mucosal surface of the upper lip has a larger surface area compared with the lower lip, which tapers in width anteriorly. The lower lip has a firm attachment to the gum between the lower canine and first premolar (interdental space). This interdental

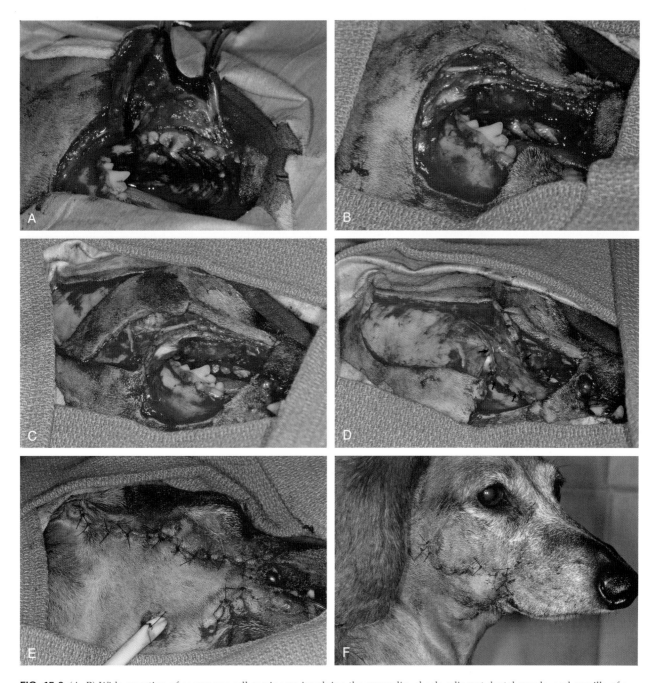

FIG. 15-9 (A, B) Wide resection of squamous cell carcinoma involving the upper lip, cheek, adjacent dental arcade, and maxilla of a dachshund.

(C, D) Closure of the mucosa defect was accomplished with oral commissure reformation, followed by inverse tube flap closure of the mucosal defect. The dorsal border of the flap was sutured to the hard palate; the ventral border was sutured to the gingival border of the mandible. Skin was advanced over the area to complete the closure.

(E, F) Labial and frontal view of the dachshund at suture removal. Functional and cosmetic results were excellent. The skin flap replaced the massive mucosal defect. (This elaborate reconstructive surgical technique is discussed in Plate 77).

attachment maintains the position of the lower lip and prevents it from sagging. When lower labial reconstruction surgery is undertaken, this tissue attachment must be substituted with appropriately placed sutures.

The lips and cheeks have two epithelial surfaces: the outer skin and inner mucosa. Between these two surfaces are two thin muscles, the outer orbicularis oris and the inner buccinator. Other facial muscles insert at this level, including the levator nasolabialis, caninus, levator labii maxillaris, platysma, zygomaticus, and sphincter colli profundus-pars palpebralis. The cheeks (buccae), which form the lateral walls of the vestibular cavity, are morphologically similar to the lips with which they are continuous.

A rich arterial and venous network supplies the skin, mucosa, and fibroelastic tissue of the lips and cheeks. The facial artery divides to form the superior labial artery, inferior labial artery, and the angularis oris artery. The infraorbital artery contributes circulation to the upper lip and cheek. The posterior, middle, and anterior mental arteries supplement circulation to the anterior aspect of the lower lip. Because of this tremendous collateral circulation, the larger flaps developed for labial and buccal defects have a high probability of survival when care is taken to incorporate one or two branches of these vessels into the flap base.

The parotid duct opens into the buccal cavity opposite the caudal margin of the fourth upper premolar or shearing tooth. On occasion, it is necessary to excise this area during tumor removal. Although the duct may be ligated, it can easily be preserved by relocating the duct through a small mucosal incision, spatulating its end and securing it to its new position with 4-0 or 5-0 absorbable sutures, using a simple interrupted pattern. In cases of severe upper labial/nasal avulsion, sutures are used to reattach soft tissues and assure the nasal passages are properly realigned. Upward septal and vomer avulsion will result in significant lateral instability of the nasal region. The paired palatine fissures can be useful in stabilizing the avulsed septum and vomer by serving as a natural opening to insert stabilizing sutures. Two suture loops can be preplaced from the oral side of one fissure, into the septum/vomer and back out the opposing foramen. The absorptive sutures can be tied within the oral cavity to improve stability. This is followed by suture apposition of the mucosal tear (Fig. 15-3).

Veterinarians should note that skin flaps can be used as substitutes for large oral mucosal defects. The ample loose skin in the facial/cervical area permits the development of advancement and transposition flaps, discussed in Chapter 11 (Fig. 15-10).

Miscellaneous Labial and Facial Procedures

Cleft Lip (Cheiloschisis, "Harelip")

Cleft lip is a congenital defect that may be the result of either a recessive or irregular dominant trait. Hormonal, nutritional, and mechanical factors also may play a role in their formation. Cleft lip is more common in brachycephalic breeds. Cleft lip (primary palate) also may be seen in conjunction with cleft palate (secondary palate). Cleft lip usually is unilateral, although bilateral cleft lip has been reported and seen by the author. Unilateral cleft lip repair is facilitated by using the opposite half of the nose as a visual guideline for tissue realignment. Textbooks vary on the ideal time to consider repair. Because cleft lip patients can eat and drink without difficulty, the author prefers to wait until the patient is 5–6 months of age (Fig. 15-11). At this age, tissues are better developed and sutures are less likely to "cut-out." Owners should be made aware of the fact that most dogs will have a slight deviation of the external nose toward the side of the cleft lip. The upper lip on the affected side may be somewhat underdeveloped when compared to the opposite side. These cosmetic imperfections are less noticeable compared to the presenting labial defect; with successful closure, owners are generally quite pleased with the overall surgical result.

Oral Commissure Advancement

Loss of a significant portion of the mandible, secondary to tumor resection or trauma, can result in loss of lateral lingual support, causing a tendency for the patient's tongue to slip or loll to the side (Fig. 15-12). The tongue slides to the corner of the mouth, displacing the buccal area caudally. Dogs usually adapt to this problem by learning to retract and lift their tongue to a variable degree. In some patients, prolonged exposure of the tongue can dry its epithelial surface, necessitating periodic application of water. Drooling and the spillage of water and food during mastication also may be noted after hemi-mandibulectomy. It is best to discuss these potential complications with the owner prior to surgery.

> The author does not routinely perform this procedure with every mandibulectomy performed. It may be more useful in large breed dogs that have greater lingual length and mass. Oral commissure advancement can be performed at a later date for those dogs with persistent overexposure.

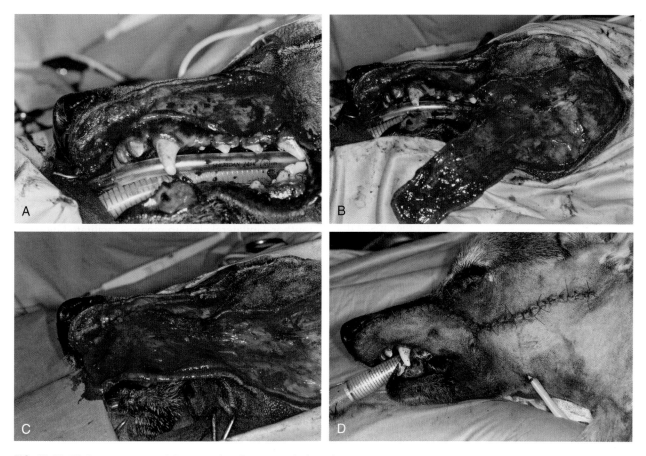

FIG. 15-10 (A) Reconstruction of the upper lip after removal of a soft tissue sarcoma.

(B) Elevation of a skin flap, with the flap base aligned with the viable oral commissure. Flap length is measured from the base of the flap to the remaining rostral labial border. Flap width equals the combined width of the labial mucosa and outer cutaneous defect.

(C) The dorsal border of the flap is sutured to the mucosal defect. The skin flap is then folded lengthwise, with the lower flap border sutured to the upper limits of the cutaneous defect.

(D) Immediate postoperative view. Postoperative swelling and gravitational pull improved subsequent coverage of the partially exposed left upper canine.

The angles of the mouth (angularis oris) where the upper and lower lips join are called the oral commissures. Resection of the labial border of the oral commissure and a variable portion of the upper and lower labial borders will allow the surgeon to suture the incised mucosal and cutaneous surfaces together. This creates a forward extension of the cheek as the oral commissure is advanced rostrally. In essence, a "sling effect" is created to support the tongue within the mouth. The length required to support the tongue is estimated at the time of surgery, which may be one-half to two-thirds the length of the lower labial border.

Cheilopexy for Drooling

In certain breeds (St. Bernards, Great Pyrenees, etc.) the overabundance of everted lower lip, rostral to the oral commissures, can impair normal retention of saliva. Excessive drooling may result in moist dermatitis of the lower labial skin. When the dog shakes its head, many owners find long strands of saliva being distributed over their furniture and house guests to be rather distasteful.

Cheilopexy is a surgical technique designed to lift and support the lower labial border by surgically attaching a portion of the everted lower lip to the mucosa of the upper lip. This technique is reportedly effective in reducing excessive drool. In patients with

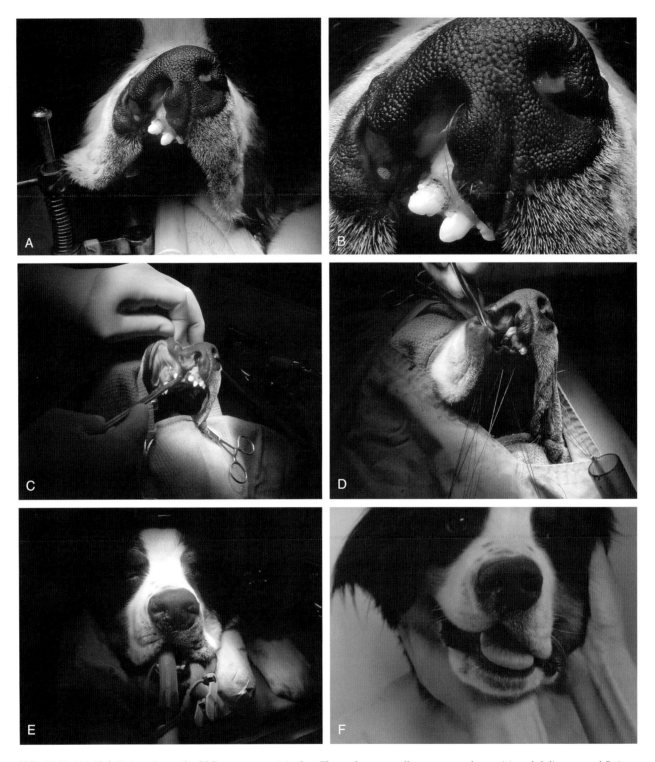

FIG. 15-11 (A) Cleft lip in a 6-month-old Bernese mountain dog. The author normally recommends repairing cleft lips around 5–6 months of age because the tissues are better able to retain sutures without tearing.

(B) Close-up view.

(C) Intraoperative view of the defect.

(D) Preplacement of sutures after creating the required surgical incisions to close the oronasal defect.

(E) Completion of the closure.

(F) View of the patient at suture removal. Note that the nose tends to tilt toward the side of the original defect in cleft lip patients. This is due to loss of normal tissue support. As in this case, you may also note the upper lip on the involved side is somewhat shorter dorsoventrally when compared to the opposite side. (See Plate 79.)

444

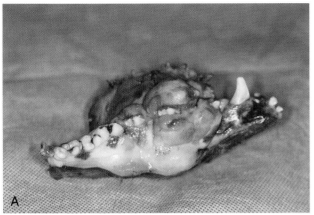

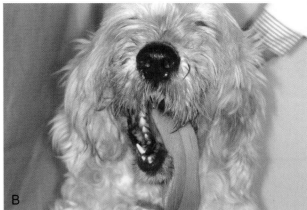

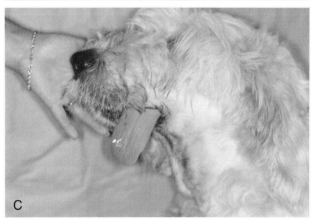

FIG. 15-12 (A) Hemimandibulectomy for osteosarcoma in an old English sheepdog.

(B, C) Front and side views of the dog. Without support from the left mandible, the tongue deviates laterally. The mass of the tongue displaces the oral commissure caudally. Most dogs will learn to retract their tongue to a variable degree; problematic cases may benefit from oral commissure advancement (See Plate 81).

nonunion mandibular fractures, cheilopexy can create a supportive sling to the affected side (see Plate 83).

> Cheilopexy is not a commonly performed procedure in veterinary practice. Most owners familiar with these breeds simply accept drooling as a part of pet ownership. Owners also may be unaware of cheilopexy as an option to control this problem.

Brachycephalic Facial Fold Surgery

Facial fold surgery in brachycephalic dogs has been advocated for two reasons: (1) fur overlying the ridge (top) of a large skin fold that causes ventromedial corneal irritation/ulceration (keratitis) and (2) chronic face fold pyoderma (chronic intertriginous infection) involving the crease or trough of a skin fold. One or two skin folds may be noted overlying the muzzle of a given brachycephalic patient. Face folds may uniformly span the width of the face or partially dissipate at the midmuzzle area.

Previous veterinary articles describe complete removal of the facial fold for these two conditions. Unfortunately, this can negatively alter the normal appearance of the patient. Partial resection of the face fold can correct these two face fold problems while still maintaining the classic facial features of the patient. In

chronic pyodermas, the skin surface underlying the crease or trough also requires removal to alleviate this problem (see Plate 82).

Suggested Readings

Howard DR, Davis DG, Merkley DF, et al. 1974. Mucoperiosteal flap technique for cleft palate repair in dogs. *J Am Vet Med Assoc* 165:352–354.

Pavletic MM. 1983. Nasal and rostral labial reconstruction in the dog. *J Am Anim Hosp Assoc* 19:595–600.

Pavletic MM. 1987. Plastic surgery of the head. In Proceedings of the American Animal Hospital Association, 392–397. Lakewood, CO: AAHA.

Pavletic MM. 1990. Reconstructive surgery of the lips and cheek. *Vet Clin No Am* 20:201–226.

Salisbury SK. 1975. Oral cavity. In: Bojrab MJ, ed., *Current Techniques in Small Animal Surgery*, 3rd ed., 151–159. Philadelphia, PA: Lea & Febiger.

Smeak DD. 1989. Anti-drool cheiloplasty: clinical results in 6 dogs. *J Am Anim Hosp Assoc* 25:181–185.

Stoll SG. 1975. Cheiloplasty. In: Bojrab MJ, ed. *Current Techniques in Small Animal Surgery*, 3rd ed., 286–292. Philadelphia, PA: Lea & Febiger.

Swainson SW, Goring RL, deHaan JJ, et al. 1998. Reconstruction of a facial defect using the ear pinna as a composite flap. *J Am Anim Hosp Assoc* 34:399–403.

Yates G, Landon B, Edwards, G. 2007. Investigation and clinical application of a novel axial pattern flap for nasal and facial reconstruction in the dog. *Austr Vet J* 85:113–118.

| Plate 68 | **Repair of Lower Labial Avulsion** |

DESCRIPTION

Avulsion wounds of the lip most commonly occur along the gingival border of the lower incisors, although they may extend caudally to involve the adjacent premolar and molar regions. Lower labial avulsion is most commonly seen in cats, with the patient presenting with the lip and lower chin hanging beneath the mandible.

SURGICAL TECHNIQUE

(A) After judicious debridement and copious pressure lavage with sterile saline, the lip is gently grasped with skin hooks or Adson-Brown thumb forceps and elevated to the level of the incisor teeth.

(B) With little or no soft tissue to which the lip can be sutured, horizontal mattress sutures are looped around the intact incisors by driving the needle as close to the mandible as possible.

(C) If teeth are missing, small holes can be driven into the border of the mandible, using a K-wire or a 1/16-inch Steinmann pin to permit passage of the suture material.

(D) Absorbable or nonabsorbable 3-0 suture material may be used. A Penrose drain can be inserted through a cutaneous stab incision to manage dead space. Drains are usually removed by the third day.

COMMENTS

Because of the excellent collateral circulation to the lips, massive tissue sloughing is uncommon. Major skin loss generally requires closure with a local skin flap.

From the author's experience, lower labial avulsions are more common in cats. They are usually the result of the animal being struck from the rear by a vehicle, driving the head downward and forward into the pavement or falling face forward from an elevated position. Although these injuries are rather gruesome to behold, they are not particularly difficult to close.

Symphyseal fractures may be seen in conjunction with lower labial avulsion wounds. Bone reduction forceps can stabilize the fracture, allowing cerclage wire (20- or 22-gauge) stabilization of the realigned mandibles before suture repair of the avulsion wound.

Plate 68

A

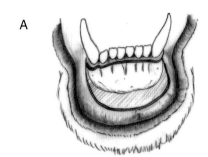

B

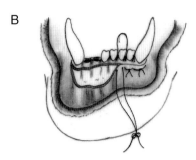

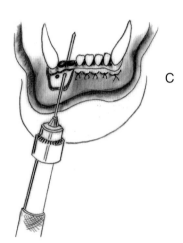

C

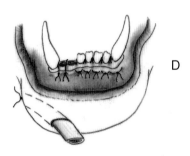

D

| Plate 69 | **Repair of Upper Lip Avulsion** |

DESCRIPTION

Avulsion of the upper lip is less common than lower labial avulsion injuries. The gingival border is pulled free of the upper incisors. Exposure of the dorsal surface of the incisive bone is noted when the nasal cartilage is grasped and gently lifted. The wound may not be readily apparent upon initial presentation as the weight of the nose returns the gingival border to its approximated anatomic position. On rare occasions, the nasal cartilage can be avulsed with portions of the upper lip.

SURGICAL TECHNIQUE

(A) After judicious debridement and copious pressure lavage, the lip is positioned in its appropriate position.

(B) Absorbable horizontal mattress (3-0) sutures are looped around the intact incisors by driving the needle as close to the incisive bone as possible. Small holes can be driven into the border of the mandible if teeth are missing, using a K-wire or a 1/16-inch Steinmann's pin to permit passage of the suture material. (See Plate 68, Repair of Lower Labial Avulsion).

(C) Sutures are tied to complete the closure.

COMMENTS

The causes of upper lip avulsion are identical to lower labial avulsion injuries. Upon impact, the nose is driven caudally and dorsally, resulting in separation of the gingival border. Suturing the lip back into position stabilizes the nasal cartilage and prevents it from being displaced by normal activities of the dog or cat. Avulsion of the nasal cartilage requires the preplacement of sutures in order to realign the left and right nostrils. As previously discussed, more severe avulsions, including the nasal septum, may require stabilizing sutures passed through the paired palatine fissures prior to closure of the remaining soft tissue margins (see Fig. 15-3).

Plate 69

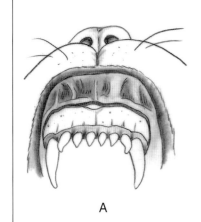

A

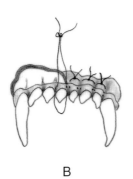

B

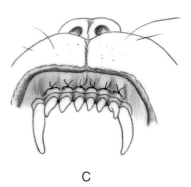

C

Plate 70   **Wedge Resection Technique**

DESCRIPTION
Wedge resection entails full-thickness excision of a lip segment. The remaining labial borders are apposed directly without the use of release/relaxing incisions to facilitate tissue apposition.

SURGICAL TECHNIQUE
(A) The size and location of the excision are determined with particular attention to obtaining adequate surgical margins in the resection of the neoplasm. A scalpel blade is used to incise through the entire thickness of the lip.

(B) The labial margins are accurately aligned with the first suture to avoid creation of an offset (stair-step) defect.

(C) Simple interrupted absorbable (3-0) sutures are placed in the submucosal layer to realign the mucosal surface.

(D) Additional sutures are used to realign subcutaneous tissues and fascia if necessary, prior to closure of the skin using 3-0 nonabsorbable suture material.

COMMENTS
Wedge resection is easy to perform, especially in the dog. Irregular defects or lacerations can be debrided and closed in this fashion. However, the surgeon should consider rectangular excision (see Plate 71) to assure adequate tissue margins are obtained with malignant tumor excision. The mouth should be manipulated intraoperatively to assure that a normal range of motion is maintained without excessive tension on the incision.

Plate 70

A

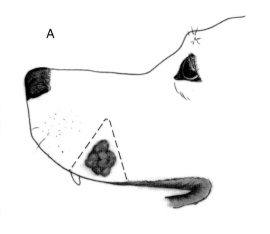

B

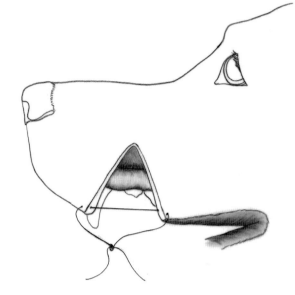

C

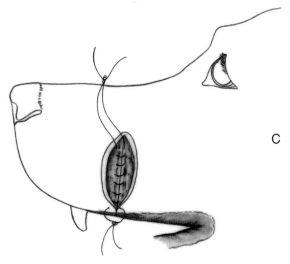

D

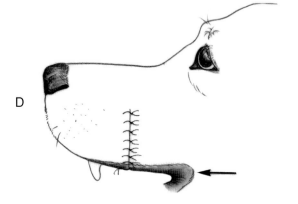

Plate 71   # Rectangular Resection Technique

DESCRIPTION

Rectangular resection entails full-thickness excision of a lip segment. The remaining labial borders are closed in a Y fashion, unlike the linear closure achieved with a wedge resection.

SURGICAL TECHNIQUE

(A) The margins of the excision are determined with particular attention to obtaining adequate surgical margins when a neoplasm is removed. A scalpel blade is used to incise through the entire thickness of the lip.

(B) Labial margins are accurately aligned with the first suture to avoid creation of an offset (stair-step) defect.

(C) The surgeon may note the oral commissure advance forward during the closure.

(D) Simple interrupted absorbable (3-0) sutures are placed in the submucosa to realign the mucosal surfaces, beginning in the upper corners of the defect. Closure progresses ventrally resulting in a Y closure.

(E) Additional sutures are used to realign subcutaneous tissues and fascia as necessary, prior to closure of the skin using 3-0 nonabsorbable sutures.

COMMENTS

Rectangular resection is easily performed in the dog and has no distinct disadvantage when compared to wedge resection. Wider surgical margins can be obtained around malignant tumors. The mouth should be manipulated intraoperatively to assure that a normal range of motion is maintained without excessive tension on the incision. This technique can be combined with partial maxillectomy. Under these circumstances, the upper mucosal margin is sutured to the palatal tissue to complete the closure of the oronasal defect.

Plate 71

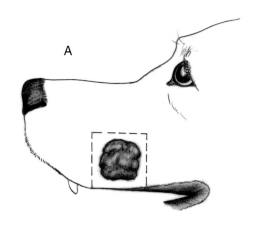

A

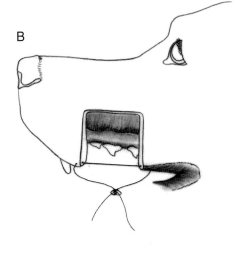

B

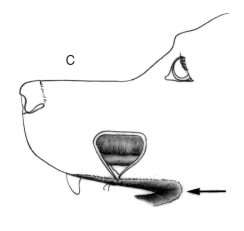

C

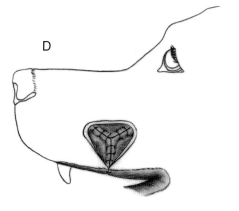

D

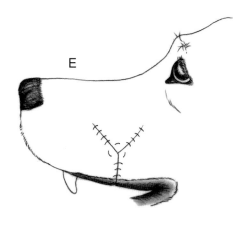

E

Plate 72	**Full-Thickness Labial Advancement Technique (Upper Lip)**

DESCRIPTION

The labial advancement flap entails complete elevation of the entire thickness of the upper lip to maximize its advancement into rostral labial defects. The superior labial artery and vein help to assure an adequate blood supply is present during this surgical maneuver.

SURGICAL TECHNIQUE

(A) This is an example of full-thickness rectangular excision of a malignant neoplasm of the upper lip.

(B) The upper lip is incised down to the mucosa. The scalpel blade is redirected slightly to leave a 5-mm strip of mucosa along the gingival border. (The mucosal strip is better able to hold sutures than the gum.) The length of the full-thickness labial advancement flap varies with the size and location of the defect, as well as the flap length required to stretch over the wound without excessive tension.

(C) Any tension bands of tissue palpated as the flap is stretched must be carefully divided at the base of the flap to avoid compromise to the blood supply. Note the rostral advancement of the oral commissure.

(D) A small, wedge-shaped area can be trimmed off the rostral border of this "composite" flap to better conform the flap to the curvature of the opposing labial margin.

(E) The mucosal surface is initially closed with 3-0 absorbable sutures in a simple interrupted pattern.

(F) The skin is closed in similar fashion with 3-0 nonabsorbable sutures. Tension sutures may be used in any area under moderate tension, if necessary. The jaw should be manipulated during closure to ensure mobility is maintained without excessive tension placed on the surgical margins.

COMMENTS

The labial advancement flap is ideal for defects involving the rostral one-third of the upper lip. It can be combined with partial maxillectomy if a neoplasm extends beyond the labial tissue. Elastic retraction of the flap can cause unilateral distortion of the nasal planum. However, this deviation usually subsides over the next 2 or 3 weeks. An Elizabethan collar is advisable until suture removal because a number of patients will attempt to paw or rub at their face during the first postoperative week.

Plate 72

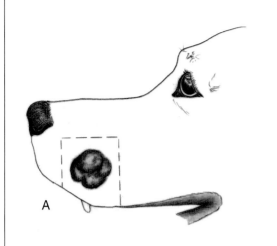

A

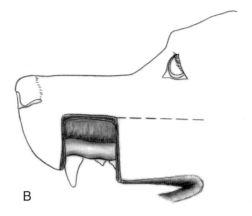

B

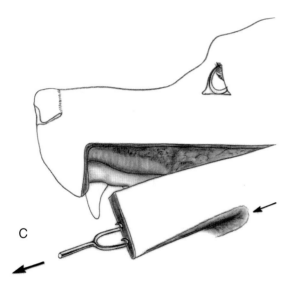

C

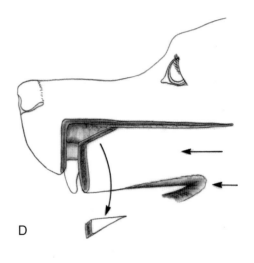

D

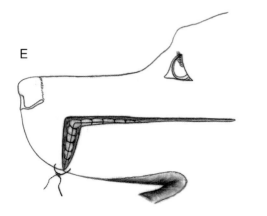

E

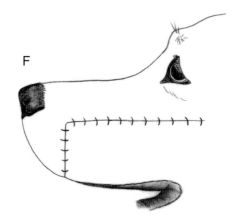

F

| Plate 73 | **Full-Thickness Labial Advancement Technique (Lower Lip)** |

DESCRIPTION

Lower labial advancement entails mobilization of the lower lip to close rostral labial defects. The inferior labial artery and vein help to assure an adequate blood supply is present during this surgical maneuver. The lower lip is easier to mobilize and advance compared to the upper lip, with the mucosa/submucosa being the major restricting tissue layer. As a result, a long skin incision is not required to maximize rostral advancement of the lip.

SURGICAL TECHNIQUE

(A) This is an example of full-thickness labial excision of malignant neoplasm.

(B) When feasible, the mucosa of the lower lip is incised 5 mm from the gingival border in a staged fashion. A skin incision of variable length is created as the lower lip is advanced forward.

(C) Rostral traction on the lower lip determines the length of the incision required to advance the mucosa and skin into the rostral defect.

(D) The mucosal incision is closed initially with 3-0 absorbable sutures. Offset placement of these sutures (by taking a suture bite along the gingival reflection rostral to the labial mucosa) can facilitate forward advancement of the lip into the defect. Sutures are used to recreate the labial attachment at the interdental space located between the lower canine and first premolar teeth to offset the tendency of the lip to sag.

(E) A 1/4-inch Penrose drain is used to control dead space prior to closure of the skin with nonabsorbable (3-0) sutures. In most cases, the drain is removed by day 3.

COMMENTS

Compared with upper labial advancement flaps, lower labial advancement flaps require less dissection. The skin, mucosa, and interposing tissue of the lower lip are not as closely joined compared to those of the upper lip; the inner elasticity of the skin of the lower lip enables the surgeon to advance it rostrally, without creating a long skin incision comparable to the length made in the mucosal surface. As noted, care must be taken to recreate the interdental attachment to prevent drooping of the lower lip. The lateral surface of the mandible is completely exposed during this procedure in the event that adjunctive surgery is required on this structure.

Plate 73

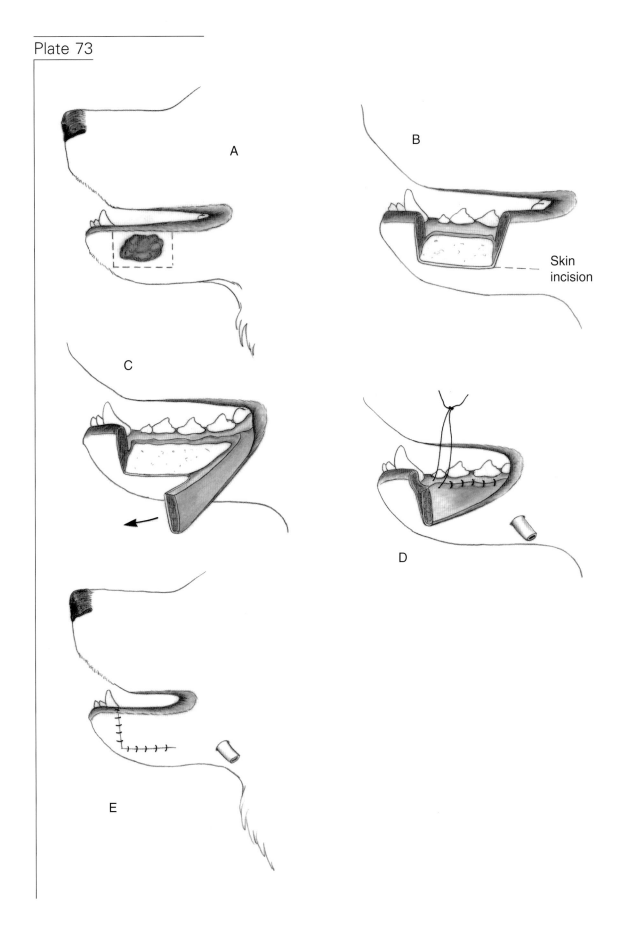

Skin incision

Plate 74   Buccal Rotation Technique

DESCRIPTION

The buccal rotation technique was developed for reconstruction of large upper lip defects in which insufficient tissues are present for effective use of the labial advancement technique.

SURGICAL TECHNIQUE

(A) This is an example of full-thickness labial excision of a malignant neoplasm. When possible, preserving a durable 5-mm mucosal margin along the gingival border is useful for suture closure of the defect.

(B) After removal of a major portion of the upper lip, wound closure is assessed by grasping and rotating the cheek margin 90 degrees.

(C) A portion of the labial border is excised of sufficient length for apposition to the rostral labial margin.

(D) Opposing gingival and labial surfaces are apposed with 3-0 absorbable sutures with an interrupted pattern.

(E) Skin is apposed with simple interrupted sutures. Areas under tension are apposed with vertical mattress sutures. In this example, a half-buried horizontal mattress suture is used on the upper corner of the flap.

COMMENTS

The buccal rotation technique is employed for reconstruction of large upper labial defects. The oral commissure advances rostrally during this surgical maneuver. However, the facial asymmetry created is not readily noticeable except by the more discriminating observer. This procedure also can be combined with simultaneous excision of the regional dental arcade and maxilla for more extensive neoplastic processes.

Although it is possible to enlarge the advanced oral commissure by incising and suturing the corresponding skin and mucosal edges, there is no practical, functional benefit to this surgical maneuver.

Plate 74

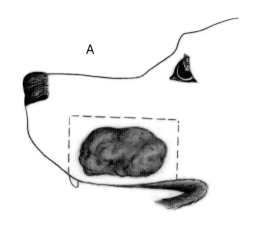

A

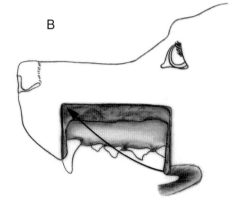

B

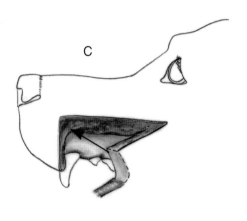

C

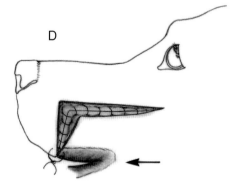

D

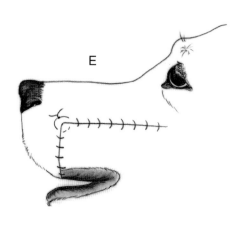

E

Plate 75	**Lower Labial Lift-Up Technique**

DESCRIPTION

The lower labial lift-up technique is used to remove masses involving the gingival and the ventral portion of the lower lip. The upper margin of the lower lip can be preserved with excellent cosmetic results.

SURGICAL TECHNIQUES

(A) The lip is incised parallel to the labial border above the mass.

(B) The bipedicle labial flap created is lifted dorsally. The diseased tissue is excised.

(C) After removal of the mass, the mucosal margins are reapposed with simple interrupted absorbable sutures.

(D) The skin is closed with simple interrupted sutures. A Penrose drain may be employed to control dead space.

COMMENTS

This technique enables the surgeon to preserve the normal labial border for optimal cosmetic results. Caution must be exercised to assure adequate tissue margins are obtained when malignant tumors are excised.

Plate 75

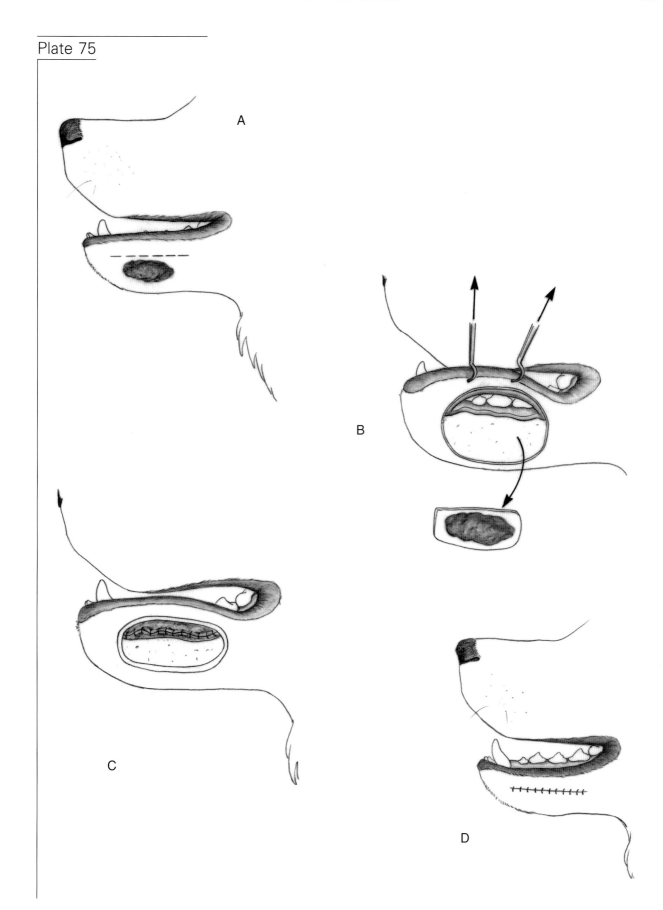

A

B

C

D

Plate 76   # Upper Labial Pull-Down Technique

DESCRIPTION

Tumors of the lateral maxilla, gingiva, and adjacent bone occasionally extend into the dorsal portion of the upper lip. Removal of a portion of the dorsal lip may be necessary. Similarly, to obtain additional exposure to this area, a full-thickness labial incision can be made parallel to the gingival area, thereby allowing the surgeon to retract or pull-down the upper lip.

SURGICAL TECHNIQUE

(A, B) Full-thickness excision of a dorsal labial lesion (dashed lines).

(C) Downward traction of the upper lip (pull-down) facilitating the surgical exposure of the area. Note that removal of the dental arcade, maxilla, and adjacent skull may be necessary to obtain margins around infiltrative neoplasms.

(D) The labial mucosa is sutured to the adjacent oral mucosal border after resection of the lesion. The labial mucosa can be sutured to the palatal tissue, when tumor extension requires resection of the adjacent facial bone and hard palate.

(E) The skin is closed with a simple interrupted suture pattern. A drain may be inserted to control dead space, if necessary.

COMMENTS

This technique permits the surgeon to preserve the labial margin and the majority of the upper lip. Caution is warranted to assure that adequate tissue margins are obtained when resecting neoplasms.

Plate 76

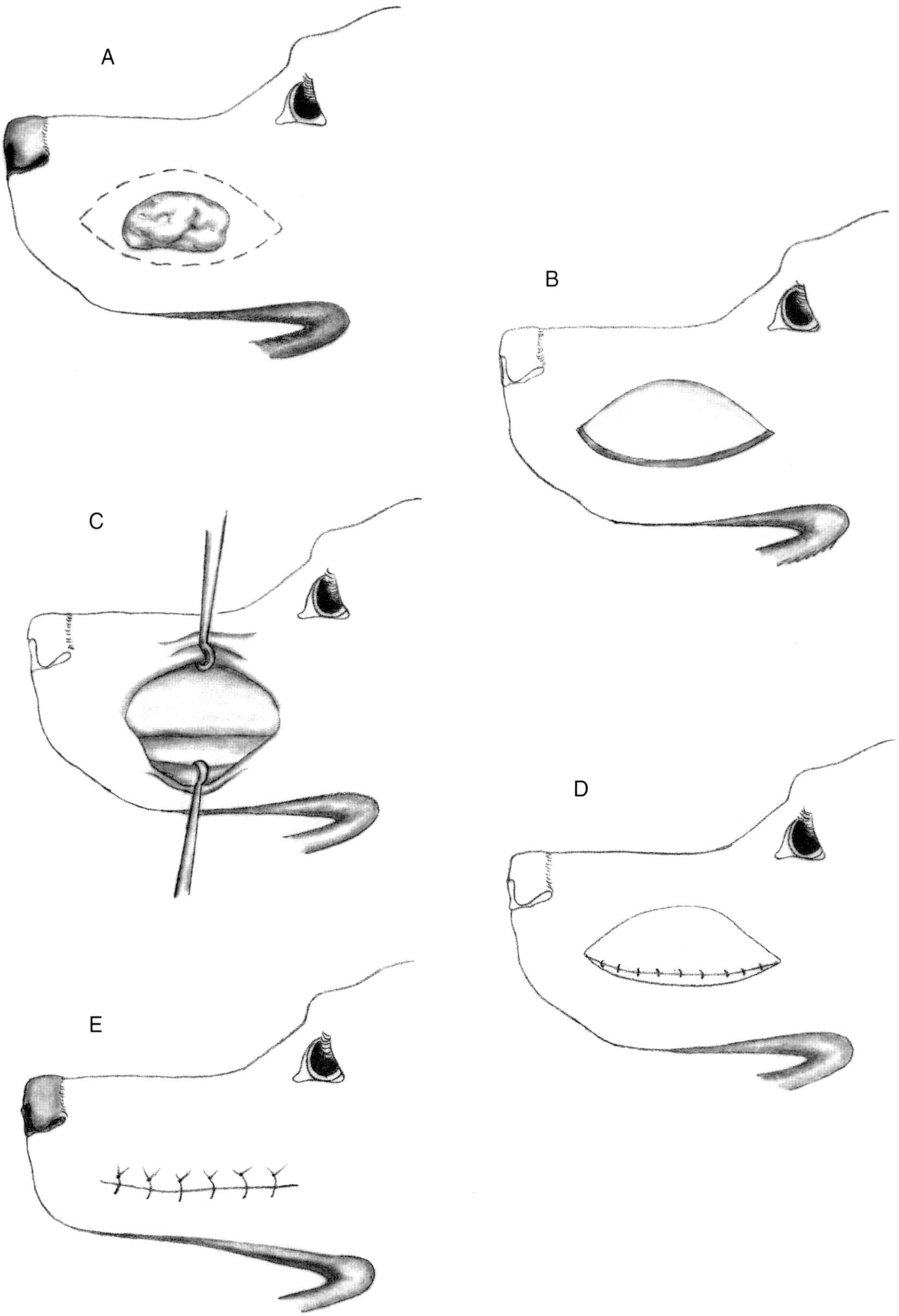

| Plate 77 | **Labial/Buccal Reconstruction with Inverse Tubed Skin Flap** |

DESCRIPTION

Occasionally, there is insufficient skin and/or mucosa available for closure of the lips or cheeks. This occurs with the removal of wider diffuse neoplasms, extensive facial trauma, and those cases in which cancer recurrence necessitates removal of additional tissue. Local transposition flaps are particularly useful to close the cutaneous surface; they also can be used to replace major mucosal defects involving the oral cavity.

SURGICAL TECHNIQUE

(A)   This is an example of full-thickness buccal and upper labial defect after tumor resection.

(B)   Partial closure of the defect is achieved by apposing remaining borders of the upper and lower lip.

(C)   A local transposition flap is carefully measured for use in replacing the remaining mucosal defect.

Plate 77

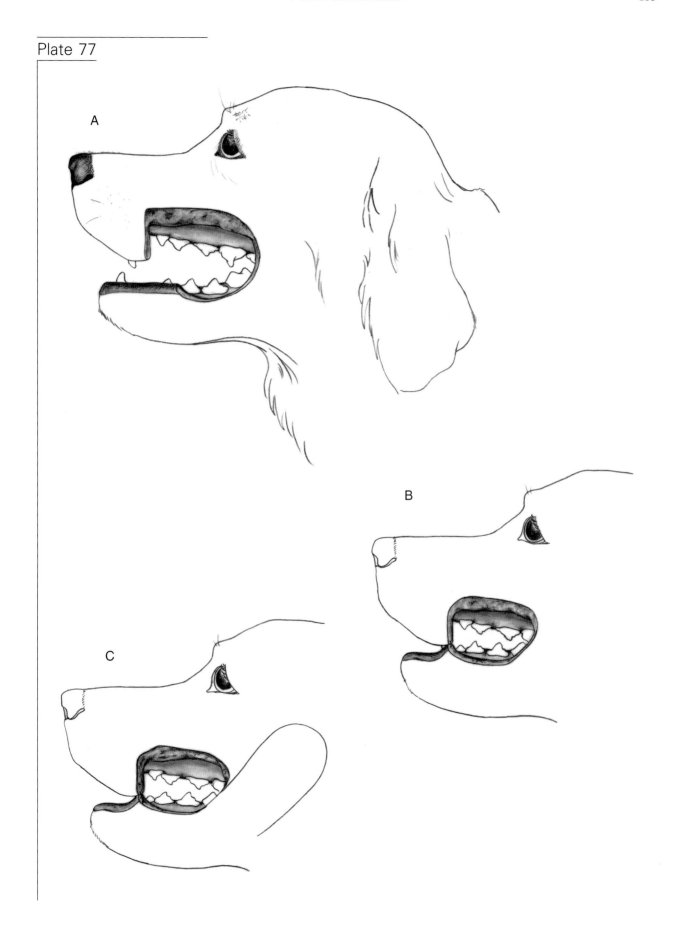

Plate 77

(Continued)

(D₁, D₂) A portion of the transposition flap is partially tubed in inverse fashion to pass the body of the flap into the oral cavity for replacement of large mucosal defects of the cheek, lip, and adjacent palate (D₁). Simple interrupted (3-0) absorbable sutures are used to secure the skin flap to the remaining mucosal borders (D₂).

(E) The skin is advanced over the transposition flap and inverse tube segment. Note the narrow opening of the epithelial lined skin tube (arrow). If necessary, this short, tubed segment can be excised when healing is complete and neovascularization to the flap is reasonably assured, that is, 4–6 weeks postoperatively.

COMMENTS

Small gaps in the mucosal surface can heal by second intention, with the exposed dermal or muscular surface serving as a vascular scaffold for the advancing epithelium. Large mucosal defects are unlikely to heal by second intention without causing significant contraction, scarring, and distortion of the overlying tissues. A skin flap can be used as a satisfactory substitute for the mucosal lining. Skin flaps also have been used successfully by the author to close oronasal fistulas when insufficient mucosa is available. This technique also can be used for closure of defects after wide tumor resection that includes partial maxillectomy (see Fig. 15-9).

Plate 77

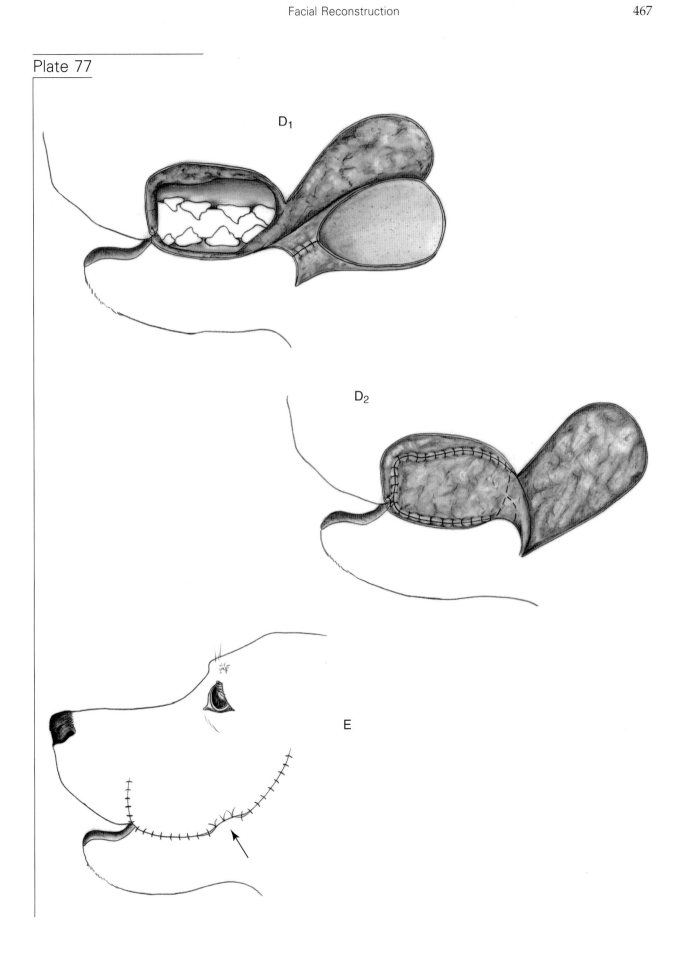

D₁

D₂

E

Plate 78	**Skin Flap for Upper Labial and Buccal Replacement (Facial Axial Pattern Flap)**

DESCRIPTION

Occasionally, major segments of the upper lip and adjacent cheek require resection for diffuse neoplasms. A cutaneous transposition flap can be used to reconstruct the skin and mucosal surfaces simultaneously. Yates, Landon, and Edwards (2007) better defined the blood supply to this flap technique and created anatomic guidelines for flap development based on this study.

SURGICAL TECHNIQUE

(A) Wide resection of this neoplasm required excision of 75% of the upper lip and adjacent cheek.

(B) Standard guidelines for transposition flap development are used. In this example, the width of the flap ideally should be twice the width of the lip excised, since "half" of the flap is required to replace the mucosal defect.

   Defined guidelines for outlining the flap are as follows: the dorsal border of the outlined flap parallels the ventral border of the zygomatic arch, and the ventral outlined border of the flap parallels the lower border of the mandible. The base of the flap incorporates the oral commissure and the adjacent upper/lower labial margins. Branches of the angularis oris vessels and interconnecting cutaneous vasculature of the labial vessels supply the base of this flap. Take care to preserve these vessels at the approach to the base of this flap during undermining. Flap length is determined by the measured distance from the base of the flap to the rostral facial defect. Flap length is normally within the defined limits of this flap design, using the vertical ear canal as the anatomic landmark as a general guideline for flap length.

(C) The upper border of the replacement flap is sutured to the remaining borders of the mucosa with 3-0 absorbable suture material, using a simple interrupted pattern.

(D) The skin flap is folded onto itself and sutured to the remaining cutaneous borders with 3-0 nonabsorbable suture material. A Penrose drain may be inserted prior to completion of the closure.

COMMENTS

Skin flap replacement of the lip and upper cheek is employed when the surgical defect is too large for the other techniques discussed in this chapter. It can be combined with partial maxillectomy when more extensive tumors are encountered. Flap dimensions can be tailored to the defect based on the general guidelines provided. The skin serves as an adequate replacement for oral mucosa, although use of mucosa is preferable whenever possible. The flap also may be used to close large cutaneous facial defects within its arc of rotation. Yates, Landon, and Edwards (2007) confirmed the efficacy of this technique for canine facial reconstruction, identifying the rich vasculature entering the base of this flap, including the angularis oris artery and branches of the superior and inferior labial arteries arising from the facial artery. The terminal end of the flap has collateral support from branches of the tranverse facial artery and masseteric artery: these branches are sacrificed during elevation of this flap.

   By definition, this skin flap qualifies as an axial pattern flap based on branches of the facial artery (facial axial pattern flap).

Plate 78

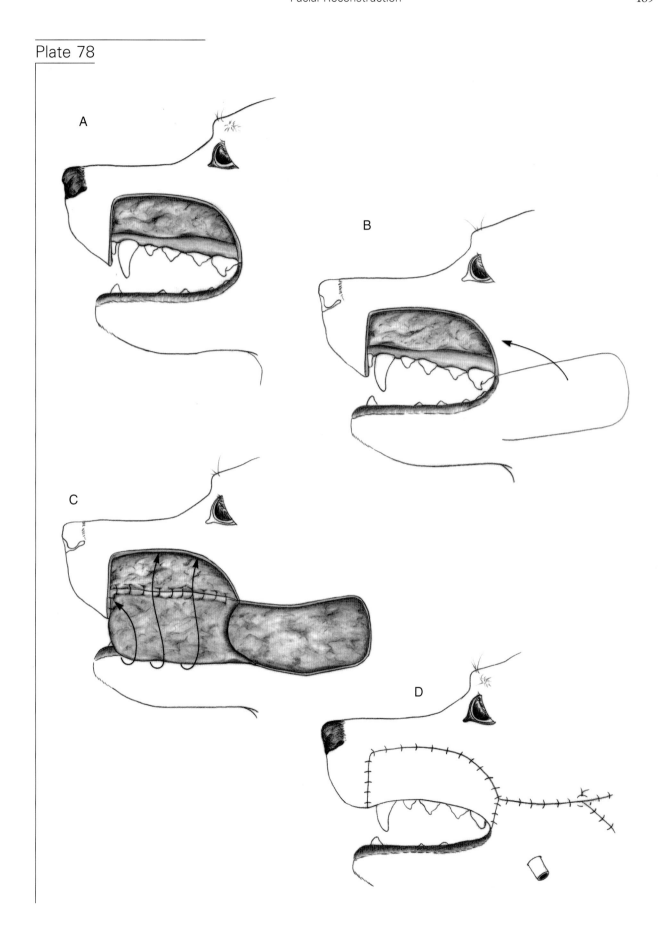

A

B

C

D

Plate 79   Cleft Lip Repair (Primary Cleft, Cheiloschisis, Harelip)

DESCRIPTION

A cleft rostral to the incisive foramina and involving the lip is termed *cleft lip*. Cleft lip can vary in depth and severity. Most cases are unilateral. Cosmetic results in the dog depend upon accurate tissue apposition in order to maintain facial symmetry, normal pigmentation, and a normal hair growth pattern comparable to the opposite side.

SURGICAL TECHNIQUE

(A) Unilateral cleft palate in a Boston terrier. The opposite half of the nose and lip serve as anatomic guidelines.

(B) Reflection of lips demonstrating oronasal communication. Malaligned incisors are occasionally present and may require extraction to facilitate closure. A mucosal incision is created (dashed line): 3-0 to 4-0 absorbable sutures are preplaced. When tied, the linear incision is folded in half to close the oronasal communication.

(C) Upon closure of the oral cavity from the nasal cavity, the epithelial borders of the labial/nasal cleft are excised.

(D) The labial mucosal surfaces are sutured with 3-0 or 4-0 absorbable sutures. The intermediate layer is closed with buried interrupted sutures in similar fashion. Accurate alignment of the labial border is completed by suturing the mucocutaneous junction, followed by the remaining cutaneous surface, with simple interrupted nonabsorbable sutures. Vertical mattress sutures may be alternated with simple interrupted sutures to offset regional tissue tension.

COMMENTS

A properly aligned closure will maintain the symmetrical curve of each lip, a straight philtrum, and the anatomic relationship of the nasal planum. Atraumatic surgical technique is mandatory for a proper repair. It is the author's experience that the more complex Z-plasty procedures and flap techniques employed in the human are completely unnecessary in the dog. There are different cosmetic considerations and anatomic variations between the face of the human and dog that obviate the necessity of more complicated closure options in most cases.

Plate 79

A

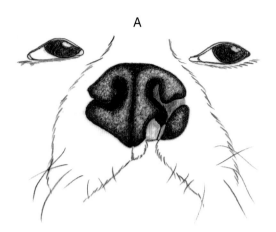

B

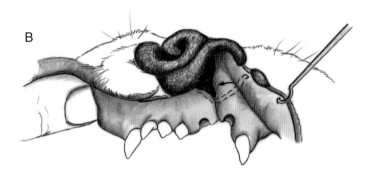

C

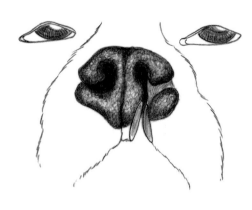

D

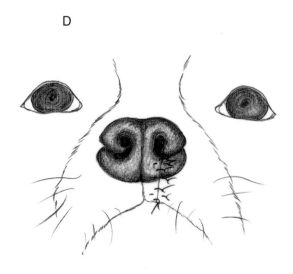

Plate 80   **Rostral Labial Pivot Flaps**

DESCRIPTION

With resection of the rostal portion of the upper lip, closure can be accomplished with labial advancement flap(s) or the rostral labial pivot flap(s) described in this plate (see Fig. 15-7). Selection is determined by regional tissue tension and which technique can more easily restore function with reasonable cosmetic results.

SURGICAL TECHNIQUE

(A) Neoplasm involving the rostral labial area.

(B) Following full-thickness resection, the lower margins are rotated dorsally (arrows).

(C) The opposing labial borders are resected in preparation for closure (dashed lines). The length resected will approximate the original length of the rostral lip.

(D) Mucosal borders are sutured, using 3-0 (slowly absorbable) sutures in a simple interrupted fashion. The dorsal labial mucosal border is sutured to the mucosa reflecting off the gingiva, followed by apposition of the opposing labial mucosal margins.

(E) Completion of the closure.

COMMENTS

A single pivot flap can be used for unilateral defects encroaching on the midline of the upper lip or bilaterally for centrally located defects as noted in this plate.

Like other facial and oral procedures, an appropriate-sized Elizabethan collar should be used to minimize pawing or rubbing at the surgical area postoperatively.

Plate 80

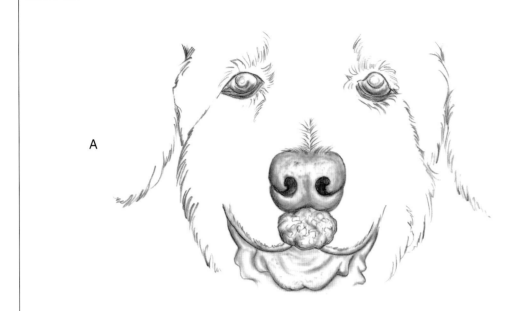

A

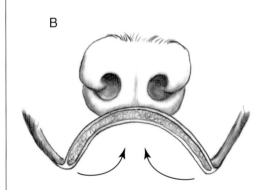

B

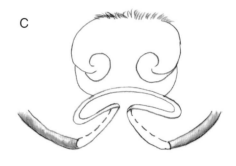

C

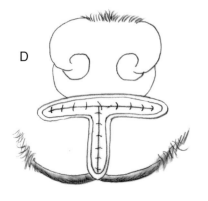

D

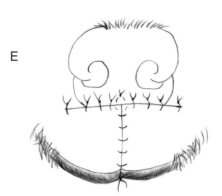

E

Plate 81	**Oral Commissure Advancement Technique**

DESCRIPTION

Oral commissure advancement is occasionally used to maintain the position of the tongue after hemi-mandibulectomy. It can be performed at the time of hemi-mandibulectomy or postoperatively as an elective surgery for those patients that would truly benefit from this procedure. It also is occasionally performed *unilaterally* or *bilaterally*, often in older patients with nonunion mandibular fractures secondary to advanced dental disease or trauma.

SURGICAL TECHNIQUE

(A) After hemi-mandibulectomy, the length and mass of the tongue has caused it to persistently shift out of the oral cavity. The patient may not have adapted to maintaining its tongue primarily in its mouth.

(B) Partial resection of the upper and lower labial margins, including the oral commissure. General guidelines for the length of the excision can be determined by the length of the tongue relative to the length of the labial borders. In general, the caudal one-half to two-thirds of the upper and lower margins may be resected to create adequate lateral support of the tongue. The base of the lingual frenulum (intermandibular attachment) also can be used as a simple anatomic landmark for the length required for commissure advancement to support the tongue.

(C) Closure is accomplished by suturing the upper and lower labial mucosal margins with 3-0 (slowly absorbable) sutures in a simple interrupted pattern.

(D) The skin is closed similarly, using a simple interrupted pattern.

COMMENTS

The dog has the remarkable ability to vary the position of the oral commissure: commissure retraction ("canine smiling") can stretch and expose the length of the upper and lower lips to a surprising degree. The decision whether or not to include this procedure at the time of hemi-mandibulectomy is based on the preference of the surgeon. It may be most useful in large dogs, where the overall size of the tongue may predispose them to lingual deviation. As noted, it also is used in older dogs that may have mandibular instability secondary to nonunion mandibular fractures. In the case of bilateral mandibular fractures, oral commissure advancement creates a supportive sling. This improves the comfort of the pet, their cosmetic appearance, and enables the patient to eat and drink more effectively.

Plate 81

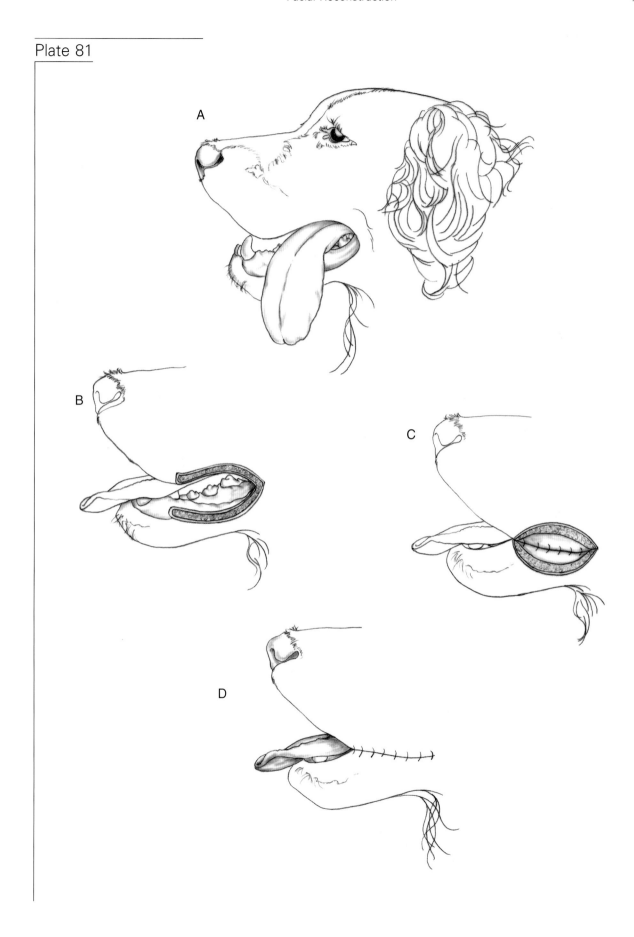

A

B

C

D

Plate 82   **Brachycephalic Facial Fold Correction**

DESCRIPTION

Brachycephalic dogs normally have one major facial fold; there can be a notably smaller facial fold rostral to the larger fold, adjacent to the dorsal nasal surface. The largest fold may uniformly cross the face or flatten to a variable degree over the middorsal nasal surface. The rostral "trough" or "valley" of the large skin fold occasionally is the location of dermatitis (intertrigo). Surgery focuses on removal of this trough and the lower, rostral portion of the largest skin fold.

There are occasions where the "ridge" of the larger skin fold and fur will rub on the patient's eyes, causing corneal irritation or ulceration. Surgical removal of a portion of the ridge can eliminate contact with the eye. This also can be accomplished by removing the rostral trough and a portion of the adjacent ridge. Upon incisional closure, the resultant linear scar is recessed in the trough or valley for a satisfactory functional and cosmetic outcome.

SURGICAL TECHNIQUE

(A) In this example, the patient has a prominent facial fold. There is a pyoderma involving the rostral trough of this large fold of skin.

(B) Elevation of the rostral surface of the fold, exposing the infected intertriginous zone. The dashed line represents the location for surgical resection of the tissue. (*Note:* The infected skin overlying the muzzle can be fibrotic, and its resection can be problematic.) A scalpel blade may be needed to tangentially "shave" or resect the skin surface in preparation for closure. (Electrocautery is needed to control the multiple small bleeding vessels when resecting chronic inflammatory tissue.)

(C) Completion of the closure. The major fold of skin is partially preserved, maintaining the normal appearance of the dog. The scar is less conspicuous, residing in the depression between the two skin folds.

COMMENTS

Various textbook illustrations have suggested complete removal of the problematic skin fold. This has the unfortunate result of dramatically changing the facial appearance of the pet. It also is unnecessary: the above reduction technique effectively corrects the two problems occasionally noted with prominent facial folds (intertrigo and corneal irritation) and better conceals the surgical scar.

Plate 82

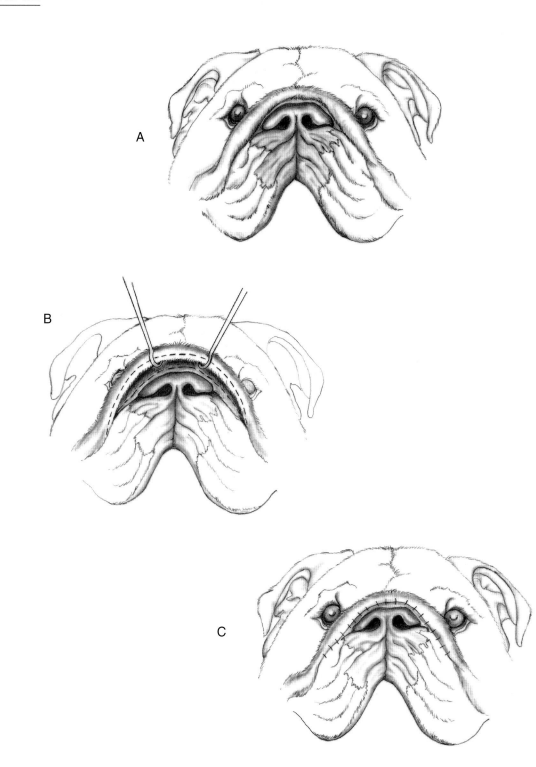

A

B

C

| Plate 83 | **Cheilopexy Technique for Drooling** |

DESCRIPTION

This technique, described by Stoll, can be used to reduce excessive drooling in the larger dogs possessing redundant labial tissue. It is a simple linear "labial pexy" of the lower labial border to the upper labial/buccal mucosal area. As a result, it lifts the lower lip, thereby creating a more effective lower labial retention barrier as saliva accumulates. In turn, the dog can swallow the saliva rather that constantly drooling on the neighboring environment.

SURGICAL TECHNIQUE

(A) The lower labial border can be assessed with the patient under anesthesia. Forceps are used to grasp the caudal aspect of the lower lip and elevate it dorsally, to get a general idea of where to create the *cheilopexy*. The mouth is opened to assure that range of motion is reasonably preserved and excessive tension is avoided after completing the cheilopexy.

  To facilitate locating the appropriate site, a line can be drawn from the medial canthus to the oral commissure (dashed line). A full-thickness labial incision is initiated immediately cranial to this guideline: the incision is 3–5 cm dorsal to the upper labial border. This incision itself is 2–4 cm long and is parallel to the labial margin. A comparable incision is made in the lower labial margin below the upper labial/buccal incision (arrow). This incision is dissected open to facilitate suturing; alternatively, a scalpel blade can be used to resect the immediate labial border. A skin hook or long-handled forceps can be used to lift the lower labial incision through the full-thickness upper labial incision.

(B) The mucosal incision of the lower lip is sutured to the labial mucosal border of the dorsal labial incision with a series of interrupted (slowly absorbable) 3-0 sutures. Large suture bites help assure adequate security of this cheilopexy.

(C) After suturing the two mucosal incisions together, the dorsal skin incision is sutured to complete the procedure.

COMMENTS

Properly positioned, the above suture closure should maintain the cheilopexy until healing is complete. Only the skin sutures require removal. More elaborate mattress suture techniques are noted in the veterinary literature and also are acceptable. Postoperatively, wrinkling of the cheek may be noted, but normally flattens over time. Local dermatitis of the lower labial skin overlapped by the upper labial mucosa appears not to be a serious problem in these patients. Should there any problem with cheilopexy, reversal of this procedure would be easy to perform.

  Few owners generally elect to have this surgery performed for two reasons: many owners are not aware of this technique and owners of these dogs generally accept the unhygienic drooling as a normal part of owning a particular breed (St. Bernard, mastiffs, Newfoundlands, etc.). It may be the first-time owner, unpleasantly surprised by this problem, who is more receptive to a discussion of corrective cheilopexy by the attending veterinarian.

Plate 83

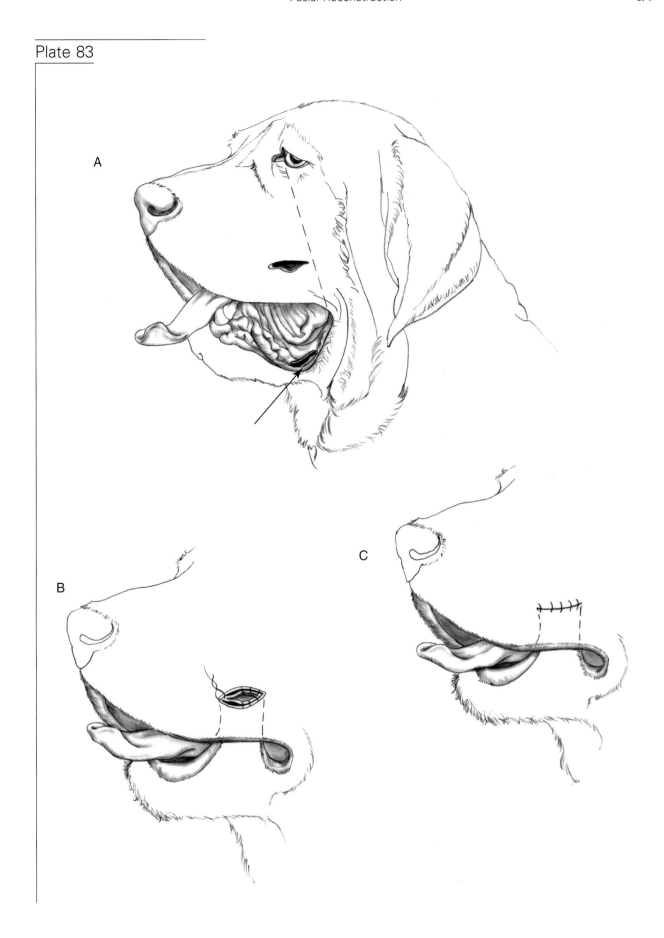

A

B

C

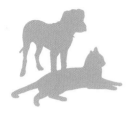

16

Myocutaneous Flaps and Muscle Flaps

INTRODUCTION

Myocutaneous (musculocutaneous) flaps are flaps in which a skeletal muscle and the overlying skin are elevated simultaneously. In humans, the intact muscle circulation supplies blood to the skin through musculocutaneous arteries exiting the muscle surface. In dogs and cats, direct cutaneous arteries exit the muscle to supply the overlying skin.

Muscle flaps and, to a lesser degree, myocutaneous flaps have clinical potential in small animal reconstructive surgery. Several individual muscles in the dog and cat are expendable without sacrificing regional function. These same muscles could be pivoted into an adjacent defect tethered by a vascular pedicle capable of maintaining circulation to the muscle unit using basic surgical instrumentation. Muscular/fascial flaps have been advocated for perineal hernia repair, soft tissue coverage, and wound closure; and for contributing circulation to fractures, promoting bone healing, and combating infection. Muscle-tendon units can be transplanted to replace essential muscle units damaged or destroyed.

Myocutaneous flaps have enjoyed considerable popularity in human reconstructive surgery because of their versatility and potential ability to transfer large skin segments in a single staged procedure. The limited amounts of loose skin available and the limited number of direct cutaneous arteries have supported the need for myocutaneous flap transfer in humans. In contrast, the dog and cat have considerable amounts of loose skin located over the trunk, and a number of direct cutaneous arteries are present for axial pattern flap development. In most cases, local flaps, axial pattern flaps, and free grafts can be used without resorting to myocutaneous flaps and the more demanding microvascular surgery occasionally used in humans to transfer them to distant locations.

MYOCUTANEOUS FLAPS

Development of a myocutaneous flap in the dog requires the presence of direct cutaneous arteries exiting the muscle surface to supply the overlying skin. Secondary myocutaneous flaps have been investigated experimentally in dogs by suturing skin onto an underlying muscle, which is later elevated and transferred to the recipient site once circulation has been established between the muscle and skin "island." These secondary myocutaneous flaps have the major disadvantage of requiring two-stage development and transfer.

The more superficial muscles in the body are best used for myocutaneous flap development. A vascular pedicle sufficient to maintain circulation is required to facilitate rotation of a muscle into potential defects within the arc of rotation. Free flap transfer using microvascular surgical technique would enable myocutaneous flap placement to distant locations, although there are far simpler techniques to close wounds in most clinical cases.

MUSCLE FLAPS

Individual skeletal muscles can be used to repair body defects beneath the skin secondary to trauma or the surgical removal of damaged or diseased tissue. Muscle-tendon units have been transposed to treat paralysis of the extensors of the carpus (radial nerve) and tarsus (peroneal nerve). Other muscles have been used for hernia repair including the transversus abdominis muscle for closure of diaphragmatic hernias, the external abdominal oblique muscle for abdominal hernia repair, the internal obturator and superficial gluteal muscles for perineal hernia repair, the temporalis muscle flap for facial defects involving the canine orbit, the rectus femoris and cranial sartorius muscle flaps for trochanteric ulcers, and semitendinosus muscle flaps for ventral perineal hernia repair and for creation of an anal sling. Flaps composed of intercostal muscle, diaphragm, sternocephalicus muscle, and sternothyroideus muscle have been used to correct strictures and defects of the esophagus. The author has used the sternothyroideus muscle for closure of entry and exit bullet wounds of the canine larynx. Muscle/fascia strips from the biceps femoris or deep gluteal muscle have been used as padding between the pelvis and femoral shaft after femoral head and neck ostectomy. Muscles are capable of contributing additional circulation to ischemic areas that are the result of trauma, poor collateral circulation, or radiation damage.

Muscle Flap Circulation and Classification

Individual muscles in the body have different vascular supplies: Mathes and Nahai (1982) have developed a classification system for muscles, based on their vascular anatomy. There are five major vascular patterns for muscles.

Type I. One vascular pedicle. Type I muscles can be elevated and pivoted on their dominant pedicle. Example: Rectus femoris muscle based on the lateral circumflex femoral vessels.

Type II. Dominant vascular pedicle(s) near the origin *or* insertion of the muscle, with minor pedicle supplying the muscle belly. Type II muscles are likely to survive despite ligation of the minor pedicles during elevation of the muscle, based on the dominant vascular pedicle. Example: Cranial sartorius muscle, based on the superficial circumflex iliac vessels.

Type III. Two dominant pedicles, supplying approximately half the muscle belly. Division of one vascular pedicle may or may not compromise that portion of the muscle supplied by the ligated pedicle: research is required to determine viability of individual muscles in this category. Example: Rectus femoris muscle based on the caudal gluteal artery and vein proximally and the distal caudal femoral artery distally.

Type IV. Smaller segmental vascular pedicles supplying the muscle between the origin and insertion. Survival may be inconsistent, depending on the vascular pedicles ligated: research is required to determine viability of individual muscles in this category. Example: Caudal sartorius muscle based on a branch of the saphenous artery and medial saphenous vein.

Type V. One dominant vascular pedicle located at the insertion of the muscle, with segmental pedicles entering near the origin. The entire muscle is expected to survive based on the dominant pedicle. Muscle survival, based on the segmental vascular pedicles alone, is questionable and would require research to determine individual viability of a type V muscle. Example: Latissimus dorsi myocutaneous flap based on the thoracodorsal artery and vein.

Preservation of muscle function and bulk will depend upon preservation of the blood supply as well as muscle innervation. The term *angiosome* describes a block of tissue (muscle or a given region, including bone, skin, fascia, etc.) that is supplied by a regional artery and vein (venae comitantes). Within a given muscle, there may be various angiosomes that are based on vessels supplying these specific areas. *True*

vascular anastomoses within the muscle occur when a major artery connects with another without changing caliber. *Choke anastomoses* are the most common, and refers to areas where arteries unite by means of a plexus of two or more reduced-caliber arteries (arterioles). As the terminology denotes, blood flow is somewhat more restricted through choke anastomoses. For example, the angiosome adjacent to a dominant pedicle is likely to survive after ligation of its segmental blood supply via collateral circulation passing through choke anastomoses. Sacrifice of the segmental blood supply to more distant angiosomes of a muscle is more likely to result in muscle necrosis: perfusion through the more distant choke anastomoses becomes increasingly tenuous. However, for reliable clinical transfer, research is needed to confirm muscle flap survival after sacrificing selective vascular pedicles.

Eight muscle flaps for clinical use will be discussed in this chapter, including the latissimus dorsi muscle, external abdominal oblique muscle, caudal sartorius muscle, cranial sartorius muscle, temporalis muscle, flexor carpi ulnaris muscle, semitendinosus muscle, and transversus abdominis muscle.

Latissimus Dorsi Muscle

The latissimus dorsi muscle is a flat triangular muscle overlying the dorsal half of the lateral thoracic wall in the dog; it is the broadest of the skeletal muscles, with the exception of the cutaneous trunci muscle. It begins as a wide tendinous leaf from the superficial leaf of the lumbodorsal fascia associated with the spinous processes of the lumbar vertebrae and the last seven or eight thoracic vertebrae. It arises muscularly from the last two or three ribs. Muscle fibers converge toward the shoulder, and the cranial border of the muscle lies under the trapezius thoracis muscle where it covers the caudal angle at the scapula. The apical end of the muscle encroaches upon the dorsal border of the deep pectoral muscle, ending in an aponeurosis medially on the triceps muscle.

The thoracodorsal and lateral thoracic arteries supply the dorsal and ventral portions of the latissimus dorsi muscle. Branches of these vessels emerge from the muscle surface to supply a portion of the cutaneous trunci muscle and the skin as short, direct cutaneous arteries. The thoracodorsal artery also sends a large direct cutaneous artery to the skin dorsally caudal to the scapula. This vessel joins the skin after passing through the craniodorsal portion of the latissimus dorsi muscle, caudal to the long head of the triceps muscle.

The intercostal arteries also supply segmental branches to the dorsal portion of the latissimus dorsi

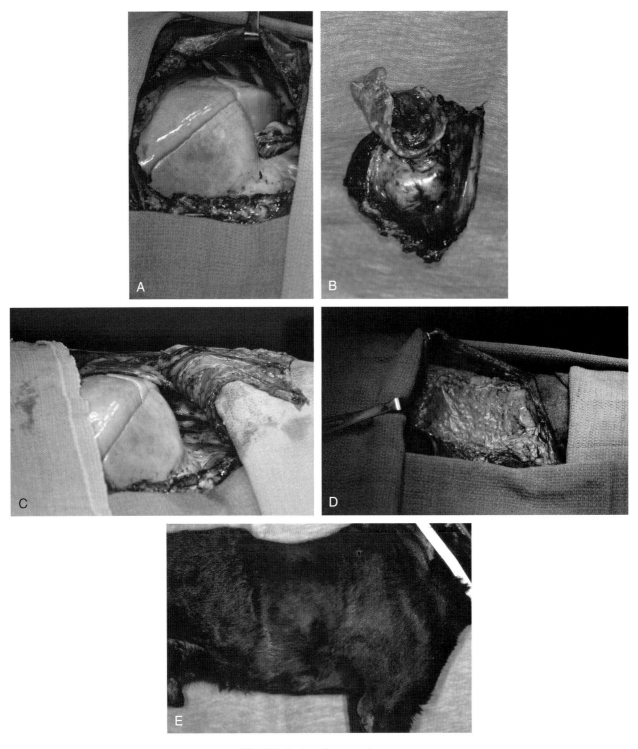

FIG. 16-1 *See legend on opposite page.*

muscle and overlying cutaneous trunci muscle. These branches perforate the latissimus dorsi muscle to supply the cutaneous trunci muscle and overlying skin as the proximal lateral cutaneous branches of the intercostal arteries. The distal lateral cutaneous branches of the intercostal arteries emerge below the ventral border of the latissimus dorsi muscle to supply the regional overlying skin (Fig. 16-1).

Cutaneous Trunci Muscle

The cutaneous trunci muscle is a derivative of the pectoralis profundus and forms a thin leaf covering most of the dorsal, lateral, and ventral walls of the abdomen in the dog. It begins in the caudal gluteal region, with muscle fibers fanning cranially and ventrally. It ends in the axilla, where it is closely associated with the underlying latissimus dorsi muscle and the caudal border of the deep pectoral muscle. The cutaneous trunci muscle causes the skin to shiver in response to external irritants over the trunk. Circulation to the cutaneous trunci muscle is from small muscular branches and direct cutaneous arteries supplying the overlying skin. Anatomic studies demonstrated that two to four short, direct, cutaneous branches of the thoracodorsal artery perforate the latissimus dorsi muscle caudal to the border of the triceps muscle and supply the cutaneous trunci and overlying skin. The subdermal plexus of the skin is closely associated with the cutaneous trunci muscles. Surgically elevating the skin and panniculus musculature together, by undermining below this muscle layer, helps preserve their circulatory relationship.

External Abdominal Oblique Muscle

The external abdominal oblique muscle is a long, flat muscle, with fibers directed caudoventrally. It consists of costal and lumbar components. The costal component originates segmentally from the fourth or fifth rib through the thirteenth rib. The lumbar component originates in the thoracolumbar fascia along the iliocostalis muscle. Ventrally and caudally, the aponeuroses of the two components contribute to the external rectus fascia, the external inguinal ring, and the prepubic tendon. The cranial branch of the cranial abdominal artery supplies the middle zone of the lateral abdominal wall and is accompanied by the cranial hypogastric nerve and a satellite vein. The deep branch of the deep circumflex artery anastomoses with the cranial and caudal abdominal arteries and is the main supply to the caudodorsal quarter of the abdominal wall. It, too, is accompanied by a satellite vein and is joined by the lateral cutaneous femoral nerve. This versatile muscle flap is technically easy to elevate and transfer (Figs. 16-2, 16-3, 16-4).

Cranial Sartorius Muscle

The cranial sartorius muscle is a long, flat, straplike muscle, arising on the iliac crest and lumbodorsal fascia. It extends to the medial surface of the thigh to pass into the medial femoral fascia above the patella. Vascular injections have demonstrated a single major vascular pedicle present at the proximal one-third of the muscle. This vascular pedicle is a branch of the femoral artery and vein, and enters all muscle specimens along its caudal border (Fig. 16-5).

Caudal Sartorius Muscle

The caudal sartorius muscle lies close beside the cranial belly on the medial surface of the thigh. It arises from the bony ridge between the two ventral spines of the ilium. Distally, it runs over the medial surfaces of the vastus medialis and stifle joint, where it forms an aponeurosis that blends with that of the gracilis muscle. Vascular injections have demonstrated a segmental blood supply with a dominant vascular pedicle off the saphenous artery and medial saphenous vein at the distal third of the muscle belly (Fig. 16-5).

FIG. 16-1 (A, B) Resection of multiple ribs to remove a chondrosarcoma.

(C) The latissimus dorsi muscle reflected backward prior to placement into the thoracic defect.

(D) Marlex mesh was used to span the defect prior to application of the muscle flap. Today, the author no longer uses mesh: the muscle alone, placed under slight tension during suturing, spans large defects quite satisfactorily.

(E) Postoperative view of the dog. Slight cavitation is noted, although clinically these patients have no issues breathing. Some paradoxical movement of the muscle can be noted over the first few postoperative days.

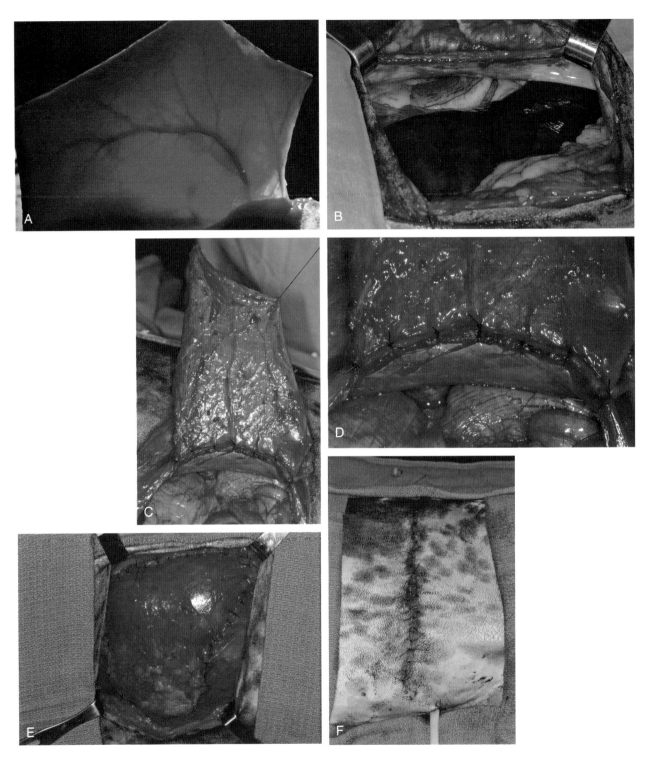

FIG. 16-2 (A) Illumination of an elevated external abdominal oblique muscle illustrating the cranial abdominal artery and vein.

(B) A 10 × 10-cm defect created in the ventrolateral abdominal wall.

(C) The overlapping base of the external abdominal oblique muscle flap is sutured to the dorsal border of the defect.

(D) Close-up view of the sutured flap base. Care is taken not to disturb the cranial abdominal vasculature.

(E) Closure is completed by suturing the remaining three sides of the muscle flap into the defect.

(F) Completion of the surgery. An access incision can facilitate the caudodorsal elevation of the external abdominal oblique muscle.

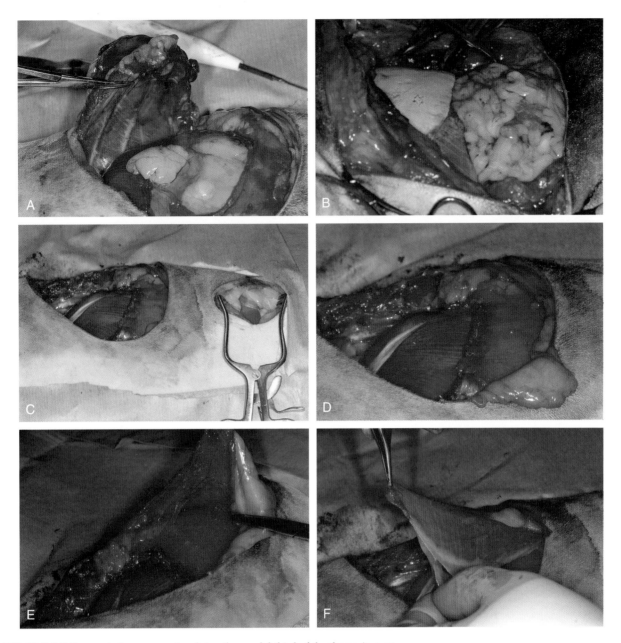

FIG. 16-3 (A) Removal of a sarcoma involving the caudal third of the thorax in a cat.

(B) The large defect exposes the left caudal lung lobe and abdominal cavity.

(C, D) Unlike in Figure 16-2, The diaphragm was sutured to the cranial border of the internal abdominal oblique and transversus muscle layer, thereby closing the abdominal cavity. Note the caudal access incision with the Weitlaner tissue retractor.

(E) The external abdominal oblique muscle separates from the underlying interabdominal oblique with minimal dissection.

(F) The muscle is pivoted into the surgical site.

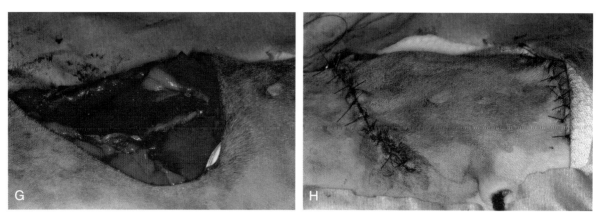

FIG. 16-3 *Continued* (G) The muscle is sutured to the remaining thoracic wall and adjacent soft tissues. (H) Completion of the surgery. The patient made a complete recovery.

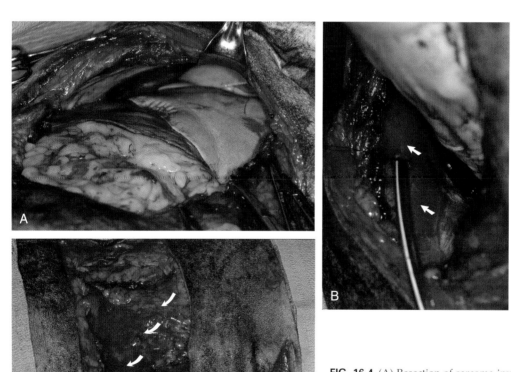

FIG. 16-4 (A) Resection of sarcoma involving the left lateral thorax and abdomen. (B) Diaphragm advancement to close the thorax. (C) Forward rotation of the external abdominal oblique muscle to close the lateral abdominal wall defect, without the need of synthetic mesh.

Miscellaneous Muscle Flap Techniques

The temporalis muscle flap (orbital defects), semitendinosus muscle (upper hind limb and perineal defects), flexor carpi ulnaris (carpal defects), and transversus abdominis muscle (large diaphragmatic defects) are less commonly used in wound repair due to their location and the relative infrequency of problematic wounds in their arc of rotation. Nonetheless, these techniques can be useful for those occasional defects in which wound healing and closure are particularly challenging.

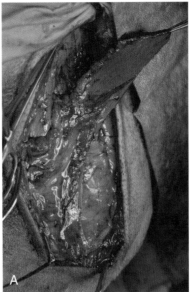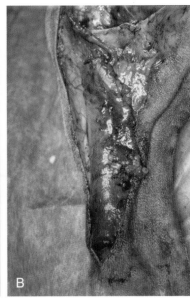

FIG. 16-5 (A) Elevation of the cranial sartorius muscle. (B) Elevation of the caudal sartorius muscle.

Suggested Readings

Alexander LG, Pavletic MM, Engler SJ. 1991. Abdominal wall reconstruction with a vascular external abdominal oblique myofascial flap. *Vet Surg* 20:379–384.

Bennett D, Vaughn LC. 1976. The use of muscle relocation techniques in the treatment of peripheral nerve injuries in dogs and cats. *J Sm Anim Pract* 17:99–108.

Bentley JF, Henderson RA, Simpson ST. 1991. Use of a temporalis muscle flap in reconstruction of the calvarium and orbital rim in a dog. *J Am Anim Hosp Assoc* 27:463–465.

Chambers JN, Purinton PT, Allen SW, et al. 1998. Flexor carpi ulnaris muscle flap for reconstruction of distal forelimb injuries in two dogs. *Vet Surg* 27:342–347.

Chambers JN, Purinton PT, Allen SW, Moore JL. 1990. Classification and anatomic categorization of the vascular patterns to the pelvic limb muscles in dogs. *J Am Vet Res* 51:305–313.

Chambers JN, Purinton PT, Moore JL, Allen SW. 1990. Treatment of trochanteric ulcers with cranial sartorius and rectus femoris muscle flaps. *Vet Surg* 19:424–428.

Chambers JN, Rawlings CA. 1991. Applications of a semitendinosis muscle flap in two dogs. *J Am Vet Med Assoc* 199:84–86.

Furneaux RW, Hudson MD. 1976. Autogenous muscle flap repair of a diaphragmatic hernia. *Fel Pract* 6:20–24.

Halfacree ZJ, Baines SJ, Lipscomb VJ, et al. 2007. Use of a latissimus dorsi myocutaneous flap for one-stage reconstruction of the thoracic wall after en bloc resection of primary rib chondrosarcoma in five dogs. *Vet Surg* 36:587–592.

Hardy EM, Kolata RJ, Earley TD, et al. 1983. Evaluation of internal obturator muscle transposition in treatment of perineal hernia in dogs. *Vet Surg* 12:69–72.

Helphrey ML. 1982. Abdominal flap graft for repair of chronic diaphragmatic hernia in the dog. *J Am Vet Med Assoc* 181:791–793.

Lesser AS, Soliman SS. 1980. Experimental evaluation of tendon transfer for the treatment of sciatic nerve paralysis in the dog. *Vet Surg* 9:72–73.

Lester S, Pratschke K. 2003. Central hemimaxillectomy and reconstruction using a superficial temporal artery axial pattern flap in a domestic short hair cat. *J Fel Med Surg* 5:241–244.

Liptak JM, Brebner NS. 2006. Hemidiaphragmatic reconstruction with a transversus abdominis muscle flap after resection of a solitary diaphragmatic mesothelioma in a dog. *J Am Vet Med Assoc* 228:1204–1208.

Mathes SJ, Nahai F. (1982). Vascular anatomy of muscle: classification and application. In: Mathes SJ, Nahai F, eds. *Clinical Applications for Muscle and Musculocutaneous Flaps*, 16–94. St Louis, MO: CV Mosby.

Pavletic MM. 1990. Introduction to myocutaneous and muscle flaps. 1990. *Vet Clin No Am* 20:127–146.

Pavletic MM. 1993. Pedicle grafts. In: Slatter DH, ed. *Textbook of Small Animal Surgery*. 3rd ed., 292–321. Philadelphia, PA: WB Saunders.

Pavletic MM, Kostolich M, Koblik P, Engler S. 1987. A comparison of the cutaneous trunci myocutaneous flap and latissimus dorsi myocutaneous flap in the dog. *Vet Surg* 16:283–293.

Peterson SL, Gourley IM. 1989. Temporal muscle fascial flap for temporomandibular joint luxation in a dog. *J Am Anim Hosp Assoc* 25:186–188.

Philibert D, Fowler JD. 1996. Use of muscle flaps in reconstructive surgery. *Compend Contin Edu Pract Vet* 18:395–405.

Puerto DA, Aroonson LR. 2004. Use of a semitendinosus myocutaneous flap for soft-tissue reconstruction of a grade IIIB open tibial fracture in a dog. *Vet Surg* 33:629–635.

Purinton PT, Chambers JN, Moore JL. 1998. Identification and categorization of the vascular patterns to muscles of the thoracic limb, thorax, and neck of dogs. *AM J Vet Res* 53:1435–1445.

Sylvestre AM, Weinstein MJ, Popovitch CA, Brockman DJ. 1997. The sartorius muscle flap in the cat: an anatomic study and two case reports. *J Am Anim Hosp Assoc* 33:91–96.

Tomlinson J, Presnell KR. 1981. Use of the temporalis muscle flap in the dog. *Vet Surg* 10:77–79.

Weinstein MJ, Pavletic MM, Boudrieau RJ. 1988. Caudal sartorius muscle flap in the dog. *Vet Surg* 17:203–210.

Weinstein MJ, Pavletic MM, Boudrieau RJ. 1989. Cranial sartorius muscle flap in the Dog. *Vet Surg* 18:286–291.

Plate 84   # Latissimus Dorsi Myocutaneous Flap

DESCRIPTION

The latissimus dorsi myocutaneous flap simultaneously transfers both muscle and skin to close a variety of defects within its arc of rotation.

SURGICAL TECHNIQUE

(A) Under general anesthesia, the patient's thorax is completely clipped and prepared for surgery. The dog is placed in lateral recumbency with the skin in its natural undistorted position relative to the underlying body mass. The forelimb is placed in relaxed extension, perpendicular to the trunk.

   The dorsal flap border (A) is drawn with a marking pen from a point ventral to the acromion (1), caudal to the border of the triceps muscle (below the origin of the thoracodorsal direct cutaneous artery) (2), and extending to the level of the head to the 13th rib (3). The ventral border of the flap (B) extends from the forelimb skin fold caudal to the lower triceps muscle's border (the lower third of the length of the humerus) (4), and extends caudodorsally to the 13th rib, parallel to the first line (5). The caudodorsal border (C) of the flap is drawn by using the level of the 13th rib border to join the dorsal and ventral flap lines.

(B) The ventral skin flap border is incised initially, and the isolated ventral border of the latissimus dorsi muscle is elevated. The skin flap incision is extended, and a latissimus dorsi muscle flap of a width equal to that of the overlying skin is elevated. As the muscle is elevated from the thoracic wall, the proximal lateral intercostal vessels are isolated, ligated, and divided below the latissimus dorsi muscle to complete the flap elevation. In this example, a bridge incision is created between the donor and recipient beds to facilitate transfer of the flap without partial tube formation.

(C) The flap is sutured into position. Penrose drains or closed suction units are used to obliterate dead space at the donor and recipient sites.

COMMENTS

Careful preoperative measurements are necessary to ensure that the flap will satisfactorily cover the defect. Note that the length of the flap decreases the more the flap is rotated. Although the latissimus dorsi myocutaneous flap is thicker, less pliable, and less elastic than the adjacent cutaneous trunci myocutaneous flap and adjacent thoracodorsal axial pattern flap, it is capable of extending down the forelimb to a variable degree, depending on the patient's body conformation. The thoracodorsal axial pattern flap and cutaneous trunci myocutaneous flaps are better suited for skin defects, whereas the latissimus dorsi myocutaneous flap, with its greater bulk, is better suited for thoracic wall defects in which the simultaneous reconstruction of the chest with muscle and skin is highly desirable.

Plate 84

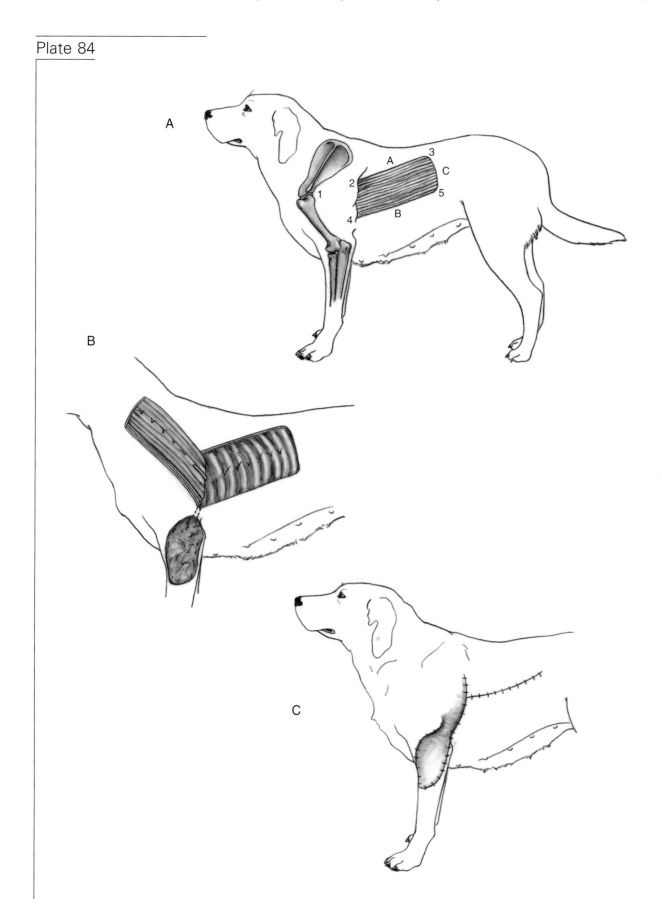

Plate 85   # Cutaneous Trunci
Myocutaneous Flap

DESCRIPTION

The cutaneous trunci myocutaneous flap is similar in shape and design to the latissimus dorsi myocutaneous flap. It is thinner than its counterpart and has slightly greater mobility within its arc of rotation.

SURGICAL TECHNIQUES

(A) The general outline for elevation of the cutaneous trunci myocutaneous flap is identical to that for the latissimus dorsi myocutaneous flap (see Plate 84). However, elevation of this flap is confined to the loose areolar fascial plane beneath the cutaneous trunci muscle.

(B) The skin is incised down to the level of the cutaneous trunci muscle, in a fashion similar to elevation of the latissimus dorsi myocutaneous flap. Branches of the proximal lateral intercostal direct cutaneous arteries (and veins) exiting the surface of the latissimus dorsi muscle require ligation and division during flap elevation. A bridge incision is used in this example to facilitate placement of the myocutaneous flap (dashed lines).

(C) Penrose drains or closed suction units are used at the donor and recipient sites to obliterate dead space during flap transfer and recipient bed closure.

COMMENTS

Careful preoperative measurement is necessary to ensure that the flap will satisfactorily cover the defect. Note that as the flap length is reduced, the more the flap is rotated. Although flap size and coverage are similar to those of the thoracodorsal axial pattern flap, the author has safely developed longer thoracodorsal axial pattern flaps in the dog, when necessary. Clinical experience, size of the flap required to cover the skin defect, and the ease of flap transplantation should be considered when selecting a flap technique.

Plate 85

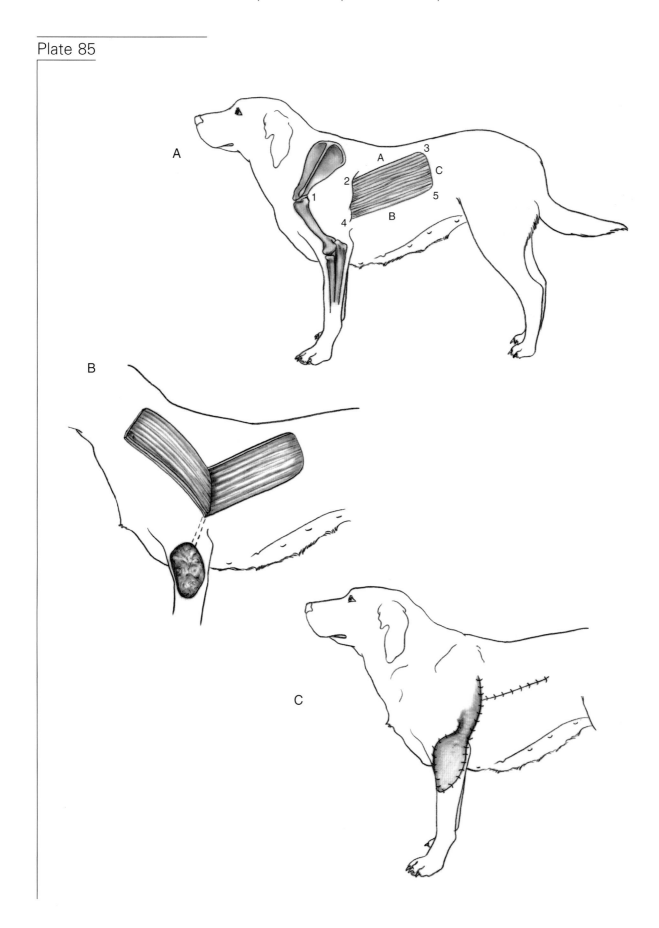

Plate 86   **Latissimus Dorsi Muscle Flap**

DESCRIPTION

The latissimus dorsi muscle is used to cover defects beneath the skin (e.g., thoracic wall) within its arc of rotation.

SURGICAL TECHNIQUE

(A) In this clinical example, a lower thoracic wall mass requires surgical resection.

(B) The neoplasm is resected. The skin margins are carefully retracted to expose the latissimus dorsi muscle.

(C) In this example, optional surgical mesh is sutured over the margins of the thoracic wall defect.

(D) The elevated muscle flap is pivoted and sutured over the mesh. Simple interrupted sutures or double-loop patterns (far-far-near-near, far-near-near-far) are sufficient for suturing the flap in position. A closed suction system is inserted prior to skin closure.

COMMENTS

Although a skin incision can be made over the muscle, parallel to its fibers, it is possible to expose the muscle through small skin incision(s), depending upon the location of the defect being closed. In many instances, the muscle can be exposed via the surgical approach required for removal of a neoplastic condition, provided that the skin can be retracted sufficiently to expose the muscle. Handheld retractors, self-retaining retractors, or large towel clamps can facilitate muscle exposure. An additional access incision can be created if required.

Given its dominant thoracodorsal vascular supply, the muscle can be rotated into adjacent thoracic wall defects. (*Important note:* In thoracic wall defects below the central body of the muscle, the terminal end of the muscle need not be detached from the terminal ribs. The dorsal and ventral muscle borders can be developed and the "bipedicle" muscle flap advanced directly into the ventral defect. This simplifies closure of the thoracic wall defect, reducing the amount of tissue dissection and operative time required to elevate the standard peninsula flap design.) The latissimus dorsi muscle has its greatest application for major thoracic wall reconstruction. The intercostal vessels entering/exiting the muscle require ligation to mobilize the muscle from the thoracic wall and overlying skin. Care must be taken to minimize trauma to the overlying skin and to preserve collateral vascular channels. The latissimus dorsi muscle can be combined with plastic mesh, adjacent composite rib flaps, or rib grafts to add rigidity to the reconstructed chest wall after multiple rib resection. However, it has been the author's experience that mesh, bone grafts, and other implants are unnecessary. The flap, sutured to the adjacent musculofascial borders of the defect, stretches over the area. Sutured under slight tension, the flap covers thoracic wall defects in a trampoline-like fashion. Muscle edges are sutured to the adjacent muscle/fascial planes bordering the defect. Postoperatively, a variable amount of (paradoxical) inward excursion of the flap can be seen during inspiration. It is self-limiting, with minimal motion noted, within a few days after surgery. A shallow depression or concavity can be seen at the flap site, but it is not recognizable in most patients after regrowth of the hair coat.

Plate 86

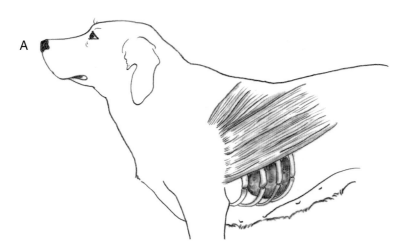

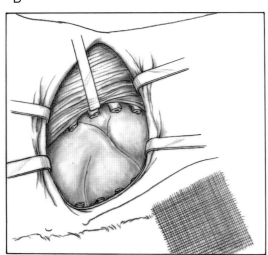

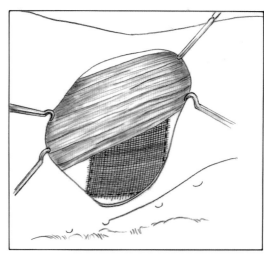

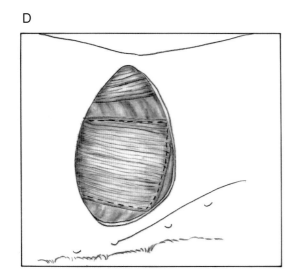

Plate 87	# External Abdominal Oblique Muscle Flap

DESCRIPTION

The external abdominal oblique muscle flap has remarkable pliability and elasticity for closure of major abdominal and caudal thoracic wall defects.

SURGICAL TECHNIQUE

(A) With the patient under general anesthesia, the entire ventral and lateral abdominal wall is clipped and prepared for surgery in standard fashion. In this example, a neoplasm involves the caudal thoracic and adjacent cranial abdominal wall.

(B) In a medium dog, a paracostal skin incision is made from the level of epaxial muscles to the ventral midline, 5.0 cm caudal to the 13th rib. However, in this clinical example, the surgical wound serves as access to the cranial portions of the muscle, while a curved access incision, cranial and parallel to the flank, provides exposure to the caudal component. The fascial edges of the lumbar external abdominal oblique are identified and divided ventrally and caudally, leaving a 1-cm margin of fascia along the muscular edge. The lumbar external oblique is undermined, and the neurovascular pedicle, consisting of branches of the cranial abdominal artery and cranial hypogastric nerve, and a satellite vein, are identified craniodorsally, caudal to the 13th rib, and preserved. The dorsal fascial attachment is divided and the lumbar external abdominal oblique muscle severed to the level of the 13th rib. The lumbar external abdominal oblique muscular/fascial island flap, tethered by its neurovascular pedicle, is pivoted into an adjacent thoracic or abdominal wall defect, based on preoperative measurements.

(C) The inner fascial surface of the flap is sutured to the overlapped defect with 2-0 or 3-0 monofilament, nonabsorbable suture material, using an interrupted mattress suture pattern. Care must be taken to avoid compromise to the vasculature of the muscle flap during suture insertion. Closure of this layer is important to prevent postoperative abdominal herniation.

(D) The remaining edges of the flap are subsequently sutured to the borders of the defect in a similar fashion. A simple interrupted suture pattern or a double-loop suture pattern (far-near-near-far, far-far-near-near) can be used to suture the flap borders. A closed suction unit is most appropriately used to manage dead space.

(E) The overlying skin and access incision are closed in routine fashion.

COMMENTS

The external abdominal oblique muscle, tethered by the dominant cranial abdominal arterial branches, can stretch and pivot to a considerable degree. This island muscle flap may be particularly well suited for closure of ventral abdominal wall and caudal thoracic wall defects. In the pilot study investigating its potential clinical use, the flap was capable of covering defects beyond the 10 × 10-cm full-thickness ventral abdominal wall defects created in medium-sized dogs.

Plate 87

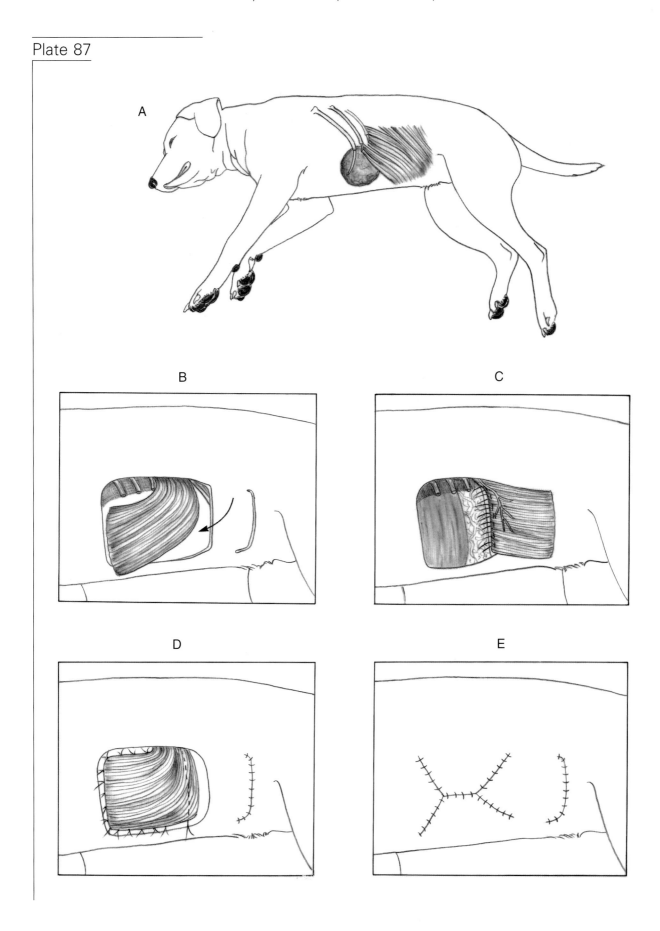

Plate 88   # Caudal Sartorius Muscle Flap

DESCRIPTION

The caudal sartorius muscle, tethered by a saphenous vascular pedicle, has considerable mobility and can extend as far distally as the metatarsal surface.

SURGICAL TECHNIQUE

(A) Under general anesthesia, the involved rear leg is clipped and prepared for surgery in standard fashion. A skin incision is made on the medial aspect of the thigh over the length of the caudal sartorius muscle. The subcutaneous tissues are dissected to expose the underlying caudal sartorius muscle.

(B) The muscle is severed proximally, approximately 4 cm distal to its origin on the ilium. The saphenous artery and medial saphenous vein are doubly ligated and transected where they join the femoral artery and vein. Care is taken to avoid damage to the saphenous vessels in the medial tibial region and more proximally, where these vessels are intimately associated with the caudal border of the caudal sartorius muscle.

(C) The muscle can be completely mobilized by transecting its insertion near the tibial crest, leaving the saphenous artery and vein at the distal end of the caudal sartorius muscle as its sole blood supply.

(D) Tethered by the saphenous artery and medial saphenous vein, the island muscle flap can be transplanted to the distal extremity by extending the skin incision and carefully freeing up the saphenous vasculature.

(E) A closed suction unit is ideally suited to manage dead space prior to skin closure.

COMMENTS

The saphenous artery and medial saphenous vein maintain the caudal sartorius muscle by reversal of circulatory flow through their distal arterial and venous anastomotic connections. Fully mobilized, the caudal sartorius muscle can extend over the metatarsal surface. It has potential clinical use for distal tibial fracture repairs, where healing is impaired by osteomyelitis or poor circulation. However, it also can be used to provide soft tissue coverage to exposed structures that it is capable of reaching. A flap or free graft can be placed over this exposed caudal sartorius muscle to provide epithelial coverage, if necessary. Angiography prior to division of the saphenous artery and medial saphenous vein would be advisable before flap elevation to ensure that the saphenous artery is not the primary source of circulation to the distal extremity; extensive trauma could have compromised the cranial tibial artery and collateral sources of circulation. Division of the saphenous vasculature from a previous medial surgical approach to the tibia or from extensive trauma would preclude its effective use.

Plate 88

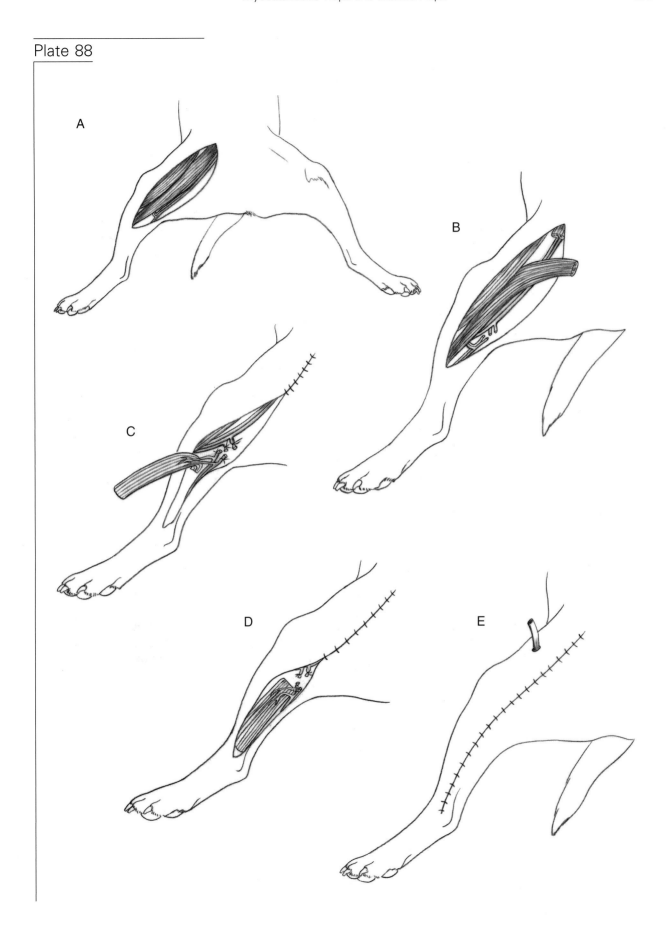

Plate 89   **Cranial Sartorius Muscle Flap**

DESCRIPTION

The cranial sartorius muscle, with its proximal base on the hind limb, can rotate into caudoventral abdominal wall defects.

SURGICAL TECHNIQUE

(A) The patient is anesthetized and the rear limb is clipped and prepared for surgery in standard fashion. A skin incision is made on the medial aspect of the thigh, overlying the length of the cranial sartorius muscle, extending proximally to the inguinal region. The subcutaneous tissue is dissected to expose the underlying cranial sartorius muscle.

(B) Muscle borders are defined by careful sharp and blunt dissection. The muscle is severed distally at its tibial insertion and elevated from the underlying tissues to the level of the proximal vascular pedicle. Care must be taken to avoid damage to the major pedicle of the cranial sartorius entering the muscle caudally and proximally.

(C) The elevated muscle can be rotated up to 180 degrees into adjacent defects. In this clinical example, the muscle flap was used for the repair of a chronic caudal abdominal hernia. Muscle borders are sutured to regional fascial planes bordering the wound.

(D) A closed suction unit is ideally suited to control dead space at donor and recipient sites.

COMMENTS

Given its base and arc of rotation, the cranial sartorius muscle may have its greatest potential use for repair of prepubic tendon rupture when tissue trauma, retraction, and fibrosis preclude adequate reapposition of the tendon to the pelvis in the dog and cat. The cranial sartorius muscle may have additional use in the repair of difficult femoral hernias. Similarly, the pectineus muscle tendon can be divided to mobilize this short muscle for femoral hernia closure or reinforcement.

Plate 89

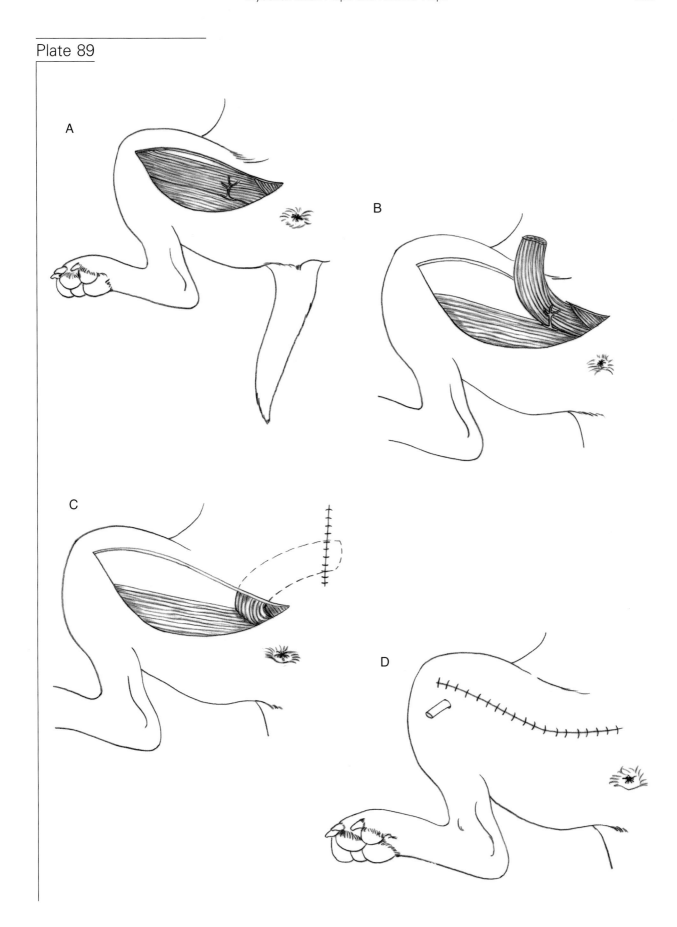

Plate 90   **Temporalis Muscle Flap**

DESCRIPTION

The temporalis muscle flap has been described for closing orbitonasal defects (trauma, tumor resection) and as a barrier for preventing skin from sagging into the orbit after orbital exenteration. A strong fascial sheet covers the muscle dorsally. The fan-shaped temporalis muscle resides in the temporal fossa and inserts on the mandibular coronoid process. More superficial circulation to the muscle is provided by the superficial temporal artery; the deep musculature is supplied by the caudal and rostral deep temporal arteries. The caudal deep temporal artery and rostral deep temporal artery both arise from the maxillary artery and course dorsally beneath the zygomatic arch where they arborize in the temporal muscle. All three arteries anastomose, forming a rich vascular network within the temporal muscle.

SURGICAL TECHNIQUE

(A) In this example, orbital exenteration has been performed, with the skin incision extended caudally to expose the temporalis muscle.
(B) This illustration highlights the two muscle bundles that make up the temporalis muscle, medial to the zygomatic arch.
(C) The skin is retracted dorsally to expose the muscle, the flap is created approximately 20% wider than the width of the orbit to offset muscle contraction after elevation of the flap. The visible superficial temporal artery is identified and protected during exposure and elevation of the flap. The muscle is incised along the margin of the sagittal crest and is elevated subperiosteally from the skull with a periosteal elevator. Care is taken to preserve the deeper vascular blood supply. The sides of the flap are developed parallel to the muscle fibers. The temporalis muscle fascia can be dissected from the zygomatic arch to improve flap mobility.
(D) The flap can be rotated on its insertion and sutured into the margins of the bony/soft tissue defect. Holes may be drilled in the bony margins to facilitate suture placement.

COMMENTS

In brachycephalic dogs, the temporalis muscles do not meet on the midline; this area is devoid of musculature. In dolichocephalic dogs, the left and right temporalis muscles join to form a middorsal sulcus. The thickness and development of this muscle layer can vary with individual dogs. Mobilization of the temporalis muscle flap to reach the rostral margin of the orbital area can be difficult in some patients. Although this muscle flap is not routinely used, it can be helpful for problematic wounds or defects located within its arc of rotation. A dorsally based flap has been described, but division of a portion of its blood supply does risk tissue ischemia and subsequent muscle necrosis/fibrosis.

Plate 90

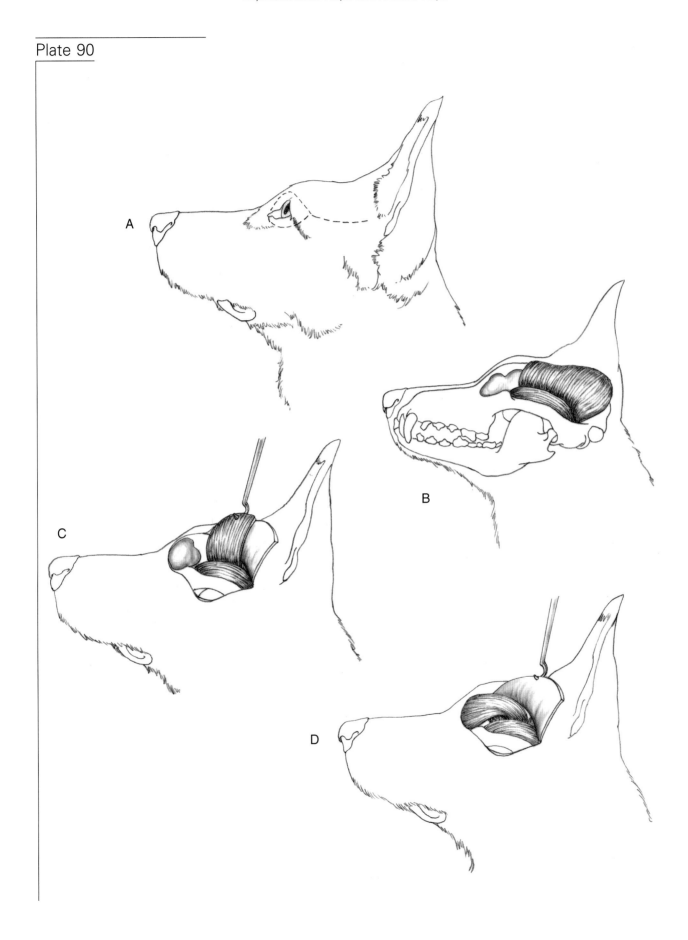

Plate 91   **Transversus Abdominis Muscle Flap**

DESCRIPTION

The transversus abdominis muscle can be elevated as a flap for closure of problematic defects of the diaphragm.

SURGICAL TECHNIQUE

(A) Anatomic outline of the diaphragm and the adjacent transversus abdominis muscle layer. A muscular branch off the phrenicoabdominal artery supplies a portion of the transversus abdominis muscle and can be incorporated into the flap during elevation. The dashed oval on the diaphragm represents the area to be replaced; the adjacent dashed line overlies the site for elevation of the transversus abdominis muscle flap.

(B) In this example, the flap is elevated in a caudal-to-cranial direction and folded forward to replace a large section of the diaphragm. The flap is secured using 2-0 or 3-0 monofilament, nonabsorbable or slowly absorbable suture materials, depending on the size of the patient. Simple interrupted sutures can be preplaced when closing the more problematic dorsal area of the diaphragmatic defect.

COMMENTS

This flap is uncommonly required for closure of diaphragmatic defects. The author has used it on two occasions to replace the right and left hemidiaphragm in long-standing chronic diaphragmatic hernias in two dogs. It also can be used in those cases of neoplasia involving the diaphragm and adjacent tissue structures. Anatomic studies (unpublished, Pavletic, Trout) highlighted the muscular branches arising from the phrenicoabdominal artery. Its inclusion into the flap is added assurance that muscle flap circulation is maintained.

Plate 91

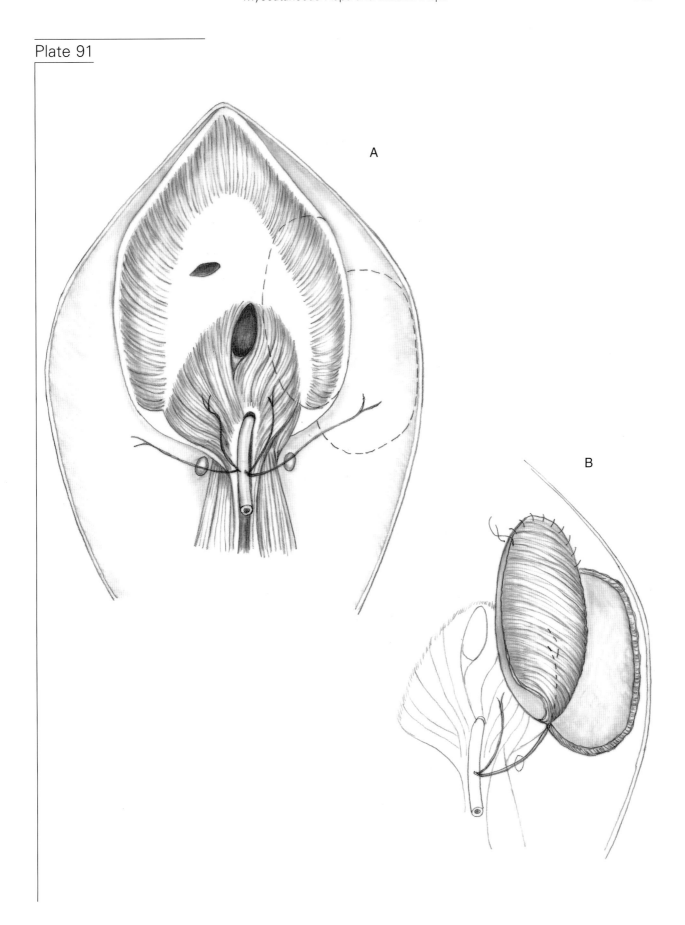

A

B

Plate 92   **Semitendinosus Muscle and Myocutaneous Flaps**

DESCRIPTION

The semitendinosus muscle has two dominant vascular pedicles (type III blood supply, see chapter text). The proximal gluteal artery supplies the upper or proximal "half" of the muscle, entering the proximal quarter of the muscle along its cranial border. The distal half of the muscle is supplied by the distal caudal femoral artery, entering the distal quarter of the muscle along its cranial surface. Because no controlled studies have been performed, it is not possible to determine whether the entire muscle can consistently survive on either vascular pedicle alone. The muscle halves can survive on separate vascular pedicles, but it is probable that larger portions of the muscle will survive on a single vascular pedicle. In one case report, the entire muscle and overlying skin segment survived as a myocutaneous flap based on the distal vascular pedicle for closure of a soft tissue defect of the tibial region.

The proximal "half" of the muscle can be used for reconstructive surgical procedures involving the perineal area (ventral perineal hernia, reinforcement of the anal sphincter for incontinence, nonhealing ulcers). The lower "half" of the muscle can be extended distally for problematic wounds of the adjacent lower extremity. It is possible to develop a myocutaneous flap based on either the proximal or distal vascular pedicle.

SURGICAL TECHNIQUE

(A₁) Outline of the proximally based semitendinosus muscle flap (left) and distally based myocutaneous flap (right) with overlying cutaneous surface (dashed lines). To expose the muscle for the proximally based muscle flap, a skin incision is made along the caudal border of the ischial tuberosity and continued distally along the caudal two-thirds to three-quarters of the length of the thigh. In this example, the muscle flap (left limb) is elevated by dividing the lower third of the muscle belly. The tendinous attachment to the ischium can be divided without compromising the circulation in order to facilitate muscle mobilization. The outline of a distally based myocutaneous flap also is illustrated (right limb).

(A₂) The dashed lines highlight the cutaneous territory of the semitendinosus myocutaneous flap based on the distal vascular pedicle. Note the width and length of the cutaneous territory approximates the major width of the muscle belly.

(B₁) In this illustration, the elevated muscle is tunneled beneath the rectum and anus for closure of a ventral perineal hernia. The muscle is secured to the ventral aspect of the anal sphincter muscle and internal obturator muscles. Exposure of the area may be facilitated with a second incision in the opposing perineal area.

(B₂) In this example, the muscle is cupped around the external anal sphincter to improve muscle tone in a fecally incontinent patient. Note the muscle attachment to the ischial tuberosity has been divided to improve flap mobility.

(C₁) The muscle has been divided distal to the ischial tuberosity and the cutaneous border of the overlying skin island incised.

(C₂) The myocutaneous flap is carefully elevated and rotated into a large defect below the caudal aspect of knee, preserving the distal vascular pedicle.

COMMENT

As noted, additional studies are required to determine whether most, if not the entire, muscle can survive on the proximal or distal vascular pedicle alone on a consistent basis. There are limited applications for the semitendinosus muscle flap and myocutaneous flap variations. However, management of problematic wounds involving the perineum and tibial region can be a challenge, and the potential accessibility of this muscle is a desirable feature.

Plate 92

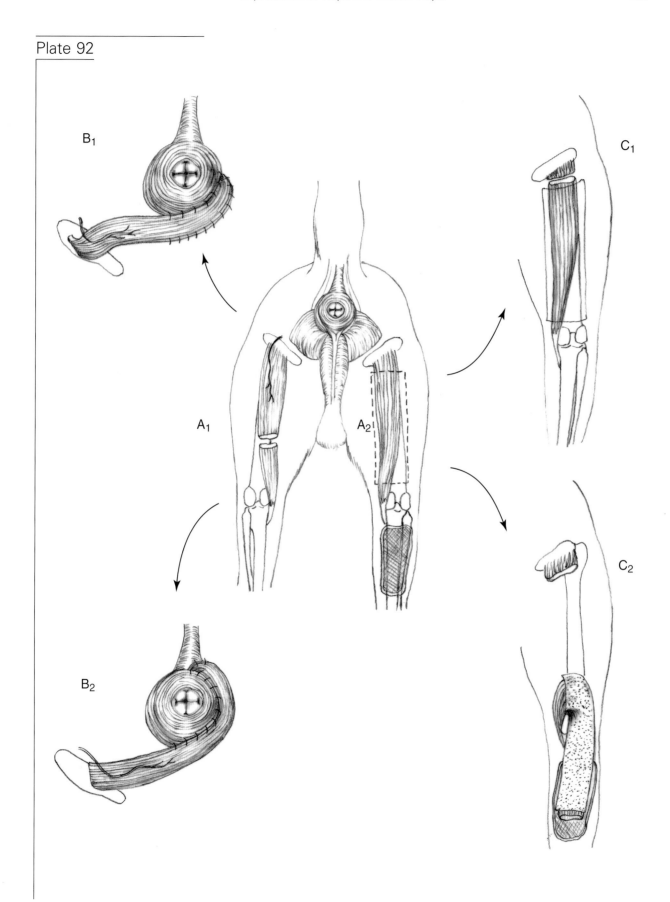

Plate 93 | **Flexor Carpi Ulnaris Muscle Flap**

DESCRIPTION

The humeral head of the flexor carpi ulnaris is supplied by a vascular pedicle primarily from the ulnar artery and, to a lesser degree, the recurrent ulnar and deep antebrachial arteries. A caudal interosseous artery enters the distal end of the humeral head of the flexor carpi ulnaris at the deep face of this muscle, near its insertion on the accessory carpal bone. Branches of this artery run proximally and anastomose intramuscularly with the descending branches of the ulnar and deep antebrachial arteries. The caudal interosseous branch is capable of supplying circulation to a variable length of this muscle after division of the proximal blood supply. The elevated muscle can be used to cover problematic carpal, metacarpal, and distal antebrachial wounds. The muscle, in turn, can support a skin graft, if additional cutaneous coverage is required.

SURGICAL TECHNIQUE

(A) The skin is incised over the caudolateral aspect of the antebrachium, extending distally 1–2 cm beyond the accessory carpal bone. The underlying antebrachial and carpal fasciae are incised, exposing the ulnar head of the flexor carpi ulnaris caudally, the ulnaris lateralis laterally, and the humeral head of the flexor carpi ulnaris located between these two muscles. The distal tendon of the *ulnar head* is transected distally and reflected to allow complete exposure of the humeral head proximally (arrow). The borders of the humeral head are dissected and a myotomy is performed at the junction of the proximal and middle third of the muscle. The borders of the muscle are carefully dissected free of the adjacent tissues in a distal direction. Caution is warranted when approaching the deep surface of the distal tendon where the caudal interosseous vascular pedicle enters the muscle. The dashed line denotes the site for a potential "bridge incision."

(B) The muscle flap can be tunneled beneath interposing skin to gain access to the wound, or a bridge incision can be created to facilitate its placement into an adjacent defect, in this case a skin wound overlying the carpal area. The flap is sutured into position.

(C) In this hypothetical example, skin was shifted over the muscle flap. Alternatively, a free graft can be applied over the surface of the muscle if insufficient skin is available for closure.

COMMENTS

The length of muscle capable of surviving on the distal vascular pedicle alone is not known. Based on limited studies, over half is likely to survive without ischemic necrosis. This length, however, may be sufficient for most defects involving the carpal area and portions of the metacarpal area. Longer muscle flaps may be attempted, and partially excised intraoperatively if bleeding and discoloration (cyanotic appearance) is noted. Alternatively, any compromised muscle can be trimmed later during postoperative assessment of the muscle flap.

Extensive trauma involving the distal muscle and caudal interosseous blood supply may preclude use of this small muscle flap without Doppler ultrasound or angiography to assess the patency of this vital vascular pedicle. This muscle flap is infrequently needed, but can be useful for ischemic wounds secondary to radiation therapy or extensive trauma. With extensive skin loss, the viable muscular surface will serve as a vascular platform for free graft application. The graft can be applied at the time of muscle transfer or delayed until viability of the muscle is assured, usually signified by the formation of granulation tissue on its surface.

Plate 93

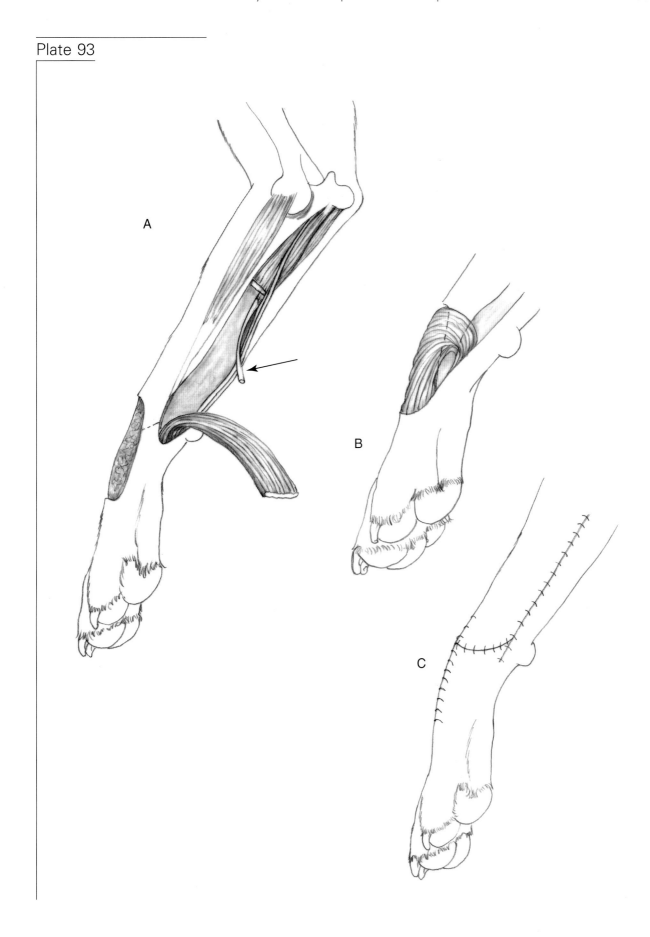

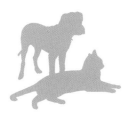

17

Oral Reconstructive
Surgical Techniques

Introduction   *512*

INTRODUCTION

Defects involving the hard and soft palate (secondary palate) can be quite difficult to close successfully. The confined space of the oral and pharyngeal cavities limits visibility and surgical manipulation of the tissues. The mucosal tissues vary in thickness and durability in the oral cavity. The "suture-holding" strength of the tissues, based on relative collagen weave and content, can vary with the age and health status of the patient.

The palatal tissues are continuously exposed to motion from lingual movement, breathing, mastication, and swallowing. This movement can result in suture "cut-out." especially when a wound closure was performed under tension. Sutures can tear through the mucosa, causing additional inflammation and fibrosis. The inherent elasticity of the mucosal tissues declines with each subsequent surgical failure.

Consistently successful closure of palatal defects requires thoughtful planning before surgery. The patient must be in good health and in a state of positive protein balance. Postoperatively, the nutritional needs of the animal must be maintained to assure that delays in healing are avoided. Tube feeding of the newborn patient is required until the animal is old enough to be fed solid food by hand. The owner and veterinarian will need to try feeding a balanced canine or feline diet by altering the size and consistency of the small portions offered and by developing an appropriate feeding schedule. Oral water may be provided by syringe, with the head tilted slightly upward. Some patients may be able to eat and drink with little or no assistance. Difficult patients may require prolonged tube feeding. Esophagostomy or gastrostomy tubes may be a practical alternative for maintaining proper nutritional intake for prolonged periods of time. Care must be taken to watch the patient carefully for signs of aspiration pneumonia or nasal impaction from food and particulate matter. The veterinarian may need to clean the nasal cavity periodically, with cotton-tipped applicators, saline flushes, and suction, with the patient under anesthesia.

Wound closure requires meticulous atraumatic surgical technique. Surgical lasers may be quite useful for optimal hemostasis and to minimize trauma during surgical closure of the wounds. Suture materials must be selected that maintain their tensile strength for a prolonged period of time. A material with a small amount of elasticity is preferred in order to adjust to the variable degree of motion most oral closures are subjected to in the postoperative period. A swaged-on reverse cutting needle is the author's preference, both for its ability to pass through tissues easily and its tendency to resist suture cut-out. Monofilament suture materials are preferred for their ability to glide through the mucosal tissues with minimal drag. In most cases, 3-0 is the most appropriate-sized material to select for the dog and cat. Although monofilament nylon and polypropylene are effective for closing palatal defects, a number of newer, slowly absorbed suture materials are practical alternatives.

Sutures should be placed beyond the 5-mm border of the wound, since collagenase activity within this healing area also can increase the possibility of suture cut-out. As a result, the author prefers to place sutures 6–10 mm from the wound border (and a similar distance apart). Because the cut borders of oral mucosa have a tendency to curl inward during suture apposition, an everting pattern is preferable to assure submucosa-to-submucosa abutment for optimal healing. The vertical mattress suture pattern is an excellent choice for its ability to resist dehiscence, evert the apposed borders, and minimally impair local microcirculation. In many cases, the author alternates vertical mattress sutures with simple interrupted sutures, since the latter pattern can help stabilize the everted wound borders during the healing process.

It must be remembered that wound closure, under *minimal tension,* is absolutely critical to a successful surgical closure. Closure under excessive tension will defeat the best suture material and pattern placement. Custom-fitted acrylic retainers have been advocated by some surgeons to protect a palate repair from postoperative motion and trauma. They may have some merit for the most difficult closures encountered. From the author's personal experience, most cleft palate repairs do not require their use or the care required to prevent food and particulate matter from accumulating between the plate and underlying incision.

This chapter includes several techniques that can be used to close the more challenging congenital and acquired defects encountered.

Cleft Palate

In the newborn puppy or kitten, palatal defects are most likely to be hereditary. Although a number of factors (nutritional, hormonal, mechanical, toxic) have been recognized as causes of palatal defects in humans, heredity is considered a major factor in animals and has been demonstrated in canine breeding studies. As a result, dogs and cats with congenital palatal defects should be spayed/neutered.

Veterinarians should always examine animals with congenital defects carefully: occasionally other anomalies may be detected.

In the human literature, there are a variety of techniques for cleft palate repair. Successful repair in humans, not only requires closure of the defect for normal eating and drinking, but also selecting a technique that will give the child the best possibility of speaking normally. In veterinary medicine, however, successful closure is measured by resumption of normal eating, drinking, and breathing. Except for extremely wide cleft palate defects, both the bipedicle flap technique and mucoperiosteal flap techniques can be used to close most of the cases presented to the veterinarian, without resorting to the more elaborate techniques used in humans. Only these two procedures are described in detail. It must be noted that both techniques, from the author's experience, work well for the "moderate-sized" gaps encountered. After using both procedures over the past two decades, the author believes the bipedicle flap is easier to execute and currently is the preferred choice for most of the cleft palate cases (congenital or acquired) managed (Fig. 17-1 and 17-2).

There are differing opinions on the optimal time to close a congenital cleft palate in small animals. Assuming the patient is healthy, well-nourished, and free of respiratory infection (secondary to possible aspiration pneumonia), the author prefers to close the defect no earlier than 4–5 months of age. Earlier closures have been advocated (64–12 weeks of age). It must be noted

that older patients have stronger tissues (greater collagen content) that are better capable of holding sutures compared to the pediatric patient. Moreover, in many cases seen, the *relative* width of the cleft narrows over time in relation to the remaining palatal tissues. As a result, there is more mucosa that can be mobilized to close the defect. Although some owners would prefer earlier closure to minimize the need to hand-feed and nurse the animal, the advantages that can be gained by delaying the closure to a later time are most significant. The surgeon must keep in mind that the *first attempt at closure is the best chance for success* in cleft palate repair.

Acquired palatal defects can be seen secondary to trauma. Cats that fall from a height or are struck by a vehicle can present with a split in the hard palate. Small fissures, a few millimeters wide, may seal with a blood clot and heal without surgical intervention. However, wider gaps may not heal and are best closed within a few day of the injury. This can be accomplished with placement of a 22-gauge wire around the root or base of opposite teeth in the midpalatal region. The wire can be placed beneath the mucosal layer of the hard palate and the wire ends gently twisted together until the bone gap is approximated. The upper and lower dental arcades should be examined to assure proper occlusion is maintained. The mucosal borders can be sutured to complete the closure. A several-day delay in repair can result in failure to compress the bony palate with a surgical wire. Under these circumstances, the use of the

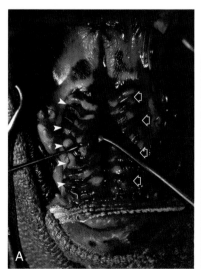 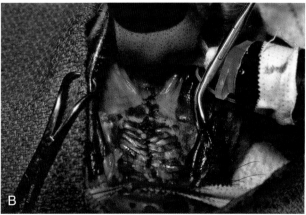

FIG. 17-1 (A) A defect of the secondary palate (hard palate and soft palate). Arrows denote the location of the lateral palate incisions. (B) Closure using bilateral, bipedicle flaps; the soft palate was closed with a conventional two-layer closure.

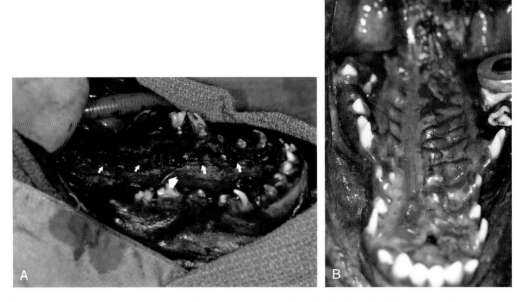

FIG. 17-2 (A) Labrador with a cleft palate closed with a mucoperiosteal flap. (B) Rapid epithelialization of the open wounds was noted within 10 days after surgery.

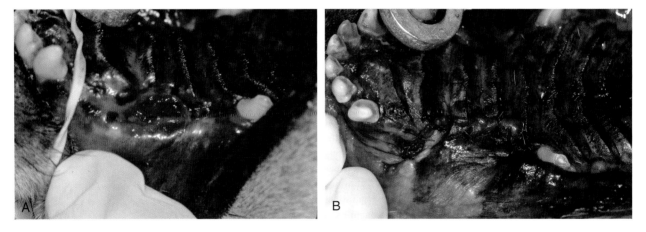

FIG. 17-3 (A) Infected, nonhealing oral defect secondary to canine tooth extraction. (B) Excision of the infected soft tissue and bone was followed by successful closure using a simple mucosal advancement flap.

bipedicle flap technique, illustrated in Plate 95 generally is successful.

Palatal Defects/Oronasal Fistulas

Most holes involving the hard palate are the result of destructive neoplasms, tumor resection with secondary dehiscence of the closure, tissue necrosis secondary to radiation therapy for neoplasms, electrical heating cord injuries, persistent openings after dental extraction, or the occasional handgun-rifle round

impacting the hard palate (Fig. 17-3). Defects adjacent to the lingual surface of the dental arcade generally are the easiest to close. Labial and buccal mucosa can be advanced or rotated into the defect after removal of the interposing teeth. The central palatal area is more problematic, especially for the larger holes in this location. Mucosal/palatal transposition flaps can be used in many of these cases. Additionally, a full-thickness labial advancement flap created perpendicular to the facial axis can be used successfully to close many of the more challenging cases (Fig. 17-4). There is one report on the successful use of a lingual flap for closure

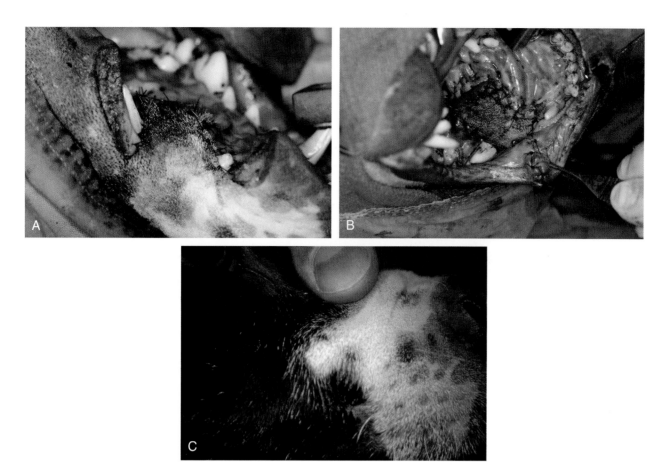

FIG. 17-4 (A) Use of a full-thickness labial flap to close a traumatic defect of the hard palate. The adjacent teeth were removed and the maxillary bone smoothed down with a Hall air drill to accommodate the labial advancement flap. The labial mucosa faces the nasal cavity; the skin surface of the flap faces the oral cavity. The labial border was trimmed and the entire flap sutured into the defect.

(B) Completion of the closure. Note that the incised labial borders were sutured together, leaving a slit opening dorsally to accommodate the base of the labial flap.

(C) The dog approximately 8 weeks later. The linear labial defect obscured by hair growth can be closed by carefully incising the cutaneous base of the flap and suturing the borders to the adjacent labial defect. Alternatively the area may be left alone if no dermatitis has been noted. (See Plate 99.)

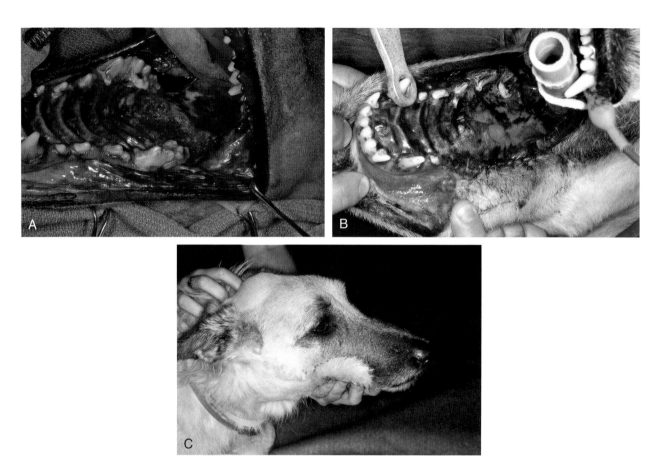

FIG. 17-5 (A) Diffuse squamous cell carcinoma involving the hard and soft palatal tissues. (B) Reconstruction with a full-thickness labial advancement flap. (C) The labial defect created by the loss of the upper lip, was replaced with a local skin flap pivoted into the area. It is advisable to consult with an oncologist to determine the best method(s) to prevent recurrence of oral neoplasms when complete surgical margins are in question.

of an oronasal fistula in a cat. More recently, a cartilaginous graft has been used to close small oronasal fistulas in cats. The angularis oris artery has also been incorporated into a flap using the adjacent buccal and lower labial mucosa for closure of problematic palatal defects.

Major reconstruction of the soft and hard palate can be problematic, and cases must be carefully selected to assure successful long-term benefits for the patient. Subtotal resection of a problematic malignancy, followed by major restorative surgery, would not be in the best interest of the patient unless adjunctive therapies are able to provide better long-term control of the neoplasm. Figure 17-5 is an example of using the upper

labial advancement flap to reconstruct the caudal hard and soft palates. A transposition skin flap was used, in turn, to reconstruct the donor (upper labial) area: the cutaneous surface faced the nasal cavity with the oral surface replaced by the labial mucosa.

Suggested Readings

Bryant KJ, Moore K, McAnulty JF. 2003. Angularis oris axial pattern buccal flap for reconstruction of recurrent fistulae of the palate. *Vet Surg* 32:113–119.
Cox CL, Hunt GB, Cadiere MM. 2007. Repair of oronasal fistulae using auricular cartilage grafts in five cats. *Vet Surg* 36:164–169.

Hammer Dl, Sacks M. 1975. The palate. In: Bojrab MJ, ed. *Current Techniques in Small Animal Surgery*, 75–85. Philadelphia, PA: Lea & Febiger.

Harvey CE. 1987. Palate defects in dogs and cats. *Compend Contin Ed Pract Vet* 9:405–418.

Howard DR, et al. 1974. Mucoperiosteal flap technique for cleft palate repair in dogs. *J Am Vet Med Assoc* 165:352–354.

Howard, DR. 1983. Palate. In: Bojrab MJ, ed. *Current Techniques in Small Animal Surgery*, 2nd ed., 109–113. Philadelphia, PA: Lea & Febiger.

Jurkiewicz MJ, Culbertson JH. 1995. *Operative Techniques in Plastic and Reconstructive Surgery: Cleft Palate Repair*. Philadelphia, PA: WB Saunders Co.

Robertson JJ, Dean PW. 1987. Repair of a traumatically induced oronasal fistula in a cat with a rostral tongue flap. *Vet Surg* 16:164–166.

Salisbury SK. 1990. Surgery of the palate. In: Bojrab MJ, ed. *Current Techniques in Small Animal Surgery*, 3rd ed., 152–159. Philadelphia: Lea & Febiger.

Smith MM. 1996. Prosthodontic appliance for repair of an oronasal fistula in a cat. *J Am Vet Med Assoc* 208:1410–1412.

Wallace LJ. 1975. An alternate procedure for repair of cleft hard and soft palate in the dog. In: Bojrab MJ, ed. *Current Techniques in Small Animal Surgery*, 85–91. Philadelphia, PA: Lea & Febiger.

Plate 94   **Mucosal Flaps**

DESCRIPTION

Upper labial and buccal mucosa can be used to close defects of the hard palate. Flaps of mucosa can be advanced or transposed to close oronasal fistulas. One of the more common fistulas occurs after canine tooth extraction.

SURGICAL TECHNIQUE

(A) Example of a chronic oronasal fistula after removal of the right upper canine in a dog.

(B) The alveolus of the canine tooth often is infected. Osteomyelitis is commonly associated with long-standing cases, as a result of food, water, and debris entering this recess. Although the alveolus can be curetted to remove debris and tissues lining the socket, a small osteotome and mallet can be used to resect the entire area, including the gingiva (circular line), in order to assure healthy tissues remain before closure with a mucosal advancement flap, outlined in the adjacent upper labial mucosa.

(C) The delicate mucosal flap is carefully undermined and advanced over the defect. Because the width of the flap tends to contract upon elevation, the author recommends the flap be wider (by 25%–30%) than the width of the defect being covered. Generally, 3-0 monofilament absorbable suture materials are used to secure the flap to the adjacent tissues.

COMMENTS

Mucosal advancement flaps are remarkably simple to perform, although the slightly more difficult 90-degree transposition flap also can be used successfully. It is important to emphasize the need to make the flaps wider than the defect to ensure closure is achieved under minimal tension.

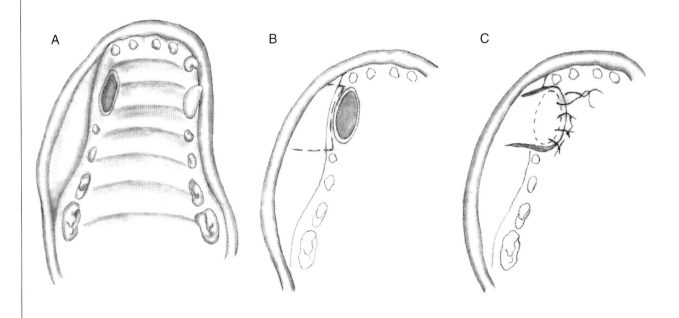

Plate 95 — Palatoplasty: Bipedicle Advancement Technique

DESCRIPTION

A classic method of closing cleft palates is the use of bilateral, bipedicle advancement flaps, using the available mucosal tissues of the hard and soft palates. The major palatine artery and vein are incorporated in these bipedicle flaps to assure adequate circulation is present during this surgical maneuver.

SURGICAL TECHNIQUE

(A) Cleft palate, extending from the hard to soft palate. Closure is attempted after 16 weeks of age, provided that the patient is healthy and well-nourished. Note the relationship of the major palatine artery with the dental arcade. The nasal cavity should be inspected for impacted food or debris, using cotton-tipped applicators, prior to preparing the mouth for surgery using povidone-iodine swabs.

(B) Two incisions are made along the lingual surface of the left and right dental arcades, creating two bipedicle flaps, upon their elevation. A small, flat, periosteal elevator is used to separate the palatal tissue from the underlying bone. Care is taken to avoid injury or division of the major palatine artery. In this example, a scalpel blade was used to resect the epithelial borders from the soft palate defect.

(C) The nasopharyngeal mucosal surface of the soft palate is apposed with slowly absorbed simple interrupted sutures. Suture bites should be approximately 8–10 mm from the defect (mucosal border). Prior to closing the oropharyngeal mucosal surface of the soft palate, release/relaxing incisions can be made (if necessary) in the mucosa, medial to the tonsillar crypts (dashed lines).

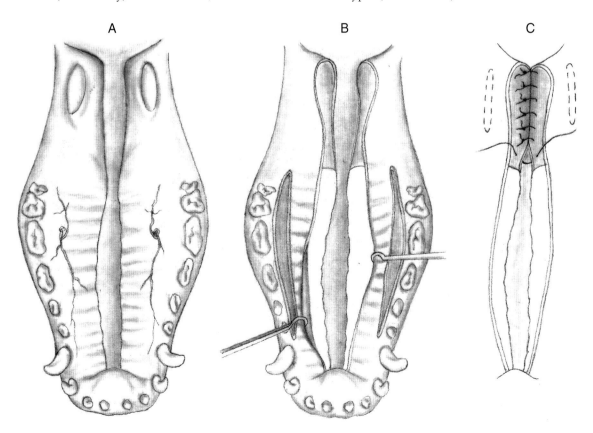

A   B   C

Plate 95

(Continued)

(D) Closure of the oropharyngeal mucosal surface of the soft palate. Vertical mattress sutures can be alternated with a simple interrupted pattern in the presence of tension.

(E) Closure of the hard palate defect with alternating simple interrupted and vertical mattress sutures. Slowly absorbable monofilament suture material, that maintains its tensile strength for a prolonged period should be selected (suture size: 3-0). Any small eversion gaps can be meticulously apposed with 4-0 simple interrupted sutures.

(F) Completion of the closure. The secondary defects created by the flap advancement will rapidly epithelialize within 2 weeks.

COMMENTS

This bipedicle palatoplasty technique can work quite well in the dog and cat, without resorting to more elaborate techniques that are reported in the human literature. Preservation of the major palatine artery is critical to complete flap survival. Meticulous, atraumatic suture technique is essential to successful closure of these challenging defects. It is not uncommon for a small rostral defect to form at the rostral tip of the hard palate closure, caudal to the upper incisors (see Fig. 17-2). In general, these small defects cause no particular problem to the patient.

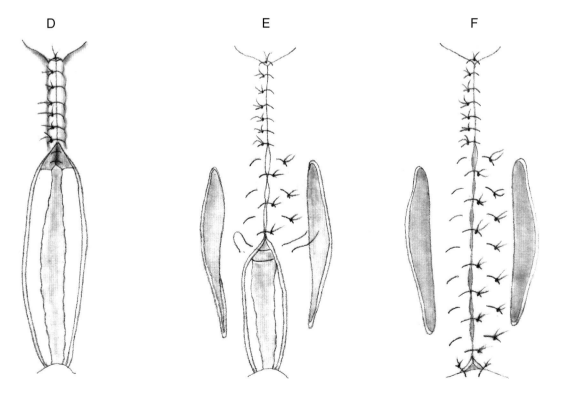

D   E   F

Plate 95

(Continued)

The vertical mattress suture is an effective tension pattern: eversion of the apposing flap borders is important to assuring that collagen can link the two connective tissue surfaces of each flap together. Inversion of the wound borders may result in failure, since the inward deviation of both epithelial borders will preclude healing. The interrupted pattern does give accurate edge-to-edge apposition and limits mild incisional "gaping" associated with the vertical mattress suture pattern used in this area. Tha author prefers suture placement 8–10 mm from the border of the defect for optimal holding power. Unlike other reports, the author does not believe a two-layer closure is feasible in many patients, nor is it necessary. A single-layer closure is quite satisfactory, provided that suture placement is precise.

Plastic plates or "retainers" have been advocated to protect the closure during the healing processes. These hard acrylic plates are wired to the dental arcade. While they may be useful in the most challenging cases, the author has not found them to be necessary. Unfortunately, food and debris can accumulate between the plate and surgical site, possibly serving as a source of infection. In most cases, failure in cleft palate closure is the result of wound closure under excessive tension, in an otherwise healthy patient.

Owners, with the assistance of their veterinarian, can tube feed patients until they are old enough to eat small pieces of solid food (balanced diet) by hand. It is useful to consult with a veterinary nutritionist should any dietary questions or problems arise. Patients should be watched closely for signs of aspiration pneumonia and treated accordingly.

The author prefers to operate on the patient no earlier than 4–5 months of age, when the tissues are better able to support suture placement. Moreover, as the patient grows and matures, the *relative* width of the palatal defect may decrease, making closure easier.

Postoperatively, animals are fed small "balls" of canned dog food the day following surgery: dogs readily swallow them whole effortlessly when fed by hand. They drink water in a normal fashion. An Elizabethan collar is advisable, especially in the days following surgery: many patients will attempt to paw at their face, likely because of the abnormal sensation in the mouth after tissue advancement.

Most cases of wound dehiscence are noted within 5 days after surgery. If the patient is doing well 72 hours after surgery, the author normally will discharge the patient and reexamine them 1 week later. Like many procedures, the surgeon's best opportunity to successfully close a palatal defect is the first surgery. Therefore, the patient must be well-nourished, in a state of positive protein balance, and healthy.

Which technique to select for closure of a cleft palate largely is a matter of preference. Over the past 20 years, the author has found that the mucoperiosteal flap and this technique work well for the wider palatal defects. For the simple, narrow defects, the bipedicle flap technique is preferable to the technically more demanding mucoperiosteal flap. Veterinarians should remember that the length of the defect is of relatively minor importance, compared to the width of the flap.

| Plate 96 | **Cleft Palate Repair: Mucoperiosteal Flap Technique** |

DESCRIPTION

The mucoperiosteal flap technique is an alternative method for closing defects of the hard palate. A medially based hinge flap is folded over the palatal defect, with the oral epithelial surface facing the exposed nasal cavity. The border of the flap is sutured beneath the opposing palatal tissue border, which is elevated as a bipedicle advancement flap.

SURGICAL TECHNIQUE

(A)   The dashed line represents the outline of the mucoperiosteal flap. Care is taken to preserve the major palatine artery.

(B$_1$)   After incising the palatal tissue with a no. 15 scalpel blade, a small periosteal elevator is used to carefully elevate the flap, leaving the palatine vasculature intact.

(B$_2$)   A cross-sectional view of the elevated flap. Note the pedicle is continuous with the nasal mucosal/periosteal surface lining the bone of the hard palate.

(C$_1$)   The palatal tissues on the opposing side of the defect are prepared as a bipedicle advancement flap while preserving the major palatine artery and vein.

(C$_2$)   Cross-sectional view of the mucoperiosteal flap and bipedicle flap, prior to suture placement.

(D$_1$)   The mucoperiosteal flap is folded over the cleft, the edge of which is tucked beneath the border of the opposing bipedicle flap. Absorbable, 3-0 PDS (polydiaxanone) sutures are used in this patient, using a mattress pattern (or vest-over-pants).

(D$_2$)   A cross-sectional view of (D$_1$).

(E)   Completion of the hard palate closure. The soft palate is closed in a conventional two-layer closure, discussed in Plate 95. Note in this example that two mucosal release incisions were made to reduce tension on closure of the soft palate defect.

COMMENTS

At one time, the author preferred to use this technique for the larger palatal defects encountered. However, the use of dual bipedicle palatal flaps and the mucoperiosteal flap, in combination with an opposing bipedicle flap, have been similarly successful for the more challenging cleft palate defects closed to date. The author feels that the mucoperiosteal flap is a slightly more demanding procedure. Complete elevation of the bipedicle flap is essential in order to assure tension on the incision line is kept to a minimum.

See Comments in Plate 95 pertaining to patient care.

Plate 96

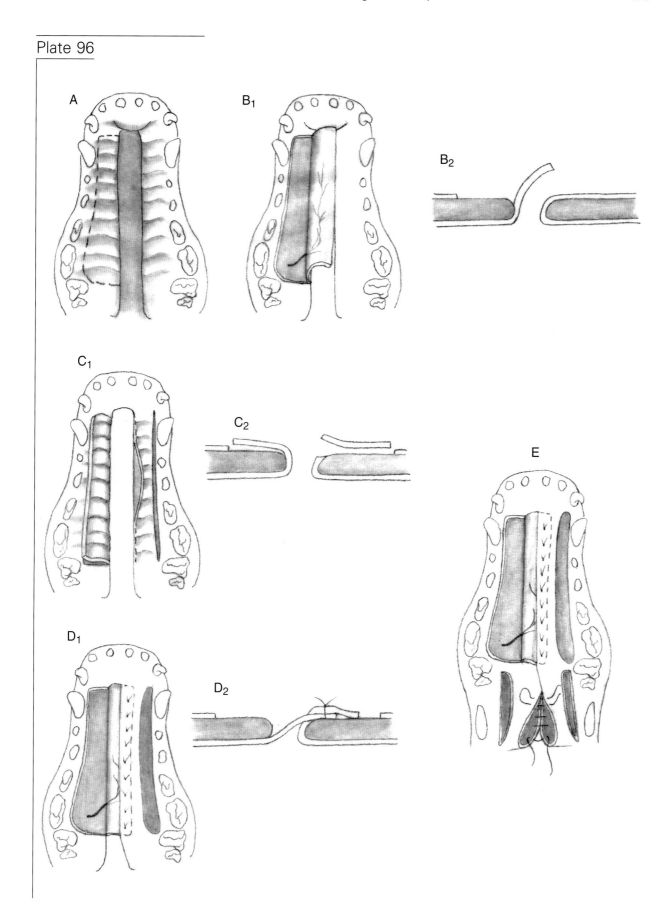

Plate 97   # Palatine Mucosal Flap

DESCRIPTION

The left and right palatine arteries course rostrally to supply circulation to a significant area of the mucosa covering the bony palate. In select cases, a mucosal transposition flap, incorporating the major palatine artery, can be used to close small- to moderate-sized oronasal fistula within its effective arc of rotation.

SURGICAL TECHNIQUE

(A) The palatine artery originates caudal and medial to the third premolar. The flap outlined in this example (dashed line) comprises two parallel incisions, one along the lingual border of the dental arcade and the second along the midline of the palate. The flap width in this illustration is sufficient to overlap the (width) borders of the oronasal fistula. The flap length is determined in the fashion noted in Plate 36, The Transposition Flap (90 degrees). The shaded area of mucosa, interposed between the donor and recipient sites, is resected to accommodate the palatine flap.

(B) Elevation of the flap. Care must be taken to avoid dividing or traumatizing the palatine artery and vein.

(C) Suturing of the palatine flap. It is highly desirable to have the flap overlap the bony border of the oronasal fistula. The ridge of bone helps to support the suture line, reducing the possibility of wound dehiscence. The donor area is not closed. The exposed viable bone and periosteum will support epithelial cell migration from the adjacent mucosal borders.

COMMENTS

Like axial pattern flaps, inclusion of an artery and vein helps assure an adequate circulation for complete survival of the flap. However, like skin flaps, smaller mucosal flaps of the hard and soft palate can be created without the need of major vessels. Effective use of the palatine flap depends on (1) preserving the integrity of the major palatine artery and vein and (2) a small- to moderate-sized defect located within the flap's effective arc of rotation.

Plate 97

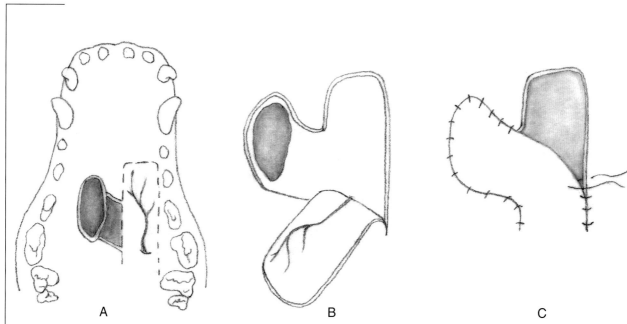

A

B

C

| Plate 98 | **Soft Palate/Pharyngeal Mucosal Flaps** |

DESCRIPTION

Significant defects of the soft palate can result in problems associated with drinking and eating. Food and water can enter the nasopharynx and nasal cavity. Direct approximation may not be possible as a result of the width of the defect. In these cases, flaps can be employed from the adjacent palatal and pharyngeal mucosa. One clinical example is illustrated.

SURGICAL TECHNIQUE

(A) This illustration demonstrates a congenital defect of the soft palate.

(B) The outline of a mucosal flap uses a portion of the soft palate. Flap dimensions should be approximately 10%–20% wider and longer than the dimensions of the defect in order to offset elastic contraction of the flap and slight shortening associated with unfolding of the flap. The mucosal border of the opposing side of the palatal defect is excised in preparation for flap application. Alternatively, the middle edge of this area can be "split" or divided with a no. 15 scalpel blade. This latter option separates the oropharyngeal and nasopharyngeal surfaces, preserving a few additional millimeters of mucosa.

(C) The flap borders are incised and the body of the flap, comprised of oropharyngeal mucosa is reflected. Note that the base or pedicle of this mucosal flap derives its circulation from the capillary network located along one border of this congenital defect. Care must be taken to minimize trauma to this delicate flap. Fine-tipped iris scissors and small skin hooks are useful for elevation of this flap. Absorbable sutures (3-0 or 4-0) are used to suture this *oropharyngeal* mucosal flap to the opposing *nasopharyngeal* mucosal border.

(D) Outline of a pharyngeal mucosal flap. See Plate 36, The Transposition Flap (90 degrees), for details on determining dimensions of this mucosal flap.

(E) The mucosal transposition flap is rotated into the oropharyngeal defect of the soft palate and secured with 3-0 or 4-0 absorbable sutures. The donor area is closed in a similar fashion, unless excessive tension precludes proper apposition.

COMMENTS

Most cases of these uncommon soft palate defects are presented to the veterinarian in "young adult" dogs. Clinical signs are more subtle than in cleft palate patients, who have notable eating difficulties as kittens or puppies. Thoracic radiographs may be advisable to rule out aspiration pneumonia prior to surgery.

Meticulous dissection and atraumatic surgical technique are essential to successful closure of this congenital defect. Tension on the closure sites should be kept to a minimum. Postoperatively, the patient is given soft food for 2–4 weeks. Exercise is kept to a minimum during this time. Reexamination of the area will require light anesthesia. Owners should be informed that closure of this and other oral defects can be difficult; dehiscence of a portion of the closure site can occur in this dynamic body region.

Plate 98

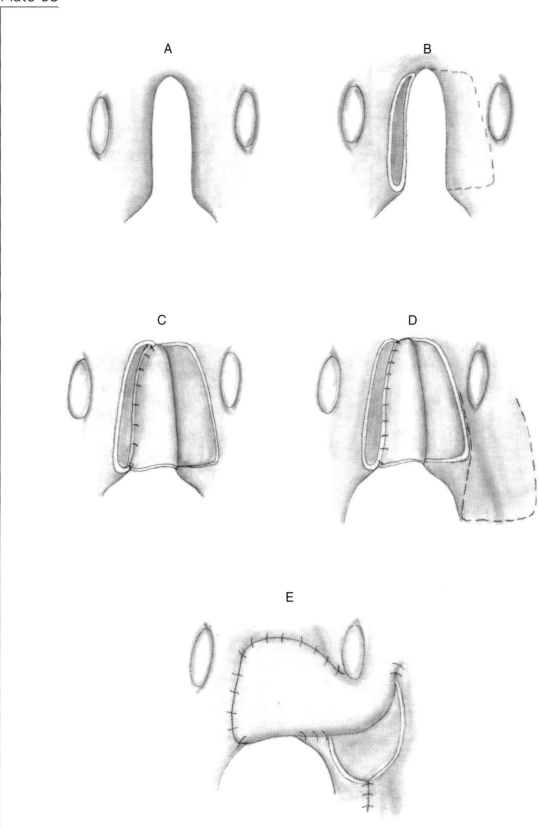

Plate 99	**Full-Thickness Labial Flap Closure of Oronasal Fistulas**

DESCRIPTION

On occasion, insufficient labial mucosa, buccal mucosa, and palatal tissue is available for closure of oronasal fistulas. Cats, in particular, lack the ample mucosal surfaces for the simple advancement closure techniques employed with dogs. A full-thickness labial advancement flap can be created perpendicular to the length of the upper lip for direct advancement into oronasal fistulas.

SURGICAL TECHNIQUE

(A) This is an example of an oronasal fistula in a cat.

(B) The width of the defect is measured rostrocaudally. The width of the flap equals this measurement. However, the author recommends making the flap 1–2 cm wider to offset elastic contraction of the flap and reduce the likelihood of incisional tension. Two full-thickness labial incisions are made and the labial border is excised. The dental arcade and gingival tissue between the oronasal fistula and base of the flap also are excised.

(C) Upon removal of the teeth and gingiva, the flap is advanced into the oronasal fistula. Inset: If additional length is required, the labial border is preserved; it is then undermined and reflected upward. This "unfolded" full-thickness labial flap is advanced over the oronasal defect.

(D) Absorbable sutures (3-0, 4-0) are employed to secure the flap into place.

(E) A notched defect is noted in the lip of the cat. See comments below.

COMMENTS

This technique results in creating a labial "notch" due to the sacrifice of a segment to close an oronasal fistula. *Note:* the incised labial margins can be reapposed over the flap to reestablish continuity to the upper lip if sufficient labial tissue is present (E, arrows). A slit or linear opening, dorsal to the apposed labial margins, remains to accommodate the flap's base or pedicle (see Fig. 17-4).

At a later date, when healing of the flap is complete, the cutaneous pedicle can be carefully incised and the edge sutured to the apposed cranial and caudal labial mucosal borders to complete the closure (dashed line in E). The author has found this to be unnecessary, since this small healed opening creates no significant cosmetic or functional problem. Hair regrowth may obscure any labial defect to achieve satisfactory cosmetic results without further surgery. This technique has been used successfully in dogs and cats.

Plate 99

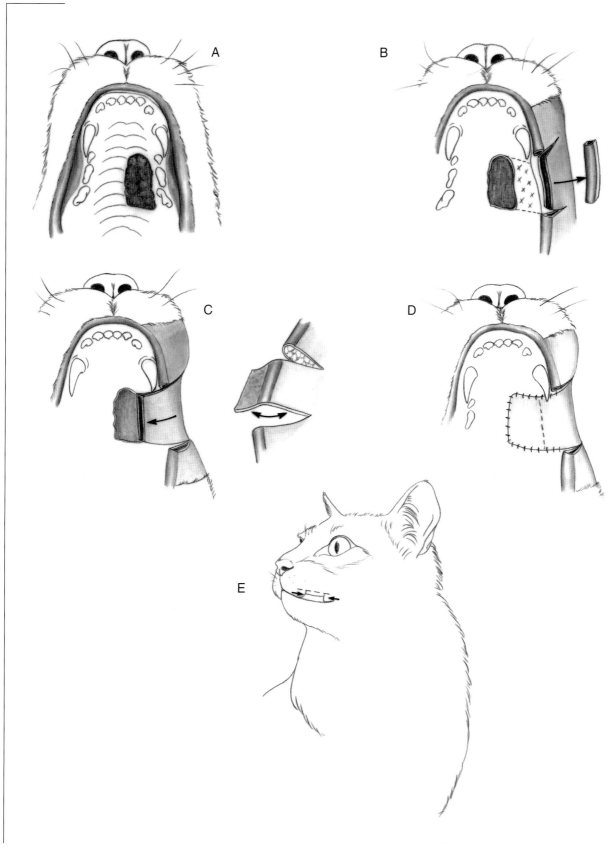

Plate 100   **Cartilage Grafts for Palatal Fistulas**

DESCRIPTION

Reported by Cox, Hunt, and Cadiere, a small cartilage graft, taken from the base of the pinna, can be used to patch small feline palatal defects; it has been successfully used both in humans and experimental dogs. The cartilage forms a tissue scaffold or platform for granulation tissue migration and subsequent epithelialization over the developed granulation surface.

SURGICAL TECHNIQUE

(A₁, A₂) Example of the area to harvest a flat piece of the conchal cartilage (scapha of the pinna) (arrow); the circular graft is harvested a few millimeters larger than the measured oral defect. (A₂) illustrates the oral defect of the caudal hard palate.

(B₁) A small periosteal elevator is used to create a pocket for the cartilage graft, between the bone and overlying soft tissue of the hard palate.

(B₂) A small rostral and caudal incision can be used to facilitate placement of the cartilage graft.

(B₃) Insertion of the cartilage graft, folding the cartilage into the small pocket created around the circumference of the defect.

(B₄) One or two sutures (minimum) of 4-0 absorbable suture material can be used to secure the small cartilage graft to the palatal tissues.

COMMENTS

Cartilage also can be harvested from the lateral ear canal (performing a lateral ear canal resection), although the curvature of this tissue makes it more problematic to lie flat during its insertion into the defect. This technique may be useful for small fistulous tracts (less than 1.5 cm) without the need to resort to more aggressive attempts at surgical closure: it is unknown if larger defects can be closed with this technique. In one case study, the cartilage graft failed, but closure with a second graft was successful. Placement of an avascular segment of cartilage into a contaminated environment does run the risk of dissolution of this tissue. Soft food is advisable during the healing process.

Plate 100

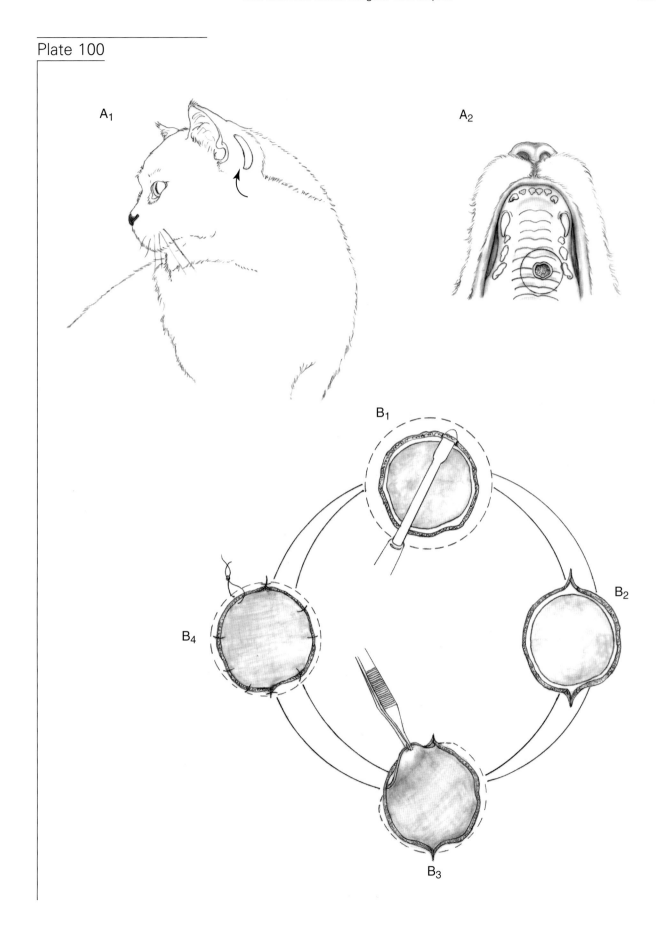

Plate 101   **Angularis Oris Mucosal Flap**

DESCRIPTION

The angularis oris artery arises from the facial artery and courses superficially from the cranial border of the masseter muscle to the ipsilateral commissure of the mouth. The pulse of the angularis oris artery can be felt by inserting the index finger into the mouth, caudal to the oral commissure. The facial artery also gives rise to the superior and inferior labial arteries, supplying the upper and lower labial tissues, respectively. Bryant, Moore, and McAnulty have described the use of a mucosal flap, based over the angularis oris vessels, for the closure of problematic palatal defects.

SURGICAL TECHNIQUE

(A) Territory of the angularis oris mucosal flap.

Inset: With the dog in lateral recumbency, a skin incision is created from the margin of the oral commissure caudally to the level of the rostral margin of the masseter muscle. The skin margins are retracted, exposing the angularis oris artery and vein. (A light source can be inserted into the oral cavity to "candle" or illuminate the vessels. A pencil Doppler probe also may be useful for locating this artery.) Two parallel incisions created dorsal and ventral to the angularis oris vessels extend through the exposed subcutaneous tissue and buccal mucosa, forming the margins of the flap (dashed lines). These incisions are extended to the caudal extent of the buccal pouch, at the level to which the angularis oris vessels extend below the cranioventral border of the masseter muscle. This mucosal flap includes the buccal mucosa to the level of the oral commissure. The flap may be "islandized" by incising the buccal mucosal base of the flap caudal to the entry of the angularis oris vessels and carefully dissecting the connective tissue to mobilize this island flap.

(B) In this illustration, the flap is being used to close a problematic palatal defect. A simple interrupted suture pattern with slowly absorbable sutures is used to appose the flap margins to the defect. The donor defect is closed by suturing the mucosal defect, followed by the overlying skin incision.

COMMENTS

This procedure was reported in two dogs. The flap has the potential of extending rostrally to the distal gingival margin of the ipsilateral canine tooth or across the palate to the contralateral dental arcade. This technique is one more option for the surgeon to consider, based on the size and location of the oral defect.

Plate 101

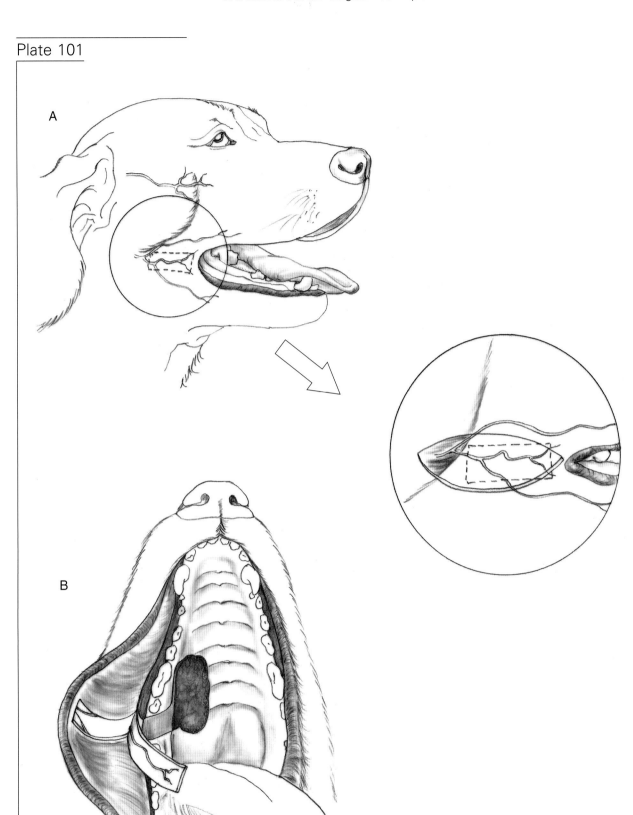

A

B

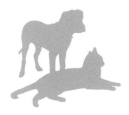

Foot Pad Reconstruction

INTRODUCTION

The foot pads of the dog include the digital pads, metacarpal pads, and metatarsal pads. They are capable of supporting the weight of the dog over a variety of surfaces. The epidermis of the pads is 1800 μm thick, considerably greater than the 25- to 40-μm thickness of the hairy skin.

The epidermis of the digital pads is elevated in a series of conical papillae. Secondary conical papillae are noted within each conical structure. This conical papillary surface provides a tough "antiskid" surface for weight bearing, whereas the underlying pad cushion serves as a shock absorber. Comprised of subcutaneous adipose tissue and collagenous and elastic fibers, the resilient pad cushion has the ability to compress, expand, and conform during activity on uniform or irregular surfaces. No other cutaneous surface can substitute completely for this highly specialized pad structure.

The center of gravity in the dog is located immediately behind the shoulder girdle, resulting in a greater force-to-body weight ratio on the front pads. The maximum vertical force on the front pads approximates the body weight of the dog, whereas the vertical force on the hind limbs is 0.8 times the body weight. Longitudinal pad force is 10 times less than vertical force. The front pad contact times can be as much as 1.5 times greater than that of the corresponding hind limb pads.

To date, options for foot pad replacement have focused on transposing or advancing digital pads to areas where their placement will provide a durable, weight-bearing surface. Careful dissection of the phalanges via a palmar or plantar incision may enable the surgeon to replace metacarpal or metatarsal pad defects (resulting from injury, tumor excision, or abnormal weight bearing secondary to musculoskeletal injuries) with one or more digital pads. Two digital pads can be employed to reconstruct the entire metacarpal or metatarsal pad. With loss of the digital pads from trauma or disease, it is possible to advance and rotate the surviving metacarpal or metatarsal pad over the end of the exposed metacarpal or metatarsal bones to provide a satisfactory weight-bearing surface.

Complete loss of all foot pads of the forelimb or hind limb in the dog is considerably more serious, since no adjacent pad tissues are available for coverage. Skin, as a pad substitute, generally lacks the durability to withstand the daily physical abuse normally sustained by foot pads in all but the smallest veterinary patients. In cats, successful skin coverage of the foot requires restricting the cat to a more sedentary existence in the house, ideally on soft surfaces to minimize trauma to the cutaneous transplant. In large dogs, amputation of the involved limb has been performed when there was no viable option for pad replacement (Fig. 18-1).

In providing a durable pad surface to the affected limb devoid of foot pads in large dogs, three potential options exist: microvascular transfer of a digital pad from another foot or free grafting of digital pad tissue from another foot. Each technique has potential advantages and disadvantages.

PAD LACERATION AND LESION EXCISION

The thick corneal pad is susceptible to abrasive and shearing forces during ambulation. The feet also are exposed to sharp objects that may result in penetrating wounds, lacerations, or shearing wounds.

Freshly lacerated wounds can be lavaged, debrided, and closed primarily. Grossly contaminated or infected wounds may require open wound management for a variable period of time prior to closure. Foot pads have relatively poor "suture-holding power." Sutures can pull out of the dermal–corneal tissues during ambulation. The displacement of the underlying pad cushion can further stress any suture line. As a result, 2-0–sized suture materials, employing vertical mattress sutures with large "bites" of pad tissue, are best employed to appose pad lacerations in medium to large canine patients. A heavily padded foot bandage, possibly with a metallic or plastic Mason metasplint, is advisable to blunt impact and minimize digital cushion spread beneath the incision in order to prevent wound dehiscence. It is strongly advisable to protect the healing pad for approximately 3 weeks to help assure proper healing. In general, sutures can be removed in about 2 weeks, barring healing complications (Fig. 18-2). On occasion, extensive damage or loss of flexor tendon support of the digits can result in abnormal weight bearing. Foot pad ulceration may be noted, especially in the larger, active dog. Successful fusion podoplasty has been reported under these circumstances. Similarly, this technique can be used for severe interdigital pyoderma cases unresponsive to therapy. This technique entails removal of all skin folds between the digits and metatarsal/metacarpal pad of the affected limbs, followed by suture apposition of the bordering pad edges.

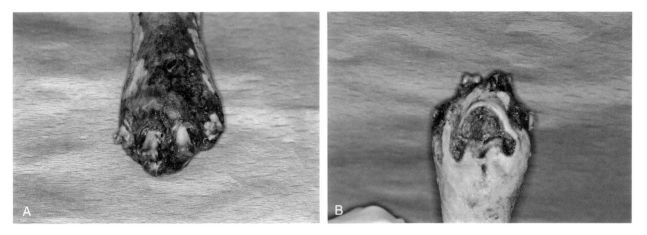

FIG. 18-1 (A) Extensive vehicular trauma to a canine paw. Complete loss of all digital pads. (B) Note loss of the metatarsal pad. A primary option for foot salvage under these circumstances is pad grafting.

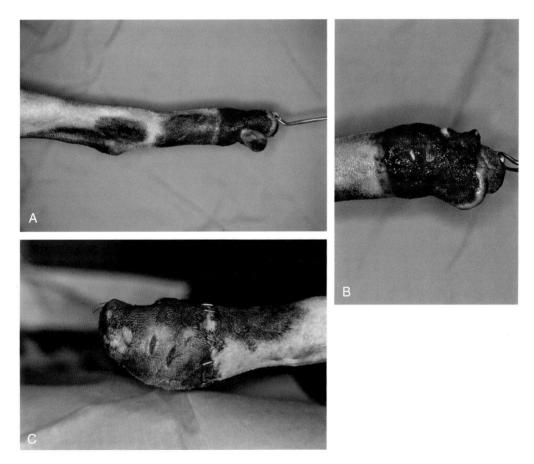

FIG. 18-2 (A) Circumferential skin loss of the hind paw in a young Dalmatian, secondary to vehicular trauma. Note partial avulsion of the metacarpal pad. (B) Close-up view of the foot. Only a portion of one digital pad survived. (C) A full-thickness mesh graft was used to resurface the circumferential skin defect. The displaced metacarpal pad was sutured into its original position. Restoration of a functional limb was achieved.

DIGITAL PAD TRANSFER

Digital pads tethered on a vascularized cutaneous pedicle can be transplanted, within their arc of rotation, to defects on weight-bearing surfaces. This is most useful when portions of the metatarsal or metacarpal pads are lost. Similarly, abnormal weight bearing as a result of limb trauma may require positioning a digital pad over an ulcerated area.

A ventral incision for removal of the first and second phalanx is preferable to a dorsal incision, thus enabling immediate placement of the flap into its new position. The veterinary surgeon will find that pads heal more slowly than other skin closures. Partial dehiscence may be noted, but the sutures can easily be replaced. A heavily padded bandage with external support is required to promote healing in this weight-bearing area (Fig. 18-3).

METACARPAL/ METATARSAL PAD TRANSFER

Loss of the digital pads from trauma or disease may require repositioning of the metacarpal or metatarsal pad to provide a durable weight-bearing surface to the limb. The destroyed digits are amputated, and a portion of the distal metacarpal/metatarsal bones may be resected to permit proper metacarpal/metatarsal pad positioning over the resultant stump. This procedure can result in a fully functional limb despite the loss of all digits (Fig. 18-4).

ACCESSORY CARPAL PAD

The small accessory carpal pad has been used to cover the stump of the front limb, when amputation was necessary, at the level of the proximal metacarpal area. Depending on the amputation site, the pad and mobile skin can be advanced, rotated into position, or incorporated into a transposition skin flap to cover the terminal end of the extremity. Significant shortening of the limb limits use of the extremity in ambulation, but may assist the animal in balance or rising from a resting position.

PAD GRAFTING

Complete traumatic loss of the pads of a foot presents a significant problem to a dog: amputation may be necessary. However, freshly severed digital and metacarpal/metatarsal pads have the potential to be grafted onto the limb. Pad-grafting options are summarized in Plates 106 and 107.

The two-staged procedure noted in Plate 106 is technically demanding (Fig. 18-5). The pad is preserved on a temporary vascular recipient site while the wound is being prepared for later flap transfer. This technique has the main advantage of providing a thick subcutaneous layer to replace the pad cushion; this cannot be achieved by direct pad application to a granulation bed. However, small pad grafts (Plate 107) have the potential advantage of preserving remaining toe pads by taking small segments without necessarily sacrificing a digit for harvesting a larger single pad graft. Grafts are ideally placed on surviving elements of the metacarpal/metatarsal pad cushion.

DIGITAL FLAPS FOR WOUND CLOSURE

Closure of distal extremity defects, secondary to trauma or tumor resection, can be problematic due to the unavailability of loose, elastic skin (Fig. 18-6). Tumor resection involving the digits and interdigital area is particularly challenging. Centrally located interdigital masses may be resected with adequate surgical margins, leaving sufficient skin to close the defect and refashion a supportive toe web (Fig. 18-7). Resection of larger and/or eccentrically located interdigital masses may necessitate wider resection. In many of these cases, the healthy skin along the lateral and palmar/plantar aspect of one digit, including the pad, may be safely preserved. Careful dissection and removal of the phalanges creates a digital flap for closure of the defect. This technique also can be useful for closure of skin defects involving digits 2 or 5, using digital flaps created from toes 3 or 4 respectively (see Plates 102 and 103). The pad tissue usually is placed in a non–weight bearing location on the paw, but closure of the defect is effectively accomplished (Fig. 18-7 and 18-8).

FUSION PODOPLASTY

Chronic pododermatitis is the result of an overall failure to control the underlying condition. In most cases, the primary pathogen is *Staphylococcus aureus*, but it may include secondary infections from *Proteus* spp., *Pseudomonas aeruginosa*, and *E. coli*. Other causes

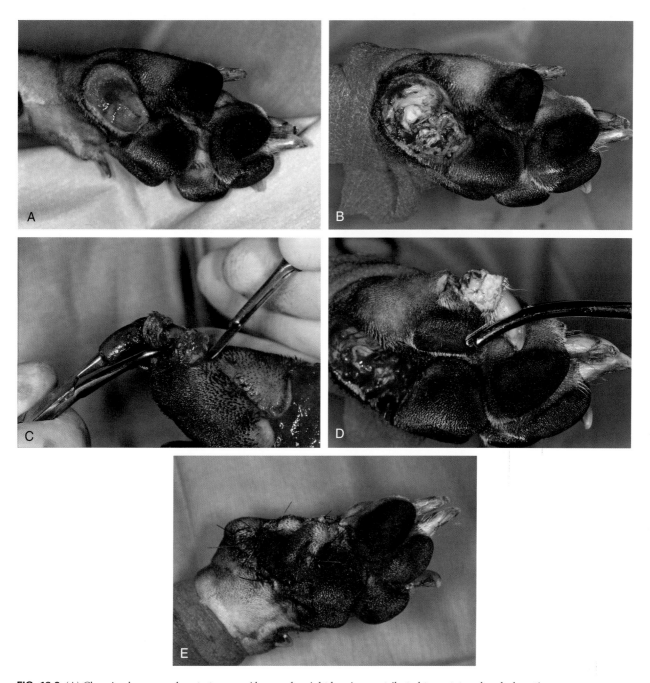

FIG. 18-3 (A) Chronic ulcer secondary to trauma. Abnormal weight bearing contributed to metatarsal pad ulceration. (B) Debridement of the ulcer. (C, D) Resection of the entire third phalanx. (E) Application of the digital pad after surgical removal of the phalanges.

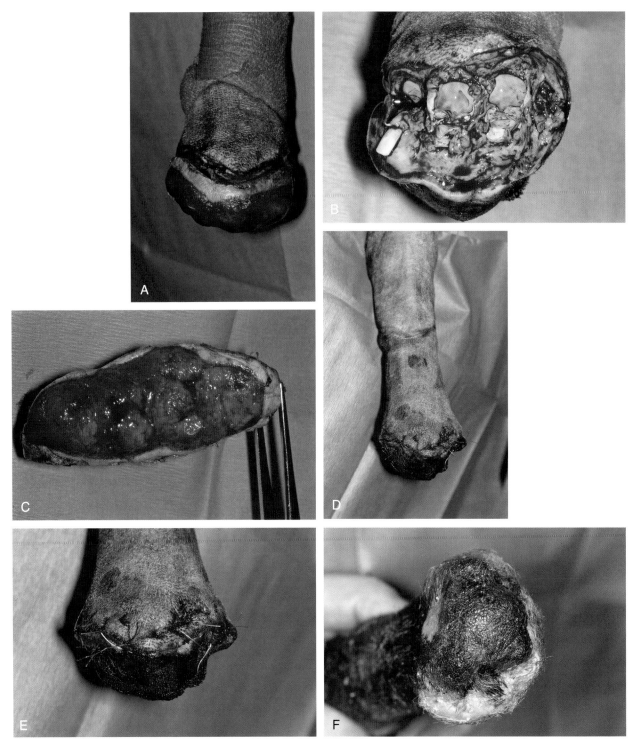

FIG. 18-4 (A) Loss of digits of the hind paw secondary to immune-mediated vasculitis (see Fig. 6-17). (B) Resection of the granulation bed. (C) The distal ends of the exposed metacarpal bones were resected. The central digits normally require partial resection. (D, E) Advancement of the metacarpal pad over the terminal stump. A functional limb was obtained. (F) The pad at suture removal.

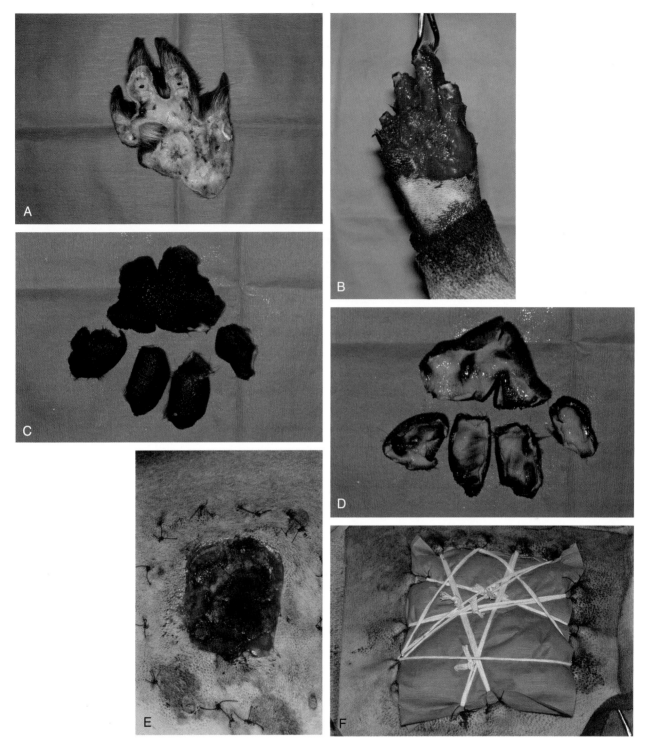

FIG. 18-5 (A, B) Left rear paw denuded of the metatarsal and digital pads, secondary to a wire snaring the paw. The patient was immediately referred to the hospital by the patient's veterinarian. The pads were immediately placed in chilled saline and neomycin, creating a 5% solution.

(C, D) The pads were separated and the digital cushions resected.

(E) The cupped pad grafts were incised to flatten their surfaces. Pads were sutured to the cutaneous trunci muscle in a predetermined location to accommodate future elevation of the denuded paw.

(F) A tie-over dressing to immobilize and protect the grafted pads.

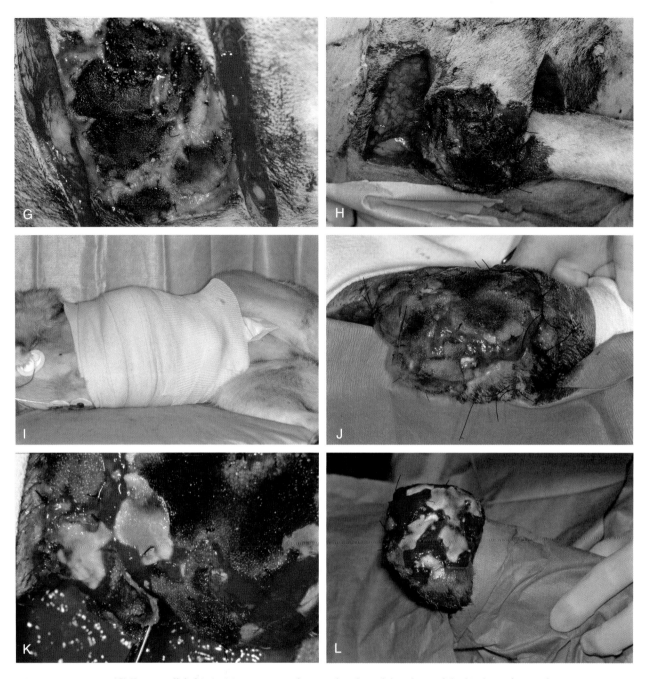

FIG. 18-5 *Continued* (G) Two parallel skin incisions were made cranial and caudal to the graft bed 7 days after application.

(H) The bipedicle flap incorporating the graft bed was undermined below the hypodermis. Skin incisions were extended to a length sufficient to accommodate the paw defect. The apposing skin and wound borders were sutured together.

(I) Cotton padding was applied between the elevated limb and abdominal wall, followed by a layer of elastic adhesive tape (Elastion, Johnson & Johnson).

(J) One week after application, the pedicles were divided in stages (one-half every 2 days). Completion of the division process.

(K) Close-up view of pad grafts reimplanted to the hind paw. The outer corneal pad layers separate, revealing the germinal epithelium.

(L) Epithelium expands over the interposing granulation tissue.

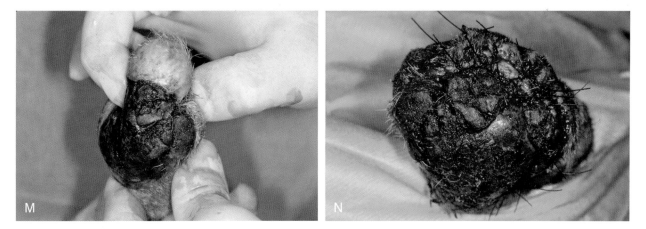

FIG. 18-5 *Continued* (M) Redundant scar tissue was resected approximately 6 weeks after completion of the pad transfer, which aligned the cornified pad surface for optimal weight bearing.

(N) Tension sutures were used to shift the pad tissue into its final location. (From Pavletic MM. 1994. Foot salvage and delayed reimplantation of severed metatarsal and digital pads using a bipedicle direct flap technique. *J Am Anim Hosp Assoc* 30:539–547.)

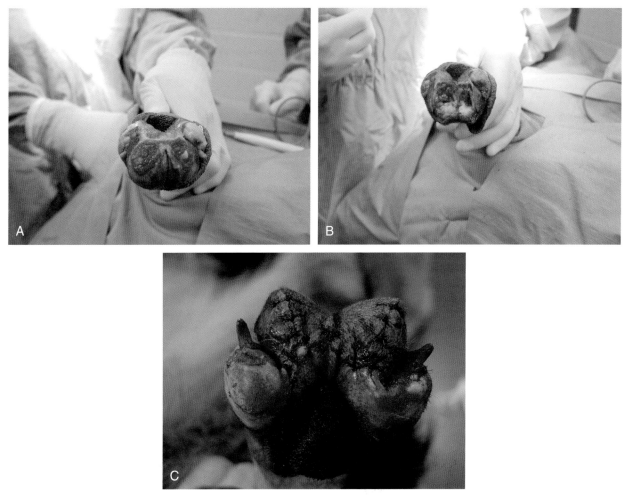

FIG. 18-6 (A) Vehicular trauma to a canine paw, with destruction of the central digital pads. (B) Excision of the granulation bed and exposed ends of the second phalanges. (C) Closure. Note that digital pads 2 and 5 were re-epithelializing and eventually formed a functional weight-bearing surface.

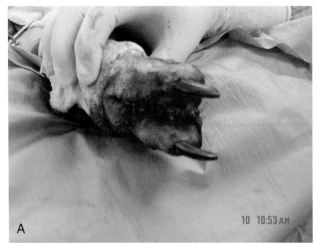
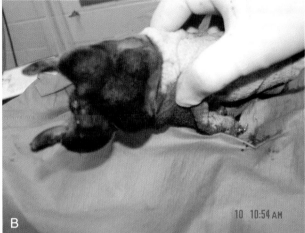
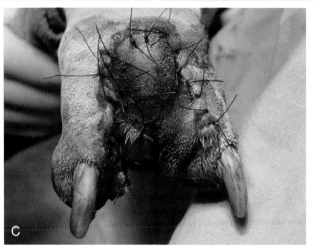

FIG. 18-7 (A) Resection of the central two toes due to neoplasia.

(B) Lower view of the foot. Restoration of a digital web helps support the remaining toes and provides a more natural cosmetic appearance.

(C) Wide resection of a soft tissue sarcoma. Resection of the lateral and plantar aspect of the adjacent digit was not required to obtain surgical margins. The phalanges were dissected free of the resultant digital flap. The flap was transposed into the defect, completing the closure.

may include allergies, mycoses, parasites, irritants, neoplasia, metabolic disease, neurological disorders, or autoimmune disease. The skin can appear as thickened, inflamed, and ulcerated. Fistulous tracts may be noted, along with a serosanguinous to purulent discharge.

Fusion podoplasty is considered for those cases of end-stage pododermatitis refractory to both medical and conservative surgical management. Fusion podoplasty refers to the obliteration of the interdigital web and palmar/plantar cutaneous space between the metatarsal/metacarpal pad and digits. Fusion podoplasty also has been used in cases where permanent flexor tendon injury has resulted in digital pad irritation and ulceration secondary to abnormal weight-bearing by the dog (see Plate 108).

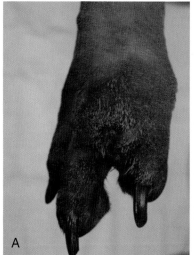
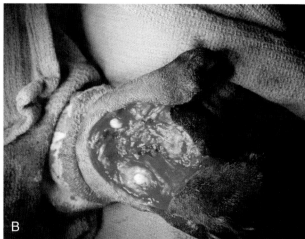
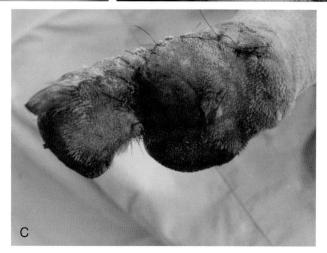

FIG. 18-8 (A) Recurrent soft tissue sarcoma referral. (B) Wide excision of the mass. (C) Closure was accomplished using the lateral digital skin and pad surface.

Suggested Readings

Barclay CG, Fowler JD, Basher AW. 1987. Use of the carpal pad to salvage the forelimb in a dog and cat: an alternative to total limb amputation. *J Am Anim Hosp Assoc* 23:527–532.

Basher A. 1994. Foot injuries in dogs and cats. *Compend Contin Edu Pract Vet* 16:1159–1175.

Basher AW, Fowler JD, Bowen CV, et al. 1990. Microneurovascular free digital pad transfer in the dog. *Vet Surg* 19:226–231.

Basher AW, Fowler JD, Bowen CV, et al. 1991. Free tissue transfer of digital foot pads for reconstruction of the distal limb in a dog. *Microsurg* 12:118–124.

Bradley DM, Scardino MS, Swaim SF. 1998. Construction of a weight-bearing surface on a dog's distal pelvic limb. *J Am Anim Hosp Assoc* 34:387–394.

Bradley DM, Shealy PM, Swaim SF. 1993. Meshed skin graft and phalangeal fillet for paw salvage: a case report. *J Am Anim Hosp Assoc* 29:427–433.

Bradley DM, Swaim SF, Alexander CN, et al. 1994. Autogenous pad grafts for reconstruction of a weight-bearing surface: a case report. *J Am Anim Hosp Assoc* 30:533–538.

Fowler JD, Miller CW. 1990. Microvascular technique: application in reconstruction surgery. *Vet Med Rep* 2:210.

Gourley IM. 1978. Neurovascular island flap for treatment of trophic ulcer in the dog. *J Am Anim Hosp Assoc* 14:119–125.

Hutton WC, Freeman MAR, Swanson SAV. 1969. The forces exerted by the pads of the walking dog. *J Sm Anim Pract* 10:71–77.

Liptak JM, Dernell WS, Rizzo SA, et al. 2005. Partial foot amputation in 11 dogs. *J Am Anim Hosp Assoc* 41:47–55.

Pavletic MM. 1994. Foot salvage and delayed reimplantation of severed metatarsal and digital pads using a bipedicle direct flap technique. *J Am Anim Hosp Assoc* 30:539–547.

Read RA. 1986. Probable trophic pad ulceration following traumatic denervation: report of two cases in dogs. *Vet Surg* 15:40–44.

Swaim SF, Bradley DM, Steiss JE, et al. 1993. Segmental paw pad grafts in dogs. *Am J Vet Res* 54:2161–2170.

Swaim SF, Garrett PD. 1985. Foot salvage techniques in dogs and cats: Options, "Do's" and "Don'ts". *J Am Anim Hosp Assoc* 21:511–519.

Swaim SF, Lee AH, MacDonald JM, et al. 1991. Fusion podoplasty for the treatment of chronic fibrosing interdigital pyoderma in a dog. *J Am Anim Hosp Assoc* 27:264–274.

Swaim SF, Milton JL. 1994. Fusion podoplasty to treat abnormalities associated with severed digital flexor tendons. *J Am Anim Hosp Assoc* 30:137–144.

Swaim SF, Riddell KP, Powers RD. 1992. Healing of segmental grafts of digital pad skin in dogs. *Am J Vet Res* 53:406–410.

Plate 102	**Digital Flap Technique:**
	Major Digital-Interdigital Defects

DESCRIPTION

The digital skin and pad can be salvaged to close problematic defects involving the paw. In this case example, the centrally located neoplasm is resected where it overlies digit 3 and the adjacent toe web associated with digit 4 (see Fig. 18-7).

SURGICAL TECHNIQUE

(A) Illustration of a neoplasm involves digit 3 with extension toward the interdigital area adjacent to digit 4. The dashed line represents the area of resection.

(B) Amputation of digit 3, the interdigital skin, and medial half of digit 4, including careful dissection and removal of the first, second, and third phalanges. In this example, the small band of skin (dashed lines) is resected to facilitate placement of the flap.

(C) The lateral and palmar/plantar cutaneous tissue, with the attached pad of digit 4, is transposed into the large surgical defect.

COMMENTS

This is a remarkably simple and effective technique for closure of surgical defects of the paw secondary to tumor resection. The lateral skin and attached pad surface of digit 4, uninvolved with the neoplasm, nicely transposes into the surgical defect. Surgical margins around any neoplasm will depend on the underlying (base) surgical margins as well as the cutaneous perimeter obtained. The surgical perimeter and base of the surgical specimen should be marked with India ink and submitted for histopathlogical examination to assess the surgical margins. (See also Plate 103.) Having this flap available for closure can give the surgeon confidence that the defect, secondary to tumor resection, can be largely or completely closed.

Dogs can have a functional limb with two or fewer toes (i.e., no digits; see Plate 105), contrary to statements in the older veterinary literature. However, a dog may favor the leg to a variable degree, especially during the first few weeks postoperatively: owners should be made aware of this probability prior to surgery. Bandage protection of the area may be necessary over a 2–3 week period to assure healing is complete.

Plate 102

A

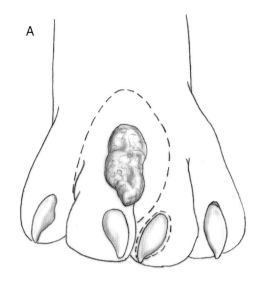

C

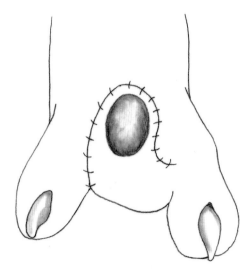

B

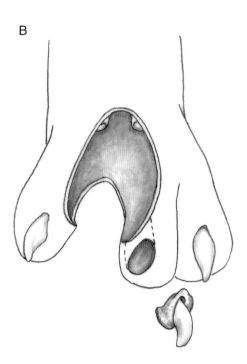

Plate 103	**Digital Flap Technique: Major Defects of Digits Two or Five**

DESCRIPTION

The uninvolved portions of the third or fourth digit, adjacent to a neoplasm involving digits 2 or 5, can be used to close the surgical defect created. Portions of the adjacent metacarpal or metatarsal bone can be resected, if needed, to achieve surgical margins (see Fig. 18-8).

SURGICAL TECHNIQUE

(A) Neoplasm involving the dorsolateral surface of the second digit. Dashed lines signify the area of excision, including a portion of the second metacarpal bone.

(B) Resection of the second digit and adjacent portion of the third digit. The phalanges of the third digit are carefully dissected and resected to preserve circulation to the remaining digital skin and pad.

(C) The skin and toe pad of digit 3 are pivoted into the surgical defect and sutured to the adjacent cutaneous borders.

COMMENTS

As also noted in Plate 102, digital flaps rely on salvaging the skin and digital pad tissues that are not involved in the disease process. Having this source of tissue available for wound closure enables the surgeon to resect tumors more aggressively, with the confidence that wound closure can be reasonably achieved in this problematic area. Dogs can have a functional limb with two or fewer toes (i.e., no digits, see Plate 105), although the dog may favor the limb to a variable degree, especially during the first few weeks following surgery. Owners should be made aware of this possibility prior to surgery in order to avoid any misunderstanding. Bandaging for a 2–3 week period is useful in helping to assure that healing occurs without complication.

Plate 103

A

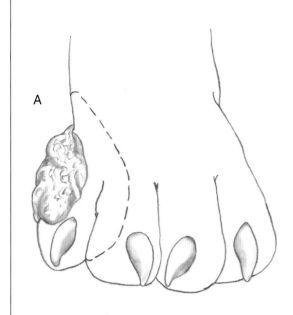

B

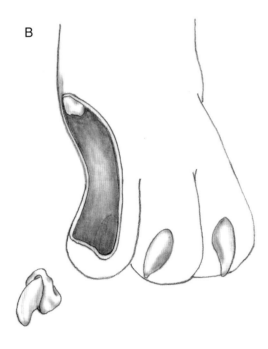

C

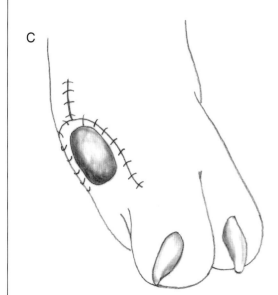

Plate 104 **Digital Pad Transfer**

DESCRIPTION

Digital pads tethered on a vascularized cutaneous pedicle can be transplanted within their arc of rotation to defects in weight-bearing surface areas. This is most evident when portions of the metatarsal or metacarpal pads are lost. Similarly, abnormal weight bearing as a result of limb trauma may require positioning a digital pad over an ulcerated area (see Fig. 8-3).

SURGICAL TECHNIQUE

(A) A no. 15 blade is used to incise around the circumference of the nail bed. The third phalanx is carefully dissected out and disarticulated.

(B) An incision is made on the underlying skin surface to gain exposure to the second and third phalanges (dotted line).

(C) The surgeon should limit dissection to the immediate periosteal surface area. Care is taken to preserve circulation to the digital pad as the phalanges are removed. A tourniquet applied proximal to the surgical area can improve tissue dissection. The circumferential access incision for excision of the third phalanx is sutured closed.

(D) The pad graft is rotated into a prepared weight-bearing defect and sutured into place with 2-0 or 3-0 nonabsorbable suture material. The opposing pad borders are trimmed to assure accurate abutment of these structures. The foot is placed in a bandage reinforced with a Mason metasplint until suture removal, approximately 3 weeks later. The bandage and support splint are changed every 3–5 days.

COMMENTS

A ventral incision is preferable to a dorsal incision, thus enabling immediate placement of the flap into its new position. The veterinary surgeon will find that pad healing is slower than other skin closures. Partial dehiscence may be noted, but the sutures can easily be replaced. A heavily padded bandage with external support is required to promote healing in this weight-bearing area.

Plate 104

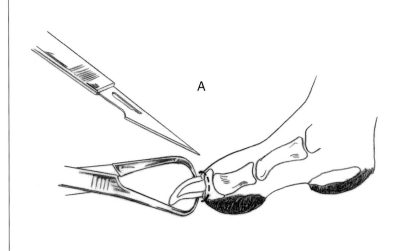

A

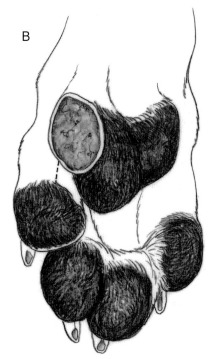

B

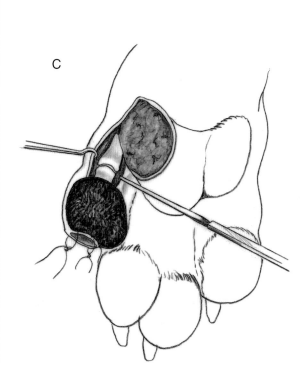

C

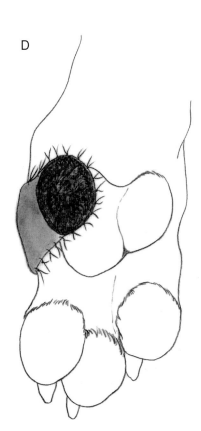

D

Plate 105	**Metatarsal/Metacarpal Pad Transfer**

DESCRIPTION

Loss of the digital pads as a result of trauma or disease may require repositioning of the metacarpal or metatarsal pad to provide for an appropriate surface for weight bearing (see Fig. 18-4).

SURGICAL TECHNIQUE

(A) Severely damaged or necrotic digits (A_1) are resected, as shown in (A_2). The wound is managed in preparation for eventual pad transfer.

(B) Metacarpal or metatarsal bones are partially resected to permit advancement of the respective metacarpal or metatarsal pad.

(C) The metatarsal or metacarpal pad is sutured into position with 2-0 monofilament, nonabsorbable sutures. A reinforced bandage is applied to protect the surgical site for up to 3 weeks after surgery.

COMMENTS

Removal of the ends of the metatarsal or metacarpal bones facilitates repositioning of their respective pads. Reduction in bone length also helps to prevent "bottoming out," in which bone deeply penetrates the cushion of the transplanted pad, increasing the likelihood of ulceration and discomfort.

Plate 105

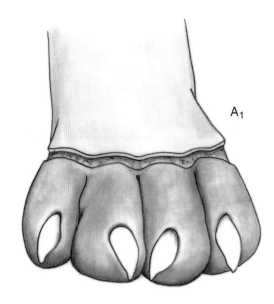

A₁

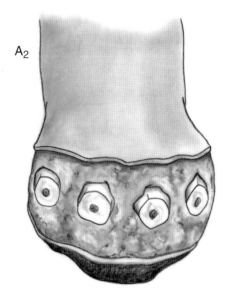

A₂

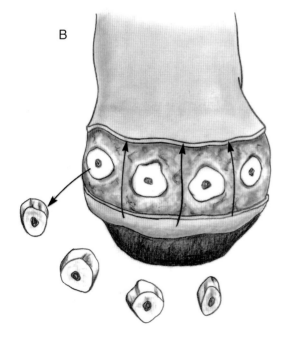

B

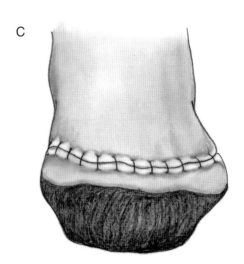

C

Plate 106   **Pad Grafting**

DESCRIPTION

Complete traumatic loss of the pads of a foot presents a significant problem to the dog: amputation may be necessary. However, several digital and metacarpal/metatarsal pads have the potential to be grafted onto the limb. The following is a case summary (see Fig. 18-5).

SURGICAL TECHNIQUE

(A) Individual foot pads in this case are separated (dotted lines; A_1). The pad cushion is excised down to the dermal layer of the avulsed or harvested digital pad or metatarsal/metacarpal pad (A_2). The pads are incised to permit their placement flatly onto the proposed bed (A_3, A_4). Each pad is sutured onto the cutaneous trunci muscle after surgical removal of the overlying skin.

(B) The temporary recipient bed for the graft is determined by placement of the injured foot up to the side of the patient (direct flap technique). A tie-over dressing is used to secure the graft for 7 days.

(C) In 7 days, a bipedicle flap incorporating the graft is elevated (see Plate 35). The injured foot is positioned beneath the flap and sutured to its edges. In 14 days, one half of each pedicle is divided (every 2 days), beginning with the ventral pedicle. Divided segments are sutured to wound borders.

(D) Several days after application, the horny pad layer will separate from the underlying germinal epithelium. These opaque epithelial islands will coalesce. The foot is supported in a heavily padded bandage reinforced with a Mason metasplint until a thick stratum corneum forms. In time, a leather or nylon hunting boot may be employed for protection. Redundant tissue may be excised to reposition the reimplanted pad for proper weight bearing.

COMMENTS

This two-staged procedure is technically demanding. The pad is preserved on a temporary vascular recipient site while the wound is being prepared for flap transfer. This technique has the main advantage of providing a thick subcutaneous layer that replaces the pad cushion, which cannot be achieved by direct pad application to the granulation bed. The feasibility of pad grafting was demonstrated by this technique. Other options for foot salvage include: (1) the microvascular transplantation of a digital pad from another foot and (2) the graft of a digital pad from another foot, in those cases in which the technique demonstrated is not feasible.

Plate 106

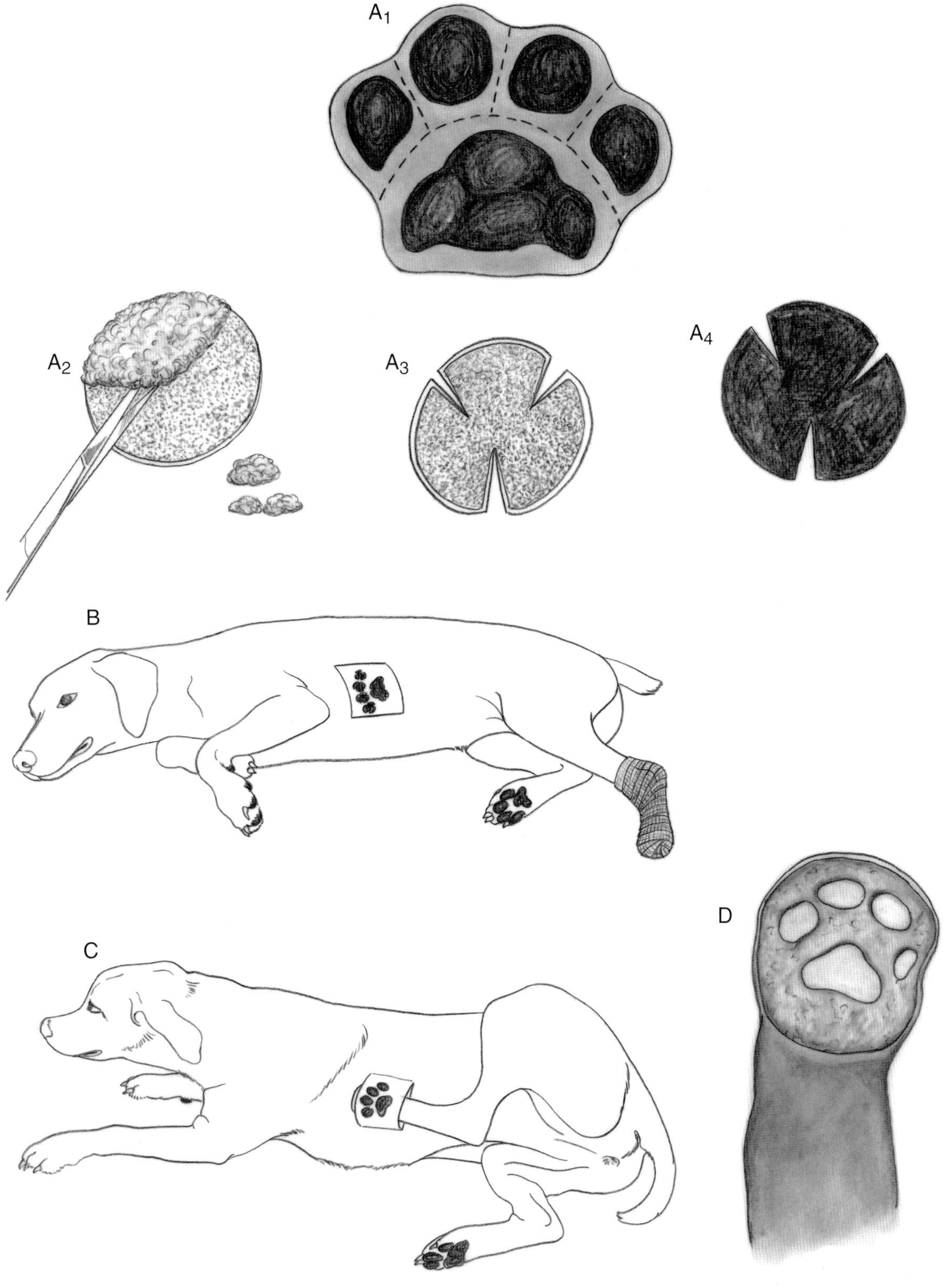

Plate 107	**Segmental Pad Grafting Technique**

DESCRIPTION

Small, rectangular segments of digital pad epithelium can be harvested as free grafts to reepithelialize large defects of the metacarpal or metatarsal pads. Development and successful use of this technique was reported by Bradley et al. (1994).

SURGICAL TECHNIQUE

(A) The digital pads of uninvolved feet can be used to harvest small pad grafts.

(B) Segmental pad grafts are harvested as small, 10- to 15-mm long, 5- to 10-mm wide grafts, depending upon the size of the dog and size of the defect to be covered. A scalpel blade (no. 11 or 15) is used to incise and elevate the grafts. Sutures can be used to approximate the donor defects.

(C) Each graft is inspected to assure that no pad cushion is covering the overlying dermal surface of each graft. A suture is placed in each graft prior to application.

(D) Example of a hind-limb injury, with loss of digits and loss of the outer portion of the metatarsal pad. Surviving remnants of the cushion layer of the metatarsal pad are covered by granulation tissue.

(E) Segmental pad grafts are sutured to the prepared granulation bed. A nonadherent dressing with ointment is secured to the graft area with skin staples or sutures, followed by application of a firm, reinforced, protective bandage.

(F) Approximately 3 weeks after graft application, epithelialization can be noted extending from the graft margins. The outer, horny layer of the graft will begin to soften and separate from the underlying, regenerative epithelium.

COMMENTS

Pad grafting for reconstruction of the metacarpal/metatarsal is best considered when all the digits have been lost. Small segmental grafts from viable digits do permit coverage of large defects of the important metatarsal/metacarpal pads, without the need to sacrifice an entire digit. However, multiple small wounds are created in several digits with this technique. The larger segmental grafts aligned along the perimeter of the defect can help assure that pad epithelium has a greater likelihood of covering the open (metatarsal/metacarpal) pad wound, rather than wound contraction and epithelialization from the wound margins. (Contact inhibition of epithelial cells from the pad grafts preclude the advancement of the cutaneous epithelium.) As noted, it is preferable to apply the grafts over the vascularized remnant of the pad cushion, which has the resiliency to absorb the forces a foot is subjected to during normal activity. It can take several weeks before these epithelial islands coalesce and, in turn, reform the thick durable pad surface. During this time, the area necessarily needs to be protected with padded bandages and splints.

    An alternative to this technique would be to sacrifice a single digit and graft the pad surface onto the recipient area. If one or more intact digits are present, the phalanges of one or two toes can be resected and the resultant digital flap(s) substituted for the missing metatarsal/metacarpal pad (plate 104): this is a preferable alternative to pad grafting.

Plate 107

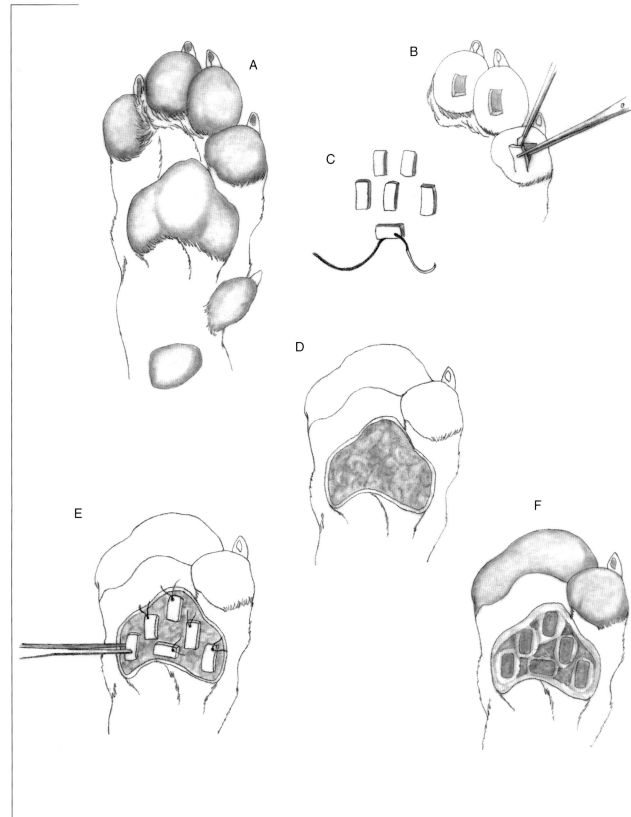

Plate 108   **Fusion Podoplasty**

DESCRIPTION

Fusion podoplasty, first reported by Swaim, is reserved for those dogs with advanced (end-stage) interdigital pyoderma (intertrigo) that has failed to respond to medical therapy. All four paws may be involved: for these patients, the forepaws may be operated on first, followed by the hind paws 1 month later.

SURGICAL TECHNIQUE

(A₁, ₂)   After surgical preparation of the paws, a marking pen (Securline [Gentian Violet] Surgical Skin Marker, Precision Dynamics Corp., San Fernando, CA) is used to outline the areas that require resection. On the palmar/plantar surface of the paw, the anterior border of the metacarpal or metatarsal pad is excised along with the interpad skin fold. Skin (2–4 mm) is preserved along the lateral and medial margins of each nail bed. Skin excisions are adjusted so that opposing interdigital skin margins align between each toe to facilitate suture alignment. Note the skin excision terminates at the midpoint of each digital pad.

(B)   After excision of the diseased interdigital and palmar/plantar interpad folds is performed, opposing pad margins are carefully trimmed with a scalpel blade to assure accurate edge-to-edge suture alignment.

(C, D)   The dorsal surface of the paw is usually sutured first, followed by closure of the palmar/plantar surfaces: skin to skin, lateral to medial digital pad borders, caudal digital pad borders to anterior border of the metacarpal/metatarsal pad.

     The end of each digit is not sutured in order to provide drainage. A strip of Penrose drain is placed in the interpad defect prior to closure of the palmar/plantar surface, with the ends of the drain segment exiting through a small stab incision in the skin, lateral and medial to the anterior border of the metacarpal/metatarsal pad. Two centimeters of the drain are exposed on each side and secured with two sutures. Bandaging and splinting of the paws is performed prior to anesthetic recovery of the patient.

COMMENTS

Although this procedure is infrequently used, it is invaluable for those patients with end-stage intertrigo of the paws. Electrocautery is required to help control hemorrhage when resecting skin with chronic pyoderma and fibrosis. Bandage care is critical to a successful surgical outcome. A metasplint (Carpal Splint, Kirschner Medical Corp., Timonium, MD; Metal Splints, Surecraft, Upton, MA) is applied to the outer bandage to reduce pressure and movement at the closure sites. Fiberglass casting materials (Scotchcast Plus, 3M Health Care, Neuss, Germany; prefabricated casting material—C-Splint, Johnson & Johnson Orthopedics, Raynham, MA) also may be fashioned into a custom-made protective splint.

    During the first week, excessive drainage may warrant daily bandage changes: absorbent pads or polyurethane foam (see Chapter 5) may be used to help retain tissue discharge between bandage changes. Broad-spectrum systemic antibiotics are advisable. Topical gentamycin ointment or silver sulfadiazine ointment may be used if a *Pseudomonas* infection is noted postoperatively. Chlorhexidine swabs may be used to clean the surgical area prior to bandage reapplication. During the second and third weeks of bandaging/splinting, changes usually can be decreased to every second or third day. The drain is removed in 7–10 days; bandaging is discontinued when healing is complete (approximately 3 weeks). A support bandage or protective boot is applied to protect each paw for a few additional weeks. Fusion podoplasty is expensive and time consuming to perform. If all four paws are involved, it will take a minimum 2-month time investment.

Plate 108

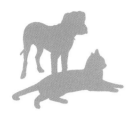

19

Major Eyelid Reconstruction

INTRODUCTION

There are numerous surgical procedures employed to remove damaged and diseased segments of the upper and lower eyelid. A number of articles and ophthalmology textbooks discuss these procedures. The techniques available for extensive loss of this structure are more limited. This chapter covers three specialized reconstructive techniques less commonly employed in veterinary surgery for major eyelid reconstruction, including the mucocutaneous subdermal plexus flap (lip-to-lid procedure), a combined mucosal graft/transposition skin flap technique, and a third eyelid–skin flap technique.

THE EYELIDS

Lesions involving the eyelids may be excised and closed directly when less than one-third of the eyelid margin is involved. The lateral canthal ligament can be divided to relieve eyelid tension during direct closure, if necessary. Cryosurgery and thermal destruction of eyelid tumors have been used with variable success in place of surgical excision.

Extensive wounds involving the cutaneous surface of the eyelid can be successfully closed with local pedicle grafts. Skin flaps alone, however, are inadequate for reconstruction of eyelid losses that include the palpebral conjunctiva, unless the remaining con-

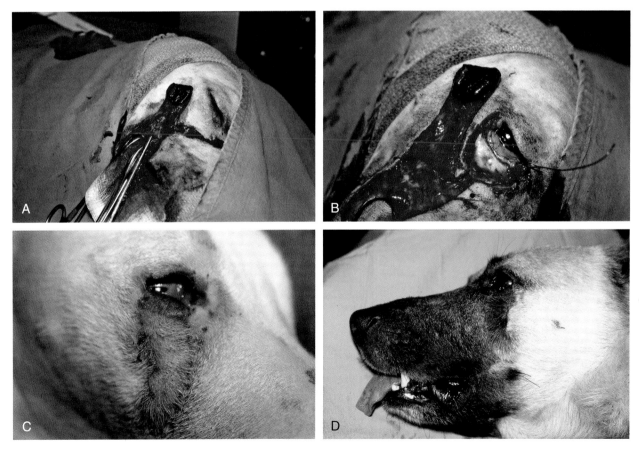

FIG. 19-1 (A) Lip replacement of the right lower eyelid. Elevation of the labial flap. (B)Resection of the lower eyelid and creation of a bridge incision for placement of the composite labial flap. (C) View of the flap, 2 weeks postoperatively. Note the prominent pigmentation of the labial margin in this white dog. (D) Note the misdirected hair growth and darker fur highlighting the flap skin (arrow).

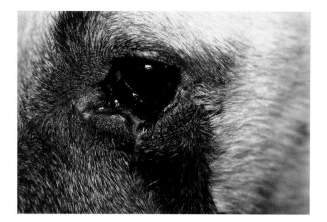

FIG. 19-2 Close-up view of lip-to-lid transplant (From Pavletic MM, Nafe LA, Confer AW. 1982. Mucocutaneous subdermal plexus flap from the lip for lower eyelid restoration in the dog. *J Am Vet Med Assoc* 180:921-926.)

junctiva can be mobilized to line the flap's dermal surface upon transfer. This can be accomplished by simple undermining and advancement of the adjacent conjunctival margins or by using conjunctival flaps from the opposing eyelid. A variation of the latter technique is the full-thickness cross-lid flap. The lower eyelid is considered a suitable donor site for large upper eyelid defects. However, the use of the upper eyelid for lower lid reconstruction is less desirable because of potential compromise to the vital function the upper eyelid normally serves for corneal protection.

Free oral mucosa and nasal mucosal grafts, including a thin layer of nasal septal cartilage, have been successfully used as a conjunctival substitute to reconstruct eyelids. The mucosal grafts are generally transplanted onto a local pedicle graft, and the resulting composite flap is transferred to the recipient site after the mucosal graft "takes." As a result, the potential hazards associated with upper eyelid "sharing" procedures are avoided. More recently, the third eyelid has been used as a conjunctival substitute for loss of the lower eyelid, with a skin flap used to restore its cutaneous surface (Plate 111).

To bypass the serious drawbacks involved with major eyelid reconstructive surgery, the author also has developed the lip-to-lid procedure whereby a portion of the upper lip is used to replace full-thickness lower and or upper eyelid defects (Figs. 19-1 and 19-2).

Plate 111 outlines the use of the third eyelid flap as a mucosal surface on which a local skin flap can be applied for lower eyelid restoration.

Suggested Readings

Hunt G. 2006. Use of the lip-to-lid flap for replacement of the lower eyelid in five cats. *Vet Surg* 35:284–286.

Pavletic MM, Nafe LA, Confer AW. 1982. Mucocutaneous subdermal plexus flap from the lip for lower eyelid restoration in the dog. *J Am Vet Med Assoc* 180:921–926.

Moore CP, Constantinescu GM. 1997. Surgery of the adnexa. *Vet Clin No Am* 27:1011–1066.

Schmidt K, Bertani C, Martano M, et al. 2005. Reconstruction of the lower eyelid by third eyelid lateral advancement and local transposition cutaneous flap after "en bloc" resection of squamous cell carcinoma in 5 cats. *Vet Surg* 34:78–82.

Plate 109   **Lip-to-Lid Procedure**

DESCRIPTION

A mucocutaneous subdermal plexus flap from the upper lip can be used to replace the entire lower lid after extensive trauma or tumor excision. It can be modified for upper eyelid reconstruction.

SURGICAL TECHNIQUE

(A) The proposed full-thickness lip incisions are drawn with a marking pen at a 45- to 50-degree angle to a line passing through the medial and lateral canthi.

(B) Elevation of the full-thickness lip flap exposes the mucosal surface. Reference incision lines slightly diverge to avoid accidental narrowing of the cutaneous pedicle. Gauze pads beneath the lip will support it when incising the lip margin.

(C) The oral mucosa is carefully split at a level sufficient to replace the missing lower lid conjunctiva. The cutaneous pedicle is carefully dissected from the oral mucosa and underlying structures, beneath the platysma muscle. Care must be exercised to avoid traumatizing the pedicle's vital subdermal plexus, to avoid severing any underlying facial structures, and to avoid the development of an unnecessarily long cutaneous transfer pedicle.

(D) The oral mucosal defect is apposed with a buried suture pattern using 3-0 absorbable sutures. A bridge incision (dashed line) is used to connect the donor and recipient beds for suture placement of the transfer pedicle. Undermining of the mucosal border of the flap should be avoided to prevent circulatory compromise.

Plate 109

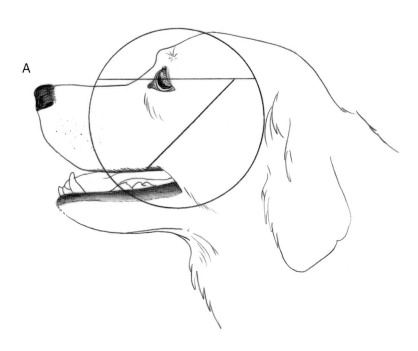

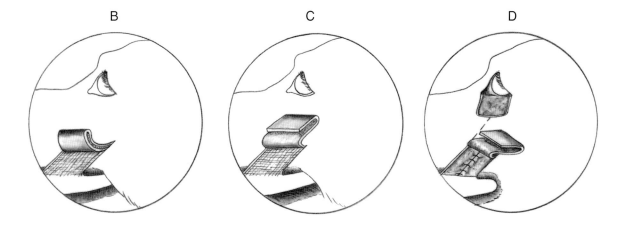

Plate 109

(Continued)

(E) The flap is initially sutured into place by apposing the oral mucosa to the remaining conjunctival edges with a buried, interrupted suture pattern using 4-0 absorbable sutures. Lastly, the cutaneous surface is sutured with a simple interrupted pattern. The cutaneous recipient bed is closed to complete the transfer. Folds and skin puckers should be left alone to avoid vascular compromise to the graft in this first stage.

(F) In 4–6 weeks, the surgeon has the option of removing the cutaneous transfer pedicle and closing the defect by simple apposition of skin edges.

(G) An optional second-stage revision procedure will improve cosmetic results. Second-stage revision can be simultaneously used to re-establish a more normal "eyelid" border in the event of partial necrosis or excessive thickness of the outer lip margin.

COMMENTS

Defects limited to the cutaneous layer of the eyelid are best restored with skin flaps. Eyelid replacement with a labial flap is reserved for wide, full-thickness defects if more conservative options for closure are unsuitable. The lip flap is a composite mucocutaneous subdermal plexus flap. Skin, oral mucosa, and portions of the orbicularis oris and buccinator muscles are used to replace the full-thickness loss of the lower eyelid. Unlike a subdermal plexus flap lined with conjunctiva or a free mucosal graft, the lip graft has a central muscular layer, thus giving more normal thickness and natural rigidity as an eyelid substitute. In addition, the wide mucocutaneous junction and hairless lip margin serve as a natural buffer zone between the cornea and the hairy skin.

The blood supply to the oral mucosa is from numerous arterial and venous anastomoses between the cutaneous subdermal plexus and the submucosal capillary network. Care must be taken to assure maintenance of adequate perfusion pressure to the terminal portion of the flap by using meticulous, atraumatic surgical technique, avoiding unnecessarily long grafts (cutaneous transfer pedicles), avoiding undermining between the graft's oral mucosal and cutaneous layers, avoiding direct placement of tissue forceps to the outer mucocutaneous border, and creating lip flaps with slightly diverging incisions to avoid accidental pedicle narrowing. No effort should be made to remove "dog ears" or tissue folds during graft transfer because that could inadvertently compromise the blood supply. As indicated, an optional revision procedure can be used in 4–6 weeks to improve the cosmetic results.

During elevation of the flap, care must be taken to avoid accidental injury to underlying structures, including the facial vein, parotid duct, and buccal nerve.

A right angle or T extension of labial mucosa can be included with the labial flap for simultaneous restoration of portions of the upper eyelid. A second surgical procedure may later be required to form or mold this larger graft for optimal cosmetic and functional results.

Plate 109

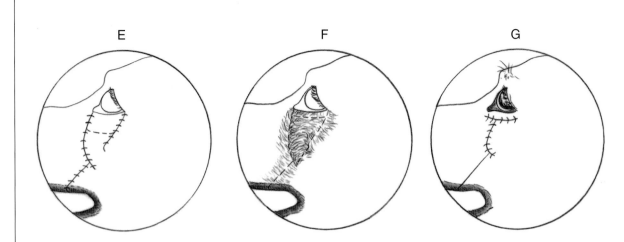

E

F

G

Plate 110 **Oral Mucosal Graft onto Skin Flap**

DESCRIPTION

The upper lip and cheek are excellent sources of mucosa for reconstructive surgical techniques requiring this unique epithelial surface. Mucosa can be grafted onto a local transposition flap that can be rotated to the eye defect 1 week after surgical graft application.

SURGICAL TECHNIQUE

(A) Example of a lower eyelid neoplasm. The solid line is the proposed outline of a transposition flap in preparation for a mucosal graft. The dashed line shows an alternate position for upper eyelid reconstruction.

(B) The upper lip is retracted to expose its mucosal surface. Stay sutures can be used to hold the lip in an elevated position; skin hooks or towel clamps also may be used. A mucosal graft is elevated from the upper lip in this example. The graft is prepared in a fashion described for full-thickness skin grafts (Plate 64). A no. 15 scalpel blade is used to elevate a premeasured segment of mucosa. It is advisable to harvest slightly larger grafts than what is measured: mucosal grafts can contract (shrink) considerably upon elevation. Minimize the amount of underlying tissue by keeping the scalpel blade close to the submucosal surface during graft elevation. Metzenbaum scissors can be used to trim any tissue adhered to the submucosal surface of the graft, as discussed in the section on skin grafting (Plate 64).

(C) The thin, prepared mucosal graft is meshed prior to application to the flap's dermal surface with fine (4-0 or 5-0) absorbable sutures.

(D) The flap is replaced in its donor bed for 4–7 days.

(E) The flap is re-elevated and placed in the donor defect after tumor removal. Borders of the mucosal graft are sutured to the borders of the remaining conjunctiva with 4-0 absorbable sutures. Completion of the closure, using 3-0 to 4-0 nonabsorbable skin sutures.

COMMENTS

For complete eyelid reconstruction, this technique or the lip-to-lid procedure (Plate 109) can be employed. The lip-to-lid procedure has some tactical advantages over mucosal onlay grafts of the transposition flap, with additional tissue bulk provided by the orbicularis oris and buccinator muscles. Moreover, the mucosal border of the lip-to-lid transfer is more mobile than the adherent mucosal graft transfer discussed in this plate. This technique can be used for mucosal graft transfer to other significant mucosal defects (e.g., prepuce, nasal cavity). Mucosal grafts can be employed for preputial reconstruction when simpler penile coverage techniques have failed.

Plate 110

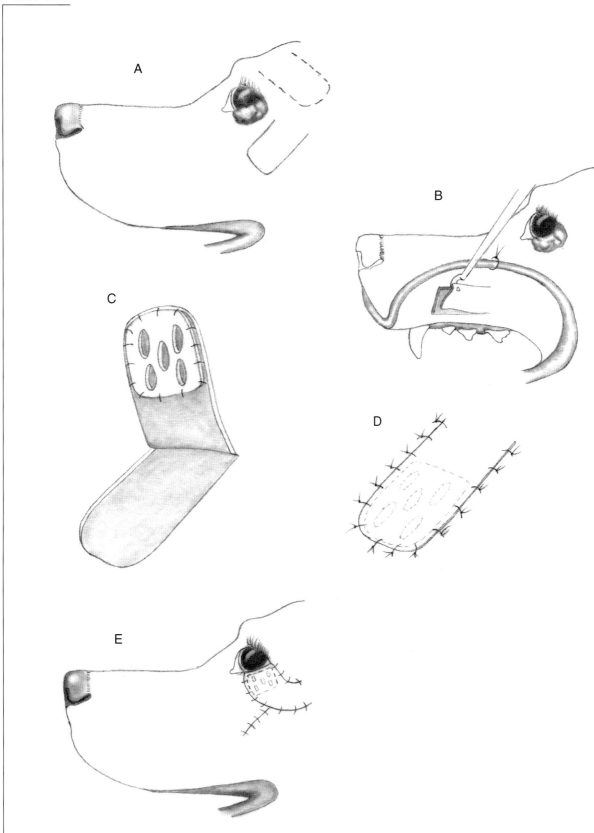

A

B

C

D

E

Plate 111   **Third Eyelid–Skin Flap Reconstruction of the Lower Eyelid**

DESCRIPTION

This is an alternative technique for lower eyelid reconstruction, using a portion of the third eyelid as a conjunctival replacement, in combination with a local transposition skin flap reported by Schmidt, Bertani, et al.

SURGICAL TECHNIQUE

(A) Example of a malignant neoplasm involving the lower eyelid.

(B) Full-thickness excision of the entire medial half of the lower eyelid.

(C) A no. 15 scalpel blade can be used to facilitate resection of the outer conjunctival surface of the third eyelid. Elevation of a 90-degree transposition flap.

(D) The flap is sutured to the dorsal margin of the third eyelid and adjacent cutaneous margins. The donor area was sutured in routine fashion.

(E) Example of the same technique used for restoration of the lateral half of the lower eyelid. This requires mobilizing and advancing the third eyelid laterally.

COMMENTS

The third eyelid flap can be used to replace the medial or lateral half of the lower eyelid. No adverse effects were reported with this technique. If necessary, a canthotomy can be performed to help restore the palpebral fissure to its normal size.

Hair should be periodically trimmed near the dorsal flap margin to prevent irritation to the cornea.

Plate 111

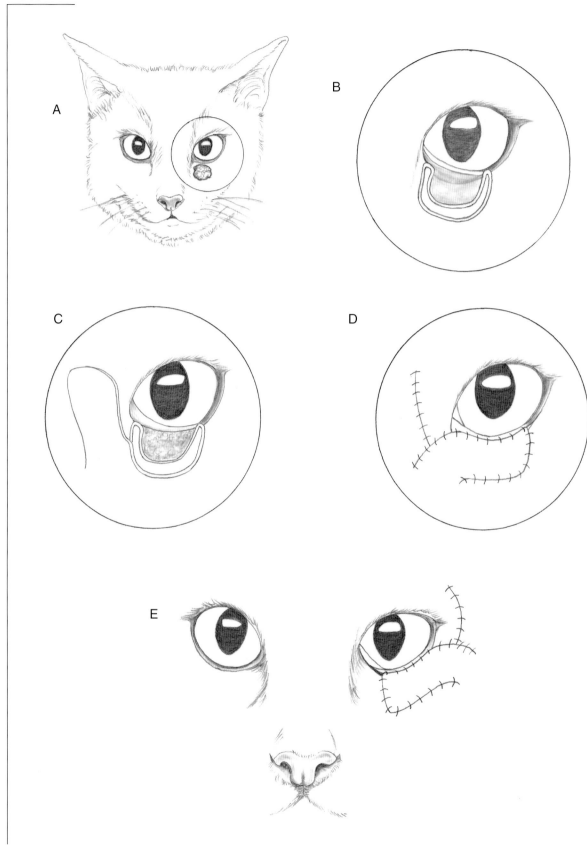

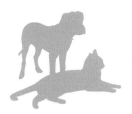

20

Nasal Reconstruction
Techniques

INTRODUCTION: NASAL ANATOMY

The external nose of the dog consists of a fixed bony case and a moveable cartilaginous framework. Muscles connected to the cartilage component permit the dog and cat to move the external nose in response to various smells and tactile stimuli. The flattened apical portion of the nose is called the *nasal plane* (planum nasale); the central groove between the nostrils is the *philtrum*.

The bony nasal aperture serves as a support frame for the nasal cartilage; dorsal and lateral nasal ligaments provide support to the dominant dorsolateral nasal cartilages. The flexible external nose is composed of several individual cartilages, including the paired dorsolateral and ventrolateral nasal cartilages, paired accessory cartilages, and a singular cartilaginous nasal septum. The ventral part of the septal cartilage is the vomeronasal cartilage. A membranous nasal septum connects the immovable caudal cartilaginous nasal septum to the mobile rostral septum described.

There are three interconnected nasal meatuses in the dog, including the dorsal meatus, middle meatus, and ventral meatus. The common nasal meatus is a longitudinal, narrow space on either side of the nasal septum: it is coextensive with these three meatuses. The nasopharyngeal meatus is an extension of the ventral nasal meatus.

The nasal cavity and external nose is supplied by an extensive capillary network, in turn supplied by an interconnecting network of arteries and veins. This extensive collateral circulation helps maintain a blood supply to these tissues despite significant trauma. Similarly, it is this outstanding circulation that enables the surgeon to manipulate these tissues during reconstructive surgical procedures with less risk of ischemic necrosis.

In general descriptive terminology, the external nose can be named according to specific anatomic regions: the central nasal region between the nostrils or *central planum*, the lateral nasal or *rolled alar cartilages*, and the lower rostral base of the nostril or *sulcus* (Fig. 20-1). The external nose is a highly specialized functional structure that contributes significantly to the general cosmetic appearance of the dog. There is no simple or practical method to precisely reconstruct large areas of this tissue lost from trauma or surgical resection. Reconstruction of the human nose secondary to trauma or tumor removal may require a single surgical technique or multiple surgeries to optimize the cosmetic outcome for the patient, depending upon the extent of the defect. The dog, however, has a hair-

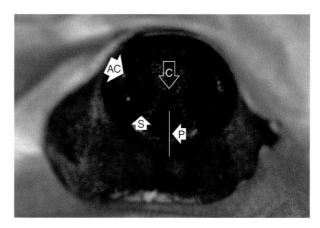

FIG. 20-1 Frontal view of the nose (nasal planum), demonstrating the rolled (lateral) alar cartilages (AC), central planum (C), sulcus (S), and philtrum (P).

less, pigmented epithelial coverage etched with polygonal-shaped indentations or grooves: replication of this surface and underlying cartilage framework can be difficult or impossible to achieve in a practical fashion, as compared with the human.

With the exception of controversial cosmetic ear-cropping and tail-docking procedures advocated for some breeds of dogs, many veterinarians have reservations about performing surgery strictly for cosmetic purposes, unless there are other benefits to the patient in correcting a given defect. The attitudes of dog owners also vary on the subject of cosmetic surgery. Many owners take particular pride in their pet's appearance. Some owners/breeders seek out cosmetic surgery to improve the appearance of their pet for dog show competition. Other owners simply are disturbed or shocked by the cosmetic outcome of a given surgery, despite the fact that patient function and comfort have been restored or maintained. In this chapter, different techniques are presented as options to help improve function to the nose while closing a given defect with the hope of achieving a more reasonable cosmetic outcome in a single surgical procedure.

TRAUMATIC WOUND MANAGEMENT

Lacerations and superficial abrasions occasionally are noted in the dog and can be managed with basic wound management techniques. Shearing wounds, usually secondary to vehicular trauma, generally are unilateral injuries from the patient tumbling to one side during impact from behind, driving the patient's rostrolateral facial area into the pavement. Management of these wounds includes control of hemorrhage, surgical debridement, and treatment of any infection present. Minor wounds can heal by second intention with basic care. More extensive wounds, which often include the rostral upper lip, may require additional surgical intervention for optimal cosmetic and functional results. Regional skin can be undermined, advanced, and sutured to the nasal mucosal and cutaneous epithelial tissue which compose the border of the defect. Alternatively, a compound upper labial advancement flap can be employed for simultaneous closure of that portion of the rostral (full-thickness) lip and nasal planum destroyed (see Plate 72).

Blunt frontal impact can result in the upward displacement of the nose, with subsequent tearing of the underlying connective tissue attachments and adjacent labial mucosa. Minor avulsion wounds may be managed by suturing the avulsed labial mucosa around the upper incisors (see Plate 69). More extensive avulsion wounds can result in the upward displacement of the nose, labial tissues, and facial skin: simply reapposing the labial mucosa may not sufficiently stabilize the nose, resulting in its lateral displacement. As discussed in Chapter 15, stabilization can be facilitated by placement of absorbable anchor sutures through one palatine fissure and into the exposed nasal septal cartilage, before passing the straight needle through the opposite foramen and into the oral cavity (Fig. 15-3). Two sutures are placed in this fashion and tied once lavage, debridement, and hemostasis are achieved. Once tied, the labial mucosal laceration is closed with a simple interrupted or continuous suture pattern. Although uncommon, trauma to the nasal cartilage can result in membranous scar tissue obstruction of the nasal opening caudal to the framework of the nasal cartilage. In one case referred to the author, a canine patient could not breathe through his nose, necessitating a ventral labial approach to gain access to the ventral nasal meatus. Scar tissue resection was followed by insertion of tubular plastic stents through the common nasal meatus, secured to each common nasal meatus with sutures for approximately 2 weeks.

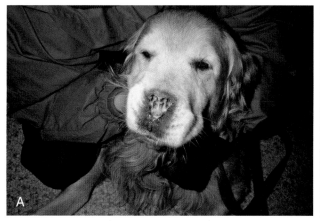
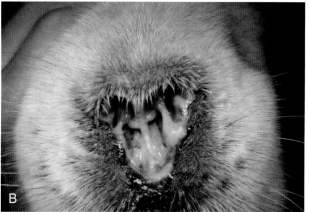
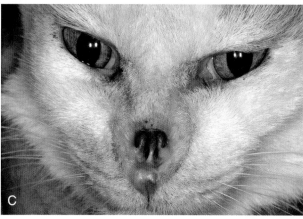
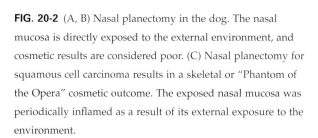

FIG. 20-2 (A, B) Nasal planectomy in the dog. The nasal mucosa is directly exposed to the external environment, and cosmetic results are considered poor. (C) Nasal planectomy for squamous cell carcinoma results in a skeletal or "Phantom of the Opera" cosmetic outcome. The exposed nasal mucosa was periodically inflamed as a result of its external exposure to the environment.

NEOPLASIA

Neoplasms involving the nasal planum are occasionally encountered in small animal practice. Squamous cell carcinoma is one of the most common neoplasms in the dog and cat. Tumor resection can be accomplished by scalpel, laser, or cryosurgery (Fig. 20-2). Radiation therapy may be an option in select cases and can be discussed with an oncologist or radiation therapist. Computer-aided tomography may be useful to better define the extent of tumor invasion. Depending on the location of the tumor, it is possible to remove tumors completely, yet preserve portions of the nasal planum to "reconstruct" the nose for better functional and cosmetic results. It also is possible to use portions of the rostral upper lip to replace areas of the nasal planum (Fig. 20-3). It is not necessary to simply resect the neoplasm and accept the less functional and less attractive cosmetic result obtained by complete nasal planectomy (Fig. 20-2).

NEOPLASMS AND SURGICAL MARGINS

Limited tumor excision, simply to achieve optimal cosmetic results and facilitate closure, likely will result in tumor recurrence within weeks after surgery. A 10- to 20-mm margin around a well-demarcated growth may be sufficient to obtain "surgical margins" in many patients, although highly invasive tumors may necessitate wider margins of healthy tissue to assure their complete removal. This basic principle of cancer surgery, however, must be tempered with avoiding unnecessarily aggressive excision of all tumors regardless of their type size, location, and classification. Tissues excised should be submitted for histopathological examination to assure that neoplastic cells do not extend to the surgical margins of the specimen. Additional resection of tissues and/or alternative cancer therapy options would be indicated under these circumstances.

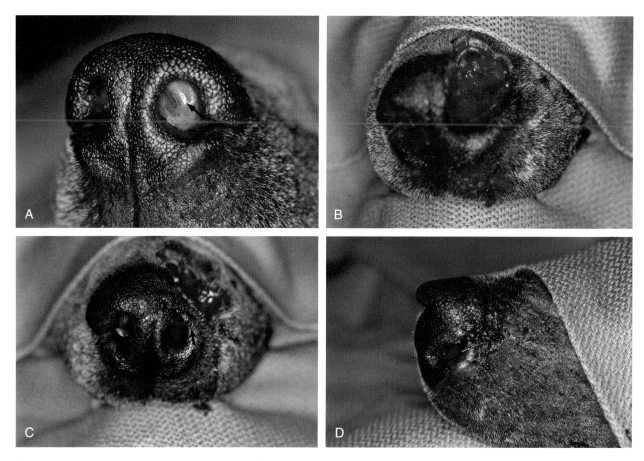

FIG. 20-3 (A) Expansile granulomatous mass (benign) involving the left alar cartilage area. (B) Complete resection of the lesion. (C) Upward rotation of the remaining nasal cartilage, recreating the left nostril. (D) Closure of the skin defect. Mild asymmetry is present from loss of the alar tissue. However, the owner was pleased with the cosmetic result and functional outcome of the patient.

NASAL RECONSTRUCTION OPTIONS

Skin Flaps

An advancement flap from the dorsal muzzle can be placed over the exposed nasal septum, improving the cosmetic appearance of the patient while protecting the nasal mucosa from irritation secondary to exposure (Fig. 20-4). See Plate 112.

Bilateral Alar Cartilage Flaps

Centrally located tumors involving the external nose can be widely excised. If the rolled alar cartilages are not involved in the disease process, each alar prominence can be carefully contoured with a scalpel blade, pivoted, and sutured together. The smaller external nasal silhouette created results in a better cosmetic outcome compared to complete planectomy. Moreover, the nasal mucosa is recessed and better protected from exposure by creation of this dorsal "cartilage" shelf (Fig. 20-5). See Plate 115.

Musculofascial Island Labial Flap

In the event that complete planectomy is required for tumor removal, the adjacent upper lip can be used to partially reconstruct the canine nose. An incision, 3 or 4 cm caudal and parallel to the rostral labial border, is made through the entire thickness of the lip. The cutaneous and mucosal surfaces are carefully excised, leaving the terminal 3 cm of skin, mucosa, and associated labial border. This musculofascial labial flap and associated island of epithelium is transposed dorsally and sutured into position. The remaining skin and labial tissues are reapposed to complete the procedure. Partial removal of the epithelial surfaces enables the surgeon to bury the pedicle beneath the skin. Although not identical to the original nose, the cosmetic appearance, judged by frontal and side views of the patient, is improved. Moreover, recreation of the dorsal nasal shelf further protects the nasal mucosa (Fig. 20-6). See Plate 116.

Labial Mucosal Inversion Technique

An alternate technique for improving nasal mucosal protection reported by Gallegos et al. (2007), uses suturing of the labial mucosa to the nasal cartilage ring after nasal planectomy. Following this, the labial borders are folded rostrally, inverting the labial mucosa, thereby partially covering the nasal opening. Segments of the lip are resected to reestablish the midline of the upper lip. The net result of this surgery is the creation of a mucosal antechamber for the nasal cavity, surrounded by pigmented labial tissue. Cosmetic results are reported to be better than those achieved by nasal planectomy alone (Plate 118).

Sulcus Flaps

Paired, small, 90-degree angle transposition flaps may be used to replace the central nasal planum after resection of lesions restricted to this area (Plate 113).

Stenosis of Reconstructed Nasal Openings

Significant gaps or loss of nasal mucosa can result in narrowing of the reconstructed nostrils. Accurate alignment of nasal mucosal tissues with the skin or adjacent mucosal tissues used in nasal reconstruction can reduce this postoperative complication. In mild cases of nasal stenosis, scar tissue may be resected and the nasal openings enlarged, apposing the available skin and mucosa. In cases of severe stenosis, mucosal grafts can be used in an attempt to create a new epithelialized opening (see Welch and Swaim 2003).

Selective Resection of Nasal Septal Tumors

In some cases, neoplasms may primarily involve the nasal septum of the external nose. An alternative to complete nasal planectomy would be selective excision of the nasal septum for those smaller tumors without clinical evidence of extensive infiltration of the planum (Plate 114). An incision can be made to elevate the dermis and epidermis of the central planum, thereby gaining exposure of the septum for wide excision. The elevated planum is resutured at the completion of tumor removal. As a result, the external cosmetic appearance of the nose can be maintained; loss of the septum causes no notable respiratory problems (Fig. 20-7).

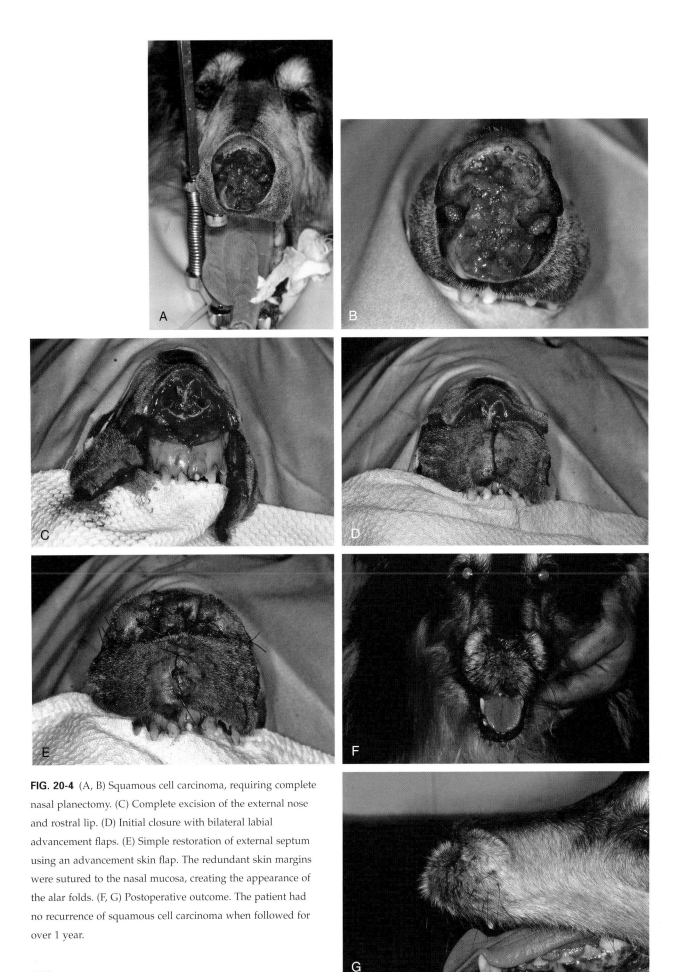

FIG. 20-4 (A, B) Squamous cell carcinoma, requiring complete nasal planectomy. (C) Complete excision of the external nose and rostral lip. (D) Initial closure with bilateral labial advancement flaps. (E) Simple restoration of external septum using an advancement skin flap. The redundant skin margins were sutured to the nasal mucosa, creating the appearance of the alar folds. (F, G) Postoperative outcome. The patient had no recurrence of squamous cell carcinoma when followed for over 1 year.

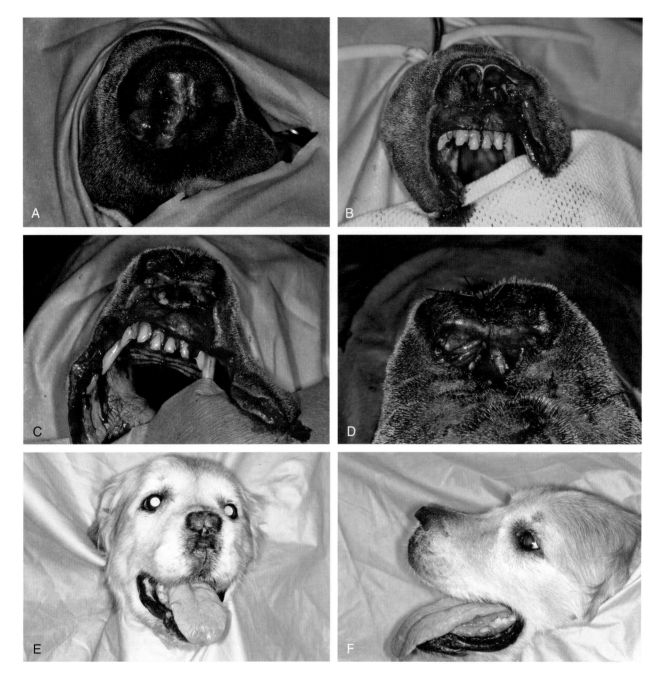

FIG. 20-5 (A) Squamous cell carcinoma of the lower nasal planum.

(B) Wide resection of the mass: the alar fold flaps were not involved in the neoplastic process and were preserved.

(C) The epithelial border of each alar fold was resected, followed by suture apposition.

(D) Final closure using bilateral labial advancement flaps.

(E, F) Postoperative views of the patient. The alar folds created the semblance of an external nose while protecting the inner nasal mucosa from exposure. No recurrence of the neoplasm after 1 year.

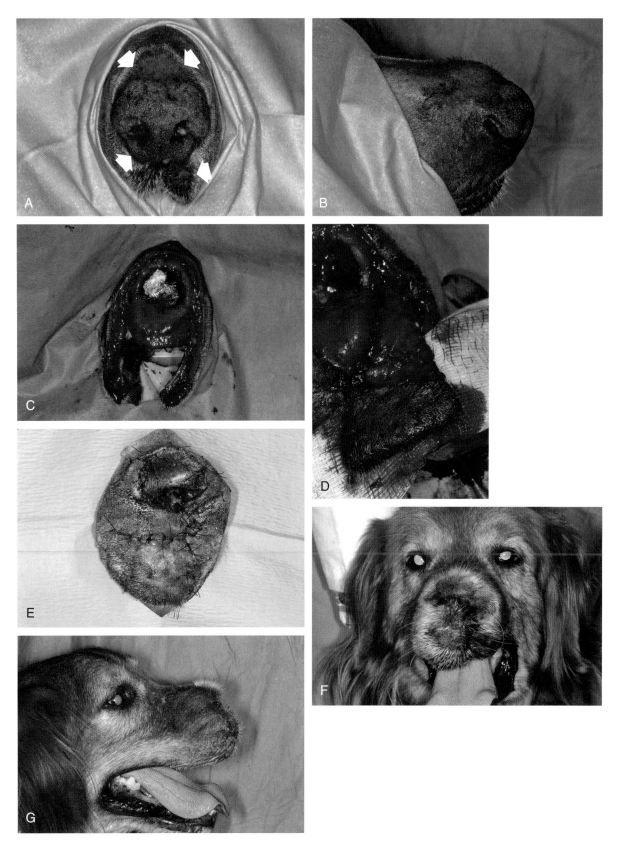

FIG. 20-6 *See legend on opposite page.*

FIG. 20-6 (A, B) Extensive squamous cell carcinoma of the nasal planum and adjacent lip.

(C) Wide excision of the neoplasm.

(D) Creation of a nasolabial island flap from the left labial tissue.

(E) Transposition of the island of labial tissue over the dorsum of the nasal opening, creating a "protective awning" to the recessed nasal mucosa. Closure of the labial defect using the remaining available labial tissues.

(F, G) Postoperative outcome. No tumor recurrence was noted after 1 year. In hindsight, resection of redundant labial tissue would have improved the cosmetic appearance in this patient. The owner was quite pleased with the results.

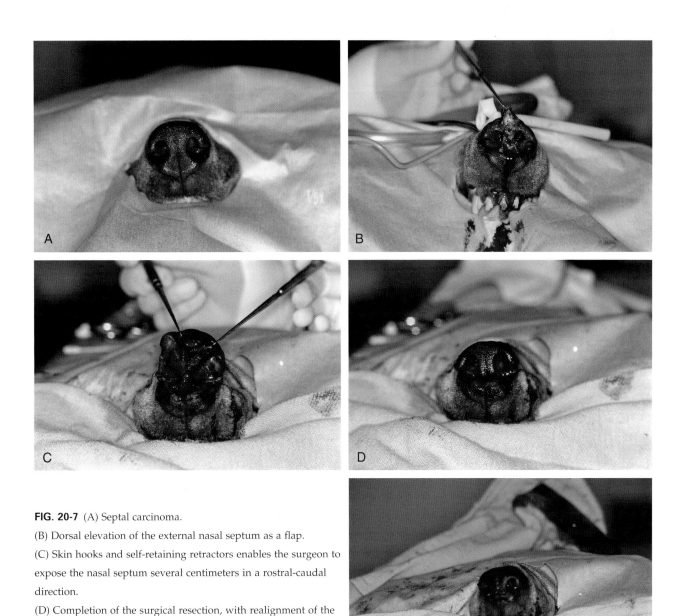

FIG. 20-7 (A) Septal carcinoma.

(B) Dorsal elevation of the external nasal septum as a flap.

(C) Skin hooks and self-retaining retractors enables the surgeon to expose the nasal septum several centimeters in a rostral-caudal direction.

(D) Completion of the surgical resection, with realignment of the external septal flap.

(E) The flap was resutured to its original position. Cosmetic and functional results were excellent, despite the extensive intranasal surgery performed.

Cantilever Suture Technique

Rostral maxillectomy can result in a loss of nasal cartilage support, with drooping of the nose postoperatively (Fig. 20-8). Breathing through the deviated external nose becomes difficult or impossible. A "cantilever" suture technique, developed by the author, can be used to elevate the nose (Fig. 20-9). See Plate 117.

Suggested Readings

Evans HE, Chrisensen GC. 1979. *Miller's Anatomy of the Dog*, 2nd ed., 507–511. Philadelphia: WB Saunders.

Gallegos J, Schmiedt, CW, McAnulty JF. 2007. Cosmetic rostral nasal reconstruction after nasal planum and pre-

maxilla resection: technique and results in two dogs. *Vet Surg* 36:669–674.

Hammer DL, Sacks M. 1975. Clefts of the primary and secondary palate. In: Bojrab MJ, ed. *Current Techniques in Small Animal Surgery I*, 75–84. Philadelphia, PA: Lea and Febiger.

Holt D, Prymak C, Evans S. 1990. Excision of tumors in the nasal vestibule of two dogs. *Vet Surg* 19:418–423.

Pavletic MM: unpublished data.

Rogers KS, Helman RG, Walker MA. 1995. Squamous cell carcinoma of the canine nasal planum: eight cases (1988–1994). *J Am Anim Hosp Assoc* 31:373–378.

Ruslander D, Kaser-Hotz B, Sardinas JC. 1997. Cutaneous squamous cell carcinoma in cats. *Comp Cont Ed Pract Vet* 19:1119–1126.

Welch JA, Swaim SF. 2003. Nasal and facial reconstruction in a dog following severe trauma. *J Am Anim Hosp Assoc* 39:407–415.

Withrow SJ, Straw RC. 1990. Resection of the nasal planum in nine cats and five dogs. *J Am Anim Hosp Assoc* 26:219–222.

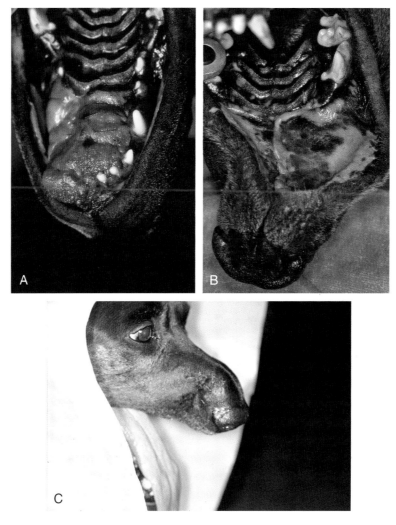

FIG. 20-8 (A, B) Rostral maxillectomy for fibrosarcoma; closure using the labial mucosa. (C) Wide resection resulted in collapse of the lower support of the external nose, causing its ventral deviation postoperatively. The patient is functional, although nasal breathing was significantly impaired.

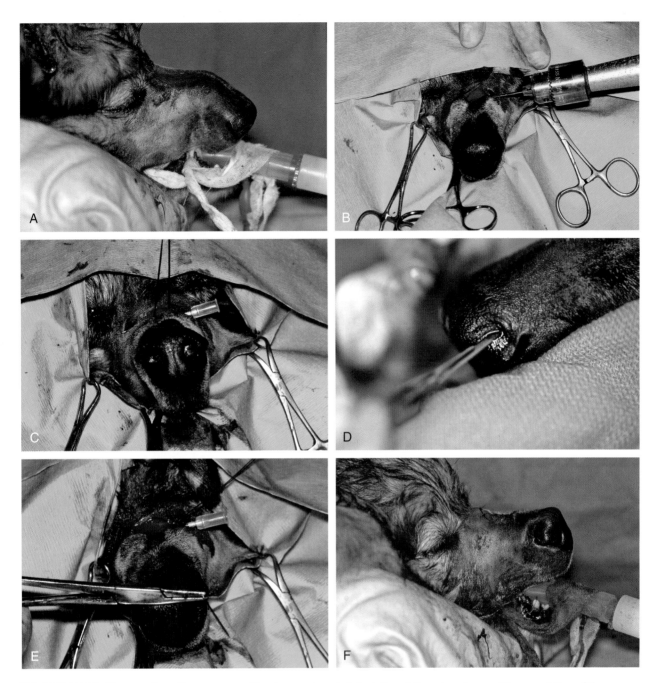

FIG. 20-9 (A) Maxillectomy for a fibrosarcoma with subsequent ventral deviation of the external nose. After completion of the maxillectomy, the patient was placed in sternal recumbency.

(B) Creation of an access tunnel in the nasal bone for the cantilever sutures using a 1/16-inch Steinman pin.

(C) Use of an 18-gauge hypodermic needle to facilitate passage of two strands of 00 monofilament nylon.

(D) Creation of small stab incisions in the lateral nasal cartilage. These stab incisions are used to facilitate passage of the cantilever sutures through the external nasal cartilage.

(E) Passage of the straight needle beneath the skin and guided out the nasal cartilage stab incision. The needle is passed through the opposite stab incision and directed back to the original skin incision.

(F) The sutures are tied under slight tension to help assure appropriate postoperative support to the external nose. The skin incision is closed to complete the procedure. Note the slight dimpling of the lateral alar cartilage as a result of the suture embedding below the epithelial surface.

Plate 112   Septal Coverage Using Cutaneous Advancement Flaps

DESCRIPTION

Complete nasal planectomy, usually secondary to wide tumor resection, results in exposure of the nasal septum and adjacent rostral nasal mucosa. This results in a poor cosmetic appearance and a variable degree of mucosal irritation secondary to exposure. A dorsal midline, single pedicle advancement flap can be advanced over the septum to improve cosmetic results and help protect the otherwise exposed mucous membranes and exposed cartilage surfaces.

SURGICAL TECHNIQUE

(A) After complete nasal planectomy, a 10- to 15-mm-wide advancement flap can be incised in increments of sufficient length to stretch forward and downward over the nasal septum (dashed lines). Slightly diverging incisions are used as the flap is incised progressively.

(B) The terminal end of the flap is sutured to the lower cutaneous border created after nasal planectomy. Fine 4-0 monofilament sutures are used to atraumatically secure the flap into position. The dermal surface of the flap usually contacts the rostral edge of the nasal septum. Note that redundant skin folds are created lateral to the flap after advancement.

(C) The remaining skin folds are sutured to the edges of the mucosa exposed after nasal planectomy. The crescent folds of skin simulate the curve of the resected lateral nasal cartilages to improve the cosmetic and functional outcome after complete nasal planectomy.

COMMENTS

Simple flap advancement, and the skin ridges created, help cover the remaining nasal septal cartilage and exposed mucosa after resection of the nasal planum. Use of this technique in part depends on the availability of skin for mobilization as a single pedicled advancement flap. The cosmetic improvements can be quite favorable compared to the classic "Phantom of the Opera" or skeletal appearance of dogs and cats after planectomy. Partial coverage of the mucosa can decrease damage to this delicate epithelial layer from desiccation and exposure to the elements. An Elizabethan collar should be used to protect the surgical site until suture removal.

Plate 112

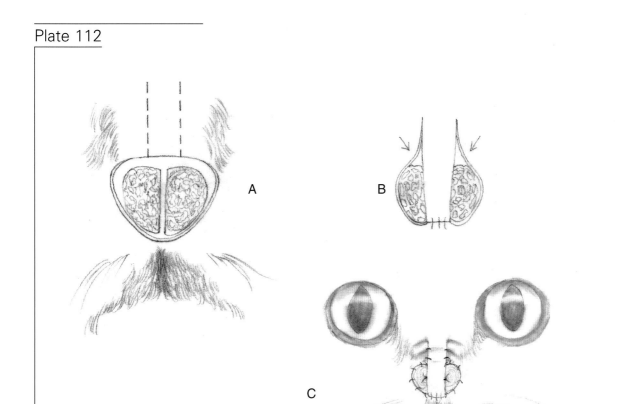

A

B

C

Plate 113   **Bilateral Sulcus Flap Technique**

DESCRIPTION

Selective resection of lesions confined to the rostral septal region can be closed with two small transposition flaps, using the left and right "sulcus" regions, along the lower borders of the common nasal meatus.

SURGICAL TECHNIQUE

(A) A lesion confined to the rostral aspect of the septal region is prepared for surgical resection.

(B) After resection of the lesion, two 10-mm flaps are outlined (dashed lines) of sufficient length to reach the dorsal border of the surgical defect. Note that the base of each 90-degree transposition flap is separated in order to avoid compromising circulation entering the pedicle of each sill flap.

(C) Each flap is rotated dorsally and sutured into position with 4-0 monofilament sutures.

(D) The shared medial borders of each flap are carefully sutured. An anchor suture may be placed along the lateral border and secured to the adjacent septal mucosa, if necessary. The donor site of each flap is closed directly.

COMMENTS

The sulcus flaps use the pigmented epithelium adjacent to the defect for optimal cosmetic results. Because these flaps are small and their capillary circulation fragile, meticulous, atraumatic surgical technique and careful suture placement are essential for an optimal outcome. This is a highly vascular area: electrocautery and topical vasoconstricting agents are useful to control hemorrhage after surgical resection of the lesion. A surgical laser unit can be very effective in minimizing hemorrhage. Postoperatively, an Elizabethan collar should be used to protect the delicate flap from rubbing and pawing by the patient. Provided that tissues are viable, small areas of dehiscence can be reinforced with additional sutures.

Plate 113

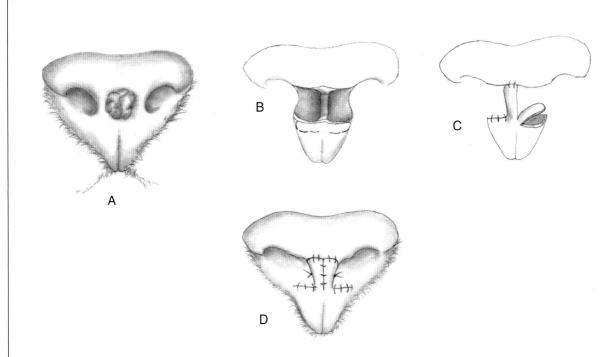

Plate 114   # Septal Resection Technique

DESCRIPTION

There are occasions in which neoplasms, such as squamous cell carcinoma, are confined to the rostral nasal septum without infiltration of the nasal planum. It is possible to elevate the central planum as a dorsally based flap, thereby preserving this tissue while gaining access to the isolated lesion.

SURGICAL TECHNIQUE

(A) The dashed line represents the site for incising the central nasal planum.

(B) The scalpel blade is angled 5–10 mm caudal to the surface of the planum. A skin hook facilitates elevation of the "hinge" flap. Hemorrhage is controlled with electrocautery, topical vasoconstrictors, and topical hemostatic agents. A laser surgical unit can be very effective in limiting hemorrhage.

(C) The diseased segment of septal cartilage is resected with a sufficient margin of normal tissue (10 mm minimum). The mass is submitted for histopathological analysis.

(D) When hemorrhage has been controlled, the flap is resutured into position using a simple interrupted suture pattern.

COMMENTS

With the use of a self-retaining retractor, aggressive excision of the cartilaginous nasal septum can be accomplished; the external cosmetic appearance after replacement of the hinge flap is often completely normal. As discussed, the number one priority is obtaining adequate surgical margins around the neoplasm. This flap technique should be considered when it is apparent that the tumor is confined to the septum but has not invaded the rostral nasal planum. Like other nasal surgical procedures, hemorrhage can be significant; smaller patients in particular may be candidates for a transfusion. A laser surgical unit may help minimize this surgical complication. An Elizabethan collar is used to protect the area from self-mutilation for approximately 2 weeks.

Plate 114

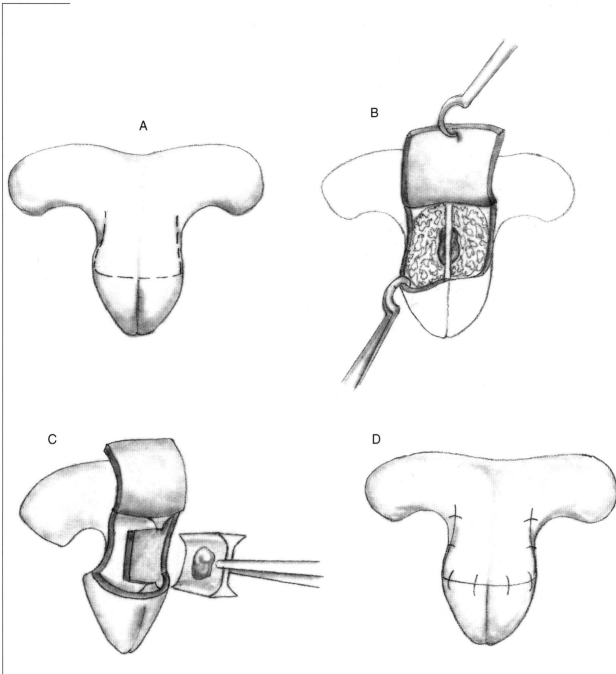

A

B

C

D

Plate 115   **Alar Fold Flaps**

DESCRIPTION

Nasal planectomy generally is reserved for the removal of invasive tumors. The lateral nasal cartilage or alar folds are not involved in the disease process in some cases. In this example, a subtotal planectomy is performed and a "nose" is fashioned from the lateral cartilages to improve cosmetic results and help shelter the exposed nasal mucosa from irritation secondary to environmental exposure.

SURGICAL TECHNIQUE

(A) Outline of resection of a malignant tumor.

(B) Complete resection of the rostral lip, philtrum, and nasal planum. The alar folds, not involved in the disease process, were preserved. The dashed lines represent the tips of the alar folds that require resection.

(C) The folds are rotated upward, the cut ends of which are sutured together.

(D) The dorsal borders of the alar folds are sutured to the adjacent cutaneous border. The dashed lines represent the site for bilateral full-thickness labial advancement flap incisions.

(E) The bilateral advancement flaps of the lip are sutured together in three layers: mucosal, musculofascial, and cutaneous surfaces independently. Note the dorsal mucosal borders of the labial advancement flaps are sutured to the mucosa along the gingival border.

(F) The skin incisions are sutured to complete the procedure.

COMMENTS

This is one option for creating some semblance of a pigmented nose for the dog. It must be stated that obtaining surgical margins is a priority in cancer surgery and should not be sacrificed at the expense of obtaining a more satisfactory cosmetic outcome. However, indiscriminate removal of tissues in the absence of clinical judgment is unsatisfactory. Computer-aided tomography may be useful to help define the limits of the tumor. An Elizabethan collar should be used to prevent rubbing and pawing of the area postoperatively. Nasal discharge should be expected: cleaning with moistened, cotton-tipped applicators should be gentle and minimized during the first 10–14 days after surgery.

Plate 115

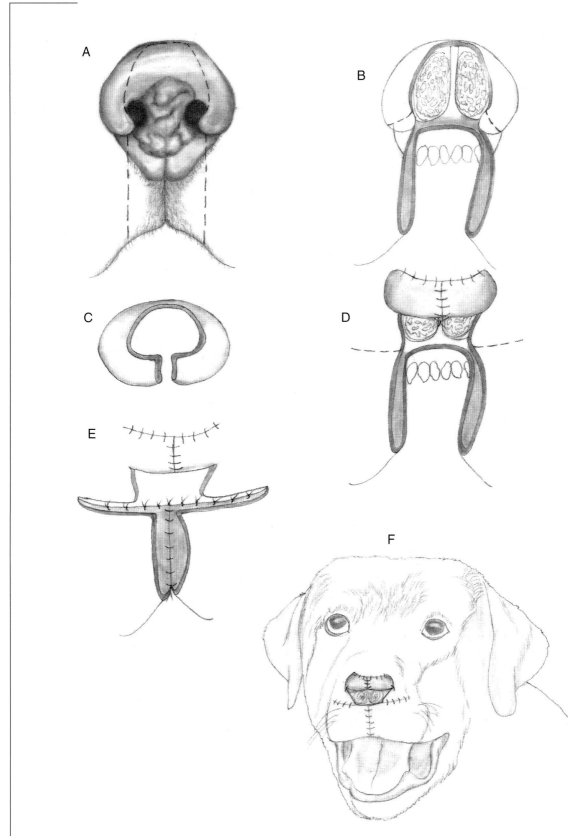

Plate 116   **Musculofascial Island Labial Flap**

DESCRIPTION

With extensive tumor invasion, the nasal planum and rostral upper labial tissues may require wide resection to achieve adequate surgical margins. Adjacent labial tissue can be used to reconstruct the nasal defect.

SURGICAL TECHNIQUE

(A) The dashed lines represent the limits of surgical removal of a neoplasm, which has extensively invaded the nasal planum.

(B) Resection of the entire nasal planum and rostral labial area.

(C) A full-thickness incision is made approximately 3–4 cm from the rostral border of the remaining (left) lip in this clinical example. The dashed lines define the area where the skin will be dissected free of the underlying musculofascial pedicle. The arrows signify the similar site for mucosal resection.

(D) A musculofascial flap is created with a terminal island of labial epithelium (skin, labial margin, labial mucosa).

(E) The musculofascial island flap is rotated upward and placed over the exposed nasal cavity. Skin borders are trimmed to create a symmetrical labial island, prior to suturing the opposing cutaneous borders (3-0 monofilament, nonabsorbable sutures). The flap's labial mucosa is sutured in a similar fashion, using absorbable sutures. The musculofascial pedicle is covered by the advancing facial skin.

Plate 116

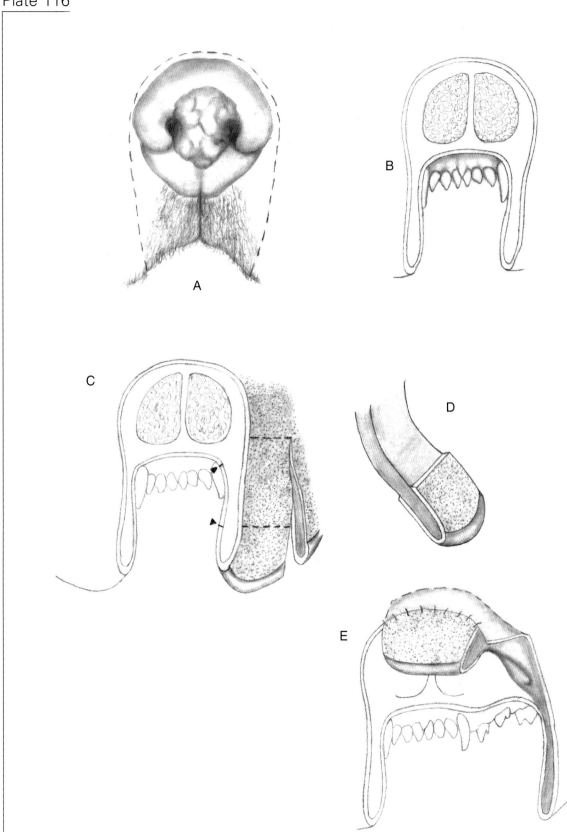

Plate 116

(Continued)

(F) Bilateral full-thickness labial advancement flaps are created (dashed lines) to close the labial defect.

(G) Mucosal borders (lip to gingiva, lip to lip) are apposed with absorbable sutures; skin is sutured with nonabsorbable sutures. The middle musculofascial layer of the lips also can be sutured to further minimize the risk of postoperative wound dehiscence.

(H) Completion of the closure. The transplanted lip now covers a single, large, common nasal opening.

COMMENTS

The island labial flap creates a protective "canopy" over the nasal mucosa and exposed cartilage borders. There is a more natural appearance both in frontal and side views of the patient. The bilateral labial advancement flaps can be trimmed of redundant skin and mucosa in order to give a more natural rostral curvature to the recreated lip. Otherwise, the reconstructed lip will be somewhat wider and straighter than the original labial silhouette. This is a somewhat minor cosmetic consideration.

Plate 116

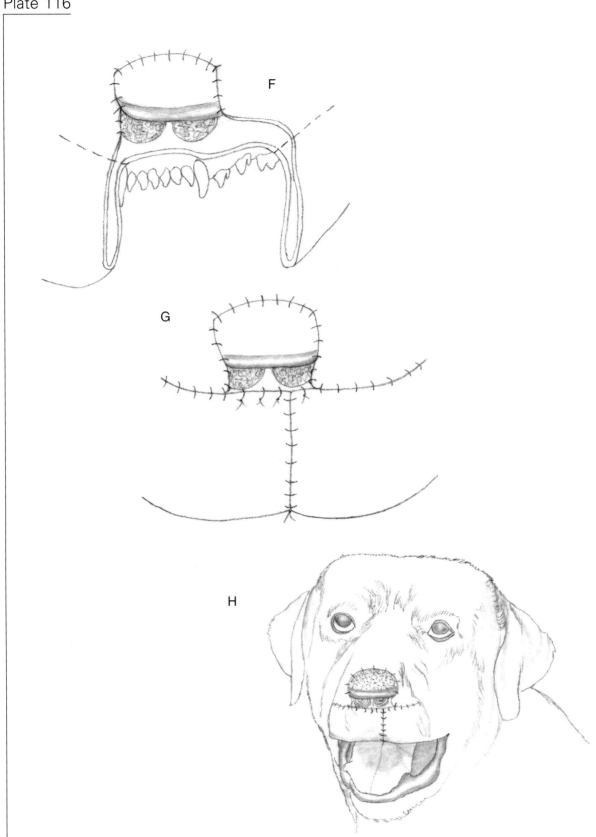

F

G

H

Plate 117 ## Cantilever Suture Technique

DESCRIPTION

Rostral maxillectomy can result in the ventral collapse or drooping of the nasal cartilage. This downward deviation can decrease the ability of the dog to breathe through each common nasal meatus. This cosmetic and functional defect can be offset by using a buried mattress suture to elevate the nasal cartilage.

SURGICAL TECHNIQUE

(A$_{1,2}$) Rostral maxillectomy for an oral neoplasm, with subsequent closure, using the upper labial mucosa. Loss of this tissue support can result in significant ventral deviation of the nasal cartilages.

(B) Downward deviation of the nasal cartilage is assessed upon completion of rostral maxillectomy. Placement of the dog in sternal recumbency and elevation of the head will enable the surgeon to determine the severity of the nasal cartilage deviation. Those patients with pronounced deviation are candidates for this technique.

(C) A midline skin incision, 3–5 cm long, is made over the muzzle, rostral to the medial canthus of each eye. The skin is undermined and retracted to expose the bone. Self-retaining retractors will facilitate exposure.

(D$_{1,2}$) A small (1/16 inch) Steinman pin is inserted into a Jacobs pin chuck. The pin is driven below the silhouette of the nasal bone to the opposite side, as illustrated. A 16- or 18-gauge needle is placed in the hole, serving as a guide for the threading of 0 or 1 monofilament polypropylene suture strands. A long, straight cutting needle is preferable. One or two sutures may be employed, depending on the size of the patient.

Plate 117

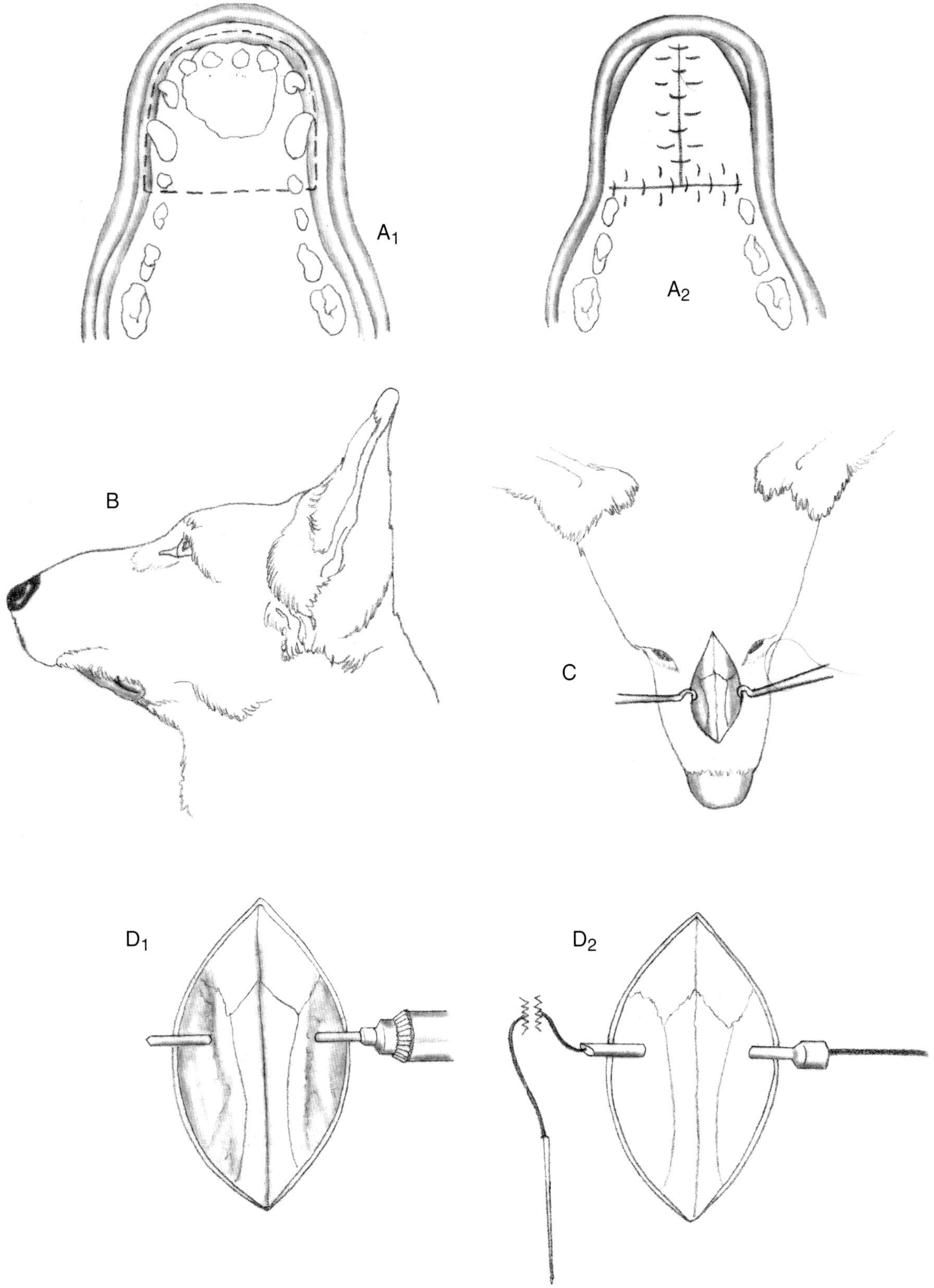

A₁

A₂

B

C

D₁

D₂

Plate 117

(Continued)

(E) A 1-cm incision is made through the epithelial surface of each lateral cartilage, as illustrated. The illustration shows the general course of the cantilever suture.

(F) A close-up view of the nasal cartilage. The straight needle is passed beneath the epithelial surface and guided out of the lateral cartilage incision(the left incision in this example). The needle is redirected across the nasal cartilage and out the opposite incision. The straight needle then is directed back to the original midline incision.

(G) The first throw of a surgeon's knot is used to help assess the most appropriate tension to apply to the cantilever suture before completing the knot.

(H) The dorsal incision is closed. The lateral nasal cartilage incisions do not require suture closure. The cantilever suture recesses into cartilage below the epithelial surface, partially collapsing these access incisions.

COMMENTS

This technique can be quite effective in elevating the nasal cartilage. However, tightening the suture will create a depression or dimple in the lateral nasal cartilages. Although this could be avoided by making deeper access incisions, there is greater purchase of cartilage by using the technique illustrated. An Elizabethan collar is advisable during the first 10–14 days after surgery.

In one clinical case, the dog struck his nose several months later, resulting in a small amount of ventral deviation of the nasal cartilage. This particular patient did not require reoperation.

Plate 117

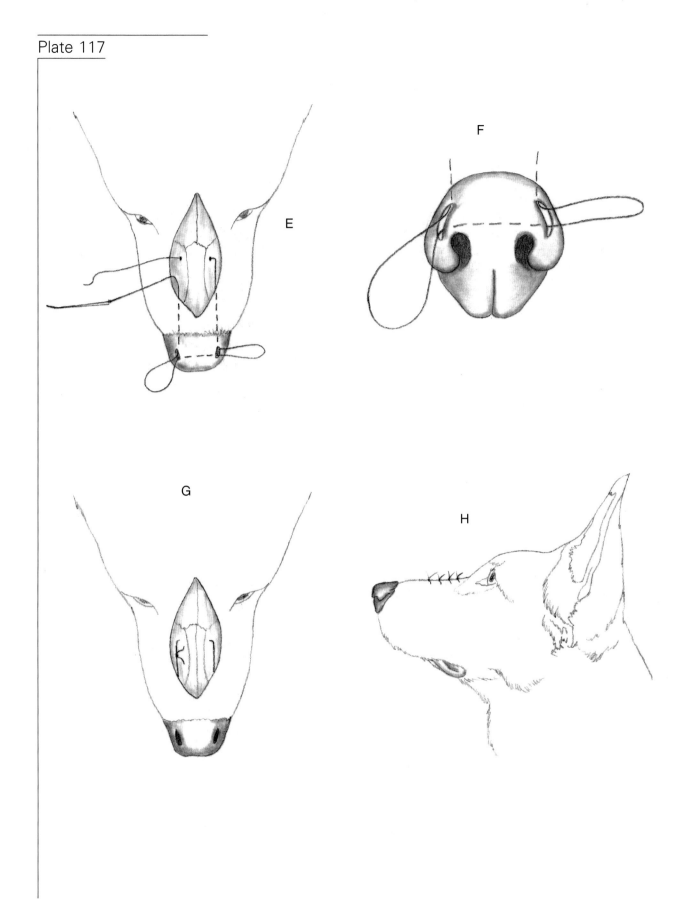

E

F

G

H

Plate 118	**Labial Mucosal Inversion Technique**

DESCRIPTION

Gallegos et al. (2007) reported a labial mucosal technique for closure of defects involving the nasal planum and adjacent rostral labial tissue in two dogs. The technique involves inverting the labial mucosa by suturing the adjacent labial mucosal borders around the circumference of the resected nasal cartilage. This is followed by apposition of the opposing labial margins. The infolded or inverted mucosa forms a recessed antechamber to the nasal cavity.

SURGICAL TECHNIQUE

(A) Resection of the external nose and adjacent labial tissue.

(B) The adjacent labial mucosal borders are secured with sutures to the circumference of the incised edge of the remaining nasal cartilage. The curved arrows denote the elevation of the incised labial mucosal margins toward the dorsal midline. The asterisks identify the final location of the incised edges of the lower labial area. See (C).

(C) The labial mucosa sutured around the circumference of the nasal cartilage border. Note a portion of the labial margins is resected (brackets): this will allow for apposition of these opposing cut surfaces to reestablish the labial midline beneath the nasal area. An incision also is created in the labial mucosa from the left to right side: the solid line represents the midpoint (M) of this mucosal incision. The dashed lines represent the location where this mucosal incision will fold on itself (curved arrows). Absorbable sutures are used to secure this mucosal incision. The closure of this mucosal incision will separate the oral and nasal compartments.

(D) The opposing (excised) labial borders are sutured together in two layers (mucosa, skin), completing the procedure. The faint dotted line represents closure of the mucosal incision described in (C). The pigmented labial margin borders the mucosal antechamber to the nasal cavity.

COMMENTS

The procedure reportedly provides a better cosmetic result than nasal planectomy alone, although other reconstructive techniques (in this chapter) also are available to improve functional and cosmetic results. The folded labial margins create a labial mucosal antechamber, cloaking the nasal cavity. This provides an elliptical labial opening, protecting the delicate nasal mucosa from direct exposure to the external environment.

Plate 118

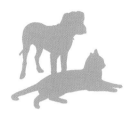

21

Cosmetic Closure Techniques

COSMETIC CONSIDERATIONS

Surface scars generally are considered secondary in importance to the successful closure of a wound. The veterinarian is frequently relieved when a large open wound finally is covered with an epithelial surface and considers the final product, in relative terms, superior to the original wound. Today, most owners are aware of the advances in human cosmetic surgery. More individuals expect a higher-quality surgical "product" for the money spent on their pet. Owners naturally take great pride in their pets' appearance. Breeders and trainers of show dogs wish to conceal scars and blemishes that detract from their canine and feline investments. Even the less particular owners occasionally judge the overall quality of a surgery by the visible component: the quality of the closure.

The author has not been a proponent of cosmetic surgery in animals for the sake of cosmetics alone. However, the veterinary surgeon should know how to minimize scarring and optimize cosmetic results when surgery is required to close a wound, excise tumors, or remove unstable scars. Indeed one of the greatest achievements of a surgeon is the successful restoration of function to a damaged area without leaving a visible scar as a reminder.

CAUSES OF SCARS

All wounds heal, to a variable degree, by scar tissue, and owners must be advised of this inevitable result. The surgeon has the potential to modify the size and severity of the scar and mask its presence. A basic understanding of the causes of excessive scar formation is necessary to help "control" this process.

As noted in Chapters 2 and 3, open wounds can heal by wound contraction and epithelialization. Initially, elastic retraction of skin edges and severe tissue trauma can make accurate assessment of the wound difficult. As inflammation and swelling subside, the true magnitude of the injury is more apparent. The subsequent decrease in skin tension enables wound contraction to proceed. If sufficient skin peripheral to the wound is available, centripetal advancement of skin over the defect proceeds over the first 6 weeks. Thereafter, the remainder of the open wound must close primarily by epithelialization. In veterinary medicine, wound contraction is largely a beneficial response when loose skin is present to promote myofibroblastic contraction. Full-thickness movement of the skin over

the wound minimizes the size of the epithelialized scar. In contrast, those processes that impede contraction result in wounds that require epithelial cell migration to complete the closure. Epithelialized scars lack the properties of normal skin. Moreover, in fur-bearing animals the poor cosmetic results are highlighted by the hairless patches that form, especially in animals that lack a dense hair coat. Gaping wounds are more likely to form visible epithelialized scars unless accurately approximated to minimize the width of the wound. In some cases, it may be more practical to resect scars upon completion of healing by second intention to improve functional and cosmetic results (Fig. 21-1).

> Scar revision is easier to perform after second intention healing is complete and regional inflammation has subsided.
> Scar excision is followed by accurate apposition of the healthy skin bordering the defect.

MINIMIZATION OF SCARRING

Surgical Technique

Meticulous atraumatic surgical technique helps to minimize scarring. Not all wounds closed by accurate approximation remain as thin scars. The elastic retraction of skin borders under tension may result in wider scars. Meticulous use of subcuticular patterns can help offset elastic retraction. W-plasty (Plate 120) and Z-plasty (Plate 17) in humans also can position a major component of the scar into a neighboring skin fold or crease, thus hiding its presence. Alteration of the angle of incision relative to tension lines also reduces visibility of the resultant scar. Relieving skin tension peripheral to a wound can help offset widening of the scar after primary closure. Carefully placed bandages can be used to protect the healing closure from external trauma or tissue disruption.

Suture Considerations

Suture patterns and suture materials and their duration of implantation can influence the severity of the scar. This is particularly true for the external skin sutures. Finer-diameter suture materials enable the surgeon to use greater numbers of sutures for meticulous skin apposition. Everting suture patterns (e.g.,

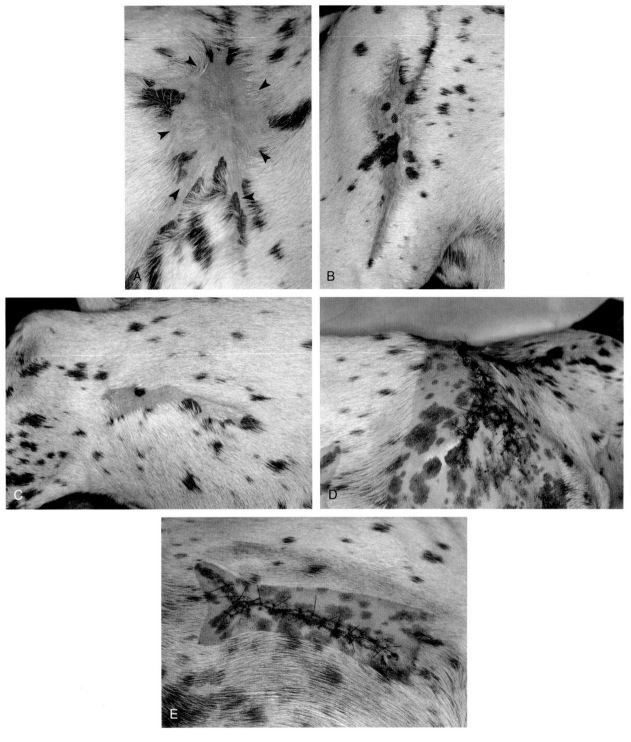

FIG. 21-1 (A, B, C) Retriever with multiple fragile scars, as a result of vehicular trauma. This large scar (arrows) was overlying the right shoulder.

(D, E) Several weeks after healing, scars were resected, and normal fur-bearing skin was apposed using a buried intradermal suture pattern followed by simple interrupted sutures (3-0 monofilament nylon). Improved cosmetic results were achieved, although selective areas had limited "scar spread" weeks after closure. Scar resection back to normal, fur-bearing skin. Hair regrowth covered the smaller surgical scars.

vertical mattress suture pattern) are preferable to patterns that invert skin edges. Inverted scars create shadows in areas with sparse hair growth. Similarly, improperly placed sutures that fail to sufficiently stabilize skin borders can result in inverted skin edges or undesirable "stair stepping," in which one skin border is elevated above the opposite skin edge. In thicker skin, split-thickness suture placement through the opposing dermal borders can accurately align skin margins and limit this displacement of cutaneous margins.

Early removal of sutures (within a week) reduces the likelihood of suture tract inflammation. The use of a fine (3-0 to 5-0) subcuticular pattern in combination with smaller-diameter skin sutures (3-0 to 5-0) provides an excellent means of supporting the skin. Alternate sutures are removed, beginning after day 5 in an uncomplicated wound. Skin tapes used to support skin wounds after early suture removal in human cosmetic surgery are not particularly well suited for use in small animals. Carefully placed bandages, however, can provide added protection to the wound, if necessary. Skin staples and surgical glues have been used for skin apposition in animals. Although a controlled study comparing cosmetic results is lacking, closure appears to be adequate for routine surgical use. Optimal apposition, however, still is best achieved by suturing by hand.

When feasible, skin incision and subsequent closure perpendicular to the direction of hair growth will cover the resultant scar more effectively. While this is likely to be irrelevant in breeds with dense and long hair coats, it is more important in patients with short hair coats because they tend to show scars much more readily. In some cases, access incisions to underlying body structures can be "hidden" by placing them into a less visible site.

Suggested Readings

Grabb WC, Smith JW. 1979. *Plastic Surgery*. Boston: Little, Brown and Co.

Swaim SF. 1980. *Surgery of Traumatized Skin: Management and Reconstruction in the Dog and Cat*. Philadelphia: WB Saunders.

Plate 119   **Scar Concealment**

DESCRIPTION

Incisions can be positioned to improve concealment of surgical scars. This is most frequently requested by owners of show dogs, especially those breeds with a short hair coat.

SURGICAL TECHNIQUE

(A) When feasible, closure of wounds perpendicular to hair growth can reduce the visibility of the resultant scar.

(B) In comparison, the linear scar from wound closure parallel to the hair growth pattern is more likely to be visible.

(C) Incisions can be placed in a less discernable area. Example: A medial arthrotomy incision is less visible compared to a lateral incision overlying the knee. Carefully undermining and retracting of the skin border still permits lateral arthrotomy.

COMMENTS

Positioning of the scar depends upon the laxity and elasticity of the skin, local skin tension, and the shape of the defect requiring closure. Concealment of scars requires careful thought and planning by the surgeon to optimize the cosmetic outcome.

Plate 119

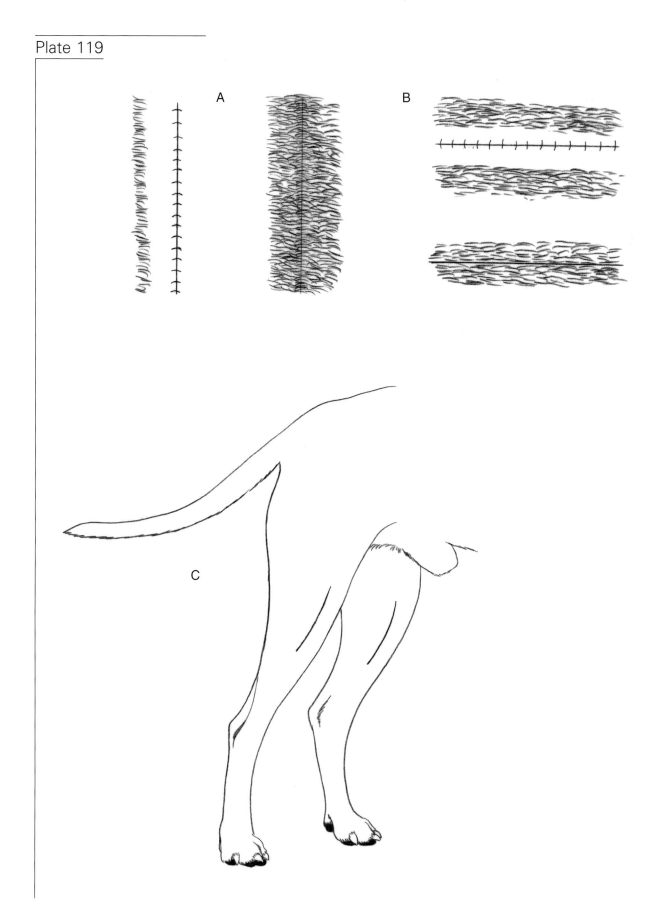

A

B

C

Plate 120   # W-Plasty

DESCRIPTION

W-plasty is a means of breaking a linear scar into a zigzag design, thereby reducing its visibility.

SURGICAL TECHNIQUE

(A) A W-plasty template is created from X-ray film, plastic, or metal. The general outline and measurements of the W-plasty template are illustrated. Equilateral triangles (60-degree angles) can be used for the sake of simplicity.

(B) A fine-point marking pen or a toothpick inserted in a vial of gentian violet or methylene blue dye is used to draw the outline of the template outside the border of the scar. Opposing patterns are offset to allow each line to interdigitate properly with an equal number of triangles. The ends of the W-plasty are in the form of Ammon's triangles to prevent "dog ears."

(C) A no. 11 or 15 scalpel blade is used to incise along the outline. A fine subcuticular pattern, 3-0 to 5-0, can be placed in the deep dermal surface in the center of each flap for initial apposition.

(D) Simple interrupted skin sutures (3-0 to 5-0) are placed in each flap to complete the closure.

COMMENTS

W-plasty has been reported to reduce scar expansion postoperatively by aligning the new zigzag scar, in part, with skin tension lines. Its use is most applicable for cosmetic scar revision rather than primary closure. It is best to avoid this technique if there is excessive tension perpendicular to the scar that would preclude proper execution of the w-plasty procedure, which requires a degree of skin laxity.

Plate 120

A

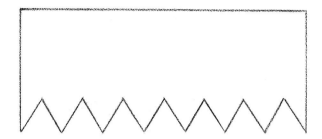

B

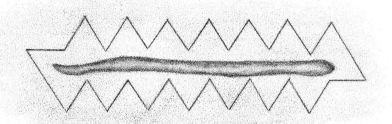

C

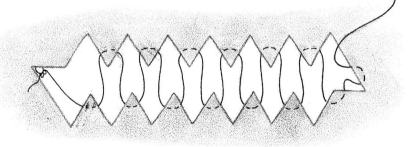

D

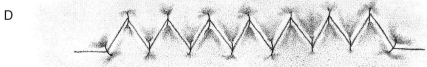

Plate 121   **Dog Ear: Surgical Correction**

DESCRIPTION

"Dog ears" are skin puckers or folds that occasionally form at the end of incisions or at the base of skin flaps. This bunching of skin usually is the result of closing the sides of the wound at too great of an angle. A dog ear also can result when one side of the ellipse is longer than the other, resulting in redundant skin (on one side) at the end of the incision. It is occasionally desirable to remove these skin folds for optimum cosmetic results.

SURGICAL TECHNIQUE

(A) Fusiform defects with a 4:1 length-to-width ratio rarely form dog ears upon closure.

(B) This is an example of excision of a dog ear formed by closure of an incision ending at a great angle. Two simple options for elliptical excision (B_1, B_2) of the redundant fold are illustrated. The dashed line denotes redundant skin excised.

(C) This is an example of correction of a dog ear resulting when one side of the incision is redundant compared to its opposing skin border. The dashed line denotes redundant skin to be excised.

COMMENTS

Many dog ears flatten without surgical excision. Thin, elastic skin is less prone to dog ear formation compared to thicker skin, especially over the back and cervical area in the dog. For symmetrical fusiform defects, a length-to-width ratio of 4:1 is reported to prevent dog ear formation. The terminal portion of a fusiform defect can be tapered to minimize skin bunching. However, adherence to such a ratio, in many instances, would create unnecessarily long incisions compared to closure and selective excision of any dog ear(s) that might form. As noted, short fusiform defects in thin, elastic skin may not result in dog ears. Dog ears that form at the base of a flap upon transfer are best left alone in order to avoid circulatory compromise of the pedicle graft from attempted removal. If they fail to flatten upon healing of the surgical area, surgical excision can be undertaken later.

Plate 121

A

B₁

B₂

C

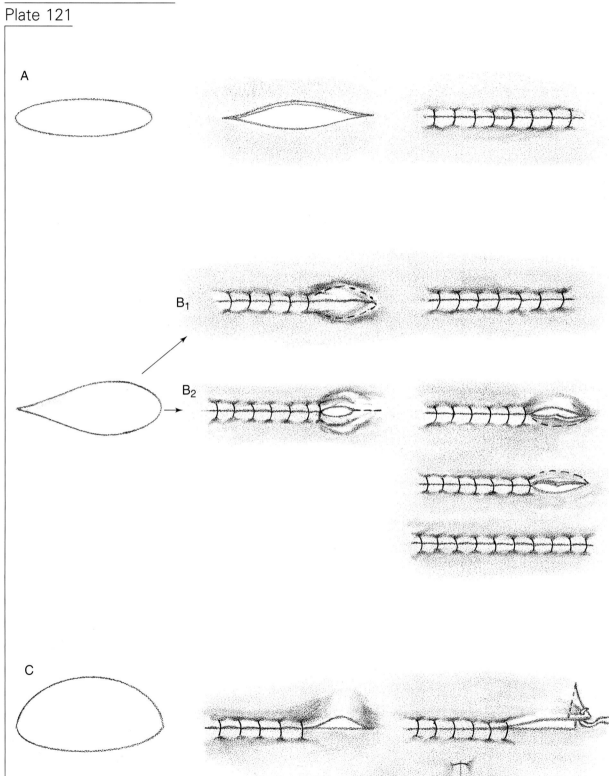

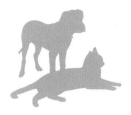

Preputial Reconstructive Surgery

INTRODUCTION

The prepuce is a tubular sheath of skin (parietal layer) lined with mucosa (inner visceral layer) that covers a portion of the penile shaft (pars longa glandis, bulbus glandis). The mucosal layer reflects off the bulbus glandis, forming a fornix, as the mucosa covers the external penis to the urethral orifice. The skin is firmly attached to and continuous with the ventral abdominal skin, forming a sling to support and protect the penis from trauma and exposure. The cranial 1–3 cm of the prepuce protrudes forward from the skin reflecting off the abdominal wall. The preputial orifice normally allows for the unimpeded extrusion and retraction of the penile shaft.

The preputial muscle, located in the hypodermis, is an extension of the cutaneous trunci muscle; it attaches to the cranial and dorsal aspect of the prepuce. The primary function of this muscle is to draw the prepuce forward to cover the glans penis after erection.

The primary source of circulation to the parietal and visceral layers is from the external pudendal artery and dorsal artery of the penis. The visceral layer also is supplied, to a lesser degree, by the artery of the bulb of the penis.

Based on its anatomy and blood supply, the prepuce is easily elevated from the abdominal wall for relocation. Similarly, a central preputial incision can be used to expose the penile shaft without compromising circulation to this structure.

SURGICAL CONDITIONS

The prepuce is susceptible to trauma, although direct trauma from automobile accidents and bite wounds, for example, are relatively uncommon from the author's clinical experience. Foreign bodies also are quite rare, although migrating awns, seeds, or fragments of plant material reportedly can imbed in the preputial cavity, causing a purulent or hemorrhagic discharge. Complete examination of the prepuce and penis can be accomplished by careful retraction and examination through the orifice. In some cases, a narrow vaginal speculum, otoscope, or forceps may be used to better visualize the preputial cavity. In more problematic cases, a midline preputial incision can facilitate examination and surgery of the penis and preputial lining. *Balanoposthitis* is common in male dogs and may mask foreign bodies as an underlying cause of this condition.

Like other anatomic structures, neoplasia is occasionally encountered, including mast cell tumors, carcinomas, papillomas, transmissible venereal tumors, melanomas, and perianal gland tumors. Similarly, tumors of the penis may extend to the prepuce or form a mechanical impediment to normal function of the prepuce and penis. Biopsies are a necessary component to the diagnosis and management of these conditions.

Congenital and acquired anomalies of the prepuce, however, are occasionally noted. This chapter will discuss surgical correction of persistent frenulum, phimosis, paraphimosis, hypospadias, and preputial urethrostomy.

Persistent Frenulum

A condition commonly seen in miniature poodles, cocker spaniels, and Pekingese, persistence of the penile frenulum may also be seen in other breeds. The frenulum normally ruptures by puberty in most dogs. This membranous tissue band connects the ventral penile shaft to the ventral mucosal surface of the prepuce.

The frenulum can prevent extrusion of the penis during physical examination. During penile erection, presence of the frenulum restricts extrusion of the penis and its ventral bowing. Persistent frenulum can contribute to urethral prolapse on rare occasions (Fig. 22-1). Persistent frenulum is easily remedied by cutting the band with a pair of scissors under light sedation. Bleeding is normally minimal.

Phimosis

Phimosis refers to the stenosis or narrowness of the preputial orifice (ostium), preventing extrusion of the penis. (In some cases, dogs may have a small penis relative to the prepuce: this is not phimosis if the penis can be manipulated out of the preputial orifice unimpeded.) The most common cause of phimosis is a small preputial orifice (congenital or acquired secondary to trauma or neoplasia). There are occasions in which neoplasms can partially obstruct the preputial orifice, including mast cell tumors and carcinomas (Fig. 22-2). On occasion, penile tumors or growths may preclude extrusion of the penis, despite a normal preputial opening (Fig. 22-3).

Basic management of phimosis is enlargement of the preputial ostium. Obstructive lesions involving the preputial orifice require removal. Penile masses normally require surgical removal.

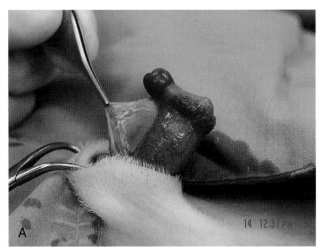
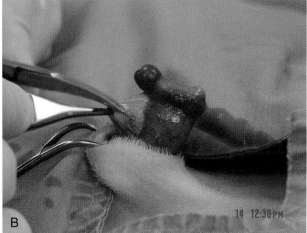
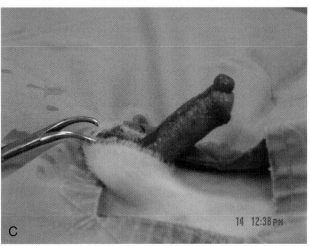

FIG. 22-1 (A) Persistent frenulum in an 8-month-old Yorkshire terrier. Chronic penile traction by the frenulum contributed to formation of urethral prolapse. (B) Simple division with scissors. Bleeding is minimal. (C) Restoration of penile mobility. The urethral prolapse was managed by laser resection and closure with 5-0 absorbable sutures, using a simple interrupted suture pattern.

> The surgical removal of the cranial preputial protrusion to remove a tumor usually does not result in significant penile exposure or paraphimosis.

Paraphimosis

In humans, paraphimosis refers to the strangulation of the glans penis due to retraction of the narrow inflamed foreskin. In veterinary medicine, paraphimosis is defined more broadly as the inability of the penis to retract into the prepuce after its extrusion from the preputial ostium. There are several causes of paraphimosis including the following.

1. Filamentous hair at the tip of the prepuce, wrapping or adhering to the exposed penile shaft. Preputial discharge can serve as a gluelike substrate.

2. Small preputial orifice that entraps the penile shaft.

3. Chronic exposure and drying of the penile surface, causing a friction or drag effect on the outer skin surface of the preputial orifice. The prepuce also may be thin and flaccid, contributing to this condition.

4. Adjacent or underlying scarring (secondary to trauma or caudal abdominal surgery) that restricts preputial coverage of the penile shaft.

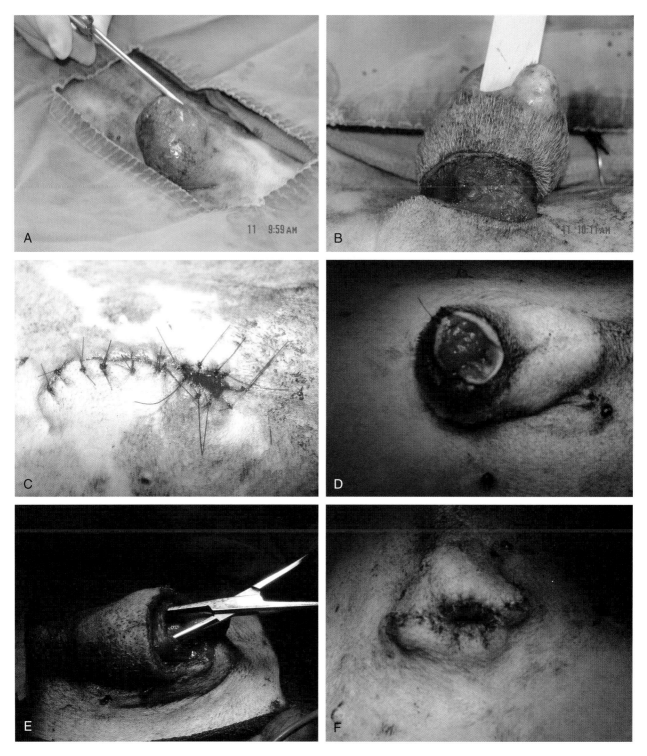

FIG. 22-2 (A) Phimosis secondary to mast cell tumor. (B) Laser resection of this neoplasm. (C) Ventral closure improved penile coverage; the penis was easily extruded through the reformed preputial orifice. (D) Resection of a preputial carcinoma, causing phimosis. (E, F) Resection with a carbon dioxide laser was followed by surgical closure.

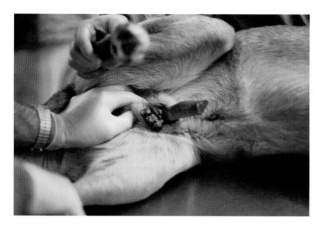

FIG. 22-3 Transmissible venereal tumor in a 6-year-old German shepherd, impairing penile extrusion. Surgical debulking was followed by vincristine chemotherapy.

5. Underdeveloped prepuce (congenital) or preputial tissue loss secondary to trauma or surgery.

6. Ineffectual retractor penis muscle. (The author is not convinced this is a significant factor contributing to paraphimosis.)

> The author does not believe shortening or imbricating the preputialis muscle is either necessary or useful in the correction of paraphimosis. Preputial advancement alone can correct most of these cases. There are other options to correct paraphimosis (below) that do not involve "corrective surgery" of the preputialis muscle.

Of particular concern is the entrapment of the penis secondary to a marginal preputial ostium. Penile erection or traumatic swelling of the extruded penis may occur with a small or inelastic preputial orifice, creating a "rubber band" effect on the penile shaft. Venous and lymphatic outflow is restricted: progressive swelling will collapse the arterial and venous circulation. Without prompt intervention, penile infarction/necrosis follows (Fig. 22-4A).

Most cases of paraphimosis do not result in penile necrosis. Smaller dogs, in particular, can present with paraphimosis despite a seemingly normal preputial opening. The preputial sheath may appear somewhat thin and flaccid, with the penis protruding. The penis can be manually replaced without difficulty, but may intermittently protrude thereafter. The exposed penile mucosa rapidly dries, with loss of its normal lubricating properties. In turn, the skin surrounding the preputial orifice literally is dragged inward as the penile shaft attempts to retract (Fig. 22-4B, C). In some cases, long-term lubrication (Quadritop Ointment [nystatin, neomycin sulfate, thiostrepton, triamcinolone acetonide], Butler Animal Health, Dublin OH) and prompt penile replacement into the preputial cavity (over a period of one month) *by an attentive owner* may allow the desiccated mucosal surface to recover, with restoration of natural lubrication. If this therapy fails, surgical advancement of the prepuce, with preputial ostium enlargement (if necessary), can correct this mild variety of paraphimosis. A second surgical option is phallopexy.

Although uncommon, pelvic trauma or restrictive surgical scars beneath the prepuce (abdominal scar after cystotomy as an example) may result in inadequate penile exposure. Division of the scar followed by preputial advancement is required to correct this cause of paraphimosis (Fig. 22-5). If the preputial orifice is also marginally small, ostium enlargement can be performed at the time of preputial advancement (Fig. 22-6).

Additional penile coverage (1 or 2 cm) can be obtained by excision of the ventral margins of the preputial orifice, creating a slinglike extension of penile coverage. Reciprocally, dorsal enlargement of the orifice will be required. Care must be taken to prevent narrowing of the preputial ostium to the point that it can potentially entrap the penis.

Phallopexy, first described in the horse, is another viable surgical option that has been reported to be effective in managing paraphimosis in dogs. This procedure entails creating a scar between the dorsal penile shaft and less mobile dorsal preputial surface via a dorsolateral preputial incision (see Plate 125). It may be used in place of, or in conjunction with, preputial advancement, depending upon the severity of the case.

Partial penile amputation, as an alternative option, is usually considered if other surgical procedures fail to completely cover the penis. In most cases, only the terminal portion of the penis, anterior to the os penis, would require resection. Intermittent bleeding may be expected for 5–7 days postoperatively.

Major preputial reconstruction has been attempted with the use of mucosal grafts and utilization of the adjacent ventral abdominal skin. These techniques are multistaged procedures that require considerable cost and effort to perform. A more practical approach is to use one or more of the techniques discussed above to improve penile coverage followed by, in many cases, partial penile amputation (if necessary). In severe

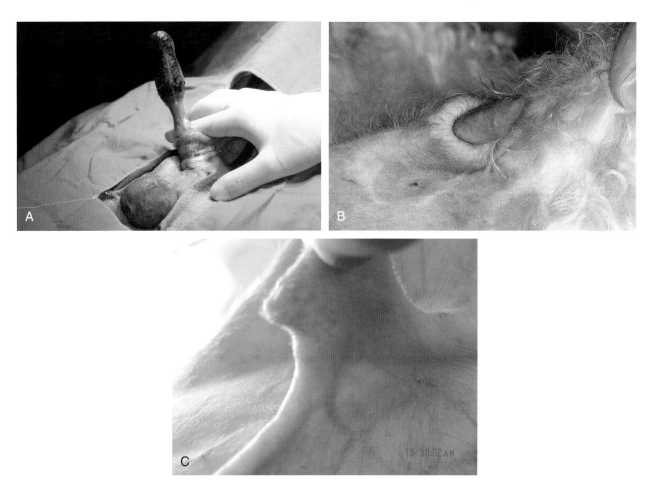

FIG. 22-4 (A) Strangulation necrosis secondary to paraphimosis.

(B) Desiccation of the penis from chronic exposure. Note the inversion of the preputial skin caused by frictional contact with the damaged penile mucosa.

(C) Note the thin, flaccid skin comprising the prepuce. The penis could be manually replaced in the preputial cavity without difficulty. In this case, application of an antibacterial ointment containing triamcinolone (Quadritop, Butler Animal Health) three times a day over the next month was curative. The owner was instructed to replace the penis every time it extruded. If conservative therapy failed, surgical correction would have been performed.

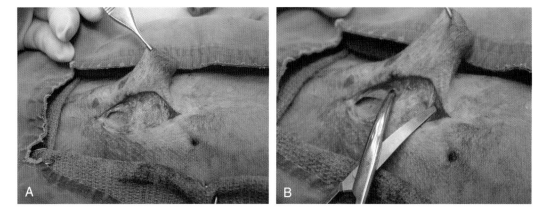

FIG. 22-5 (A) Scar tissue between the base of the prepuce and abdominal wall as a cause of paraphimosis. The dog had previous cystotomies for bladder stones.

(B) Division of the scar. A midline cystotomy was performed to remove stones, followed by preputial elevation and advancement.

620

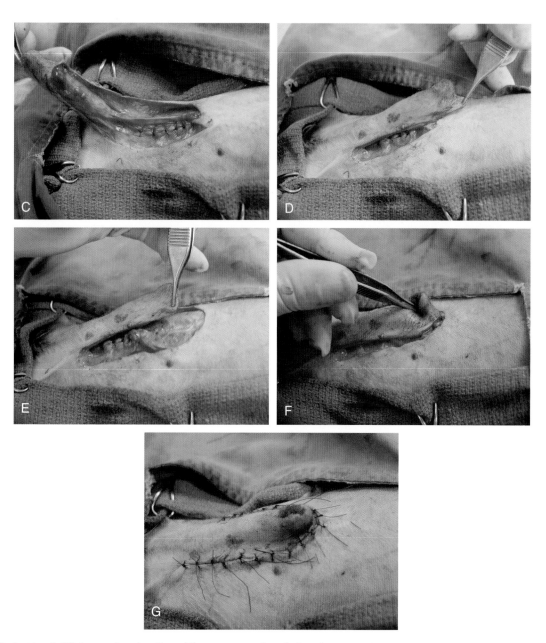

FIG. 22-5 *Continued* (C) Aggressive elevation of the prepuce and penis for advancement.

(D) After preputial elevation, the base of the prepuce is grasped and advanced to determine its new forward location.

(E) Resection of the skin in preparation for preputial advancement.

(F) Intradermal, monofilament nylon sutures were used to secure the prepuce to the fascia of the external abdominal oblique muscle.

(G) Closure of the skin incision, completing the surgery. The preputial orifice was normal diameter and required no corrective enlargement.

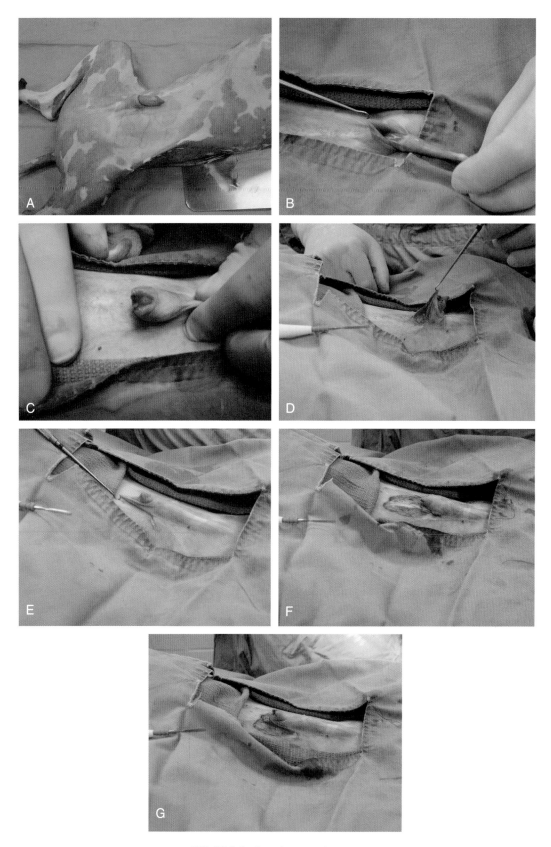

FIG. 22-6 *See legend on opposite page.*

FIG. 22-6 (A) Penile mucosa desiccation secondary to long-term exposure.

(B) Note the delineation between the unexposed and exposed penile mucosa.

(C) A dorsal "release" incision and closure was required to enlarge the preputial orifice.

(D) Following preputial enlargement, the prepuce was advanced.

(E) Forward intraoperative advancement to determine the appropriate location for preputial advancement.

(F) Resection of skin to accommodate the prepuce.

(G) Following securing the cranial base of the prepuce to the external abdominal oblique muscle, the skin incision was closed to complete the procedure.

---

cases, penile amputation with a scrotal or prescrotal urethrostomy is a viable option to consider.

Hypospadias

Embryologically, hypospadias is a failure in fusion of the urogenital folds, resulting in the premature involution of the interstitial cells of the developing testes. The loss of androgen production results in incomplete masculinization of the external genitalia. It has been reported to be most common in the Boston terrier, although the author has seen it in a variety of breeds, including large breed dogs (German shepherds, mixed-breed dogs, Newfoundlands). It is exceedingly rare in the cat (Fig. 22-7). Undescending testicles and renal anomalies have been reported in humans, with one report in the veterinary literature of a renal aplasia and cryptorchidism in an 8-month-old beagle. Urinary incontinence also has been reported in the dog: this has not been noted by the author to date.

Hobson et al. (1978) have described five basic areas in which an abnormal urethral meatus may occur in hypospadias: glandular, penile, scrotal, perineal (subanal), and anal. Of these forms, subanal urethral openings are the greatest concern due to the high incidence of lower urinary tract infections. An abnormal meatus involving the glans or penile shaft (Fig. 22-8) is uncommon and may be noted as an incidental finding. More extensive changes of the external genitalia can be seen with the other forms of hypospadias, with incomplete formation or agensis of the penis and prepuce (Fig. 22-9). A dog with a scrotal or lower perineal urethral meatus essentially urinates in a fashion similar to patients that have had a scrotal or prescrotal urethrostomy. As noted, a urethral meatus adjacent to the ventral anal margin is exposed to fecal

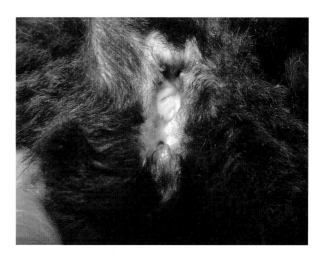

FIG. 22-7 A rare example of hypospadias in a black domestic long-haired cat. The cat had a history of recurrent urinary tract infections due to the proximity of the abnormal urethral orifice to the anus. This was surgically corrected by increasing the distance between these two structures.

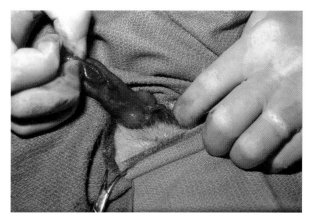

FIG. 22-8 Example of penile hypospadias in a Dalmatian.

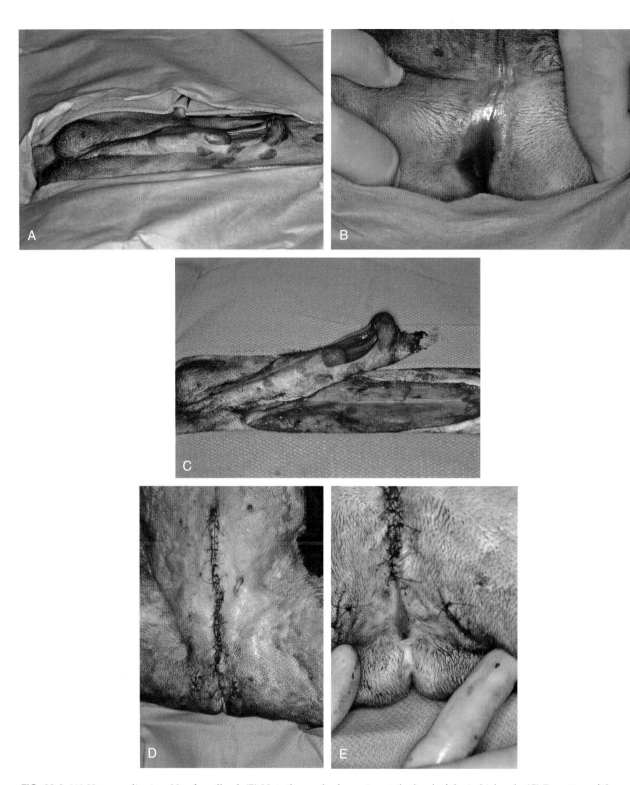

FIG. 22-9 (A) Hypospadias in a Newfoundland. (B) Note the urethral opening at the level of the ischial arch. (C) Resection of the rudimentary penis and prepuce. (D) Closure of the surgical defect. (E) Close-up view of the urethra. Note the two separate incisions required to castrate this dog.

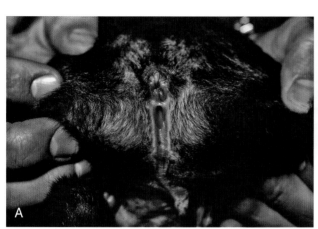
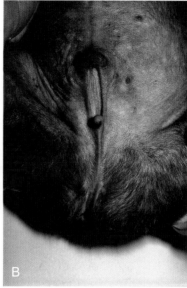

FIG. 22-10 (A) Hypospadias in the perineal area, immediately below the anus. (B) Note the incomplete formation of the penis and prepuce.

contamination, and recurrent bacterial cystitis is commonly seen in these patients (Fig. 22-10). Castration is recommended at the time of corrective surgery for hypospadias (Fig. 22-11).

SURGICAL TECHNIQUES

Preputial Urethrostomy Techniques

In the event of penile necrosis involving the penis at the level of the preputial fornix, the preputial urethrostomy technique is an alternative to prescrotal or scrotal urethrostomy (see Plate 127). The urethral end, after amputation, is anastomosed to the adjacent preputial mucosa. Use of a ventral midline preputiotomy incision will greatly facilitate this surgical technique (Fig. 22-12).

Emergency Enlargement of the Preputial Orifice: Paraphymosis

In those cases of paraphimosis with lymphatic and circulatory compromise to the penis, immediate enlargement of the prepuce may be accomplished with a ventral or dorsal incision (a ventral incision is the easiest to perform). Sedation or the use of a local lido-

caine block may be considered. However, because of the extreme penile swelling and circumferential tension of the preputial orifice, a quick cut with sharp scissors or a scalpel blade may be used to provide immediate tension relief. The lubricated end of a Bard-Parker scalpel handle may be partially inserted between the penis and preputial orifice to protect the penile shaft when a scalpel blade is used. In general, a 10- to 20-mm incision will release the circumferential tension. The exposed penis can be treated with topical lidocaine to reduce local discomfort. K-Y lubrication can be applied to the penis to permit its replacement into the prepuce. Conservative management for paraphimosis includes the application of ointment to prevent desiccation of the exposed penis; systemic corticosteroids also may be considered to reduce edema. Topical 50% dextrose also may be used as a hyperosmotic agent to reduce edema after performing the preputiotomy. Cold compresses may be used to help decrease swelling, but may not be well tolerated by the patient without the adjunctive use of analgesics and sedatives.

The penis is assessed for viability; extensive necrosis usually is associated with a deep purple to black appearance to the entrapped penile shaft. However, hemorrhage, venous stasis, and a mottled appearance of the penile shaft may warrant a conservative "wait and reassess" approach over the next 5–7 days. In many cases, even dramatic swelling of the penile shaft can resolve, provided that extensive tissue necrosis is not present. Patchy areas of mucosal necrosis on the

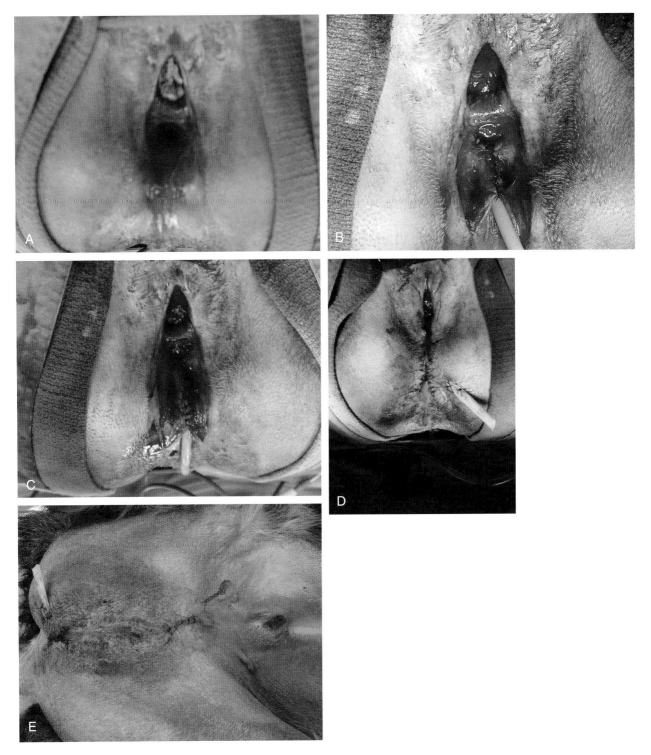

FIG. 22-11 (A) German shepherd with urethral opening immediately below the anus.

(B) Creation of a urethral tube extension with an inversed tubed skin flap.

(C) Completion of the inverse tube.

(D) The skin margins were advanced over the tube flap, completing the procedure.

(E) Abdominal view of rudimentary penis. A small area of irritated epithelium was resected. (From Pavletic MM. 2007. Reconstruction of the urethra by use of an inverse tubed bipedicle flap in a dog with hypospadias. *J Am Vet Med Assoc* 231:71–73.)

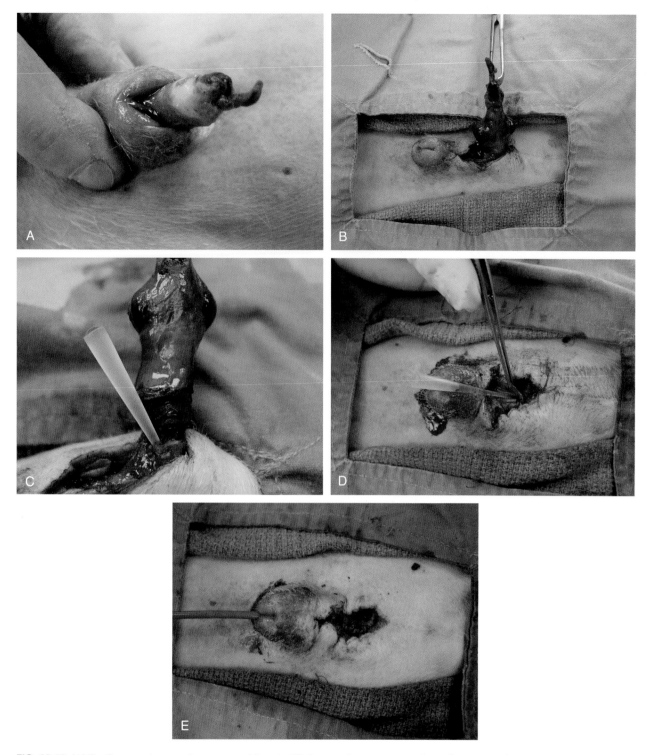

FIG. 22-12 (A) Penile necrosis secondary to paraphimosis. (B) A preputiotomy was performed to expose the necrotic penile shaft. (C) Carbon dioxide laser resection of the necrotic penile segment. (D) Anastomosis of the urethra to the preputial mucosa. (E) Closure of the preputial mucosa. Closure of the skin completed the procedure. (From Pavletic MM, O'Bell SA. 2007. Subtotal penile amputation and urethrostomy in a dog. *J Am Vet Med Assoc* 230:375–77.)

penile surface normally heal by second intention. A urinary catheter may be required if swelling has obstructed the urethra.

Extensive necrosis of the penis is managed by partial penile amputation. *Note:* Although the preputial shortening surgery has been advocated for dogs undergoing partial penile amputation, it has *not been the author's experience that this procedure is at all necessary.* Urine passes through the prepuce unimpeded, without irritation of its mucosal lining.

Permanent Enlargement of the Preputial Ostium

Permanent treatment of phimosis or paraphimosis normally requires enlargement of the preputial orifice. A dorsal incision of approximately 10–15 mm is made through the entire thickness of the prepuce. The incision can be increased in small increments until the penis can be easily extruded. The skin is sutured to the apposing mucosa with 4-0 absorbable sutures, thereby creating a permanent triangular or "pie-shaped" notch. If an emergency ventral preputiotomy incision was performed prior to this procedure (see above), it may be sutured at this time (see Plate 122).

Ventral Preputial Ostium Closure to Improve Coverage to the Penile Tip

If 1–2 cm of additional ventral penile coverage is still required despite aggressive preputial advancement, the mucocutaneous junction of the ventral preputial orifice can be resected: the mucosa and skin are sutured together to give better ventral penile coverage. However, a reciprocal dorsal preputial incision is required to enlarge the prepuce, as discussed above (Plate 123). Ventral preputial closure also can be used in a dog with an excessively large ostium.

Preputial Advancement: Coverage of the Chronically Exposed Penis

Preputial advancement is accomplished by creating a U-shaped incision anterior to the cranial base of the prepuce and advancing the prepuce in a more cranial position. There are a few key points that need to be followed for successful used of this surgical technique. (See Plate 124.)

Phallopexy

Pallopexy was originally reported for use in equine patients. In dogs, a dorsal penile mucosal incision is sutured to a reciprocal dorsal preputial mucosal incision in a position to maintain permanent caudal traction on the penile shaft (see Plate 125). There are insufficient case numbers to determine whether phallopexy or preputial advancement is the superior procedure. These two techniques also may be combined in more challenging cases.

Surgical Management of Hypospadias

Surgical management of hypospadias depends upon the location and severity of the anomaly. Incomplete formation of the penis, prepuce, and scrotum is common, and the abnormal urethral opening will vary in location. The testicles are usually located beneath separate skin or scrotal pouches divided by a rudimentary band of mucosal epithelium between them. If the urethral opening is located anterior to the ischial arch (scrotal or prescrotal area), the patient can urinate relatively normally, in a fashion similar to a dog with a scrotal or prescrotal urethrostomy. If the urethral opening is located in the perineum, a variable degree of urine scalding may be expected. If the urethral opening is immediately below the anus, ascending urinary tract infections are fairly common and may necessitate creation of a urethral tube extension using the available hairless skin and uroepithelium present. This procedure will divert urine ventral to the anus, thereby reducing the potential of fecal contamination; local skin irritation will be noted from urine contact to the adjacent skin unless the area is kept groomed and cleaned. Topical antibiotic ointments may be used to control occasional bouts of dermatitis.

Many articles advise removal of the rudimentary penis and prepuce at the time of castration. Presence of these tissues may be a source of irritation to the dog. However, in many cases, these tissues cause no problem and their removal is not mandatory. Castration, however, is advisable.

Ventral Diversion of the Urine Stream in the Male Dog

Although rare from the author's experience, male dogs may inadvertently urinate on their front legs (unpublished data). This usually is the result of the anatomic

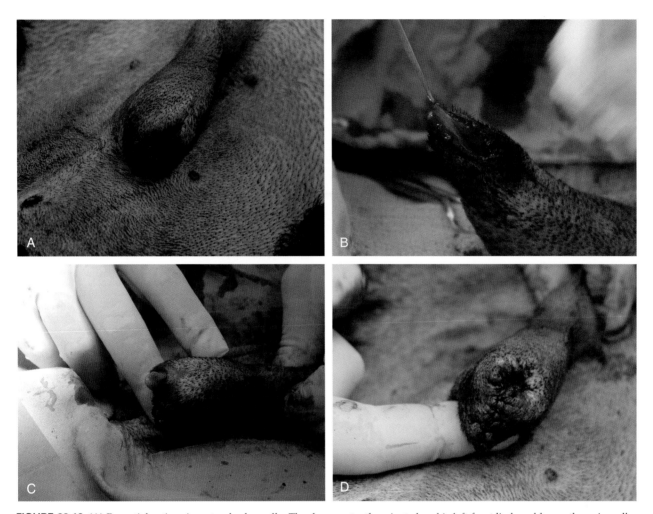

FIGURE 22.13 (A) Preputial ostium in a standard poodle. The dog constantly urinated on his left front limb and lower thoracic wall, at the level of the xiphoid process.

(B) Excision of the mucocutaneous junction of the upper half of the preputial ostium. Absorbable interrupted sutures (4-0) are used to close the mucosa, followed by the skin.

(C) Partial closure of the ostium is followed by enlarging the ostium ventrally, using a midline ventral incision of sufficient length to allow normal extrusion of the penis.

(D) The V-shaped notch created by this incision is closed by suturing the individual mucosal and cutaneous borders separately. The urine stream will strike the closed dorsal ostium site, curving or rerouting flow in a ventral or downward direction.

conformation of the patient's trunk and prepuce. A prominent dome-shaped thorax and unusually elevated (tucked-up) abdominal wall can result in the urine stream exiting the prepuce, striking the lower thorax and/or forelimb. This condition is problematic for the patient and owner, necessitating bathing the urine-soaked area after each urination.

Surgical diversion of the urine stream can be accomplished by altering the preputial ostium. The craniodorsal 50%–60% of the ostium can be closed side-to-side after resection of the mucocutaneous junction in a fashion noted in Plate 124. Absorbable suture (4-0) is used to appose the preputial mucosa and skin. Reciprocal enlargement of the preputial ostium is performed by incising the ventral midline of the ostium sufficiently to easily extrude the penis. The mucosa and skin are sutured in the fashion discussed in Plate 122. As a result, the urine stream strikes the closed cranial preputial ostium, with the stream diverted ventrally (Fig. 22-13).

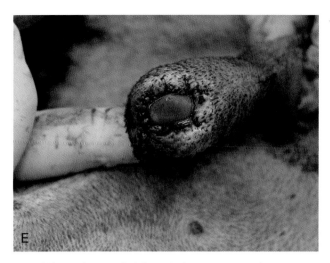

FIG. 22-13 *Continued* (E) The penis could be easily extruded through the new preputial ostium. Postoperatively, the urine stream went directly downward, to the relief of the frustrated owners. (From Pavletic MM, Brum DE. 2009. Diversion of the urine stream by surgical modification of the preputial ostium in a dog. *J Am Vet Med Assoc* [in press].)

Suggested Reading

Ader PL, Hobson HP. 1978. Hypospadias: a review of the veterinary literature and a report of three cases in the dog. *J Am Anim Hosp Assoc* 14:721–727.

Booth HW. 2003. Penis, prepuce, and scrotum. In: Slatter D, ed. *Textbook of Small Animal Surgery*, 3rd ed., 1531–1541. Philadelphia, PA: Saunders Elsevier Sciences.

Fowler JD. 1998. Preputial Reconstruction. In: Bojrab MJ, ed. *Current Techniques in Small Animal Surgery*, 4th ed., 534–537. Philadelphia, PA: Lea and Febiger.

Hobson HP. 1990. Surgical procedures of the penis. In: Bojrab MJ, ed. *Current Techniques in Small Animal Surgery*, 3rd ed., 423–430. Philadelphia, PA: Lea and Febiger.

Pavletic MM. 2007. Reconstruction of the urethra by use of an inverse tubed bipedicle flap in a dog with hypospadias. *J Am Vet Med Assoc* 231:71–73.

Pavletic MM, O'Bell SA. 2007. Subtotal penile amputation and preputial urethrostomy in a dog. *J Am Vet Med Assoc* 230:375–377.

Pope ER, Swaim SF. 1986. Surgical reconstruction of a hypoplastic prepuce. *J Am Anim Hosp Assoc* 22:73–77.

Proescholdt TA, DeYoung DW, Evans LE. 1977. Preputial reconstruction for phimosis and infantile penis. *J Am Anim Hosp Assoc* 13:725–727.

Sarierler M, Kara ME. 1998. Congenital stenosis of the preputial orifice in a dog. *Vet Rec* 143:201.

Schumacher J. 1999. The penis and prepuce. In: Auer JA, Stick JA, eds. *Equine Surgery*, 546–547. Philadelphia, PA: Saunders.

Smith MM, Gourley IM. 1990. Preputial reconstruction in a dog. *J Am Vet Med Assoc* 196:1493–1496.

Somerville ME, Anderson SM. 2001. Phallopexy for treatment of paraphimosis in the dog. *J Am Anim Hosp Assoc* 37:397–400.

Suann CJ, Korney FD. 1983. Surgical treatment of paraphimosis in a pony. *Can Vet J* 11:341–342.

Plate 122   **Preputial Ostium Enlargement**

DESCRIPTION

Enlargement of the preputial orifice or *ostium* is normally performed to correct phimosis and those cases of paraphimosis where the size of this orifice is marginal.

SURGICAL TECHNIQUE

(A$_1$, A$_2$) Cranial and lateral views of the preputial orifice. The dorsal midline incision is created in small increments; the penis is extruded after each progressive incision to assure the penis can easily enter/exit the ostium.

(B$_1$, B$_2$) The penis can be extruded and replaced without difficulty into the prepuce.

(C$_1$, C$_2$) The opposing skin and mucosal borders are sutured with 4-0 absorbable sutures, creating a permanent V-shaped notch.

COMMENTS

In those urgent/emergent cases of paraphimosis with penile entrapment, the ventral ostium is more assessable for temporary emergency enlargement by creating a linear incision using blunt-tipped scissors. A scalpel blade also can be used, but insertion of a lubricated Bard-Parker scalpel handle inside the ostium is advisable, providing a protective shield to the enlarged penis. Provided that the penile viability is maintained, permanent ostium enlargement is performed as illustrated above.

Plate 122

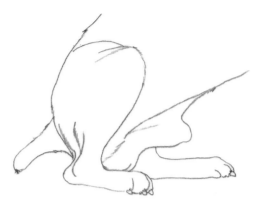

A₁ 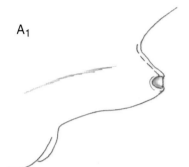   A₂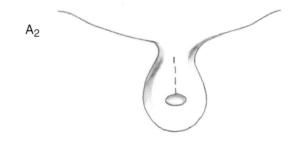

B₁ 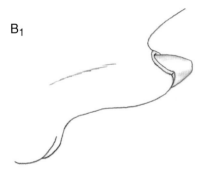   B₂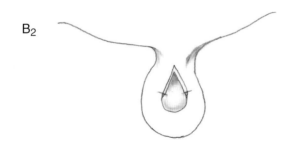

C₁ 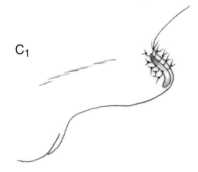   C₂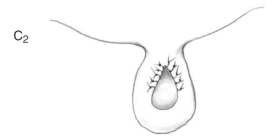

Plate 123 **Preputial Ostium Reduction**

DESCRIPTION

Ventral reduction in the size of the ostium is used for two purposes: correction of an excessively large ostium to prevent penile exposure or to create a ventral sling cover in conjunction with preputial advancement (Plate 124) for moderate to severe cases of paraphimosis. In the latter case, a reciprocal enlargement of the orifice is required (Plate 122).

SURGICAL TECHNIQUE

(A_1, A_2) Lateral and frontal view of the ostium and exposed penile tip.
(B_1, B_2) Excision of the ventral "third" of the mucocutaneous junction of the ostium.
(C_1, C_2) Apposition of the mucosal surface with absorbable 4-0 sutures.
(D_1, D_2) Closure of the cutaneous margins.

COMMENTS

Partial ventral closure of the orifice alone, as a primary treatment for paraphimosis, must be done with caution: should the dog have an erection, strangulation of the exteriorized penis is possible. Intraoperatively, the penis is extruded after surgically manipulating the ostium to help assure this orifice is the appropriate size. The author normally reserves this technique as an adjunct to preputial advancement to gain an additional 1–2 cm of coverage of the penile tip, with reciprocal enlargement of the dorsal portion of the ostium. As noted, phallopexy (Plate 125) also is a surgical option to consider for those challenging cases of paraphimosis.

Plate 123

A₁

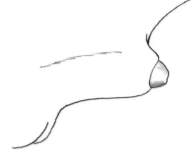

A₂

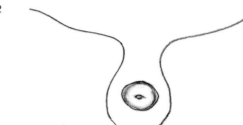

B₁

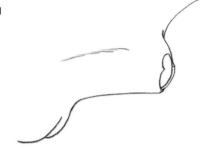

B₂

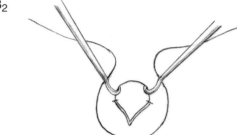

C₁

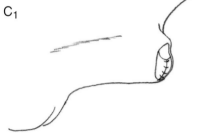

C₂

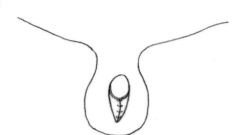

D₁

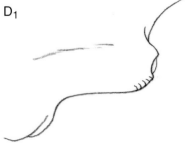

D₂

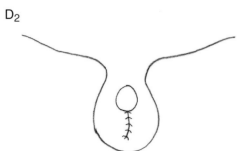

Plate 124   **Preputial Advancement Technique**

DESCRIPTION

Preputial advancement is the most common surgical technique employed for managing paraphimosis. Enlargement of the preputial orifice or *ostium* can be performed if necessary (see Plate 122). An alternative to preputial advancement is a modification of the Bolz phallopexy technique, described in Plate 125.

SURGICAL TECHNIQUE

(A) Example of paraphimosis. The surgeon can initially assess preputial advancement by grasping the prepuce with forceps and applying forward traction.

(B) A curved incision is created from this cranial point in a caudal direction: the width of the curve will approximate the width of the prepuce and attached cutaneous skin margin. A second curved incision is created anterior to the base of the prepuce and extends caudally a few centimeters along the junction of the prepuce and ventral abdominal wall. The skin within this area (dashed lines) is resected.

Plate 124

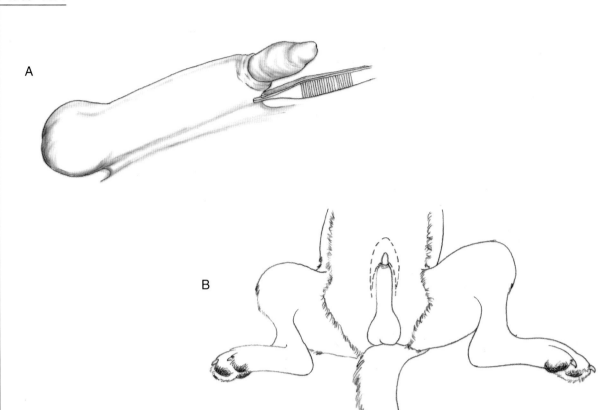

A

B

Plate 124

(Continued)

(C) Skin hooks or stay sutures applied to the incised skin border are ideally suited for forward traction to the undermined prepuce. The prepuce is undermined and the lateral incisions extended to facilitate advancement as needed. The prepuce is ideally advanced to the point at which the penis retracts into the preputial cavity 1–2 cm from the ostium. (It is the author's experience that overcompensation does not create a problem.) Three or four nonabsorbable (monofilament nylon or prolene) or slowly absorbable sutures are used to secure the cranial dermal border of the prepuce to the external abdominal oblique muscle fascia (3-0 or 4-0, depending on the patient size and skin thickness). The hind limbs can be manipulated (flexed and extended) to assure penile coverage is complete. The remaining incision can be closed with an intradermal suture pattern.

(D) This is followed by closure of the skin with a simple interrupted suture pattern (3-0 or 4-0).

COMMENTS

Positioning of the patient's rear legs can affect the outcome of this procedure. The author normally places the legs in a neutral to slightly extended position to promote penile extrusion. Unless this is done, the surgeon may underestimate the forward advancement required to properly cover the penis.

The entire penis and prepuce can be completely elevated from the abdominal wall without compromising their circulation. This would suggest that surgeons can be more aggressive in elevating the prepuce prior to advancement. Any restrictive scar bands that underlie the prepuce must be divided to facilitate preputial advancement.

A key to effective preputial advancement is often overlooked in the veterinary literature: securing the dermal surface of the advanced preputial border to the external abdominal oblique muscle fascia. Otherwise, the elastic skin of the abdomen can stretch, negating the penile coverage gained by this surgical technique. Securing the lead dermal border of the prepuce to the abdominal wall dramatically reduces tension on the skin anterior to the point of advancement.

It has been the author's experience that imbrication or shortening of the preputialis muscle alone cannot correct paraphimosis. Preputial advancement alone can correct paraphimosis without the need to operate on this thin muscle. Simply put, surgical manipulation of the preputialis muscle is not necessary.

If, after maximal advancement, there is persistent exposure of the penile tip, the ventral border of the preputial ostium can be closed to improve ventral coverage. Reciprocally, a small dorsal incision can be made to enlarge the ostium (see Plates 122 and 123).

Partial penile amputation is considered only in those cases where preputial advancement, ventral ostium closure, and/or phallopexy (alone or combined) cannot adequately cover the penis. In this case only a portion of the penis, anterior to the os penis, normally requires removal.

Preputial advancement can be problematic in small dogs with a prominent dome-shaped thorax. Preputial advancement over the more dorsally "tucked" abdominal wall of a dog can result in the urine stream striking the lower curvature of the caudal thorax. This can be remedied by closure of the dorsal ostium, described in Fig. 22-13. Under these circumstances, phallopexy (Plate 125) may be a better surgical alternative in patients with this body conformation.

Surgeons have been concerned about overcompensating for paraphimosis, causing the penis to be displaced too far caudally in the preputial cavity. The fear is that urine irritation will cause balanoposthitis. From the author's clinical experience, this is not a cause for concern. The mucosal lining of the prepuce routinely tolerates urine exposure. Preputial shortening, advocated in some textbook articles after partial penile amputation, is considered unnecessary.

Plate 124

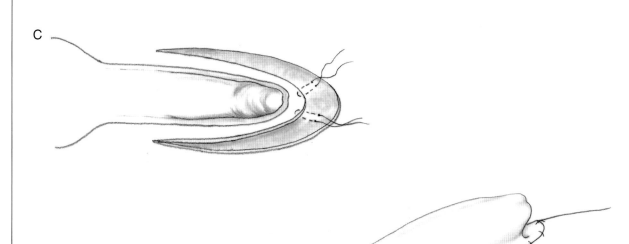

C

D

Plate 125   **Phallopexy**

DESCRIPTION

Phallopexy creates a permanent adhesion between the inner preputial lining and adjacent penile surface to prevent recurrent paraphimosis. It may be used as an alternative to the preputial advancement technique discussed in Plate 124, depending upon the severity of the condition. This is based on the technique published by Somerville and Anderson (2001).

SURGICAL TECHNIQUE

(A)   A 2–4 cm incision is made along the junction of the prepuce and dorsal body wall, approximately 3 cm caudal to the preputial ostium. The incision is extended through the parietal preputial layer, exposing the penile shaft. The excision can be enlarged to facilitate surgical exposure. Small self-retaining retractors are inserted to facilitate visualization.

(B)   A 1.5- to 2-cm incision is created along the dorsal midline of the preputial cavity beginning 3 cm caudal to the preputial ostium: a 5-mm strip of mucosa can be resected to facilitate suture placement. To expose the dorsal penile surface, the penile shaft can be exteriorized through the preputial orifice. It may be possible to exteriorize the penis through the preputial access incision created. (It is the author's experience that it is easier to exteriorize the penis through the preputial access incision created.) Once exposed, a superficial reciprocal penile incision/mucosal strip is created approximately 2 cm from the tip of the penis.

(C)   A trial interrupted suture (3-0 or 4-0, slowly absorbable) is placed at the anterior aspect of the apposed incisions. Exteriorization of the penis is attempted through the preputial orifice. If the penis can be exposed, the dorsal preputial incision can be extended caudally, and the penis resutured to a more caudal portion of the dorsal preputial incision. If complete exteriorization of the penis cannot be performed manually, several (6 to 8) interrupted absorbable sutures are used to appose the dorsal preputial and penile mucosal incisions, completing the phallopexy.

(D, E) Closure of the preputial mucosa is followed by closure of the cutaneous access incision, completing the surgery. Castration can be performed prior to or after phallopexy.

COMMENTS

This is a variation of the Bolz phallopexy technique used to treat paraphimosis in horses. Somerville and Anderson (2001) reported that the dorsal preputial wall is less mobile than its ventral counterpart, possibly providing a better anchor for phallopexy. They also noted that the penile urethra is more superficial ventrally. The author has found, however, a ventral phallopexy is easier to perform using the basic guidelines provided; however, the ventral penile incision is placed approximately 1 cm lateral to the ventral midline of the glans penis to avoid injury to the urethra. The penile mucosal incision is sutured to the ventral preputial mucosal incision used to expose the penis.

   Somerville and Anderson (2001) expressed concern that excessive penile retraction could result in urine pooling with secondary balanoposthitis. The author's experience has indicated this potential complication does not occur, and the risk of this problem has been grossly overstated (or perpetuated) in the veterinary literature. It is for this reason that preputial shortening after partial penile amputation is unnecessary.

Plate 125

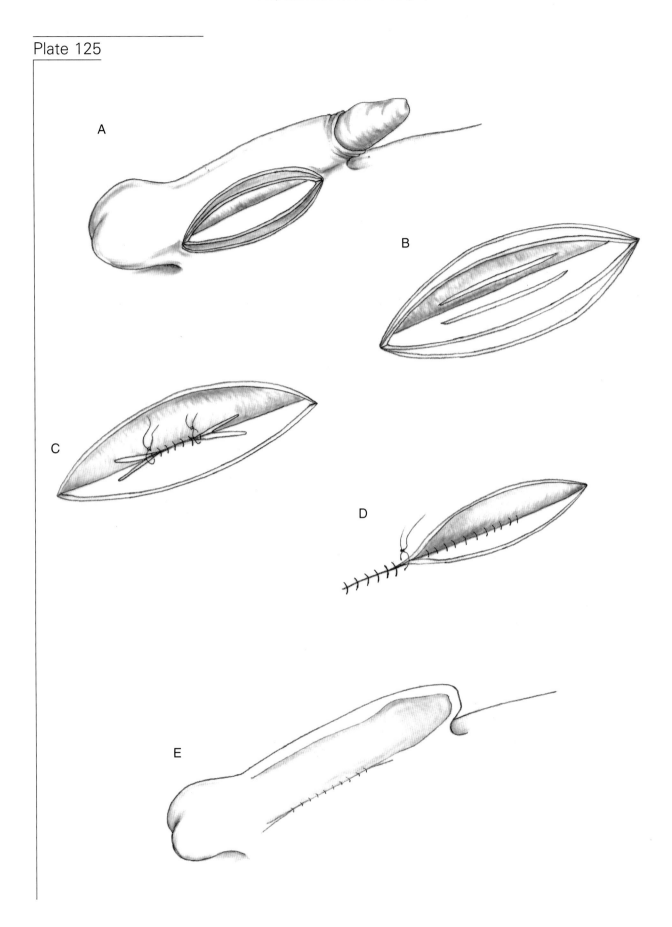

A

B

C

D

E

Plate 126	**Urethral Reconstruction for Subanal Hypospadias**

DESCRIPTION

Perineal (subanal) hypospadias predisposes patients to recurrent ascending urinary tract infections. Reconstruction of a urethral extension can separate the terminal urethra from the anal orifice, dramatically reducing bacterial contamination and secondary cystitis.

SURGICAL TECHNIQUE

(A) Illustration of perineal (subanal) hypospadias.

(B) Insertion of a Foley catheter, approximating the diameter of the terminal urethra. The circumference of the urethra can be calculated by multiplying the diameter of the intact urethra times 3.14 (π). (If the terminal urethra is 15 mm in diameter, then the circumference is 47.1 mm.) The arms of the U incision, in this example, would be 47.0 mm apart, with the curvature of the U incision dorsal to the urethral orifice. Incisions are extended ventrally 4–7 cm, depending on the size of the dog.

(C) The skin is gently undermined and folded inward: the opposing skin borders are sutured with a series of simple interrupted absorbable sutures (3-0, 4-0). The upper portion of the U is sutured, creating a Y closure.

(D) The outer skin borders are advanced and sutured over the "inverse urethral tube."

COMMENTS

The Foley catheter can be connected to a closed collection system if postoperative swelling is anticipated and removed as tissue edema subsides (3–5 days as a suggested guideline). Premature removal of the Foley, in face of postoperative tissue swelling, can impair normal urination. Long hair should be trimmed around the oriface to help prevent future irritation from urine contact with the adjacent skin.

Plate 126

A

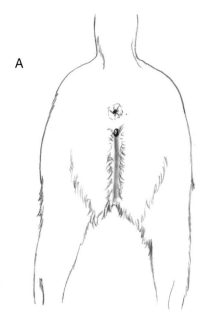

B

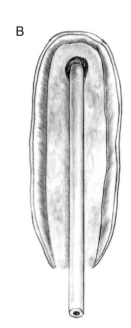

C

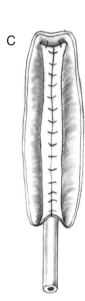

D

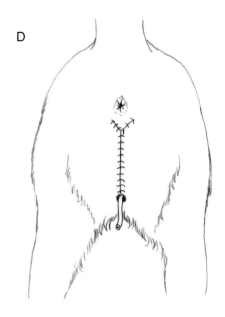

Plate 127   **Preputial Urethrostomy Technique**

DESCRIPTION

Penile amputation secondary to trauma or disease will dictate the location of a urethrostomy. In those cases of penile resection at the level of the preputial fornix, anastomosis of the terminal urethra to the preputial mucosa can result in a simple and effective permanent urethrostomy. Urine exits the preputial ostium in a steady stream, eliminating urine irritation and scalding occasionally noted with prescrotal urethrostomies. A ventral preputiotomy incision simplifies penile amputation and urethral anastomosis to the inner preputial mucosal lining.

SURGICAL TECHNIQUE

(A) Full-thickness ventral preputiotomy incision. The penis is extruded and penile amputation of the necrotic penis (secondary to strangulation necrosis secondary to paraphimosis) is performed caudal to the os penis in this example. A carbon dioxide laser may be used to reduce hemorrhage.

(B) The terminal urethra is sutured to the caudal border of the preputial mucosa. Absorbable suture (4-0 or 5-0) is used for the anastomosis. (It is also possible to anastomose the terminal urethra via a small circular incision created in the adjacent preputial mucosal surface.)

(C) Continuation of the suturing of the urethra to the preputial mucosa. (*Note:* If tension is noted during anastomosis, a release incision can be made cranial to the anterior base of the prepuce: this facilitates the caudal displacement of the prepuce. Upon completion, the release incision can be closed.)

(D) After anastomosis, the preputial access incision is closed, first by closure of the mucosal layer.

(E) The cutaneous preputiotomy incision is closed completing the procedure.

COMMENTS

The preputial cavity serves as a satisfactory conduit for urine passage from the urethrostomy site. Postoperative use of a urinary catheter may not be necessary, unless postoperative swelling at the anastomotic site is noted, resulting in straining to urinate with secondary urinary bladder enlargement.

Plate 127

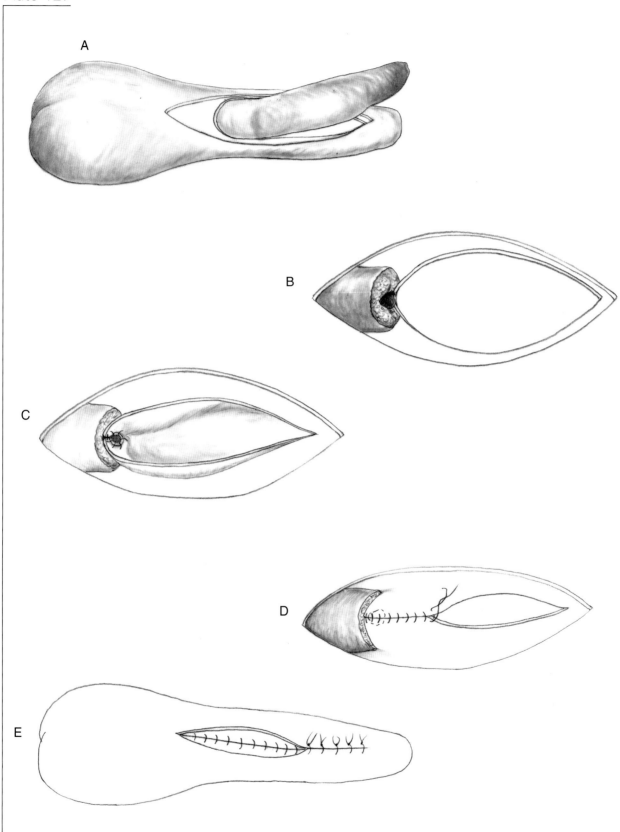

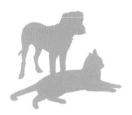

Miscellaneous Reconstructive Surgical Techniques

This chapter was designed to introduce surgical techniques that fail to fit neatly into the standard surgical categories described in the preceding chapters of this atlas. The omentum and scrotum, and their potential uses in reconstructive surgery, are described. Surgical management of tail fold and vulvar fold intertrigo are also discussed. Lastly, simple flap options for pinnal defects are discussed.

OMENTUM

An understanding of the basic anatomy of the omentum is useful for determining how best to mobilize this tissue for wound closure. The omentum is subdivided into the greater and lesser omentum. The greater omentum (epiploon or *omentum majus*) is a lacy apron extending from the greater curvature of the stomach to the level of the urinary bladder. It covers the intestinal tract ventrally and on the sides. The greater omentum appears to be a single layer, but is actually is a double peritoneal sheet (that reflects or folds back on itself distally). It is composed of connective tissue and streaks of fat that surround fine arteries passing through this tissue. The omentum is nearly transparent due to its thinness. The greater omentum is further subdivided anatomically into a large *bursal portion* and a smaller *splenic* and *veil portion*.

The bursal portion of the omentum attaches cranioventrally to the greater curvature of the stomach. Distally, it reflects on itself and returns to the region dorsal to the stomach. The ventral layer and the deeper dorsal layer can be separated by gentle manual traction. Between these two surfaces is a potential pocket or cavity called the *omental bursa* or *lesser peritoneal cavity*. Except for this large constant opening, the epiploic foramen, the omental bursa is a closed pouch. The epiploic foramen is bounded ventrally by the peritoneum covering the portal vein and dorsally by that covering the caudal vena cava.

The *splenic portion* of the omentum is also referred to as the *gastrosplenic ligament*. The *veil portion* contains the left extremity and caudal margin of the left lobe of the pancreas.

Surgical Applications

The omentum has been used for the following surgical applications

- Closure of problematic abdominal hernias
- Closure of diaphragmatic defects
- Omentalization of prostatic, hepatic, and pancreatic abscesses and cysts
- Omentalization of abcesses and cysts within the abdominal cavity
- Omental overlay of gastrointestinal incisions
- Omental overlay of urinary bladder to prevent adhesions and leakage
- Omental flap transfer for thoracic wall defects
- Thoracic omentalization for pleural effusion
- Omental overlay of the caudal esophagus
- Closure of feline indolent axillary wounds
- Closure of problematic external wounds

The omentum can reach most areas within the abdominal cavity and outer abdominal wall (Fig. 23-1). The omentum in some patients may not reach the caudal aspects of the abdominal and pelvic cavities without surgically lengthening this tissue. Similarly, lengthening procedures are required for transferring the omentum to the anterior thoracic and axillary areas. (See Plate 128.)

The omentum can be useful for closure of problematic defects by improving (donating) circulation to ischemic or compromised tissues. For example, a chronic radiation burn, lacking circulation, would potentially benefit from a muscle or omental flap. Each can provide a source of circulation to the area, not only to improve healing but to potentially serve as a vascular surface for skin graft application. The major limitation in using omentum is its relative fragility and lack of "bulk" for closing larger defects. Overextension of the omental flap can result in circulatory compromise to the more distal portion of this tissue. However, within its normal arc of rotation or advancement, the omentum can be gathered or folded to improve its bulk for defects involving the abdominal wall or diaphragm. Synthetic mesh can be used for added rigidity.

In thoracic wall reconstruction, the latissimus dorsi muscle flap is superior to the use of Marlex mesh and omentum, based on the tissue bulk provided and simplicity of elevation and transfer. Nonetheless, omentum and mesh can be used in those cases in which the use of this muscle is not possible.

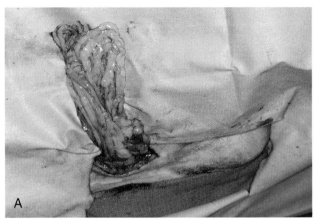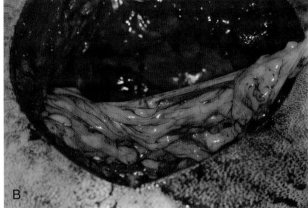

FIG. 23-1 (A) Omentum elevated out of the abdominal cavity through a midline laparotomy. This mobile tissue can be used for a variety of problematic wounds within its normal arc of rotation.

(B) Resection of the caudal thoracic wall for osteoscaroma in a 2-year-old golden retriever. A portion of the diaphragm attached to the tumor was resected. Note how easily the omentum can be passed through the diaphragm and into the thoracic cavity.

SCROTUM

The scrotum is a multilayered tissue enveloping the testicle; each testicle is separated by a connective tissue septum. The septum blends with the abdominal fascia dorsal to the testicles. Residing beneath the thin scrotal skin is the *dartos*, a layer comprising connective tissue, elastin fibers, and smooth muscle. Smooth muscle contraction of the dartos layer draws the testicles closer to the abdominal wall. Around each testicle is an outer parietal tunic and the visceral tunic enveloping the testicle. The cremaster muscle, derived from the internal abdominal oblique muscle (or occasionally the transversus abdominis muscle) inserts on the parietal vaginal tunic at the level of the testis. Contraction of the cremaster draws the testicles closer to the body (Fig. 23-2).

The principal blood vessel to the scrotum is the external pudendal artery. The cremasteric artery arises from the femoral or deep femoral artery. The scrotal arteries run along the cranioventral surface of the testis, superficial to the common vaginal tunic. The perineal branches of the external pudendal artery supply the scrotum, in part. The draining veins follow the same course in reverse.

Surgical Application

The scrotum has been described in humans as a simple advancement style flap for closing defects of the adja-

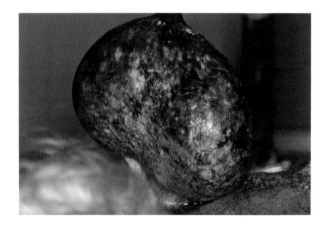

FIG. 23-2 Scrotum with enlargement secondary to a large Sertoli cell tumor. Note the capacity for the scrotum to stretch to underlying expansile masses.

cent inner thigh. Matera et al. (2004) describe the use of the scrotal skin for closure of similar cutaneous defects, after its dissection from the underlying dartos layer (see Plate 129). The elevated skin can be advanced or transposed into adjacent cutaneous defects.

The surface area of the scrotum varies in the male, depending on the age of the dog, the size of the testicles, and the variable effects of gravity. The scrotum has a tendency to shrink after castration, whereas the scrotum tends to have a greater surface area in the intact male dog. The author also has used the scrotum for local wound closure on a limited basis, leaving the dartos attached to the overlying skin surface.

TAIL FOLD INTERTRIGO (SCREW TAIL)

Intertrigo (skin fold dermatitis) is an inflammatory condition associated with skin creases or depressions. Deeper creases or folds have a natural tendency to accumulate moisture; skin-to-skin contact can create local irritation contributing to the formation of pyoderma. While diligent conservative treatment with skin-cleansing solutions and topical antibiotic agents by pet owners may palliate this condition in assessable areas, ventral tail fold pyoderma is often impossible to maintain in this fashion (Fig. 23-3).

"Screw tail" is a descriptive slang term for the corkscrew-like deviation of the tail most commonly seen in English bulldogs. On occasion, it can be seen in French bulldogs, pugs, and Boston terriers. This condition also has been called "ingrown tail." In some cases, the ventral skin fold can be several centimeters deep when

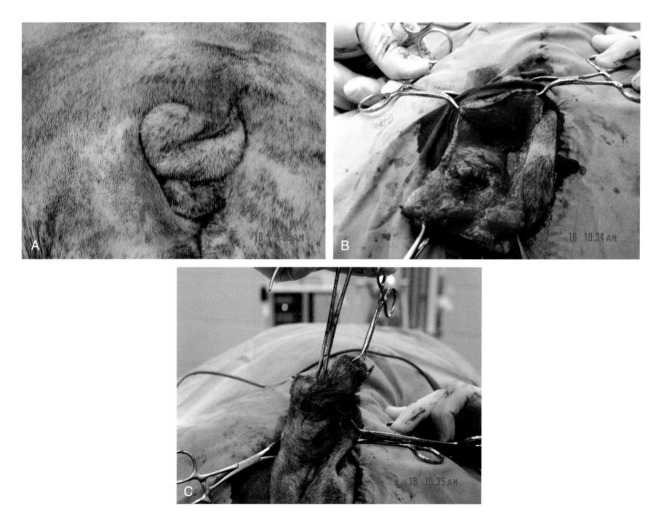

FIG. 23-3 (A) Tail fold pyoderma and severe ventral deviation of the tail over the anus.

(B) After amputation of the tail via a dorsal T incision, firm traction of the skin fold and the tail helps remove the ventral fold. The skin dorsal to the anus is incised to complete the resection. The skin fold in this case was firmly adhered to the ventral surface of the deviated tail.

(C) Note the depth or surface area of this ventral fold and the large mat of hair that accumulated in this cutaneous trough. Preservation of the major dorsal fold creates a symmetrical appearance of a short tail stump (see Fig. 23-5).

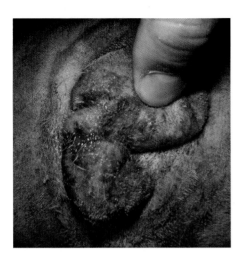

FIG. 23-4 Dorsal skin folds occasionally present with intertrigo. Topical medical therapy can be attempted to control this condition, unlike many of the ventral skin folds seen in these patients.

assessed by the insertion cotton tipped applicators. The deformed tail can take a ventral bend that partially or completely covers the anus, further contributing to the problem. Intraoperatively, the dorsal surface of the deep skin fold can adhere firmly to the undersurface of the deviated coccygeal vertebrae, making surgical resection of the inverted skin fold a greater challenge. On occasion, the dorsal tail fold(s) also may develop intertrigo, but it is more amenable to conservative treatment (Fig. 23-4).

Clinical signs of tail fold intertrigo usually include the dog rubbing or scooting its rear on the floor or carpeting. The owners may note a foul odor around the tail base or note fecal accumulation beneath the distal tail segment.

Surgical Correction

Standard textbooks normally show one or two basic approaches to caudectomy for tail fold intertrigo: a dorsal linear incision over the tail or the creation of a horizontal elliptical incision around the entire tail area. Following amputation of the tail anterior to the initial point of coccygeal deviation, the skin fold and redundant skin is resected. Preservation of the major dorsal skin fold enables the surgeon to create a semblance of a short symmetrical tail with satisfactory cosmetic results (Fig. 23-5). The author's preferred approach is described in Plate 130.

VULVAR FOLD PYODERMA

The infolding of the vulva below the adjacent skin surface may be of a congenital or acquired nature. Hypoplasia of the vulva may result in its recession deeper to the adjacent skin. Slight angular deviation of the vulva also has been noted in conjunction with hypoplasia. The recessed vulva in turn can result in moisture accumulation and dermatitis. Bacterial infection normally follows this sequence. Most cases of vaginal fold pyoderma are acquired in nature. Subcutaneous fat accumulation dorsal to the vulva stretches the skin to a variable degree with the assistance of gravity. The redundant skin drapes over the vulva (Fig. 23-6). Urine scalding and moisture accumulation secondary to chronic dermatitis perpetuates the pyoderma. In long-standing cases, the skin lateral and ventral to the vulva also may appear to be thin, hairless, and somewhat shiny due to long-standing dermatitis. The upper thighs may contact each other, creating another crease for frictional contact and dermatitis.

Although many dogs with this condition do not present with a bacterial cystitis, vulvar fold pyoderma may be a source of recurrent urinary tract infections in some canine patients. Surgery is considered the acceptable standard for correcting vulvar fold pyoderma (Fig. 23-7).

Neoplasia of the vulva is occasionally noted in older dogs, including squamous cell carcinoma and mast cell tumors (Fig. 23-8). Most of these neoplastic conditions do not present as typical vulvar fold pyoderma.

> When in doubt, biopsy.

Tumor enlargement and ulceration is often associated with the vulva, rather than the skin dorsal to this structure. Partial or complete vulvar resection can be performed in these cases, with care taken to identify and preserve the urethral tubercle. Owners are warned that local urine scalding is a possibility, in part depending on how the patient squats to urinate (Fig. 23-8). Postoperatively, the fur should be trimmed to reduce moisture accumulation and facilitate cleaning the area after urination. Commercially available disposable baby wipes are convenient for this purpose.

Surgical Technique

Surgery is focused on removal of the redundant skin and the area of intertrigo using connecting inverted U ("Dutchman's pants," inverted horseshoe) incisions.

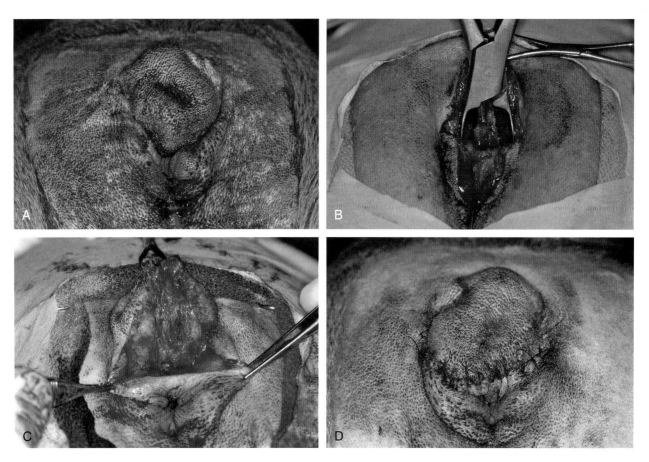

FIG. 23-5 (A) A typical case of tail fold intertrigo.

(B) A skin incision caudal to the large anterior dorsal fold of the tail is followed by a central incision directed caudally, forming a T incision. The T incision simplifies dissection around the deviated tail segment, followed by its amputation with bone-cutting forceps. The ventral skin fold is resected.

(C) Following control of bleeding vessels with electrocautery and ligatures, the dead space can be closed with the application of absorbable sutures. Note the elevated tail fold.

(D) The elevated fold is sutured to the ventral incision, creating the illusion of a short tail stump.

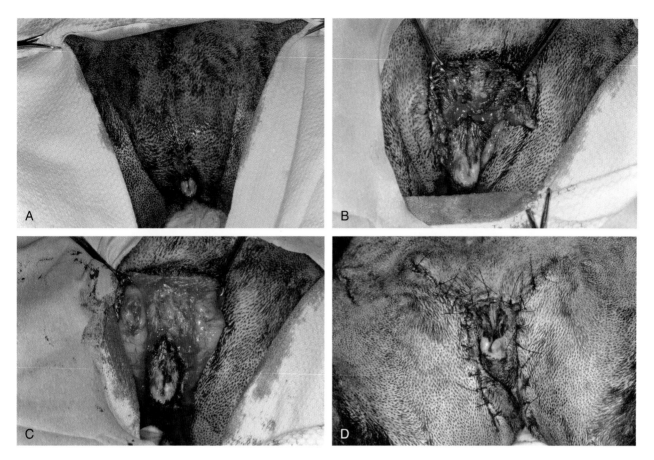

FIG. 23-6 (A) Vaginal fold pyoderma or intertrigo. Note the prominent subcutaneous fat dorsal to the obscured vulva.

(B) Traction of the skin rim dorsal to the vulvar fold, demonstrating the chronic dermatitis.

(C) Resection of the excessive skin and subcutaneous fat.

(D) Because of the mismatch in the paired curved incisions, the skin was closed with two dorsal lateral incisions. Note the lower thigh incisions: a small amount of skin was removed ventral and lateral to the vulva bilaterally, creating a "thigh tuck." This maneuver slightly separates the thigh skin and improves skin aeration ventral and anterior to the vulva, where chronic moist dermatitis also is noted.

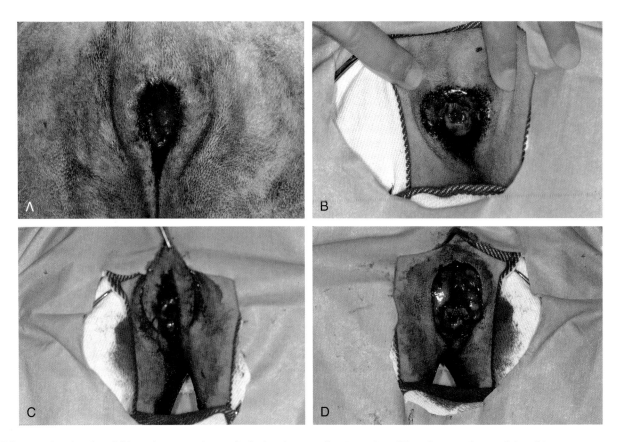

FIG. 23-7 (A, B) Vulvar fold pyoderma can be overlooked, unless an effort is made to lift and retract the overlying skin. (C, D) Excision of the redundant skin is followed by removal of the excess subcutaneous fat noted below the skin.

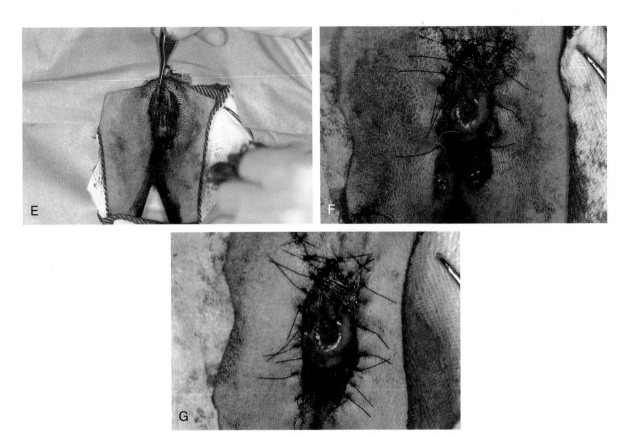

FIG. 23-7 *Continued* (E) The dorsal midpoint of the vulva is lifted to the dorsal skin border. Sufficient skin was removed to prevent recurrence of the skin fold. Absorbable interrupted sutures are used to close the defect, followed by simple interrupted skin sutures. (F) An additional amount of caudal thigh skin is resected below the vulva, creating a "thigh tuck." (G) Compare this case to the canine patient in Figure 23-6. Note how slight separation below the vulva improved exposure of the chronically inflamed skin below and anterior to the vulva.

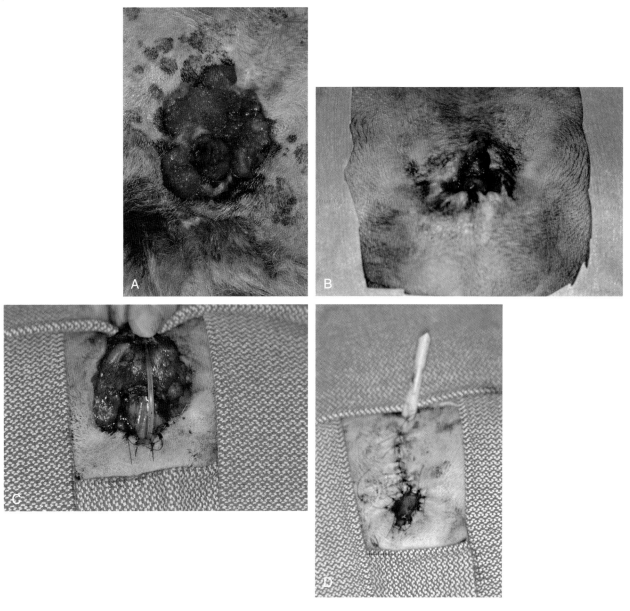

FIG. 23-8 (A) Squamous cell carcinoma involving the vulva with the patient in sternal recumbency for this photograph.

(B) A second case example of squamous cell carcinoma, with the patient in dorsal recumbency.

(C, D) View of the patient after resection of the vulva and ajoining skin. The urethral papilla is preserved. The author prefers to perform this particular surgery with the patients in dorsal recumbency.

Removal of redundant subcutaneous fat is important for correcting this condition and facilitating closure (Fig. 23-6). The lateral skin incisions can be extended below the lower vulvar margin. A small amount of skin can be resected at this location to create a "thigh tuck," which better separates the inner thigh tissues for those patients in whom chronic dermatitis extends ventral and cranial to the vulva. Care must be taken to avoid excessive skin resection dorsal to the vulva (Figs. 23-6C, D and 23-7F, G). Wound dehiscence secondary to excessive tension can create a perineal defect that can be quite difficult to close (Plate 131).

CLOSURE OPTIONS FOR DEFECTS OF THE PINNA

Pinnal skin defects secondary to tumor resection or trauma can present a closure challenge to the veterinarian. In some cases, veterinarians may consider amputation of major portions of the pinna when no practical surgical option appears to be available. However, the loose skin around the base of the ear provides a donor area for a variety of transposition flap options.

Surgical Technique

Plate 132 demonstrates several options for closing defects involving the pinna. Flaps are especially useful for defects involving the lower half of the pinna, although some flaps are capable of covering large areas of the pinnal surface, depending on the length of the ear for a given patient.

Suggested Readings

Omentum
Bray JP, White RAS, Williams JM. 1997. Partial resection and omentalization: a new technique for management of prostatic retention cysts in dogs. *Vet Surg* 26:202–209.

Bright RM, Birchard SJ, Long GG. 1982. Repair of thoracic wall defects in the dog with an omental pedicle flap. *J Am Anim Hosp Assoc* 18:278–282.

Bright RM, Thacker HL. 1982. The formation of an omental pedicle flap and its experimental use in the repair of a diaphragmatic rent in a dog. *J Am Anim Hosp Assoc* 18:283–289.

Brockman DJ, Pardo AD, Conzemius MG, et al. 1996. Omentum-enhanced reconstruction of chronic nonhealing wounds in cats: techniques and clinical use. *Vet Surg* 25:99–104.

Campbell BG. 2004. Omentalization of a nonresectable uterine stump abscess in a dog. *J Am Vet Med Assoc* 224:1799–1803.

Evans HE, Christensen GC.1979. *Miller's Anatomy of the Dog*, 467–471. Philadelphia, PA: Saunders.

Friend Ej, Niles JD, Williams JM. 2001. Omentalisation of congenital liver cysts in a cat. *Vet Rec* 149:275–276.

Hill TP, Odesnik BJ. 2000. Omentalization of a nonresectable uterine stump abscess in a dog. *J Sm Anim Pract* 41:115–118.

Hoelzler MG, Bellah JR, Donofro MC. 2001. Omentalization of cystic sublumbar lymph node metastasis for long-term palliation of tenesmus and dysuria in a dog with anal sac adenocarcinoma. *J Am Vet Med Assoc* 219:1729–1732.

Hosgood G. The omentum—the forgotten organ. Physiology and potential surgical application in dogs and cats. *Compend Contin Educ Pract Vet* 12:45–50.

Jerram RM, Warman CG, Davies ESS, et al. 2004. Successful treatment of a pancreatic pseudocyst by omentalisation in a dog. *N Z Vet J* 52:197–201.

Johnson MD, Mann FA. 2006. Treatment for pancreatic abscesses via omentalization with abdominal closure versus open peritoneal drainage in dogs: 15 cases (1994–2004). *J Am Vet Med Assoc* 228:397–402.

LaFond E, Wierich WE, Salisbury SK. 2002. Omentalization of the thorax for treatment of idiopathic chylothorax with constrictive pleuritis in a cat. *J Am Anim Hosp Assoc* 38:74–78.

Lascelles BDX, Davison L, Dunning M, et al. 1998. Use of omental pedicle grafts in the management of non-healing axillary wounds in 10 cats. *J Sm Anim Pract* 39:475–480.

Lascelles BDX, White RAS. 2001. Combined omental pedicle grafts and thoracodorsal axial pattern flaps for the reconstruction of chronic, nonhealing axillary wounds in cats. *Vet Surg* 30:380–385.

Ross WE, Pardo AD. 1993. Evaluation of an omental pedicle extension technique in a dog. *Vet Surg* 22:37–43.

Smith BA, Hosgood G, Hedlund CS.1995. Omental pedicle used to manage a large dorsal wound in a dog. *J Sm Anim Pract* 36:267–270.

White RAS, Williams JM. 1995. Intracapsular prostatic omentalization: a new technique for management of prostatic abscesses in dogs. *Vet Surg* 24:390–395.

Willliams JM, Niles JD. 1999. Use of omentum as a physiologic drain for treatment of chylothorax in a dog. *Vet Surg* 28:61–65.

Scrotum
Evans HE, Christensen GC. 1993. The urogenital system. In: *Millers Anatomy of the Dog*, 494–558. Philadelphia, PA: Saunders.

Matera JM, Tatarunas AC, Fantoni DT, et al. 2004. Use of the scrotum as a transposition flap for closure of surgical wounds in three dogs. *Vet Surg* 33:100–101.

Tail Fold and Vulvar Fold Pyodermas
Bellah J. 2006 Tail and perineal wounds. *Vet Clin No Am* 36(4):913–929.

White RAS. 2003. Surgical treatment of specific skin disorders. In: Slatter D, ed. *Textbook of Small Animal Surgery*, 3rd ed., 39–42. Philadelphia, PA: Saunders.

Plate 128   **Omental Flap Options**

INTRODUCTION

The omentum is a thin, lacy, mesothelial membrane with a rich capillary and lymphatic network. In reconstructive surgery, the tissue can be mobilized to close body wall defects and facilitate the revascularization and closure of problematic wounds. The omentum is essentially an anatomic purse, with the epiploic foramen serving as the opening into the omental bursa. The dorsal and ventral surfaces of the omentum can be unfolded and divided to increase its length, enabling it to reach more distant areas of the patient.

SURGICAL TECHNIQUE

(A) The surgeon's view of the omentum through a midline laparotomy.
(B) Stage 1: The omentum is lifted upward and cranially, exposing the dorsal surface of the omentum. Scissors are used to divide its dorsal pancreatic attachment. A few small branches of the splenic artery are ligated during this maneuver.
(C) This first-stage maneuver doubles the length of the omentum.
(D) Stage 2: Further lengthening can be accomplished by creating an inverted L incision using scissors, beginning on the left side of the omentum caudal to the gastrosplenic ligament. Omental branches are ligated during this maneuver. The initial incision crosses one-half to two-thirds of the width of the omental sheet created. The caudal portion of the incision extends two-thirds the length of the omental sheet, completing the stage 2 extension of the omentum.

COMMENTS

The omentum has been used for decades to close and reinforce defects in the abdominal cavity, adjacent abdominal wall, and diaphragm. "Omentalization" has become a code word for packing omentum into abscesses or cystic cavities to obliterate dead space: the omentum also provides an alternative source of circulation and the essential components required to promote the healing processes. Improving circulation also assists in the control of infection. Most intra-abdominal and abdominal wall defects can be closed without lengthening the omentum. The omentum may be of sufficient length for advancement into the thoracic cavity and pelvic canal, without stage 1 lengthening. This can be performed if the intact omentum is required to reach the cranial thoracic cavity or thoracic wall. Omentum can be used in thoracic wall reconstruction using a synthetic mesh. This technique is considered inferior to the use of the latissimus dorsi muscle flap due to the simplicity of the latter technique and the greater bulk the muscle provides without the need for mesh reinforcement.

Stage 1 extension of the omentum can be performed with little likelihood of significant circulatory compromise. Further lengthening (stage 2) includes the added risk of circulatory compromise since collateral vascular channels within the omentum are necessarily divided. Caution is required during its transfer to distant body regions. When tunneled beneath the skin to reach the recipient area, care must be taken not to compress or overly stretch this delicate tissue: collapse of the capillary circulation will result in omental necrosis.

Plate 128

A

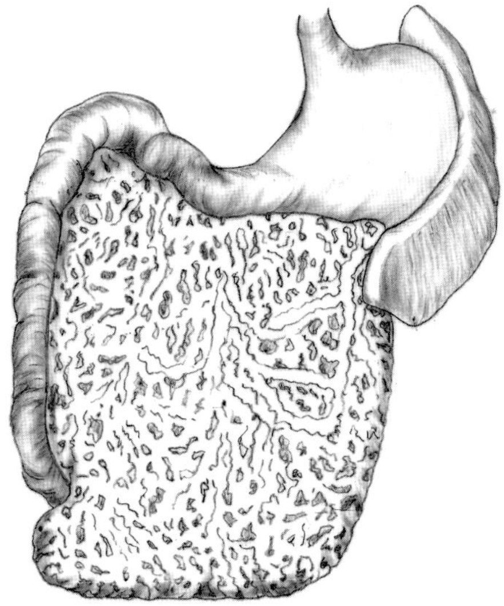

B

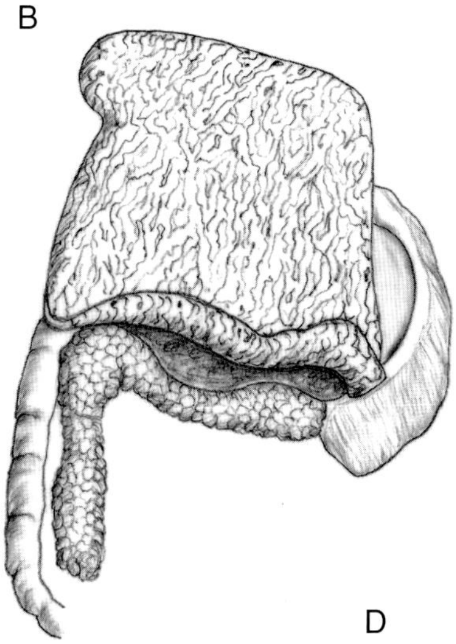

C

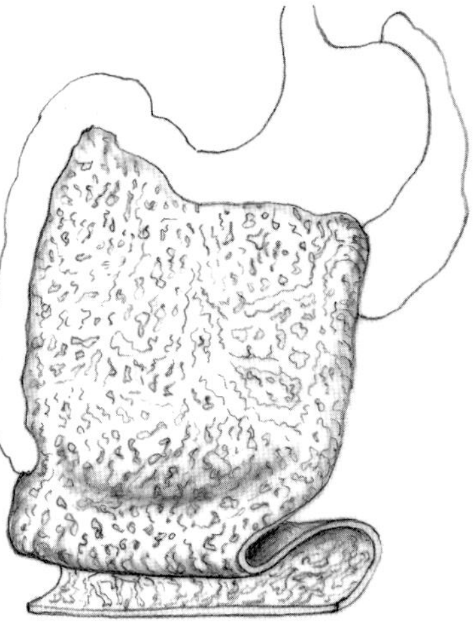

D

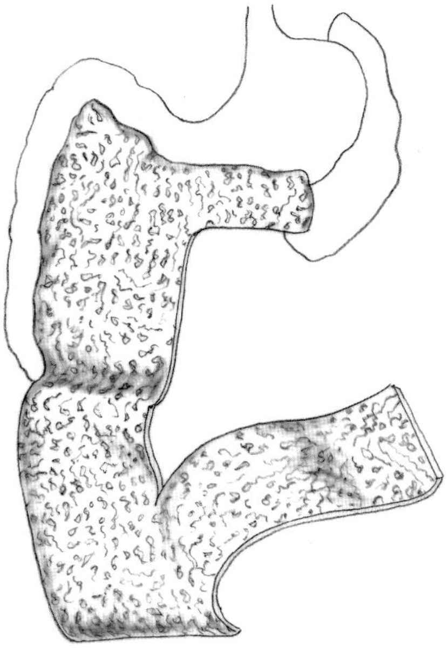

Plate 129 — Scrotal Flap Technique

DESCRIPTION

The surface area of the scrotum varies considerably in individual dogs. In older intact males, the scrotum can be pendulous, whereas in younger castrated dogs, the surface area can be relatively small. The scrotum can be advanced as a flap into adjacent problematic skin defects. The vascular supply to the scrotum is derived from the collateral cutaneous blood supply, perineal branches of the external pudendal artery, and cremasteric artery. The ventral scrotal artery and dorsal scrotal artery anastomose to supply the overlying scrotal tissue. These vascular branches course along the cranioventral surface of the testis, superficial to the common vaginal tunic. Branches of the scrotal artery can be identified and preserved during flap elevation.

SURGICAL TECHNIQUE

(A) Ventral view of the scrotum and adjacent inguinal area. A skin defect is noted lateral to the scrotum.

(B) Close-up view of the scrotum and adjacent cutaneous wound. An incision is made at the adjacent base of the scrotum. To preserve circulation, at least one-quarter of the circumference should be preserved. Preservation of vascular branches supplying the scrotal tissue also is desirable. In this illustration, the small area of skin interposed between the flap and wound bed (large dashed lines) can be excised to facilitate scrotal advancement.

(C) Progressive elevation of the scrotal flap. The dartos and fascia can be carefully dissected from the scrotal skin if necessary to improve flap advancement and coverage of the skin defect.

(D) Completion of the closure.

COMMENTS

The use of the scrotum as a source of skin for wound closure has been reported in the human literature. Although castration can be performed using a prescrotal incision, elevation of the scrotal flap will give the surgeon direct access to each testicle. This technique should be kept in mind when a problematic wound involves the adjacent perineum, inner thigh, or cutaneous region anterior to the scrotum.

Plate 129

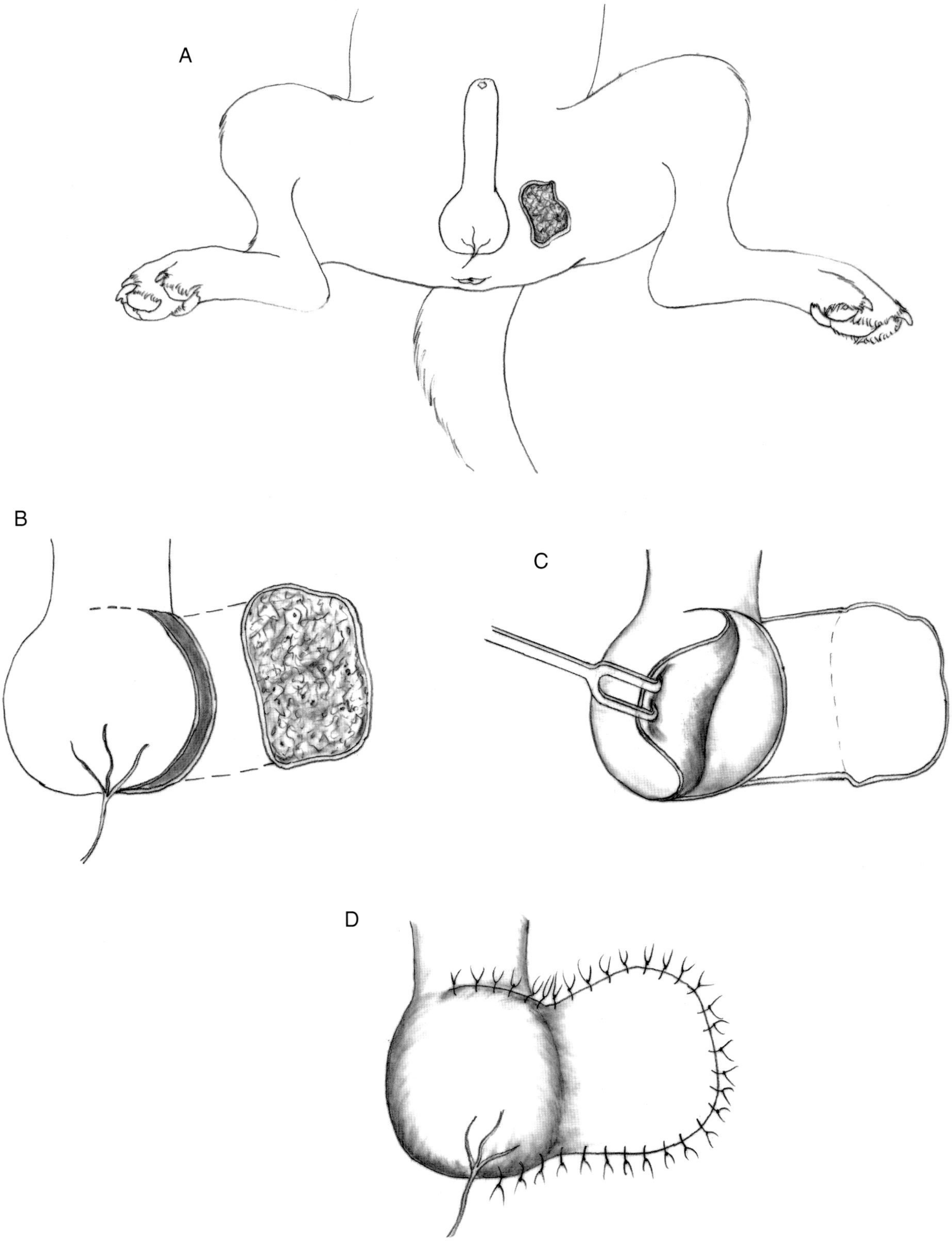

| Plate 130 | **Caudectomy for Tail Fold Intertrigo** |

DESCRIPTION

English bulldogs, French bulldogs, and Boston terriers occasionally present with a somewhat fixed, deformed tail. A fold or crease beneath the tail is prone to chronic dermatitis or intertrigo. A cotton-tipped applicator can be used to assess the depth of this fur-lined crease: occasionally, it is several centimeters in depth. The deviated tail can cover the anus, making routine defecation problematic and cleansing of the area difficult. Dogs often present with a history of scooting secondary to the dermatitis; owners may note an unpleasant odor as a result of the debris accumulation and bacterial infection.

Surgery is primarily directed at (1) resecting the abnormal coccygeal vertebrae and (2) removing the ventral crease or fold. Redundant tail skin is removed in the process, but the most cranial dorsal skin fold is preserved to fashion a new tail silhouette.

SURGICAL TECHNIQUE

(A) A T incision is created caudal to the cranial skin fold at the base of the tail (dashed lines).

(B) The triangular skin flaps created by the T incision are retracted, curved, and dissection is directed to exposure of the coccygeal vertebrae anterior to the point of tail deviation. A Carmalt clamp can be directed beneath the tail to protect the underlying dorsal rectal wall.

(C) Bone cutters are then used to cut directly through or between the exposed vertebra. (Alternatively, some surgeons will use a scalpel to divide between individual coccygeal vertebrae.) Electrocautery is normally used to control bleeding vessels: vascular clips or ligatures may be used for larger vessels.

(D) With successful division of the vertebra, the loose terminal tail segment is grasped with forceps. Firm traction is applied in a dorsal direction; this facilitates eversion of the invaginated or recessed ventral cutaneous fold. Metzenbaum scissors can be used to undermine and mobilize the ventral skin fold. A curved incision is made at the ventral base of the tail fold (dashed line), completing the resection of the tail and ventral skin crease.

(E) After resection of the tail and associated ventral skin folds, the area is lavaged and examined for any remaining bleeding vessels prior to closure. Absorbable sutures may be used to close dead space prior to approximating the skin margins with absorbable interrupted intradermal sutures. Simple interrupted skin sutures are used to complete the skin closure. The large preserved cranial skin fold forms a prominent peak, giving the semblance of a short, symmetrical tail.

COMMENTS

As noted, several textbooks advocate complete removal of the entire tail and associated folds. Preserving the large cranial fold achieves a pleasing cosmetic tail silhouette that better represents the appearance of the breed. During amputation, care is taken to avoid deeper dissection that may perforate the dorsal rectal wall. Dividing the tail with bone cutters is notably faster than attempting to dissect between individual vertebrae with a scalpel blade.

Plate 130

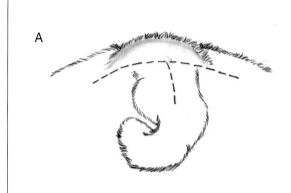

A

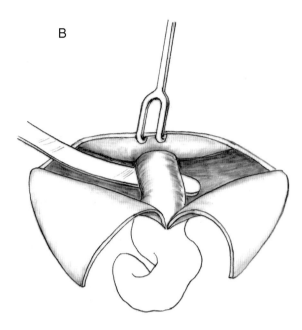

B

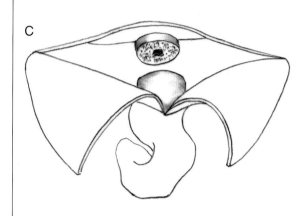

C

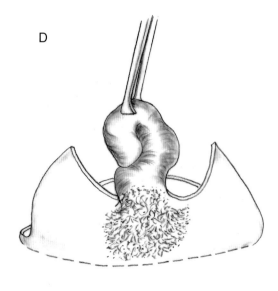

D

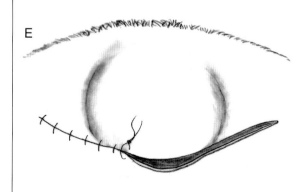

E

Plate 131   **Episioplasty**

DESCRIPTION

Episioplasty involves the resection of the redundant skin fold and subcutaneous fat dorsal and lateral to the vulva. It is commonly performed in the management of chronic dermatitis (intertrigo), which forms in the skin crease created by the overlapping skin. In some patients, the skin infection promotes lower urinary tract infections.

SURGICAL TECHNIQUE

(A) General outline of the episiotomy (dashed line). A purse-string suture is used to prevent fecal contamination. The ends of this suture can be looped around the base of the tail and held with needle holders or hemostats. This serves as a visual reminder to remove the purse string when surgery has been completed. (Use of a purse string may also be recorded on the anesthesia sheet as an added reminder to remove this suture at the completion of the surgery.)

(B) The dorsal midline border of the vulva is grasped with forceps and elevated to determine the appropriate point for relocating the vulva. The scalpel blade can be used to nick or mark the skin at this point. Two curved incisions are created: the dorsal incision encompasses the mark created; the second, smaller, curved incision is created dorsal to the vulvar midline. The two incisions arc downward; the dorsal incision is curved inward to meet the ventral incision. The hatched area can be resected to draw the thigh skin ventral to the vulva apart. The resultant "thigh tuck" will reduce dermatitis associated with skin contact at this level (arrows denote area of skin contact).

It is important to remove the exposed redundant subcutaneous fat dorsal to the vulva prior to closure of the surgical site. Electrocautery is used to control hemorrhage. (The author also has found the carbon dioxide laser useful in resecting this redundant skin and subcutaneous tissue.)

(C) Absorbable intradermal, interrupted sutures are used to appose the cutaneous margins, followed by a simple interrupted skin suture pattern. Note how the skin resected (hatched area in B) creates slight skin traction, thereby reducing skin contact (dermatitis) below the vulva and inner thigh area (arrows).

(D) Completion of the surgery is followed by removal of the purse-string suture. Sutures are normally removed 10–14 days postoperatively.

COMMENTS

Standard textbook articles fail to address the dermatitis that is occasionally noted below and anterior to the vulva, especially in the larger dogs. Removal of a small amount of skin (B above) can separate the inner thigh skin enough to better control the intertrigo occasionally noted.

Excessive removal of skin dorsal to the vulva can, in turn, create excessive tension on skin closure. Wound dehiscence in the perineal area can result in a problematic defect due to the relative lack of mobile skin.

The interrupted, intradermal suture pattern provides an added measure of security when closing the skin, reducing the risk of dehiscence. An Elizabethan collar is advisable to prevent licking at the surgical incision.

Plate 131

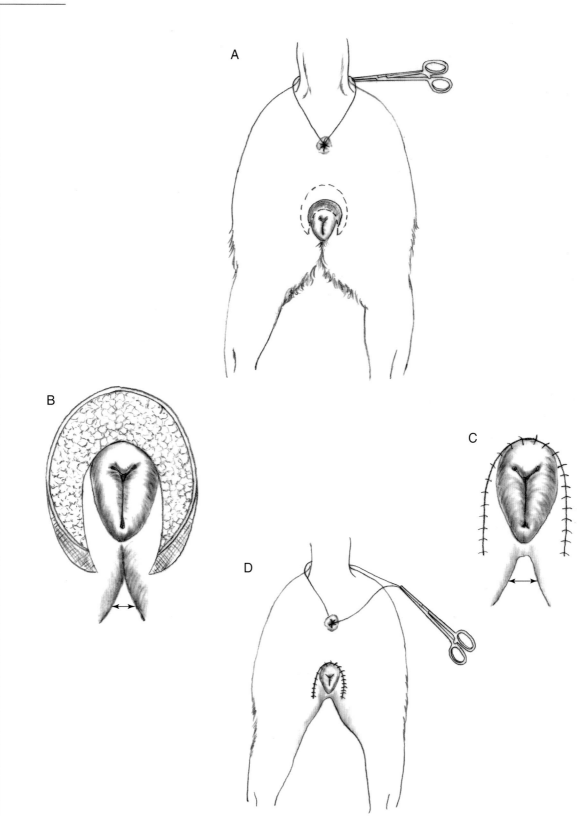

Plate 132 — **Closure Options for Select Pinnal Defects**

DESCRIPTION

Ninety-degree transposition flaps can be used to close a variety of cutaneous defects involving the pinna of the dog and cat. The various flap options illustrated should be kept in mind for closure of problematic skin defects involving this structure.

SURGICAL TECHNIQUE

(A) Dorsal view of two transposition flap options to close defects involving the rostral and caudal border of the pinna. The flaps can extend along the length of the ear to a variable degree, depending on the length and conformation of the pinna.

(B) Examples of two additional transposition flap options, rostral and caudal to pinnal defects. The body of the flap can be folded, cupping a defect that involves both cutaneous surfaces of the pinna.

(C) In this example, a transposition flap is used to resurface a large skin defect involving the pinna. (Note that the auricular axial pattern flap can be used to resurface the majority of the pinna. See Plate 57.)

(D) Pinnal defects can be tucked beneath the adjacent skin using a bipedicle or single pedicle flap technique in the adjacent facial skin. This is a variation of a "distant direct" skin flap technique. In approximately 2 weeks, the base(s) of the flap can be incised in a staged fashion and sutured to complete the transfer. In this illustration note the dotted line denotes the potential to create a "second" flap to close the opposing surface of a pinnal defect. The first flap would overlap the border of the cartilaginous defect to assure its revascularization prior to the staged elevation of this second small flap.

COMMENTS

Flap coverage depends on the location and size of the pinnal defect. There is ample skin around the perimeter of the ear to facilitate local flap elevation and transfer. Larger flaps used in closure occasionally become edematous postoperatively, and the increased weight of the flap can cause the ear to occasionally sag. Over a few weeks, swelling resolves as circulation improves. Keep in mind that the skin flap can be thicker than the original cutaneous surface of the pinna requiring coverage. Hair growth also will vary. Nonetheless, preserving the pinna is cosmetically more pleasing to the owner than resection of a large segment of the pinna. In smaller mast cell tumors, excision of the underlying cartilage border may provide a suitable base margin; the defect, in many cases, can be closed with a local transposition flap.

Plate 132

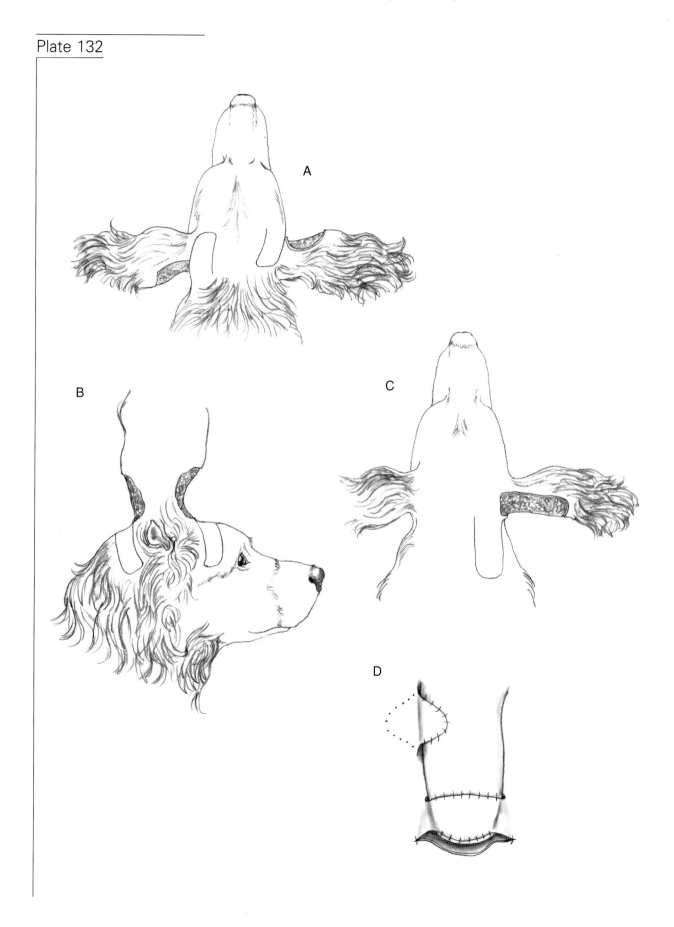

Index